T0225626

Nanomedicine in Drug Delivery

Nanomedicine in Drug Delivery

Edited by

Arun Kumar | Heidi M. Mansour
Adam Friedman | Eric R. Blough

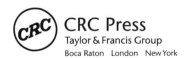

CRC Press
Taylor & Francis Group
Boca Raton   London   New York

CRC Press is an imprint of the
Taylor & Francis Group, an **informa** business

CRC Press
Taylor & Francis Group
6000 Broken Sound Parkway NW, Suite 300
Boca Raton, FL 33487-2742

First issued in paperback 2017

© 2013 by Taylor & Francis Group, LLC
CRC Press is an imprint of Taylor & Francis Group, an Informa business

No claim to original U.S. Government works

Version Date: 20130412

ISBN 13: 978-1-138-07261-9 (pbk)
ISBN 13: 978-1-4665-0616-9 (hbk)

This book contains information obtained from authentic and highly regarded sources. Reasonable efforts have been made to publish reliable data and information, but the author and publisher cannot assume responsibility for the validity of all materials or the consequences of their use. The authors and publishers have attempted to trace the copyright holders of all material reproduced in this publication and apologize to copyright holders if permission to publish in this form has not been obtained. If any copyright material has not been acknowledged please write and let us know so we may rectify in any future reprint.

Except as permitted under U.S. Copyright Law, no part of this book may be reprinted, reproduced, transmitted, or utilized in any form by any electronic, mechanical, or other means, now known or hereafter invented, including photocopying, microfilming, and recording, or in any information storage or retrieval system, without written permission from the publishers.

For permission to photocopy or use material electronically from this work, please access www.copyright. com (http://www.copyright.com/) or contact the Copyright Clearance Center, Inc. (CCC), 222 Rosewood Drive, Danvers, MA 01923, 978-750-8400. CCC is a not-for-profit organization that provides licenses and registration for a variety of users. For organizations that have been granted a photocopy license by the CCC, a separate system of payment has been arranged.

Trademark Notice: Product or corporate names may be trademarks or registered trademarks, and are used only for identification and explanation without intent to infringe.

Library of Congress Cataloging-in-Publication Data

Nanomedicine in drug delivery / editors, Arun Kumar ... [et al.].
    p. ; cm.
  Includes bibliographical references and index.
  ISBN 978-1-4665-0616-9 (hbk. : alk. paper)
  I. Kumar, Arun (Professor)
  [DNLM: 1. Drug Delivery Systems. 2. Nanomedicine--methods. 3. Nanoparticles--therapeutic use. 4. Nanotechnology--methods. QV 785]

RS403
615.1'9--dc23   2013013507

Visit the Taylor & Francis Web site at
http://www.taylorandfrancis.com

and the CRC Press Web site at
http://www.crcpress.com

Contents

Preface.. vii
Editors.. ix
Contributors.. xiii

1. Nanoparticles in Drug Delivery Systems...1
   Emilio Castro and Arun Kumar

2. Synthesis and Characterization of Nanoencapsulated Drugs 23
   Arun Kumar, Ashley E. Saienni, and Niketa Dixit

3. Nanoparticle Lung Delivery and Inhalation Aerosols for
   Targeted Pulmonary Nanomedicine 43
   Heidi M. Mansour, Chun-Woong Park, and Don Hayes, Jr.

4. Biological Systems for the Delivery of Nanoparticles..........................75
   Niketa Dixit, Mark Glaum, Arun Kumar, and Don F. Cameron

5. Nanodermatology: The Giant Role of Nanotechnology in
   Diagnosis and Treatment of Skin Disease..89
   Adam Friedman

6. Nanoparticles for Drug Delivery of Small Molecules........................ 131
   Ana Sofia Macedo and Eliana B. Souto

7. Nanoparticle Therapies for Wounds and Ulcer Healing.................... 143
   *Chiara Gardin, Letizia Ferroni, Luca Lancerotto, Vincenzo Vindigni,
   Chiara Rigo, Marco Roman, Warren R. L. Cairns, and Barbara Zavan*

8. Nanoparticles in Bioimaging 187
   Javier L. Pou Ucha

9. Nanoparticles in Anticancer Drug Delivery... 213
   Frederic Lagarce

10. Formulations of Nanoparticles in Drug Delivery 239
    Sushama Talegaonkar, Mohammad Tariq, and Zeenat Iqbal

11. Nanoparticles for Ocular Drug Delivery...287
    Jaleh Barar and Yadollah Omidi

12. Toxicology of Nanoparticles...337
      Siva K. Nalabotu and Eric R. Blough

**13. Animal and Cellular Models for Use in Nanoparticles Safety
      Study** 355
      Kevin M. Rice and Eric R. Blough

Index...423

Preface

The use of nanoscale technologies to design novel drug delivery systems and devices is a rapidly developing area of biomedical research that promises breakthrough advances in therapeutics and diagnostics. Over the last few years, numerous breakthroughs in nanotechnology have made great impact on different fields of scientific research. Out of these many breakthroughs, some of them have proved to be very promising for diagnosis and treatment of diseases. The term "nanomedicine" describes the applications of nanotechnology in medicine for treatment and diagnosis of diseases. There is an unambiguous need for the discovery and development of innovative technologies to improve the delivery of therapeutic and diagnostic agents in the body. The goal of nanomedicine is to deliver drugs, therapeutic proteins to local areas of disease or to tumors to maximize clinical benefit while limiting unwanted side effects. This book brought together different aspects of nanomedicine to give an overview which will be highly helpful to design and develop some of the unique approaches for research in nanomedicine.

Arun Kumar, PhD
University of Delaware

Editors

Arun Kumar, PhD, is an assistant professor in the Department of Medical Laboratory Science and the Department of Biomedical Engineering at the University of Delaware.

Dr. Kumar received his PhD from the University of Delhi, India in 2003 in chemistry with the emphasis on the development of clinical biosensors. Before moving to the United States he was associated with many laboratories of the Council of Scientific and Industrial Research (CSIR) of India, such as the Indian Institute of Chemical Technology, Institutes of Genomic and Integrative Biology, and National Physical Laboratories. In 2003, Dr. Kumar associated with Professor Joseph Wang's Research group at New Mexico State University where his research was focused on the microchip technology and nanofiber-based biosensor development. In 2004, Dr. Kumar joined the University of South Florida as a research assistant professor at Nanomaterial Nanomanufacturing Research Center (NNRC). Later, in 2005 he was appointed as faculty in the College of Health Sciences, Department of Internal Medicine where his main research focused on nanomedicine, immunology, and cancer. Further, Dr. Kumar was appointed in 2010 as director of the Nanomedicine Division at the Center for Diagnostics Nanosystems at Marshall University, West Virginia. In 2011, he worked as an assistant professor in the Department of Medical Laboratory Science at University of Delaware, where he also holds a joint appointment with the Department of Biomedical Engineering at University of Delaware. Dr. Kumar has received top referee of the year award in 2006 and 2007 from Elsevier and the editor of *Biosensor and Bioelectronics*. Dr. Kumar is also a charter member of the Academy of Innovation at University of South Florida. Dr. Kumar's research is currently focused on how nanotechnology can be used for solving clinical problems related to cancer, cardiology, and tissue engineering. Dr. Kumar has filled in more than 26 patents on his research related to biosensors and nanotechnology. He has presented his work at more than 60 international conferences worldwide, published more than 35 peer-reviewed research articles and two book chapters, and is an editorial board member of *Sensors and Transducers Journal*. He mentored several PhD, master, and undergraduate students on nanomedicine-related research. Dr. Kumar's work has been covered by many different media outlets including news agencies in Florida and West Virginia and Nanotechnology now. He also served at many study sections at the National Science Foundation, National Institutes for Health, and other federal grant agencies in the United States. In August 2012, he organized and served as chair of an international conference on nanomedicine in drug delivery and cancer diagnosis at University of Delaware.

Heidi M. Mansour, PhD, RPh, is an assistant professor of Pharmaceutics & Drug Delivery, UK College of Pharmacy, a faculty associate at the UK Center of Membrane Sciences, and a graduate faculty at the University of North Carolina-Chapel Hill (UNC-Chapel Hill).

Dr. Mansour currently holds faculty appointments and graduate appointments at the University of Kentucky (UK) College of Pharmacy, the UNC-Chapel Hill, and is faculty associate of the UK Membrane Center. She is a faculty mentor in the UK Engineered Bioactive Interfaces and Devices Program funded through the National Science Foundation Integrative Graduate Education Research Training (NSF IGERT) Program and the NSF Research Education for Undergraduates (NSF REU) Training Program joint with the UK College of Engineering. She is also a faculty mentor in the National Cancer Institute-Cancer Nanotechnology Training Center (NCI-CNTC). Previously, she was an instructor (both in the graduate and PharmD programs) and a postdoctoral fellow at UNC-Chapel Hill School of Pharmacy receiving the 2007 UNC-Chapel Hill Postdoctoral Award for Research Excellence from the Office of the Vice-Chancellor and the 2007 American Association of Pharmaceutical Scientists (AAPS) Postdoctoral Fellow Award in Research Excellence, in addition to other honors and awards. She has a BS in pharmacy (highest honors and distinction) and a PhD in pharmaceutical sciences with a PhD major in drug delivery/pharmaceutics (School of Pharmacy—2003) and a PhD minor in advanced physical and biophysical chemistry (Department of Chemistry—1999) from the University of Wisconsin-Madison. She serves on the editorial advisory boards of eight journals in drug delivery and nanomedicine, the NIH U.S. Pediatric Formulations Initiative New Drug Delivery Systems Aerosols Working Group, and is a delegate to the United States Pharmacopeia (USP). Dr. Mansour has published more than 40 peer-reviewed scientific publications, invited papers, 5 book chapters, more than 80 abstracts, and is coeditor of this book on nanomedicine drug delivery by Taylor & Francis/CRC Press. Her research program enjoys funding from federal sources (NIH, NSF, FDA) and the pharmaceutical industry. Dr. Mansour has been an invited speaker at numerous national and international scientific conferences. She leads a multi-disciplinary group of postdoctoral scholars, visiting scholars, visiting professors, graduate students, physician-scientist fellows, and undergraduate students.

Eric Blough, PhD, is an associate professor and director of Pharmacology and Toxicology at Marshall University.

Dr. Blough received a BS in biology from Michigan Technological University in 1990, his MS in exercise physiology from Southern Illinois University in 1992, and a PhD in exercise physiology at the Ohio State University in 1997. After his PhD he completed a postdoctoral fellowship in the Department of Physiology and Biophysics at the University of Illinois.

In 2003, he joined the faculty at Marshall University as an assistant professor in the Department of Biological Sciences with a joint appointment in the Department of Physiology and Toxicology in the Joan C. Edwards School of Medicine. Dr. Blough has also held adjunct faculty positions in the Biotechnology program at West Virginia State University and the Exercise Physiology program at Marshall University. In 2006, Dr. Blough was promoted to the rank of associate professor of biological sciences and since 2010 he has also been an adjunct clinical assistant professor of cardiology in the Joan C. Edwards School of Medicine at Marshall. In 2010, Dr. Blough founded the Center for Diagnostic Nanosystems. A prolific researcher and publisher, Dr. Blough and his colleagues have received over $11,000,000.00 in research awards since 1998 and published over 150 scientific manuscripts, technical reports, and abstracts—all while maintaining a strong focus on student development and mentoring in his teaching. Dr. Blough has awarded the 2005 Marshall Distinguished Artists and Scholars Award (Jr. Level), the 2009 Marshall Distinguished Artists and Scholars Award (Sr. Level), and the 2009 John and Frances Rucker Outstanding Graduate Advisor Award. Furthermore, Dr. Blough has been nominated for multiple teaching, research, and advising awards nearly every year since joining the faculty at Marshall.

Adam Friedman, MD, FAAD, is an assistant professor of medicine (dermatology) and physiology and biophysics, and currently serves as director of Dermatologic Research and Associate Residency Program at the Unified Division of Dermatology of Montefiore Medical Center—Albert Einstein College of Medicine.

Dr. Friedman graduated Magna Cum Laude from the University of Pennsylvania and received his MD with distinction in dermatology research from Albert Einstein College of Medicine. He was trained in medicine at New York Hospital Queens, affiliated with NY Presbyterian Hospital/Weil-Cornell Medical Center and completed his dermatology residency as chief resident at the Albert Einstein College of Medicine.

Dr. Friedman is currently investigating novel nanotechnologies that allow for controlled and sustained delivery of a wide spectrum of physiologically and medicinally relevant molecules, with an emphasis on treating infectious diseases, accelerating wound healing, immune modulation, and correcting vascular dysfunction. He holds several patents derived from these investigations, and has published over 80 papers/chapters on both his research as well as a variety of clinical areas in dermatology with an emphasis on emerging medical therapies.

Dr. Friedman lectures extensively in both national and international forums, currently serves as the dermatology expert for healthguru.com, and is the vice president of the Nanodermatology Society, and for his work on nanotechnology, has been featured on the online forums DermMatters,

Nanotechnology Thought Leaders, and Dermquest. He has received awards from multiple organizations such as the American Academy of Dermatology, American Society for Dermatologic Surgery, Dermatology Foundation, and the La Roche Posay North American Foundation. Dr. Friedman has appeared on television news programs such as Good Morning America, and has been quoted in numerous leading publications, including WebMD, MSN.com, Good Housekeeping, and Women's Day.

Contributors

Jaleh Barar
Tabriz University of Medical Sciences
Tabriz, Iran

Eric R. Blough
Center for Diagnostic
    Nanosystems
and
Department of Internal Medicine
Joan C. Edwards School of Medicine
and
Department of Pharmaceutical
    Science
School of Pharmacy
and
Cell Differentiation and
    Development Center
and
Department of Pharmacology
    Physiology, and Toxicology
Joan C. Edwards School of Medicine
and
Marshall University
Huntington, West Virginia

Warren R. L. Cairns
Institute for the Dynamics
    of Environmental
    Processes-CNR
Venice, Italy

Don F. Cameron
Department of Cell Biology and
    Pathology
University of South Florida
Tampa, Florida

Emilio Castro
3B's Research Group–
    Biomaterials Biodegradables
    and Biomimetics
University of Minho
Guimarães, Portugal
and
ICVS/3B's-PT Government
    Associate Laboratory
Guimarães, Portugal

Niketa Dixit
Department of Psychology
College of Arts and Science
University of Delaware
Newark, Delaware

Letizia Ferroni
Department of Biomedical
    Sciences
University of Padua
Padua, Italy

Adam Friedman
Department of Medicine, Division
    of Dermatology
and
Department of Physiology and
    Biophysics
Albert Einstein College of Medicine
Bronx, New York

Chiara Gardin
Department of Biomedical
    Sciences
University of Padua
Padua, Italy

Mark Glaum
Department of Internal Medicine
University of South Florida
Tampa, Florida

Don Hayes
Departments of Pediatrics and
    Internal Medicine
The Ohio State University
and
The Ohio State University
Davis Heart & Lung Research
    Institute
Columbus, OH

Zeenat Iqbal
Department of Pharmaceutics
Jamia Hamdard Deemed University
New Delhi, India

Arun Kumar
Department of Medical
    Laboratory Science
University of Delaware
Newark, Delaware

Frederic Lagarce
Department of Biopharmacy and
    Pharmaceutical Technology
Lunam University
Angers, France

Luca Lancerotto
Department of Neurosciences
University of Padua
Padua, Italy

Ana Sofia Macedo
Fernando Pessoa University
Porto, Portugal

Heidi M. Mansour
Department of Pharmaceutical
    Sciences-Drug Development
    Division
University of Kentucky
Lexington, Kentucky

Siva K. Nalabotu
Center for Diagnostic Nanosystems
School of Pharmacy
Marshall University
Huntington, West Virginia

Yadollah Omidi
Research Center for Pharmaceutical
    Nanotechnology,
Tabriz University of Medical
    Sciences
Tabriz, Iran

Chun-Woong Park
Chungbuk National University
Cheongju, Republic of Korea
and
University of Kentucky
Lexington, Kentucky

Javier L. Pou Ucha
Department of Nuclear Medicine
University Hospital Complex
    of Vigo
Vigo, Spain

Kevin M. Rice
Center for Diagnostic Nanosystems
and
Department of Internal Medicine
Joan C. Edwards School of Medicine
and
Cell Differentiation and
    Development Center
and
Marshall University
Huntington, West Virginia

Chiara Rigo
Institute for the Dynamics
    of Environmental
    Processes–CNR
Dorsoduro
Venice, Italy

Marco Roman
Institute for the Dynamics of
    Environmental Processes–CNR
Venice, Italy

Ashley E. Saienni
Department of Medical Laboratory
    Science
University of Delaware
Newark, Delaware
and
Georgia Institute of Technology
Atlanta, Georgia

Eliana B. Souto
Fernando Pessoa University
Porto, Portugal
and
Institute of Biotechnology
    and Bioengineering
Centre of Genomics
    and Biotechnology
University of Trás-os-Montes
    and Alto Douro (IBB/
    CGB-UTAD)
Vila Real, Portugal

Sushama Talegaonkar
Department of Pharmaceutics
Jamia Hamdard Deemed
    University
New Delhi, India

Mohammad Tariq
Department of Pharmaceutics
Jamia Hamdard Deemed University
New Delhi, India

Vincenzo Vindigni
Department of Neurosciences
University of Padua
Padua, Italy

Barbara Zavan
Department of Biomedical Sciences
University of Padua
Padua, Italy

1

Nanoparticles in Drug Delivery Systems

Emilio Castro and Arun Kumar

CONTENTS

1.1 Nanoparticles: Small Size, Big Advantages 2
1.2 Numerous Types of Nanoparticles 4
    1.2.1 Inorganic Nanoparticles 4
    1.2.2 Lipid Nanoparticles...7
    1.2.3 Polymeric Nanoparticles...8
1.3 Further On: Hybridization and Multifunctionality 13
1.4 The Journey of a Nanoparticle in the Body 14
1.5 Drug Release in Action 17
1.6 The Big Impact of Nanoparticles..19
Acknowledgments...20
Suggested Readings..20

Drug delivery systems (DDS) are designed to improve the pharmacological and therapeutic properties of drugs administered in vivo, and DDS include particle carriers that can function as drug reservoirs. Drug carrier systems allow for the controlled release of drugs at the desired sites, thus altering the pharmacokinetics and biodistribution of the drugs. In this sense, nanoparticles are intrinsically advantageous over conventional particles. The pharmacokinetics of particle DDS is largely affected by splenic filtration, which occurs at the interendothelial cell slits (<200 nm) in the walls of venous sinuses. Furthermore, vesicles larger than 100 nm must be designed to prevent surface opsonization processes, which lead to phagocytic uptake of the particles in the liver. Taken together, nanoparticles can be a long-circulatory drug carrier. Based on the enhanced permeability and retention effect, this kind of DDS is useful for cancer chemotherapy.

Among the DDS reported so far, liposomes have entered the market and polymeric micelles are currently in clinical trials. In addition, polymeric nanoparticles have received increased attention. All of these DDS are organic nanoparticles consisting of lipids or synthetic polymers. Compared with the rapid progress in developing DDS using organic particles, less progress has been made in developing inorganic nanoparticle-based drug delivery systems (NDDS). However, recent progress in the field of nanotechnology and nanofabrication has led to the production of various inorganic nanoparticles, including iron oxide nanoparticles, gold nanoparticles, and fullerenes, as attractive vehicles for drug delivery. There are several advantages to using these inorganic nanoparticles as drug carriers. First, they are easy to prepare with a defined size. More interesting, they often exhibit multiple functions useful in medicine, for example, as exothermic reactors and contrast agents; in contrast organic nanoparticles, such as liposomes and micelles, serve only as drug reservoirs. Nevertheless, both organic and inorganic NDDS, due to their diminute size, can penetrate barriers through small capillaries to enter individual cells, allowing efficient drug accumulation at the targeted locations in the body. As a result, the therapeutic agent toxicity is reduced, the drug side effects are decreased, and the treatment efficacy is enhanced.

Precise drug release into highly specific targets involves miniaturizing the delivery systems to be much smaller than their targets. It is highly expected that these minute DDS can be realized through the advances in nanobiotechnology. The integration of nanotechnology products, such as nanoparticles, with therapeutic agents, has recently created a new therapeutic trend that would not otherwise be possible.

1.1 Nanoparticles: Small Size, Big Advantages

Nanoparticles are nanosized materials (diameter 1–100 nm) that can carry multiple drugs and imaging agents. Owing to their high surface-area-to-volume ratio, it is possible to achieve high ligand density on the surface for targeting purposes. Nanoparticles can also be used to increase local drug concentration by carrying the drug within and controlling its release when nanoparticles are bound to targets.

Nanoparticles exhibit size-related properties that differ significantly from those observed in bulk materials. Nanoparticles are devices and systems produced by chemical or physical processes with specific properties. The reason why nanoparticles are attractive for such purposes is based on their important and unique features, such as their surface-to-mass ratio, which is much larger than that of other materials, as well as their ability to absorb and carry other compounds.

The composition of nanoparticles varies. Source materials may be of biological origin, such as phospholipids, lipids, lactic acid, dextran, and chitosan, or the materials may have more "chemical" characteristics, such as various polymers, carbon, silica, and metals. The ways nanoparticle interacts with cells vary widely depending on whether the source materials are biological components, such as phospholipids, or whether the components are nonbiological, such as gold and cadmium. Especially in the area of engineered nanoparticles of polymer origin there is a vast area of possibilities for the chemical composition. Although solid nanoparticles may be used for drug targeting, when reaching the intended diseased site in the body, the drug carried needs to be released. So, for drug delivery biodegradable nanoparticle formulations are needed because the intention is to transport and release the drug.

Nanoparticles have unusual properties that can be exploited to improve drug delivery. Because of their minute size, they are often taken up by cells, whereas larger particles would be excluded or cleaned from the body. Recent strategies have included using polyethylene glycol (PEG) to increase circulation time and using PEG in competition with binding groups to reduce nonspecific attachment or uptake.

We made a systematic search in Scopus to identify the number of publications made in this area of research (see Figure 1.1). From 1990 to 2000, only several hundred research papers were published on "NDDS"; however, between 2000 and 2010, many thousands of research papers have been published.

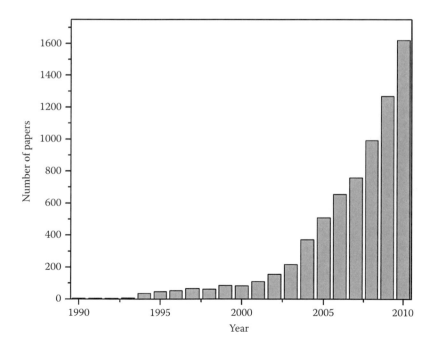

FIGURE 1.1
Number of scientific papers published from 1990 to 2010 involving DDS using nanoparticles.

1.2 Numerous Types of Nanoparticles

Nanoparticles have been developed using a number of materials, including polymers, metals, and ceramics. Based on the manufacturing method and material, the nanoparticles can take various shapes and sizes and have distinct properties. The family of nanoparticles includes, among others, polymeric nanoparticles, solid lipid nanoparticles, liposomes, micelles, dendrimers, carbon nanotubes, and metal nanoparticles (see Figure 1.2).

1.2.1 Inorganic Nanoparticles

For drug compounds with poor water solubility, grinding them into nano scale crystals increases the surface area, which leads to a faster dissolution rate. Elan Pharmaceutical NanoCrystal® Technology, one of the best-known cases, uses nanoparticles smaller than 1 μm in diameter and produced by milling the drug using a wet-milling technique. The result is an aqueous dispersion of the drug, with only a thin coating composed of a surfactant or a combination of surfactants behaving like a solution that can be processed into finished dosage forms for all routes of administration. Problems typical of poorly soluble drugs, like including reduced bioavailability, improper

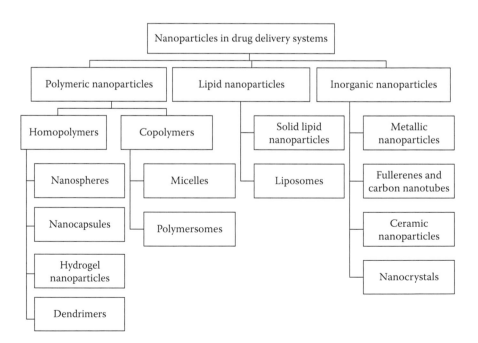

FIGURE 1.2
Classification of NDDS.

absorption pattern, and problems in preparing the parenteral dosage form may be resolved through formulating the drug as nanocrystals. Only a minimum quantity of surfactants needs to be added for safe and effective passage through capillaries. The potential of nanocrystals as NDDS can be inferred by the FDA approval of Rapamune®, containing sirolimus (an immunosuppressant drug to prevent graft rejection in children after liver transplantations) and Emend®, which contains aprepitant (MK 869) and is used to treat emesis associated with cancer chemotherapy.

Ceramic nanoparticles are typically composed of inorganic nanomaterials, such as silica and alumina. However, the nanoparticle core is not limited to just these two materials; metals, metal oxides, and metal sulfides can also be used to produce myriad nanostructures with varying sizes, shapes, and porosities. Moreover, the nanoparticles may be porous and provide a physical encasement to protect an entrapped molecular payload from degradation or denaturation. Hollow silica nanoparticles, such as calcium phosphate-based nanoshells, have been prepared with surface pores leading to a central reservoir. In contrast, mesoporous silica material contains a complex, worm-like network of channels throughout the interior of the solid nanoparticle. Generally, inorganic nanoparticles may be engineered to evade the reticulo-endothelial system by varying size and surface composition.

The most commonly investigated ceramic materials for drug delivery are porous silicon and silica. Porous hollow silica nanoparticles are fabricated in a suspension containing sacrificial nanoscale templates, such as calcium carbonate. Silica precursors, such as sodium silicate, are added into the suspension, which is then dried and calcinated creating a core of the template material coated with porous silica shell. Creating drug carriers involves mixing the porous hollow silica nanoparticles with the drug molecules and subsequently drying the mixture to coalesce the drug molecules to the surface of the silica nanoparticles. Porous nanoparticles exhibit a more desirable gradual release than other types of nanoparticles.

Silica nanoparticles may be prepared by sol–gel or microemulsion-based methods, such as an organic–aqueous biphasic system. Solvent cages formed within the microemulsion direct the size and aggregation properties of the growing silica nanoparticles. MCM-41 is an example of a mesoporous silica nanoparticle. Silica nanoparticles are typically synthesized via sol–gel processes in the presence of a surfactant such as C_{12}-trimethylammonium bromide or C_{16}-trimethylammonium bromide. The relative ease of synthesis and functionalization make silica nanoparticles attractive targets for drug delivery; however, the lack of information on their biodegradation remains a noteworthy limitation.

Emerging evidence indicates metallic nanoparticles are good carriers for DDS and biosensors. Although nanoparticles composed of various metals have been made, silver and gold nanoparticles are of prime importance for biomedical use. Their surface functionalization is very easy. A large number of ligands have been linked to nanoparticles, including sugars, peptides, proteins, and DNA. These ligands attached to metallic nanoparticles have been used for delivery of bioactive agents, drug discovery, bioassays, detection, imaging, and many other applications because of the surface functionalization capability of this type of nanoparticles.

Preparing gold nanoparticles commonly involves the chemical reduction of gold salts in aqueous, organic, or mixed solvent systems. However, the gold surface is extremely reactive, and aggregation can occur as a result. To circumvent this issue, gold nanoparticles are regularly reduced in the presence of a stabilizer that binds to the surface and precludes aggregation via favorable cross-linking and charge properties. Several stabilizers exist to passivate a gold nanoparticle surface, including citrate, thiol-containing organic compounds, encapsulation within microemulsions, and polymeric coatings. Several synthetic strategies also exist, such as the two-phase liquid–liquid method initially described by Faraday in 1857 as a way to create metal colloidal suspensions. Faraday reduced an aqueous gold salt with phosphorous in carbon disulfide to obtain a ruby-colored aqueous suspension of colloidal gold particles. Using the Brust–Schiffrin method further optimized this two-phase liquid–liquid system with gold salts being transferred from water to toluene using tetraoctylammonium bromide as the phase transfer reagent, with reduction by aqueous sodium borohydride in the presence of dodecanethiol. Using modifications of this method, gold nanoparticles have been synthesized with numerous biomolecular coatings (see Figure 1.3).

Two nanostructures that have received much attention in recent years are hollow, carbon-based, cage-like architectures: nanotubes and fullerenes, also known as buckyballs. Single-wall nanotubes, multiwall nanotubes, and C_{60} fullerenes are common configurations. The size, geometry, and surface characteristics of these structures make them appealing as drug carrier. Single-wall nanotubes and C_{60} fullerenes have diameters of 1 nm, about half the diameter of the average DNA helix.

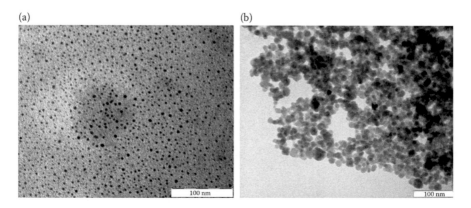

FIGURE 1.3
Transmission electron microscope images of inorganic nanoparticles: (a) gold and (b) magnetite.

In 1990, physicists W. Krätschmer and D. R. Huffman for the first time produced isolable quantities of C_{60} by causing an arc between two graphite rods to burn in a helium atmosphere and using an organic solvent to extract the carbon condensate. Using C_{60} for drug delivery is becoming more common, and we forecast these interesting nanomaterials will be used for a wide variety of applications in the field of health sciences.

Carbon nanotubes were discovered in 1991 by S. Iijima. Currently, the physical properties are still being discovered and disputed. What makes the task so difficult is that nanotubes have a broad range of electronic, thermal, and structural properties that change depending on the different kinds of nanotubes (defined by their diameter, length, and chirality, or twist). Multiwall nanotubes have diameters ranging from several to tens of nanometers depending on the number of walls in the structure. Fullerenes and carbon nanotubes are typically fabricated using electric arc discharge, laser ablation, chemical vapor deposition or combustion processes. Surface-functionalized carbon nanotubes can be internalized within mammalian cells and may one day be used to deliver drugs.

Several synthetic strategies exist to prepare superparamagnetic iron oxide nanoparticles. In particular, a water-in-oil microemulsion system with reverse micelles has been used extensively. For maghemite (γ-Fe_2O_3) and magnetite (Fe_3O_4) nanoparticles, this precipitation technique requires alkalization of a solution of metal salt with subsequent hydrolysis in microemulsions. Additionally, biosynthetic routes using magnetic bacteria exist; the resulting nanoparticles typically range from 50 to 100 nm in diameter. Further, iron oxide nanoparticles have been synthesized through chemical coprecipitation, sonochemical decomposition, and thermal decomposition of iron pentacarbonyl followed by oxidation. When optimized, these methods will result in monodisperse nanoparticles with sizes ranging from 3 to 20 nm for magnetite and 4–16 nm for maghemite. Another benefit of iron oxide nanoparticles is they are capable of fairly easy surface modifications, which presents an attractive prospect for direct drug payload attachment. Recently, ultrasmall, peptide-coated magnetite nanoparticles have been used to target integrin-rich tumor cells.

1.2.2 Lipid Nanoparticles

Liposomes, discovered in 1961 by Alec D. Bangham, are concentric, bilayered vesicles in which an aqueous volume is entirely enclosed by a membranous lipid bilayer mainly composed of natural or synthetic phospholipids (see Figure 1.4). Liposomes are characterized in terms of size, surface charge, and number of bilayers. Liposomes have a number of advantages, including amphiphilic character, biocompatibility, and ease of surface modification, rendering liposomes suitable for use in delivery systems for biotech drugs. Using liposomes greatly alters the pharmacokinetic profile of loaded drugs, especially in the cases of proteins and peptides, and liposomes can easily be modified through surface attachment of polyethylene glycol, thus increasing the circulation half-life.

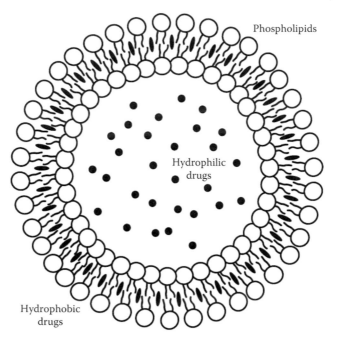

FIGURE 1.4
Structure of liposomes.

Liposomal formulations were the first NDDS introduced to market; the Doxil® PEGylated liposomal formulation for doxorubicin was the first product based on liposomes. The liposomes used in such formulations are called "stealth" liposomes because of the size <200 nm and the hydrophilic (PEG) surface. These long circulating liposomes target tumor tissue through a mechanism known as enhanced permeation and retention. Hence, liposomal formulations of doxorubicin considerably reduced the cardiotoxicity of doxorubicin. Many other liposomal products are in various phases of clinical trials.

Solid lipid nanoparticles consist of a solid lipid matrix, in which the drug is normally incorporated, with an average diameter below 1 μm. To avoid aggregation and to stabilize the dispersion, different surfactants are added. The main reason solid lipid nanoparticles were developed is they result in a combination of advantages from different carrier systems, including liposomes and polymeric nanoparticles. Solid lipid nanoparticles have been investigated for parenteral, pulmonic, and dermal application routes.

1.2.3 Polymeric Nanoparticles

Polymers are the most commonly explored materials for constructing NDDS. A polymer used in controlled drug delivery formulations must be chemically inert, nontoxic, and free of leachable impurities. The polymer must also have an appropriate physical structure, with minimal undesired aging, and be readily indictable. Polymeric nanoparticles can be made from synthetic polymers, including poly(lactic acid) and poly(lactic-*co*-glycolic acid), and from natural polymers, such as chitosan and collagen. Additionally, they may be used to encapsulate drugs without chemical modifications. The drugs can be released in a controlled manner through surface or bulk erosion, by diffusion through the polymer matrix, through swelling followed by diffusion, or in response to the local environment. In comparison to solid lipid nanoparticles and nanocrystals, polymeric nanoparticles consist of biodegradable polymer. The advantages of using polymeric nanoparticles in drug delivery are numerous, the most important of which is that they generally increase the stability of any volatile pharmaceutical agents and that they are easily and cheaply fabricated in large quantities by a multitude of methods. Also, polymeric nanoparticles may be engineered specially, allowing them to deliver a high concentration of pharmaceutical agent to a desired location (see Figure 1.5). Concerns about using polymeric nanoparticles include the inherent structural heterogeneity of polymers, reflected, for example, in a high polydispersity index.

Polymeric nanoparticles are a broad class composed of both vesicular systems (nanocapsules) and matrix systems (nanospheres). Nanocapsules are systems in which the drug is confined to a cavity surrounded by a unique polymeric membrane, whereas nanospheres are systems in which the drug is dispersed throughout the polymer matrix. Several natural polymers, such as gelatin, albumin, and alginate, are used to prepare the nanoparticles; however, natural polymers have some inherent disadvantages, including poor batch-to-batch reproducibility, a tendency to degrade,

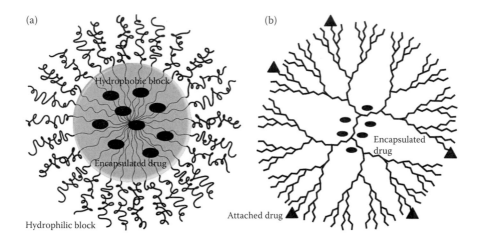

FIGURE 1.5
Two examples of polymer nanoparticles used in drug delivery systems: (a) block copolymer micelles and (b) dendrimers.

and the potential for antigenicity. Synthetic polymers used for nanoparticle preparation include preformed polymers, including polyesters such as polycaprolactone and poly(lactic acid), and monomers that can be polymerized *in situ*, such as polyalkyl cyanoacrylate. The drug is dissolved, entrapped, attached, or encapsulated throughout or within the polymeric shell/matrix. Depending on the method of preparation, the release characteristic of the incorporated drug can be controlled. Polymeric nanoparticulate systems are attractive modules for intracellular and site-specific delivery. Nanoparticles can be made to reach a target *in situ* because of their size and because their surface can be modified and functionalized with a specific recognition ligand (see Figure 1.6).

Abraxane® was the first polymeric nanoparticle-based product marketed by American Pharmaceutical Partners and American Bioscience. The product approved in 2005, consists of albumin-bound paclitaxel nanoparticles. The product is free of toxic solvents, such as cremophor-EL, which was previously used to solubilize paclitaxel so the drug could be administered to patients intravenously. Cremophor-EL is known to cause life-threatening allergic reactions. The success of Abraxane shows that nanotechnology can result in many exciting products that overcome hurdles in formulation science.

Polymeric micelles are supramolecular self-assemblies of synthetic macromolecules in which individual block copolymers (unimers) are held together

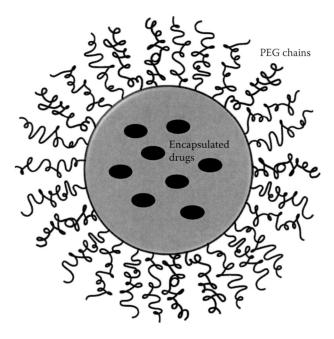

FIGURE 1.6
Structure of polymeric nanoparticles.

by noncovalent interactions. Block copolymer micelles possess a typical core–shell structure. The cores of the micelles solubilize drugs, and the coronas allow for the suspension of the micelles in aqueous media. To obtain spherical micelles with hydrophobic cores, the molecular weight of the corona-forming blocks should not exceed that of the core-forming parts of the block copolymer. The defining properties of micelles include critical micellization concentration, aggregation number, size, and shape. Typical block copolymer micelles will have low critical micellization concentration values, >100 individual polymer chains, hydrodynamic radii of 25–50 nm, and a largely spherical shape. The polymer that forms the blocks of the micelles can be classified into amino acids, polyesters, and poloxamers. These micelles have a fairly narrow size distribution and are characterized by their unique core–shell architecture.

Polymeric micelles have been an excellent DDS because of their high and versatile loading capacity, stability in physiological conditions, slower rate of dissolution, high accumulation of drug at the target site, and capability to functionalize the end group for conjugation of the targeting ligands (see Figure 1.7). Polymeric micelles belong to a group of amphiphilic colloids that can be formed spontaneously from amphiphilic molecules through using certain concentrations and temperatures. The hydrophilic surface of polymer micelles protects their nonspecific uptake by the reticuloendothelial system. An example of a polymeric micelle under clinical evaluation is NK911, which consists of a bound doxorubicin fraction for metastatic pancreatic cancer treatment. Another micellar DDS is NK105, a micelle containing paclitaxel; this NDDS was evaluated for pancreatic, colonic, and gastric tumor treatment.

Dendrimers are synthetic, branched macromolecules that form a tree-like structure; the size and shape of dendrimers can be precisely controlled. The well-defined structure, monodispersity of size, surface functionalization capability and stability are properties of dendrimers that make them attractive drug carrier candidates. Drug molecules can be incorporated into dendrimers via either complexation and encapsulation. Dendrimers used in drug delivery studies typically incorporate one or more of the following

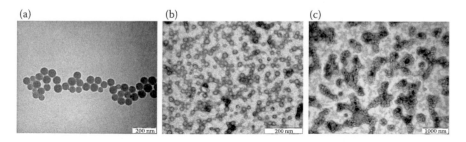

FIGURE 1.7
Transmission electron microscope image of organic nanoparticles: (a) polymer nanoparticles, (b) micelles, and (c) polymersomes.

polymers: polyamidoamine, melamine, poly(L-glutamic acid), polyethylene-imine, poly(propyleneimine), and poly(ethylene glycol).

In late 1970s, scientists Fritz Vögtle, at the University of Bonn (Germany), and Donald A. Tomalia, then working for Dow Chemical in Michigan, started to build the first of dendrimers. Dendrimers are fabricated from monomers using either convergent or divergent step-growth polymerization. The manufacturing process involves a series of repetitive steps, starting with a central initiator core. Each subsequent growth step represents a new "generation" of polymer with a larger molecular diameter, twice the number of reactive surface sites, and approximately double the molecular weight of the preceding generation. Vivagel® is the first NDDS based on dendrimers and is in Phase 1 clinical trial.

Polymersomes are mainly composed of amphiphilic block copolymers that are held together in water because of the strong physical interactions between the insoluble hydrophobic blocks, thus forming bilayer morphology or, in the case of triblock copolymers, a bilayer-like morphology. Polymersomes have been found to be considerably less permeable than liposomes, even though the membrane thickness may be only a few nanometers. This characteristic can be attributed to the increased length of the amphiphile and its conformational freedom, which allows for greater toughness and reduced permeability compared to natural amphiphiles. This reduced permeability may enhance the polymersome's benefits in drug delivery by decreasing the rate of release.

Polymersomes can be turned to achieve sizes close to that of liposomes (which is important for selective drug administration), better mechanical stability because of a thicker membrane, low permeability, and the capability to tune the membrane properties through the copolymer chemistry. In addition, shell-forming hydrophilic flexible polymeric blocks reduce the interaction between vesicles and macrophages thus conveying surface-protective properties to the drug carrier. Considering all these factors, these polymeric carriers can be designed to achieve physical, chemical, and biological functions in the desired formulations. Polymersome preparation is similar to that of liposomes, usually using the film rehydration technique, solvent method, or direct dissolution. Despite the benefits of using polymersomes, there are still no clinically approved strategies that use active cellular targeting for polymersome-based DDS.

Hydrogel nanoparticles use hydrophobic polysaccharides to encapsulate and deliver drugs. A novel system using cholesterol pullulan shows great promise. In this system, four cholesterol molecules gather to form a self-aggregating hydrophobic core with pullulan outside. The resulting cholesterol nanoparticles stabilize entrapped proteins by forming this hybrid complex. These nanoparticles stimulate the immune system and are readily taken up by dendritic cells.

Stimuli-responsive hydrogels have been prepared; they respond to changes in pH and temperature, and they have been found to be tissue compatible. Recently, a novel type of temperature-responsive oxygen carrier was prepared using poly(*N*-isopropyl acrylamide) hydrogel nanoparticles that encapsulate bovine hemoglobin; this formulation might benefit tissue hypoxia caused by decreased body temperature. Hydrogel nanoparticles have been used to effectively deliver antigens, DNA, and oligonucleotides. Cross-linked hydrogel nanoparticles that are 35–50 nm in diameter and composed of natural polymers allow intracellular sites to be targeted; they also have good acceptability because of the higher water content.

1.3 Further On: Hybridization and Multifunctionality

Presently, considerable interest exists in inorganic–organic hybrid nanoparticles because of the excellent properties that result from combining inorganic and organic materials. For example, because of the unique superparamagnetic properties found in hybrids but not found in other materials, the functionalization and surface modification of magnetite nanoparticles has attracted special attention in medicine and other fields. If magnetite nanoparticles are coated with polymers, the hybrid magnetic nanoparticles gain the advantage of good dispersion and high stability against oxidation, and the functional groups at the surface can be used for further functionalization. Recently, magnetite-polymer hybrid nanoparticles have been drawing great attention in drug delivery because they can be manipulated by an external magnetic field gradient to control a targeted delivery. If fluorescence groups can be linked to magnetite–polymer hybrid nanoparticles, as a result of the enrichment of fluorescence molecules, these nanoparticles can serve as efficient tracers of drug carriers to study the magnetic-targeting effect of magnetic nanoparticles, allowing them to be more extensively applied in targeted DDS.

Because of the potential benefits of multimodal functionality in biomedical applications, researchers would like to design and fabricate multifunctional magnetic nanoparticles. Currently, there are two strategies to fabricate magnetic nanoparticle-based multifunctional nanostructures. The first strategy is molecular functionalization. Biofunctional molecules (e.g., antibodies, ligands, and receptors) coat the magnetic nanoparticles and make them interact with a biological entity with high affinity, thus providing a controllable means of "tagging." After molecular functionalization, the biofunctional magnetic nanoparticles confer high selectivity and sensitivity for many biological applications. The second strategy is to combine magnetic nanomaterials and other functional nanostructures by sequential growth or coating, which produces a single entity conferring multiple functions in nanoscale. For example, using magnetic nanoparticles as seeds, the growth of semiconducting chalcogenides produces core–shell or heterodimer nanostructures with both magnetic and fluorescent properties, leading to the demonstration of intracellular manipulation of nanoparticles. Integrating magnetic and metallic nanoparticles forms heterodimer structures that offer two distinct surfaces and properties to allow different kinds of functional molecules to attach to the specific parts of the heterodimers, which may bind to multiple receptors or act as agents for multimodality imaging. The encapsulation of a potential anticancer drug by iron oxide nanoshells results in yolk-shell nanostructures, which promise novel nanodevices for controlled drug delivery.

Multicomponent hybrid nanoparticles can exhibit multiple functionalities for applications that are difficult (or even impossible) to achieve with single-component nanoparticles. For example, hybrid noble metal/iron oxide nanoparticles exhibit not only unique optical properties but also magnetic responses. The large-scale synthesis of such hybrid nanoparticles is a challenge. Multifunctional hybrid nanoparticles combine some of the unique physical and chemical characteristics of two or more classes of materials, such as polymers, metals, and ceramics, to create a versatile and robust new class of nanoparticles. Combining multiple nanomaterials make use of the strengths of one material to improve on the weaknesses of another material, expanding the functionality of single-component systems. Hybrid nanoparticle platforms provide unique opportunities in cancer therapy, specifically in the treatment of multidrug-resistant cancer.

1.4 The Journey of a Nanoparticle in the Body

The body's clearance mechanisms for colloids depend on their size, shape, and surface characteristics. Contemporary chemistry and material science now allow in-depth control over these properties. As a result, the number of potentially different NDDS has become virtually unlimited. Therefore, with the plethora of available nanomaterials, specific applications must be used to dictate the optimization of nanoparticle characteristics. The development of efficient nanomedicines requires a thorough understanding of the body characteristics. To potentiate progress at each step of the NDDS development process, it is necessary to completely characterize the interactions of nanoparticles with biological milieus, as well as make critical comparisons with data from existing systems. For example, the concept of long-circulation time differs greatly from one NDDS to another. Hence, each new nanoparticle must be positioned according to previously established standards. Similarly, routine integration of head-to-head comparisons between novel systems and other formulations will shed more light on the technical advances achieved with each innovation. Efficient and safe formulations will mature only when clinical considerations are taken into account early in the process of developing materials. The implications of nanotechnological achievements can sometimes eclipse the remote perspective of therapeutic applications. Nevertheless, when the final objective is to deliver active agents, fabricating complex nanostructures should never occult important biological considerations. The true challenge of nanomedicines is conciliating innovative nanomaterial advancements with a realistic clinical perspective.

Although NDDS can enter the body via different routes (e.g., pulmonary or oral), the most reproducible way to deliver drugs is usually through peripheral intravenous injection. From the injection site, the drugs are transported directly to the heart via the venous network. Blood is delivered to the right ventricle and continues into pulmonary circulation; the entire cardiac output passes through pulmonary circulation. Lung capillaries are among the smallest blood vessels in the body, with diameters between 2 and 13 μm in humans. Physiologically, the small diameter of the capillary lumen facilitates exchanges with the extravascular milieu and restricts passage from blood components. This size restriction allows qualitative control of the cell population in the lungs: highly deformable red blood cells transit very rapidly, and the passage of larger and more rigid white blood cells is delayed. Large, rigid NDDS can be sequestered in the lungs. These NDDS are trapped very rapidly upon their first passage through pulmonary circulation. Rigid NDDS with a diameter of 10 μm remain permanently trapped; particles with a diameter of 3–6 μm are initially caught in lung capillaries, but eventually escape to reach the systemic circulation, while smaller particles (<3 μm) avoid pulmonary retention. Rigid aggregates arising from physicochemical instability or interactions with blood components can also result in the sequestration of the carrier in the lung capillaries. Once they have passed the pulmonary capillaries, NDDS return to the left ventricle of the heart via the pulmonary veins and are pumped into the systemic circulation (see Figure 1.8).

Blood is the connective tissue responsible for transporting oxygen, nutrients, and waste products. Blood consists of cells suspended in a solution of

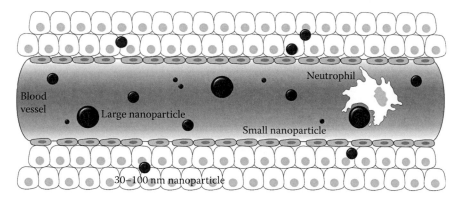

FIGURE 1.8
Nanoparticles in a blood vessel.

proteins and low molecular weight solutes, called plasma. It is the connective pathway for NDDS between organs. Intravascular interactions of blood cells with pathogens and NDDS are uncommon; NDDS interact with plasma proteins in the bloodstream. These interactions are guided by the physicochemical properties of NDDS, and the interactions highly influence the circulation time as well as the deposition in tissues.

Upon NDDS injection, rapid and nonspecific interactions with albumin occur through ionic and hydrophobic interactions. Although early deposition of albumin on the surface of NDDS can protect them from further opsonization with other proteins, these contacts are transient, and albumin can be easily displaced by other less-abundant proteins with higher affinities. Indeed, NDDS with physically adsorbed albumin have only marginally increased circulation times. The more abundant clinical experience comes from albumin-coated paclitaxel nanoparticles commercialized in 2005 (Abraxane).

The complement activation by NDDS depends on the surface properties of the nanoparticle; negative or positive charges and highly hydrophobic or irregular surfaces promote the adhesion of complement proteins. Similarly, the low radius of curvature of larger particles (>200 nm) facilitates the deposition of opsonins and their assembly into bulkier complexes. The sheathing of NDDS with hydrophilic polymers, such as poly(ethylene glycol), decreases nonspecific protein deposition and complement activation. PEGylation still remains the gold standard for imparting NDDS with long circulating times. Even so, the hydrophilic coating never totally abrogates protein deposition and complement activation (see Figure 1.9).

Other plasma proteins have been shown to interact with NDDS. The deposition of immunoglobulins (IgM and IgG) on nanoparticles enhances their

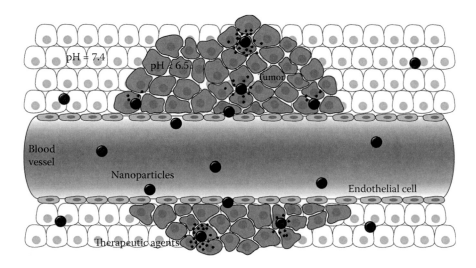

FIGURE 1.9
Passive tumor targeting of nanoparticles using the enhanced permeability and retention effect.

clearance through cooperative effects with complements. These proteins can recognize specific surface epitopes and adsorb through hydrophobic interactions. Although immunoglobulins are constitutively present in blood, their secretion is usually induced through immunogenic reactions. Other constitutive proteins (fibronectin, fibrinogen, or C-reactive protein) could play a role in the blood clearance and biodistribution of colloids through receptor-mediated internalization. In the case of PEG-*block*-poly(lactic acid) micelles, interactions with blood proteins (globulins) and cell membranes have been found to destabilize micelles and facilitate the release of their payload. For these reasons, early kinetic, qualitative, and quantitative evaluations of NDDS-protein interactions should help identify potential negative effects of blood protein adsorption on a nanoparticle's performance. During such evaluative studies, the nature of the biological fluid used should also be carefully chosen because the end result will be affected by the sampling conditions. Plasma contains anticoagulants, which can interfere with complement cascade activation and deplete serum of coagulation proteins (fibrinogen and others).

Most NDDS are too large to be filtered without prior biodegradation. Exceptions include quantum dots, which have been shown to be filtered for diameters up to 5.5 nm, and carbon nanotubes. The unique shape of carbon nanotubes might cause a favorable orientation in the blood flow or cause a distinctive transport mechanism, promoting their renal clearance.

1.5 Drug Release in Action

It is important to consider both drug release and polymer biodegradation when developing a nanoparticle-based DDS. In general, the drug release rate depends on (a) drug solubility, (b) desorption of the surface-bound or adsorbed drug, (c) drug diffusion through the nanoparticle matrix, (d) nanoparticle matrix erosion or degradation, and (e) the combination of erosion and diffusion processes. Hence, solubility, diffusion, and biodegradation of the particle matrix govern the release process.

In the case of nanospheres, where the drug is uniformly distributed, drug release occurs by diffusion or erosion of the matrix. If the diffusion of the drug is faster than the erosion of the matrix, then the mechanism of release is largely controlled by a diffusion process. The rapid, initial release, or "burst," is mainly attributed to a drug weakly bound to or adsorbed by the relatively large surfaces of nanoparticles. If the nanoparticle is coated with polymer, the release is controlled by diffusion of the drug from the polymeric membrane. The membrane coating acts as a drug-release barrier. Therefore, drug solubility and diffusion in or across the polymer membrane has become determining factors in drug release.

   A key goal of delivery systems is to discharge their payloads specifically at the diseased tissue. Two approaches to achieve this goal are passive and active targeting. Active targeting requires the therapeutic agent to be achieved by conjugating the therapeutic agent or carrier system to a tissue-specific or cell-specific ligand. Passive targeting is achieved by incorporating the therapeutic agent into a macromolecule or nanoparticle that passively reaches the target organ. Drugs encapsulated in nanoparticles and drugs coupled with macro-molecules can passively target tumors through the enhanced permeability and retention effect. Alternatively, catheters can be used to infuse nanopar-ticles to the target organ or tissue (see Figure 1.10).

   Liposomes have been demonstrated to be useful for delivering pharma-ceutical agents. Such systems use contact-facilitated drug delivery, which involves the liposomes binding to or interacting with the targeted cell mem-brane. This binding or interaction permits enhanced lipid–lipid exchange with the lipid monolayer of the nanoparticle, which accelerates the convec-tive flux of lipophilic drugs (e.g., paclitaxel) to dissolve through the outer lipid membrane of the nanoparticles to targeted cells. Such nanosystems can serve as drug depots, exhibiting prolonged release kinetics and long persis-tence at the target site.

   We will use Doxil as an example; although it is an effective carrier for deliv-ering doxorubicin to the tumor tissue, only a modest increase in antitumor activity has resulted. The major reason is the low rate of release of the drug both in blood circulation and in the tumor tissue. High-level tumor accumu-lation resulting from the nanoparticle formulation does not directly correlate with the bioavailability of the drug to the tumor; the bioavailability is more dependent on the rate of drug release. Moreover, Doxil causes side effects,

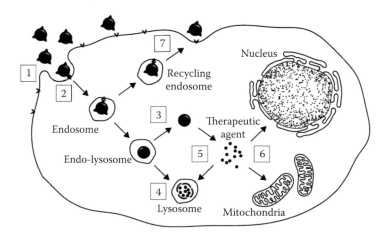

FIGURE 1.10
Active internalization of surface-modified nanoparticles through receptor-mediated endo-cytosis. The numbers 1–7 represent the order in which the active internalization of surface-modified nanoparticles through receptor-mediated endocytosis occurs.

including hand–foot syndrome and mucositis, possibly because of the slow release of the drug. Although Doxil has not been shown to cause acute cardiotoxicity, the side effects limit the maximum tolerated dose. Another typical example is the liposomal Cisplatin® formulation. In clinical trials, it has been found to accumulate substantially in the tumor tissue and to have no antitumor effects. Cisplatin cannot diffuse through the intact liposomal membrane; thus, it predominantly stays inside the PEGylated liposome and displays little activity.

1.6 The Big Impact of Nanoparticles

Nanoparticle-enabled DDS are forecast to dramatically reshape the way existing drugs are delivered. The growing range of NDDS is poised to change the way new compounds are formulated and to extend the life cycle of existing compounds. But that is just the beginning; after 2015, NDDS are expected to take the lion's share of the market, composing nearly 90% of the drug delivery market—a complete transformation of the way DDS are formulated.

The benefits of using NDDS will be dramatic for both doctors and patients, providing lower drug toxicity, more specific targeting, and reduced costs of treatments. At present, many drugs fail clinical trials because the compound cannot be delivered to the site where it is needed without having some interaction with the human body on the way. The result can range from triggering a severe immune system response to toxic side effects. Effectively delivering the active compound where it is needed is one of the holy grails in the treatment of diseases, from inflammation to cancer.

The global pharmaceutical industry has been developing compounds for over a century, but many of the compounds never get to the market. The acceptance of new drug formulations is expensive and slow, taking up to 15 years to obtain accreditation, with no guarantee of success. Compounds that are highly effective, such as Taxol® in treating cancer, are also toxic to healthy cells, and current delivery methods are unable to target just the diseased cells, leading to side effects. As a result, drug formulation companies are seeking to make use of drugs already in use and to find better ways to deliver the drug to their targets.

The development of NDDS has not been restricted to large pharmaceutical companies. Many new, small companies have developed novel methods of exploiting nanotechnologies in drug delivery, and many more methods are in incubation. Unlike other markets in which nanotechnology is merely projected to have an impact, the NDDS market has already represented a $3.39 billion market. But we are just seeing the tip of the iceberg. In 2012, the total market for NDDS is expected to rise to $26 billion, representing a compound annual growth rate of 37%. After 2012, things are expected to become really interesting: the value of NDDS is projected to sky rocket, reaching $220 billion by 2015.

Beyond just the economics, the use of nanoparticles will transform medical treatment. Practitioners will be able to use drugs to target specific areas of the body without concerns about side effects or toxicity because of the ability to concentrate the drugs where needed and thus use smaller doses. The potential to improve human health and quality of life through using nanoparticles in drug delivery is enormous.

Acknowledgments

This work has been carried out in the context of the Andalusian Initiative for Advanced Therapies. Special thanks to Dr. Vega Asensio (http://www. NorArte.es) and her beautiful scientific illustrations for this chapter.

Suggested Readings

Arruebo, M., Fernández-Pacheco, R., Ibarra, M.R. et al. 2007. Magnetic nanoparticles for drug delivery. *Nano Today* 2:22–32.

Bertrand, N. and Leroux, J.-C. 2011. The journey of a drug-carrier in the body: An anatomo-physiological perspective. *J. Controlled Release* doi:10.1016/j. jconrel.2011.09.098.

Bianco, A., Kostarelos, K., and Prato, M. 2005. Applications of carbon nanotubes in drug delivery. *Curr. Opin. Chem. Biol.* 9:674–679.

Blanco, E., Hsiao, A., Mann, A.P. et al. 2011. Nanomedicine in cancer therapy: Innovative trends and prospects. *Cancer Sci.* 102:1247–1252.

Bottini, M., Rosato, N., Gloria, F. et al. 2011. Public optimism towards nanomedicine. *Int. J. Nanomed.* 6:3473–3485.

Cho, K., Wang, X., Nie, S. et al. 2008. Therapeutic nanoparticles for drug delivery in cancer. *Clin. Cancer Res.* 14:1310–1316.

De Jong, W.H. and Borm, P.J.A. 2008. Drug Delivery and nanoparticles: Applications and hazards. *Int. J. Nanomed.* 3:133–149.

De, M., Ghosh, P.S., and Rotello, V.M. 2008. Applications of nanoparticles in biology. *Adv. Mater.* 20:4225–4241.

Duncan, R. and Gaspar, R. 2011. Nanomedicine(s) under the microscope. *Mol. Pharmaceut.* 8:2101–2141.

Faraji, A.H. and Wipf, P. 2009. Nanoparticles in cellular drug delivery. *Bioorg. Med. Chem.* 17:2950–2962.

Foldvari, M. and Bagonluri, M. 2008. Carbon nanotubes as functional excipients for nanomedicines: II. Drug delivery and biocompatibility issues. *Nanomedicine* 4:183–200.

Ganta, S., Devalapally, H., Shahiwala, A. et al. 2008. A review of stimuli-responsive nanocarriers for drug and gene delivery. *J. Controlled Release* 126:187–204.

Ghosh, P., Han, G., De, M. et al. 2008. Gold nanoparticles in delivery applications. *Adv.Drug Delivery Rev.* 60:1307–1315.

Hamidi, M., Azadi, A., and Rafiei, P. 2008. Hydrogel nanoparticles in drug delivery. *Adv. Drug Delivery Rev.*60:1638–1649.

Harper, T. 2011. *Nanotechnology in Drug Delivery 2011–2021.* London: Cientifica Ltd.

He, Q. and Shi, J. 2011. Mesoporous silica nanoparticle based nano drug delivery systems: Synthesis, controlled drug release and delivery, pharmacokinetics and biocompatibility. *J. Mater. Chem.* 21:5845–5855.

Kataoka, K., Harada, A., and Nagasaki, Y. 2001, Block copolymer micelles for drug delivery: Design, characterization, and biological significance. *Adv. Drug Delivery Rev.* 47:113–131.

Kumar, A., Jena, P.K., Behera, S. et al. 2010. Multifunctional magnetic nanoparticles for targeted delivery. *Nanomedicine* 6:64–69.

LaVan, D.A., McGuirre, T., and Langer, R. 2003. Small-scale systems for *in vivo* drug delivery. *Nat. Biotechnol.* 21:1184–1191.

Letchford, K. and Burt, H. 2007. A review of the formation and classification of amphiphilic block copolymer nanoparticulate structures: Micelles, nanospheres, nanocapsules and polymersomes. *Eur. J. Pharm. Biopharm.* 6:259–269.

Li, S.-D. and Huang, L. 2008. Pharmacokinetics and biodistribution of nanoparticles. *Mol. Pharmaceut.* 5:496–504.

Liu, T.-Y., Hu, S.-H., Liu, D.-M. et al. 2009. Biomedical nanoparticle carriers with combined thermal and magnetic responses. *Nano Today* 4:52–65.

Liu, Z., Tabakman, S., Welsher, K. et al. 2009. Carbon nanotubes in biology and medicine: *In vitro* and *in vivo* detection, imaging and drug delivery. *Nano Res.* 2:85–120.

Malam, Y., Loizidou, M., and Seifalian, A.M. 2009. Liposomes and nanoparticles: Nanosized vehicles for drug delivery in cancer. *Trends Pharmacol. Sci.* 30:592–599.

Muller, R.H. and Keck, C.M. 2004. Challenges and solutions for the delivery of biotech drugs—A review of drug nanocrystal technology and lipid nanoparticles. *J. Biotechnol.* 113:151–170.

Müller, R.H., Mäder, K., and Gohla, S. 2000. Solid Lipid nanoparticles (SLN) for controlled drug delivery: A review of the state of the art. *Eur. J. Pharm. Biopharm.* 50:161–170.

Najlah, M., Freeman, S., Attwood, D. et al. 2007. *In vitro* evaluation of dendrimer prodrugs for oral drug delivery. *Int. J. Pharm.* 336:183–190.

Neuberger, T., Schöpf, B., Hofmann, H. et al. 2005. Superparamagnetic nanoparticles for biomedical applications: Possibilities and limitations of a new drug delivery system. *J. Magn. Magn. Mater.* 293:483–496.

Nishiyama, N. and Kataoka, K. 2006. Current state, achievements, and future prospects of polymeric micelles as nanocarriers for drug and gene delivery. *Pharm. Ther.* 112:630–648.

Onaca, O., Enea, R., Hughes, D.W. et al. 2009. Stimuli-responsive polymersomes as nanocarriers for drug and gene delivery. *Macromol. Biosci.* 9:129–139.

Panyam, J. and Labhasetwar, V. 2003. Biodegradable nanoparticles for drug and gene delivery to cells and tissue. *Adv. Drug Delivery Rev.* 55:329–347.

Peer, D., Karp, J.M., Hong, S. et al. 2007. Nanocarriers as an emerging platform for cancer therapy. *Nat. Nanotechnol.* 2:751–760.

Pissuwan, D., Niidome, T., and Cortie, M.B. 2011. The forthcoming applications of gold nanoparticles in drug and gene delivery systems. *J. Controlled Release* 149:65–71.

Savic, R., Eisenberg, A., and Maysinger, D. 2006. Block copolymer micelles as delivery vehicles of hydrophobic drugs: Micelle–cell interactions. *J. Drug Targeting* 14:343–355.

Singh, R. and Lillard, J.W. Jr. 2009. Nanoparticle-based targeted drug delivery. *Exp. Mol. Pathol.* 86:215–223.

Slowing, I.I., Trewyn, B.G., Giri, S. et al. 2007. Mesoporous silica nanoparticles for drug delivery and biosensing applications. *Adv. Funct. Mater.* 17:1225–1236.

Slowing, I.I., Vivero-Escoto, J.L., Wu, C.-W. et al. 2008. Mesoporous silica nanoparticles as controlled release drug delivery and gene transfection carriers. *Adv. Drug Delivery Rev.* 60:1278–1288.

Soppimath, K.S., Aminabhavi, T.M., Kulkarni, A.R. et al. 2001. Biodegradable polymeric nanoparticles as drug delivery devices. *J. Controlled Release* 70:1–20.

Sung, J.C., Pulliam, B.L., and Edwards, D.A. 2007. Nanoparticles for drug delivery to the lungs. *Trends Biotechnol.* 25:563–570.

Upadhyay, K.K., Bhatt, A.N., Mishra, A.K. et al. 2010. The intracellular drug delivery and anti-tumor activity of doxorubicin loaded poly(γ-benzyl-glutamate)-b-hyaluronan polymersomes. *Biomaterials* 31:2882–2892.

Wissing, S.A., Kayser, O., and Müller, R.H. 2004. Solid lipid nanoparticles for parenteral drug delivery. *Adv. Drug Delivery Rev.* 56:1257–1272.

Zhou, L., Cai, Z., Yuan, J. et al. 2011. Multifunctional hybrid magnetite nanoparticles with pH-responsivity, superparamagnetism and fluorescence. *Polym. Int.* 60:1303–1308.

Zhou, L., Yuan, J., Yuan, W. et al. 2009. Synthesis and characterization of multifunctional hybrid magnetite nanoparticles with biodegradability, superparamagnetism, and fluorescence. *Mater. Lett.* 63:1567–1570.

2

Synthesis and Characterization of Nanoencapsulated Drugs

Arun Kumar, Ashley E. Saienni, and Niketa Dixit

CONTENTS

2.1   Introduction 24
2.2   Synthesis of Nanoencapsulated Drugs 24
     2.2.1   Chemical Methods 25
           2.2.1.1   Emulsion Polymerization 25
           2.2.1.2   Interfacial Polymerization 26
     2.2.2   Physical Method 26
           2.2.2.1   Plasma Methods 26
           2.2.2.2   Vapor Deposition Methods 27
           2.2.2.3   Hydrothermal Synthesis 28
           2.2.2.4   Spray Synthesis 29
2.3   Tools for Characterizations of Nanoencapsulated Drugs 29
     2.3.1   Electron Microscopy 29
     2.3.2   Transmission Electron Microscope 30
           2.3.2.1   How to Prepare Biological Sample for Nanoparticles Visualization 31
     2.3.3   Scanning Electron Microscope 31
     2.3.4   Atomic Force Microscope 33
     2.3.5   Dynamic Light Scattering 34
     2.3.6   X-Ray Photoelectron Spectroscopy 35
     2.3.7   Powder X-Ray Diffraction 36
     2.3.8   Fourier Transform Infrared Spectroscopy 36
     2.3.9   Matrix-Assisted Laser Desorption/Ionization Time-of-Flight Mass Spectrometry 37
     2.3.10 Ultraviolet–Visible Spectroscopy 37
     2.3.11 Dual Polarization Interferometry 38
     2.3.12 Nuclear Magnetic Resonance 38
References 39

2.1 Introduction

Several methods are used for the synthesis and characterizations of nanoencapsulated drug particles; these methods vary with the development of new technologies and techniques. As the use of nanomaterials is becoming more popular, its applications are widely spreading throughout several fields and are motivating scientists to develop new approaches for synthesis and characterizations. Different applications demand different properties of nanomaterials that lead to the expansion of methods for nanoparticle assembly and dispersion in various media. The principles of nanoparticle fabrication and functionalization transcend their eventual applications [1,2].

Characterization is crucial for establishing an understanding and control over the synthesis of nanoparticles and its potential applications. An assortment of techniques is used with several different functions, all with varying benefits and drawbacks. It is important for researchers to understand the potential and proper usage of all instruments to successfully identify nanoparticles and their properties. A majority of characterization techniques originate from materials science, a field dependent on these instruments. The most common techniques include, but are not limited to, electron microscopy (transmission electron microscopy [TEM]), scanning electron microscopy (SEM), atomic force microscopy (AFM), dynamic light scattering (DLS), x-ray photoelectron spectroscopy (XRS), powder x-ray diffraction (XRD), Fourier transform infrared spectroscopy (FTIR), matrix-assisted laser desorption/ionization time-of-flight mass spectrometry (MALDI–TOF), ultraviolet–visible spectroscopy (UV-Vis), dual polarization interferometry (DPI), and nuclear magnetic resonance (NMR). The applications of these techniques for nanomaterials will be reviewed and described in the following sections.

2.2 Synthesis of Nanoencapsulated Drugs

Nanoparticles are receiving considerable attention for the delivery of therapeutic drugs. The literature emphasizes the advantages of nanoparticles over microparticles and liposomes. The submicron size of nanoparticles offers a number of distinct advantages over microparticles, including relatively higher intracellular uptake compared with microparticles. In terms of intestinal uptake, apart from their particle size, nanoparticle nature and charge properties seem to influence the uptake by intestinal epithelia. Uptake of nanoparticles prepared from hydrophobic polymers seems to be higher than that of particles with more hydrophilic surfaces; thus, more hydrophilic particles may be rapidly eliminated. Nanoencapsulation of drugs involves forming drug-loaded particles with diameters ranging from 1 to 1000 nm. Nanoparticles are defined as solid-, submicron-sized drug carriers that may or may not be biodegradable [1,2]. The term nanoparticle is a collective name for both nanospheres and nanoencapsules. Nanoencapsules technically should be within the range of 1–100 nm in size but many encapsulated drugs exceed their size beyond 100 nm. Nanospheres have a matrix type of structure and drugs may be absorbed on their surface or may be encapsulated within the sphere. Some nanocapsules are vesicular systems in which the drug is confined to a cavity consisting of an inner liquid core surrounded by a polymeric membrane. In this case, the active substances are usually dissolved in the inner core but may also be adsorbed to the capsule surface. Generally, nanoparticles synthesized from hydrophobic polymers such as poly(styrene), uncharged, and positively charged, provide an affinity to follicle-associated epithelia as well as to absorptive enterocytes, whereas negatively charged poly(styrene) nanoparticles only show low affinity to any type of intestinal tissues. In contrast, nanoparticles based on hydrophilic polymers, negatively charged, show a strong increase in bioadhesive properties and are absorbed by both microfold cells (*M* cells) and absorptive enterocytes. A combination of both nanoparticle surface charges and increased hydrophobicity of the matrix material seem to affect the gastrointestinal uptake in a positive sense [3,4]. The various approaches to synthesize nanoparticles are divided broadly into chemical methods and physical methods based on the techniques used to synthesize them [5–15].

Synthesis of nanomaterials:

A. Chemical methods
    a. Emulsion polymerization
    b. Interfacial polymerization
B. Physical methods
    a. Plasma methods
    b. Vapor deposition methods
    c. Hydrothermal synthesis
    d. Spray synthesis

2.2.1 Chemical Methods

2.2.1.1 Emulsion Polymerization

Emulsion polymerization is one of the fastest methods for nanoparticle preparation and is readily scalable. The method is classified into two categories, based upon the use of either an organic or aqueous continuous phase. The continuous organic phase methodology involves the dispersion of a monomer into an emulsion or inverse microemulsion, or into a material in which the monomer is not soluble (nonsolvent). Polyacrylamide nanospheres were produced by this method [16,17]. The methods for the production of nanoparticles by using surfactants or protective soluble polymers can be used to prevent aggregation of nanoparticles at the early stages of polymerization. This procedure has become less important, because it requires toxic organic solvents, surfactants, monomers, and initiator, which are subsequently eliminated from the formed particles. Owing to the nonbiodegradable nature of this polymer as well as the difficult procedure, alternative approaches are developed. The poly(methylmethacrylate) (PMMA), poly(ethylcyanoacrylate) (PECA), and poly(butylcyanoacrylate) nanoparticles can be produced by dispersion method by using surfactants in solvents such as cyclohexane, *n*-pentane, and toluene as the organic phase. Some of the drugs that are encapsulated with this system are triamcinolone, fluorescein, pilocarpine, and timolol. In the aqueous continuous phase, the monomer is dissolved in a continuous phase that is usually an aqueous solution, and the surfactants or emulsifiers are not needed. The polymerization process can be initiated by different mechanisms; the initiation can occur when a monomer molecule dissolved in the continuous phase collides with an initiator molecule that might be an ion or a free radical [12,18]. Alternatively, the monomer molecule can be transformed into an initiating radical by high-energy radiation, including g-radiation, or ultraviolet or strong visible light. Chain growth starts when the initiated monomer ions or monomer radicals collide with other monomer molecules according to an anionic polymerization mechanism. Phase separation and formation of solid particles can take place before or after termination of the polymerization reaction. The PMMA nanoparticles synthesized using these approaches are suitable adjuvants for vaccines and gene delivery [17,19].

2.2.1.2 *Interfacial Polymerization*

One of the advantages of poly(alkylcyanoacrylate) nanoparticles synthesis is their rapid polymerization process that occur in seconds and can be initiated by ions present in the medium itself. Cyanoacrylate monomer and drug were dissolved in a mixture of an oil and absolute ethanol. This mixture was then slowly extruded through a needle into a well-stirred aqueous solution, with or without some ethanol or acetone-containing surfactant. Nanocapsules are formed spontaneously by polymerization of cyanoacrylate after contact with initiating ions present in water. The resulting colloidal suspension can be concentrated by evaporation under vacuum [19,20]. The polymers poly(isobutylcyanoacrylate) and poly(isohexylcyanoacrylate) can be used for the synthesis of nanoparticles by a similar approach as the example of the drug encapsulated by these methods is insulin [21].

2.2.2 Physical Method

2.2.2.1 *Plasma Methods*

Thermal plasma method has been used for the synthesis of Ti and Si nanoparticles. This technique can deliver the energy necessary to cause evaporation of Ti and Si and can produce small micrometer-sized particles. The thermal plasma temperatures are in the order of 10,000 K, so that solid powder easily evaporates and nanoparticles are formed upon cooling while exiting the plasma region. The main types of the thermal plasma torches used to produce nanoparticles are dc plasma jet, dc arc plasma, and radio frequency (RF) induction plasmas. In the arc plasma reactors, the energy necessary for evaporation and reaction is provided by an electric arc that is formed between the anode and the cathode. For example, silica sand can be vaporized with arc plasma at atmospheric pressure. The resulting mixture of plasma gas and silica vapors can be rapidly cooled by quenching with oxygen, thus ensuring the quality of the fumed silica produced. In RF induction plasma torches, energy coupling to the plasma is accomplished through the electromagnetic field generated by the induction coil. The plasma gas does not come in contact with electrodes, thus eliminating possible sources of contamination and allowing the operation of such plasma torches with a wide range of gases, including inert, reducing, oxidizing, and other corrosive atmospheres. The working frequency is typically between 200 kHz and 40 MHz. The laboratory units run at power levels in the order of 30–50 kW while the large-scale industrial units have been tested at power levels up to 1 MW. As the residence time of the injected feed droplets in the plasma is very short, it is important that the droplet sizes are small enough to obtain complete evaporation. The RF plasma method has been used to synthesize different nanoparticle materials, for example, synthesis of various ceramic nanoparticles such as oxides, carbours/carbides, and nitrides of Ti and Si [22,23]. Another approach, inert-gas condensation is frequently used to make nanoparticles from metals with low melting points. The metal is vaporized in a vacuum chamber and then supercooled with an inert gas stream. The supercooled metal vapor condenses into nanometer-sized particles, which can be entrained in the inert gas stream and can be deposited on a substrate or studied *in situ*.

2.2.2.2 Vapor Deposition Methods

The vapor deposition is used to create thin films and coatings for various applications and it is also widely used to grow nanoscale particles [24]. The synthetic processes in many cases produce nanoparticles of irregular shape, which have a size of a few hundred nanometers. Particle properties such as particle density, size, size distribution, shape surface topography, surface energy, and surface hardness affect the flow performance of powders. However, omnipresent adhesion and cohesion forces, that is, van der Waals forces between particle surfaces are the main factors to affect the separation of particles. The modification of dry-particle surfaces is important to optimize particle delivery. These attractive forces need to be minimized for successful drug delivery into the lungs. This can be done by minimizing the contact area between adjacent particle surfaces. Mainly, a curved surface with small asperities and lowered surface energy has been proved to be effective for drug delivery [25]. The current surface-modification techniques such as powder blending and spray drying are based on lowering the surface energy of particles with excipient materials such as lecithin, or magnesium stearate. In powder blending, the excipient material occupies high-energy sites on particle surfaces, and hence, only the remaining low-energy sites are used for drug–carrier adhesive interaction. In spray drying, the formation of the surface layer relies largely on the properties of excipient materials to accumulate onto air–solvent interface of droplets before drying takes place. Such interfacial active materials might also affect the morphology of particles to result in furrowed- and corrugated-particle surfaces. Improved dispersion of such powders can be improved by reducing the area of contacts and increased separation distance between the particles can also provide better distribution. The interaction forces can be further reduced by reducing the size of the particles [10,11,26]. The small particles can absorb more drugs or biomolecules on the surface as compared to micron-sized particles. The adsorptions of nanoparticle glidants on large particles are strong and sufficient for glidants and provide better surface roughness. Consequently, the contact area of interacting particle surfaces decreases. In addition to contact area, the separation of particles also depends on the contact distance between particles, that is, the size of glidant particles [23].

Vapor-phase fabrication: The vapor-phase fabrication processes are typically conducted in vacuum under elevated temperatures, that is, via pyrolysis or chemical vapor deposition [27].

The steps involved in the formation of nanoparticles are

    i. Precursor vaporization (as a catalyst)
   ii. Nucleation
  iii. Growth stage

The effective methods for nanoparticle fabrication is out-of-vapor phase, that is, methods that are simple, inexpensive, and operate continuously with high product yield, are aerosol spray methods. In spray pyrolysis, the solution is dispersed as droplets into a carrier gas and then sprayed into a drying chamber that is heated above the vaporization temperature of the solvent used as a carrier. The solid particles are then collected via electric field precipitator [25,28].

2.2.2.3 Hydrothermal Synthesis

Hydrothermal techniques are extensively used in many chemical processes, including materials processing, crystal growth, and waste treatment. Hydrothermal synthesis is a crystal synthesis or a crystal growth under high-temperature and high-pressure water conditions from substances that are insoluble in water at ordinary temperature and pressure (<100°C, <1 atm). Since the ionic product (Kw) has a maximum value of around 250–300°C, hydrothermal synthesis is usually carried out below 300°C. The critical temperature and pressure of water are 374°C and 22.1 MPa, correspondingly. The supercritical water gives a favorable reaction field for particle formation, the augmentation of the reaction rate, and large supersaturation based on the nucleation theory, due to lowering the solubility [29]. In recent years, techniques of hydrothermal synthesis have been further developed by the collective use of electrode reactions and crystallization. While there have been many applications of hydrothermal techniques in the preparation of metal-oxide nanoparticles, only a few of them are reported and explored for hydrothermal synthesis of metal nanoparticles. For example, the Fe_3O_4 nanoparticles can be synthesized using hydrothermal approach. Further, to use metal-oxide nanoparticles for the therapeutic application require metal oxide, that is, Fe_3O_4 nanoparticles should have narrow size distribution, superparamagnetic behavior, and specific surface modification. The surface modification of metal-oxide nanoparticles can improve the biocompatibility and agglomeration of the bare particles due to improved magnetostatic interaction [30,31].

2.2.2.4 Spray Synthesis

Spray pyrolysis is a physical method, which is relatively simple, reproducible, size controllable, low cost, and continuous for synthesis of some nanometal oxides, mixed metal oxides, and metals on metal oxides [32]. Nanoparticle powders prepared by this method, compared with those from chemical methods are more crystalline and less agglomerated with higher purity and also have large specific surface areas [16]. Metal acetate, chloride, and nitrate precursor solutions are used to synthesize metal-oxide nanoparticles by spray pyrolysis methods [32]. Since the chloride and nitrate precursor compounds produce acid gases, which are environmental pollutants and corrosive, metal acetate is a more preferable solution for synthesis. Furthermore, metal acetate precursors produce fine-grained, high-specific surface area, and aggregate-free powders due to their exothermic decomposition in the reaction whereas nitrate precursors produce strongly aggregated nanoparticle powders [33].

2.3 Tools for Characterizations of Nanoencapsulated Drugs

2.3.1 Electron Microscopy

Electron microscopy involves a high-powered electron beam for the analysis of nanoparticles and other specimens. This instrumentation is an upgrade from the traditional light microscopy, and its increased function allows for greater application. The diffraction effects restrict the resolution of optical microscopy; therefore, structures cannot be observed with light. The development of electron microscopes has resulted in instruments that are capable of consistently producing magnifications of the order of 1 million and can disclose details with a resolution of up to 0.1 nm.

There are two main types of electron microscopy, both functioning in similar fashion. An electron beam interacts with a specimen, multiple measurable signals are generated, and then electrons can be transmitted, backscattered, or diffracted. TEM uses the transmitted electrons to form a sample image, and the SEM utilizes backscattered electrons and secondary electrons emitted from the sample to form an image. The activity of the electrons is what allows the images to form and be analyzed. Depending on the specimen thickness, transmitted electrons can pass through without significant energy loss. The transmitted electrons form a two-dimensional projection of the sample because the abating of the electrons depends significantly on the density and thickness of the sample. Particles can also be used for diffraction, as electrons in the primary beam can collide with atoms in the specimen and can be scattered back or can remove more electrons from these atoms. The removed electrons are referred to as secondary electrons. The backscattering and generation of secondary electrons become more effective as the atomic number of the atoms being sampled increases.

2.3.2 Transmission Electron Microscope

The TEM is a commonly utilized electron microscopy that operates on the same basic principles as the light microscope, but with a few key differences. The TEM uses electrons instead of light to magnify images, which is more effective. The power of a light microscope is limited by the wavelength of light, restricting its magnifying capacity being up to 2000 times [34]. Electron microscopes are able to produce much more highly magnified images because the beam of electrons has a smaller wavelength, therefore increasing the resolution of the images (Figure 2.1).

This instrument uses a particle beam of electrons to visualize specimens and generate highly magnified images. Samples can be magnified by up to 2 million times its original size [32]. To process the specimen, a high-voltage electron beam is used to create the resulting image. An electron gun at the top of the microscope emits electrons that travel through the microscope's vacuum tube. Instead of using a glass lens to focus the light, as employed by light microscopes, the TEM utilizes an electromagnetic lens that focuses the electrons into a very fine beam, which then passes through the specimen. The specimen should be cut very thin, enabling electrons to pass through the cells. The electrons then scatter or hit a fluorescent screen at the bottom of the microscope. The image produced on the screen depicts assorted parts of the specimen, and are highlighted in different shades according to its density. The image can be studied directly within the TEM or can be photographed.

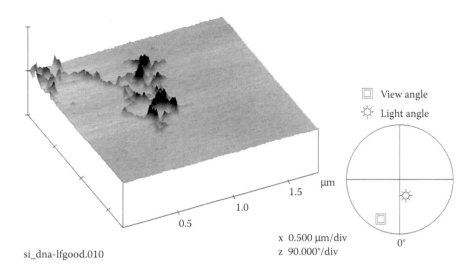

si_dna-lfgood.010

x 0.500 μm/div
z 90.000°/div

FIGURE 2.1
Three dimensional atomic force microscope (AFM) picture of deoxyribose nucleic acid (DNA) fragment on mica.

2.3.2.1 How to Prepare Biological Sample for Nanoparticles Visualization

The biological sample for TEM can be prepared for visualizing nanoparticles or detailed analysis of the tissue or cell structure; the most important factor is the thinness of the specimen, as previously stated. An ultramicrotome is commonly used to cut the tissue or materials into thin slices, which must be put in a chemical-preserved solution to maintain the cell structure. The tissues must also be dehydrated, and once properly preserved, the samples are placed in a hard, clean plastic, which supports the tissue as it is being cut by the ultramicrotome. Sections are cut and mounted onto grids and a solution of lead is used to stain the particles. The lead provides a contrast by staining particular cell parts, and allows the electrons to be scattered once placed in the TEM. The areas left dark in the final image produced are where the electrons were unable to penetrate the particles. The TEM of a nanoparticle alone can provide more detailed morphology of the nanoparticle's surface (Figure 2.2).

2.3.3 Scanning Electron Microscope

SEM uses electrons instead of light to form an image. SEM was developed in the early 1950s, allowing researchers to examine a much bigger variety of specimens. SEM has higher resolution than a traditional microscope, allowing closely spaced specimens to be magnified at much higher levels. The SEM uses electromagnetic lenses rather than glass lenses, which allows more control over the greater degree of magnification. The SEM provides another example of common electron microscopy used for the characterization of

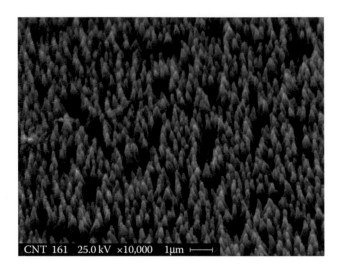

CNT 161   25.0 kV ×10,000   1μm ⊢──┤

FIGURE 2.2
The transmission electron microscope (TEM) picture of carbon nanotube.

nanoparticles. This microscopy was developed in the early 1950s, and allowed researchers to examine a much larger variety of specimens. The SEM utilizes a focused beam of high-energy electrons to produce a variety of signals at the surface of solid specimens or nanoparticles. These signals reveal information about the sample, including external morphology, chemical composition, crystalline structure, and orientation of materials [35]. A two-dimensional image is generated, which displays spatial variations of these properties. Since the SEM has a greater depth of field, it allows more of a specimen to be in the focus at one time. Conventional SEM techniques use magnification resolution ranging from 20 to 30,000 times, with a spatial resolution of 50–100 nm. It has a higher resolution than that of a traditional microscope, which allows closely spaced specimens to be magnified at much higher levels.

The function of the SEM is characteristic of other electron microscopes. A beam is produced at the top of the microscope by an electron gun. The electron beam follows a vertical path through the microscope that is held within a vacuum. The beam travels through the electromagnetic fields and lenses, which focus the beam down toward the specimen. Once the beam hits the sample, electrons and x-rays are ejected from the sample. The detectors collect the x-rays, backscattered electrons, and secondary electrons and convert them into a signal that is transferred to a screen that visualizes the final image [36].

Just before the preparation of nanoparticle specimen for an SEM, special provisions are necessary because of the fundamental vacuum conditions and the use of the electrons to form an image. The sample must be dehydrated, as the water would vaporize in the vacuum and all materials must be made conductive using some type of conducting material. The metallic nanoparticles are conductive and require no preparation before being analyzed, but nonmetals must be made conductive by covering the sample with a thin layer of conductive material [7,14,15].

2.3.4 Atomic Force Microscope

AFM is categorized under the Scanned Probe Microscopy family of instruments, and unlike other microscopy techniques that only offer images in two dimensions, this instrumentation allows for individual particles and groups of particles to be visualized in three dimensions. AFM was invented in 1985 by Binnig, C.F. Quate, and Ch. Gerber [37]; the AFM can distinguish between different materials providing spatial distribution information on composite materials. Specifically, physical properties such as morphology and surface texture can be measured, along with size information such as length, width, and height [38]. Nanocomposites can also be analyzed for dispersion of particulate matter, and material inhomogeneity can be viewed on a topographically flat organic film.

To analyze these properties, in an AFM, a constant force is maintained between the probe and the sample while the probe is raster scanned (a technique using parallel lines) across the surface. By monitoring the movement of the probe as it is scanned across the sample surface, a three-dimensional image of the surface is constructed. AFM utilizes the attractive or repulsive forces encountered by a probe tip when in close proximity to a sample surface (<200 nm). The AFM is a versatile instrument, as it operates both in air or in water, and does not require a current between the sample surface and the tip, which allows the examination and movement into potential regions of a sample [39]. The AFM can measure the surface or interface properties (such as mechanical, magnetic, electric, optical, thermal, or chemical characteristics) of insulators, organic materials, biological macromolecules, polymers, ceramics, and glasses all in different environments, such as liquids, vacuums, and at low temperatures (Figure 2.3).

There are two types of AFM: contact mode and dynamic force mode. In contact mode, the probe tip is brought to a distance at which repulsive forces dominate the tip–sample interaction and a very soft cantilever tip is mechanically contracted with the sample surface at an applied force [39]. In this mode, ionic repulsion forces take the leading role as the AFM measures hard-sphere repulsion forces between the tip and the sample, which maintains close contact as the scanning proceeds. The only major drawback of the contact mode is that large lateral forces on the sample exist as the tip is dragged over the specimen. In the dynamic force mode, the microscope is operated with a stiff cantilever that is oscillated near its resonant frequency. This mode is also divided into two subgroups: noncontact AFM and tapping/intermittent contact mode. In a noncontact AFM, the

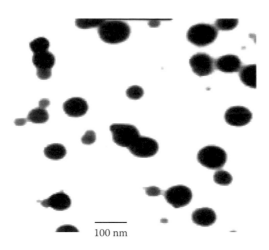

FIGURE 2.3
The transmission electron microscope (TEM) picture of magnetic nanoparticles Fe_2O_3 coated with polyethylene glycol (PEG 400).

cantilever vacillates above the surface of the sample at such a distance that there is no longer a repulsive regime of intermolecular force. The cantilever oscillates with a low amplitude (<5 nm), near its resonance frequency, and the applied force is measured by comparing this frequency relative to the driving signal [40]. The tapping/intermittent contact mode technique is typically used for samples with soft surfaces, as it operates in the repulsive force region, but touches the surface only for a minimal period of time that reduces potential damage to fragile samples. The tip lightly taps on the surface, coming in contact with the sample through the absorbed fluid layer during each oscillation [37].

It is important to recognize that all AFM used for particle characterization have a relatively high resolution, compared to traditional microscopes that are capable of only one measure of resolution, which is in the focal plane of an image. AFMs have two measures of resolution: one in the plane of measurement and the other in the direction perpendicular to the surface. The in-plane resolution is dependent upon the geometry of the probe used in the instrumentation for scanning, and the vertical resolution of the direction perpendicular to the surface is determined by relative vibrations of the probe above the surface, which can be maximized by minimizing the vibrations [40].

2.3.5 Dynamic Light Scattering

DLS is most commonly used to analyze nanoparticles but it also has other applications. The basis of this technique focuses on the idea that particle size can be determined by measuring random changes in the intensity of light scattered from a suspension or a solution [39]. These fluctuations are the result of interference effects arising from the relative Brownian movements of an ensemble of a large number of particles within a sample. DLS is also frequently referred to as photon correlation spectroscopy (PCS) or quasi-elastic light scattering (QELS). All these instruments are best used for submicron particles and can be used to measure particles with less than 1 nm in size [39].

The operation of the DLS begins with light from the laser light sources and illuminates the sample within a cell or other medium [6]. The scattered light signal is collected with one of the two detectors, either at a right angle of 90° or 173° scattering back angle. Both detectors allow for more flexibility in choosing measurement conditions, depending on the applications and sample materials. Particles can be scattered in a variety of liquid, but the liquid refractive index and viscosity must be identified to accurately interpret the measurement data. The resulting optical signal represents random changes due to the randomly changing relative position of the particles. The signal is analyzed in terms of an autocorrelation function, as the incoming data is processed in real time [39]. Compared to other laser diffraction methods, DLS measurements are typically made at a single angle, although data at various angles can be beneficial. DLS is also a noninvasive technique, which allows particle motion to continue whether or not it is being examined or probed by the instrumentation [41].

2.3.6 X-Ray Photoelectron Spectroscopy

XPS is predominantly used for the investigation of the surface chemistry of electrically conducting and nonconducting samples. This technique is used for analysis of nanoparticles, as well as depth profiling on surfaces, identification and measurement of surface contamination and organic overlayers, identification of counterfeit products, catalysis and corrosion studies, and the characterization of other materials [42]. XPS provides data on the elemental composition with up to 0.1% sensitivity, chemical state information, thickness measurement of overlayers of up to 8 nm on a specimen, surface chemical imaging with a resolution of 8 μm, thickness and depth distribution of chemical species, and depth profiling utilizing an ion gun to sputter away the surface during analysis [42]. Ultraviolent photoelectron spectroscopy (UPS) is a similar characterization technique that is often available in the same instrumentation that provides information on the density of the valence band and electron work functions [43].

The basic function of XPS begins with the surface of the sample being irradiated with x-rays, typically Al Kα or Mg Kα, within a vacuum. An x-ray photo hits and transfers this energy to a core-level electron, and then is emitted from its initial state with a kinetic energy dependent on the incident x-ray and binding energy of the atomic orbital that it originated [16]. The intensity and energy of the emitted photoelectrons are interpreted to determine and identify the concentrations of the elements present in the sample [42]. These photoelectrons originate from a depth of less than 10 nm; therefore, the data received is from within the depth of the sample at nanometer scale.

2.3.7 Powder X-Ray Diffraction

Powder XRD is a rapid analytical technique primarily used for phase identification of crystalline material and can provide data on unit cell dimensions [44]. Max von Laue discovered in 1912 that crystalline substances act as three-dimensional diffraction gratings for x-ray wavelengths similar to the spacing of planes in a crystal lattice. This leads to the development of the XRD instrumentation and the fundamental principle that the broadening of reflections in a powder diffraction pattern contains much information on crystalline strain, shape, and stacking faults [45]. Recently, applications have expanded to new studies [10,14,43], including the determination of the crystal structure and the extraction of three-dimensional microstructural properties. Various nanocrystalline materials can be characterized from XRD, including inorganics, organics, drugs, minerals, zeolites, catalysts, metal, and ceramics [55]. The amount of data that is possible to extract depends on the sample's microstructure (such as crystallinity, structure imperfections, crystallite size, and texture), the complexity of the crystal structure (the number of atoms in the asymmetric unit cell, unit cell volume), and the quality of experimental data (such as instrumental performances, counting statistics) [46].

2.3.8 Fourier Transform Infrared Spectroscopy

Fourier transform infrared spectroscopy (FTIR) is the standard and preferred method of infrared spectroscopy used to study nanoparticles coupled with molecules to use them for drug delivery or for targeting strategy or for bioimaging purpose. This technique has been used for material analysis for over 70 years, and can be applied to the analysis of solids, liquids, and gases [47]. FTIR is primarily used for identifying unknown materials, determining the quality of consistency of a sample, and quantitating the amount of a component in a mixture [48]. FTIR can be used to identify chemicals in spills, paints, polymers, coatings, drugs, and contaminants, making it an especially useful technique in nanomedicine and drug delivery. This instrument is computerized, making it faster and more sensitive compared to older, dispersive methods.

To identify the types of chemical bonds or functional groups, FTIR analyzes the wavelength of the light absorbed by the sample at specific wavelength. By examining the infrared absorption spectrum, the chemical bonds in a molecule can be determined. FTIR analyses of pure compound are so unique that they can be described as "molecular finger prints," with each one unlike any other [46]. Inorganic compounds typically have rich, detailed spectra, compared to inorganic compounds that are visually more simplistic. For common materials, the spectrum of an unknown sample can be determined by comparison to the library of known compounds, but to identify less common samples, FTIR is often combined with NMR, mass spectroscopy, emission spectroscopy, x-ray diffraction, and/or other techniques [46].

The strength of the sample light absorption can also be examined through quantitative analysis, which has determined it to be proportional to substance concentration. Depending on the element and type of bond, molecular bonds vibrate at different frequencies, and according to quantum mechanics, these frequencies correspond to the ground state (lowest frequency) and several excited states (higher frequencies) of the molecules.

2.3.9 Matrix-Assisted Laser Desorption/Ionization Time-of-Flight Mass Spectrometry

Matrix-assisted laser desorption/ionization time-of-flight mass spectrometry (MALDI–TOF–MS) is an emerging technique featuring fast and accurate determination of multiple polymer characteristics [49]. It is a popular and versatile technique to analyze a range of particles and biomolecules in complex samples, including cells, tissue, peptides, proteins, oligosaccharides, and oligonucleotides. The MALDI–TOF–MS is characterized by high accuracy and sensitivity, with a wide mass range of 1–200 kDa. This method was first introduced in the late 1980s when Tanaka and Karas and Hillenkamp first demonstrated a successful MALDI biochemical analysis [50]. This instrumentation has become commercially available since 1991, and though relatively young compared to other analytical techniques using mass spectroscopy, there has been a significant increase in the usage and publication of MALDI methods and applications in literature for two reasons [8].

2.3.10 Ultraviolet–Visible Spectroscopy

To characterize nanoparticles, ultraviolet–visible spectroscopy (UV–Vis) is a technique used to quantify the light that is absorbed and scattered by a sample. This quality is referred to as extinction, or the sum of absorbed and scattered light [46].

The function of UV–Vis spectroscopy incorporates a beam of light from a visible or ultraviolet light source, which is divided into its component wavelengths by a prism or other diffraction grating. Each monochromatic beam is then separated into two equivalent intensity beams by a half-mirrored instrument. One beam, the sample beam, passes through a transparent cuvette containing a solution of the nanoparticle being studied in a transparent solvent. The reference beam passes through an identical cuvette containing only the solvent [51]. The intensities of these two beams are then measured and examined by electronic detectors, with the intensity of the reference beam having suffered little or zero-light absorption. The UV–Vis spectrometer automatically scans all the component wavelengths through the previously described process over set intervals. The UV region is scanned in standardized 200–400 nm, and the visible portion for analysis is 400–800 nm [46].

2.3.11 Dual Polarization Interferometry

Dual polarization interferometry (DPI) is a characterization method that was introduced in 2003, and was used by researchers in life and physical sciences, particularly in nano- and biological science studies [46]. Its main purpose is to measure and characterize molecular conformation at a sub-atomic resolution. The most recent generation of instruments can measure and analyze molecular phase transitions, including a protein melt under conditions of a temperature of 65°C. DPI is also commonly used for characterizing kinetics and affinity of interactions at different temperatures, quantifying free energy, enthalpy, and entropy of binding or conformational changes, and direct measurement of affinity, kinetics, and thermodynamics [52]. DPI is a growing technique, as it addresses many of the shortfalls of other optical methods. The inability is to differentiate the changes in sample layer thickness for some instrumentation, and this limitation hinders the proper study of membrane interaction analysis and molecular aggregation [56]. DPI provides a solution to this problem, as it analyzes thin films to acquire the date of optogeometrical properties, such as density, mass, thickness, and refractive index [53].

2.3.12 Nuclear Magnetic Resonance

Nuclear magnetic resonance (NMR) is a characterization technique in which the nuclei of particular atoms are immersed in a static magnetic field and exposed to a second oscillating magnetic field [54]. NMR spectroscopy is the study of interactions of electromagnetic radiation with matter, specifically the use of NMR phenomenon to study physical, chemical, and biological properties of matter, including nanoparticles and nanoencapsulated drugs. This technique produces two different types of images, each with a specific functionality. The one-dimension technique is used to study the chemical structure, whereas the two-dimensional technique is used to determine the structure of more complicated molecules. NMR spectroscopy replaces x-ray crystallography for determination of protein structure [46]. This technique is very helpful when we are more interested in knowing the information about particle size *in situ*, which opens the possibility, for example, of studying how the size and environment of nanoparticles change during catalytic reactions [50].

References

1. Hall, J. B., Dobrovolskaia, M. A., Patri, A. K., and McNeil, S. E. 2007. Characterization of nanoparticles for therapeutics. *Nanomedicine (London)*, 2(6), 789–803.
2. Huang, T. and Nancy Xu, X.-H. 2010. Synthesis and characterization of tunable rainbow colored colloidal silver nanoparticles using single-nanoparticle plasmonic microscopy and spectroscopy. *Journal of Material Chemistry*, 20, 9867–9876.
3. Wang, Y., Dave, R. N., and Pfeffer, R. 2004. Polymer coating/encapsulation of nanoparticles using a supercritical anti-solvent process. *Journal of Supercritical Fluids*, 28, 85–99.
4. Boras, L., and Gatenholm, P. 1999. Surface composition and morphology of CTMP fibers. *Holxforschung*, 53(2), 188–194.
5. Usón, I. and Sheldrick, G. M. 1999. Advances in direct methods for protein crystallography. *Current Opinion in Structural Biology*, 9(5), 643–648.
6. Karas, M. and Hillenkamp, F. 1988. Laser desorption ionization of proteins with molecular masses exceeding 10,000 daltons. *Analytical Chemistry*, 60, 259–280.
7. Bunshah R. 1994. (Ed.), *Handbook of Deposition Technologies for Films and Coatings: Science Technology and Applications*. Noyes Publications, Blue Ridge, NJ.
8. Marvin, L. F., Roberts, M. A., and Fay, A. B. 2003. Matrix-assisted laser desorption/ionization time-of-flight mass spectrometry in clinical chemistry. *Clinica Chimica Acta*, 337, 11–21.
9. Reverchon, E. and Adamia, R. 2006. Nanomaterials and supercritical fluids. *Journal of Supercritical Fluids*, 37, 1–22.
10. Wakayama, H., Hatanaka, T., and Fukushima, Y. 2004. Synthesis of Pt-Ru nanoporous fibers by the nanoscale casting process using supercritical CO_2 for electrocatalytic applications. *Chemistry Letters*, 33, 658.
11. Wadley, H. N. G. Zhou, X. Johnson, R. A., and Neurock, M. 2001. Mechanisms, models and methods of vapor deposition. *Progress in Material Science*, 46, 329–377.
12. Chan, C. S. 2006. Emulsion polymerization mechanisms and kinetics. *Progress in Polymer Science*, 31, 443–486.
13. Hiemenz, P. C. and Rajagopalan, R. 1997. *Principles of Colloid and Surface Chemistry*, Marcel Dekker, New York.
14. Zhang, X. Chan-Yu-King, R., Jose, A., and Manohara, S. K. 2004. Nanofibers of polyaniline synthesized by interfacial polymerization. *Synthetic Metals*, 145, 23–29.
15. Ramanuja, N., Levy, R.A., Dharmadhikari, S.N., Ramos, E., Pearce, C.W., Menasian, S.C., Schamberger, P.C., and Collins, C.C. 2002. Synthesis and characterization of low pressure chemically vapor deposited titanium nitride films using $TiCl_4$ and NH_3. *Materials Letters*, 57, 261–269.
16. Cao, G. 2004. *Nanostructures and Nanomaterials: Synthesis, Properties and Applications*, Imperial College Press, London, UK.
17. Nomura, M., Tobita, H., and Suzuki, K. 2005. Emulsion polymerization: Kinetic and mechanistic aspects. *Advances in Polymer Science*, 175, 1–128.

18. Dixon, D. J., Johnston, K. P., and Bodmeier, R. A. 1993. Polymeric materials formed by precipitation with a compressed fluid antisolvent. *AIChE Journal*, 39, 127.
19. Chen, W., Liu, X., Liu, Y., Bang, Y., and Kim, H.-I. 2010. Synthesis of PMMA and PMMA/PS nanoparticles by microemulsion polymerization with a new vapor monomer feeding system. *Colloids and Surfaces A: Physicochemical Engineering Aspects*, 364, 145–150.
20. Korikov, A. P. Kosaraju, P.B., and Sirkar, K.K. 2006. Interfacially polymerized hydrophilic microporous thin film composite membranes on porous polypropylene hollow fibers and flat films. *Journal of Membrane Science*, 279, 588–600.
21. Furtado, S., Abramson, D., Burrill, R., Olivier, G., Gourd, C., Bubbers, E. et al. 2008. Oral delivery of insulin loaded poly(fumaric-co-sebacic) anhydride microspheres. *International Journal of Pharmaceuticals*, 347(1–2), 149–155.
22. Shigeta, M. and Watanabe, T. 2007. Growth mechanism of silicon-based functional nanoparticles fabricated by inductively coupled thermal plasmas. *Journal of Physics, D: Applied Physics*, 40, 2407–2419.
23. Shigeta, M. and Watanabe, T. 2008. Numerical investigation of cooling effect on platinum nanoparticle formation in inductively coupled thermal plasmas. *Journal of Applied Physics*, 103, 074913.
24. Gomez, M. V., Guerra, J., Myers, V. S., Crooks, R. M., and Velders, A. H. 2009. Nanoparticle size determination by 1H NMR spectroscopy. *Journal of American Chemical Society*, 131, 14634–14635.
25. Kima, B. K. and Choia, C. J. 2001. Fabrication of nanostructured powders by chemical processes. *Scripta Material*, 44, 2161–2164.
26. Eastoe, J., Hollamby, M. J., and Hudson, L. 2006. Recent advances in nanoparticle synthesis with reversed micelles. *Advances in Colloid and Interface Science*, 128–130, 5–15.
27. Yahya, R. B., Hayashi, H., Nagase, T., Ebina, T., Onodera, Y., and Saitoh, N. 2001. Hydrothermal synthesis of potassium hexatitanates under subcritical and supercritical water conditions and its application in photocatalysts. *Chemistry of Materials*, 13, 842–847.
28. Noboru, I., Yoshiharu, O., and Seiichiro, K. 1988. *Superfine Particle Technology*, Springer-Verlag, London, p. 79.
29. Hawa, C. Y., Mohamed, F., Chia, C. H., Radiman, S., Zakaria, S., Huang, N. M., and Lim, H. N. 2010. Hydrothermal synthesis of magnetite nanoparticles as MRI contrast agents. *Ceramics International*, 36, 1417–1422.
30. Unruh, K. M., and Chien, C. L. 1996. In: Edelstein, A. S., and Cammarata, R. C. (eds.) *Nanomaterials: Synthesis, Properties and Applications*, Institute of Physics Publishing, Bristol, UK, Magnetic and electron transport properties of granular films, p. 374.
31. Adschiri T., Hakuta, Y., and Arai, K. 2000. Hydrothermal synthesis of metal oxide fine particles at supercritical conditions. *Industrial and Engineering Chemistry Research*, 39(12), 4901.
32. Tok, A. I. Y., Boey, F. Y. C., Du, S. W., and Wong, B. K. 2006. Flame spray synthesis of ZrO_2 nanoparticles using liquid precursors. *Materials Science and Engineering*, B 130, 114–119.
33. Calderon-Moreno, J. M. and Yoshimura, M. 2001. Hydrothermal processing of high-quality multiwall nanotubes from amorphous carbon. *Journal of American Chemical Society*, 123, 741.

34. Egerton, R. F. 2005. *Physical Principles of Electron Microscopy: An Introduction to TEM, SEM, and AEM.* Springer Adis US, LLC., New York, NY, p. 202.
35. Suzuki, E. 2002. High-resolution scanning electron microscopy of immunogold-labelled cells by the use of thin plasma coating of osmium. *Journal of Microscopy,* 208(3), 153–157.
36. Reimer, L. 1998. Scanning Electron Microscopy: *Physics of Image Formation and Microanalysis.* Springer Adis US, LLC., New York, NY, p. 527 .
37. Trad, T., Donley, K., Look, D., Eyink, K., Tomich, D., and Taylor, C. 2010. Low temperature deposition of zinc oxide nanoparticles via zinc-rich vapor phase transport and condensation. *Journal of Crystal Growth,* 312(24), 3675–3679.
38. Vasenka, J., Manne, S., Giberson, R., Marsh, T., and Henderson, E. 1993. Colloidal gold particles as an incompressible AFM imaging, standard for assessing the compressibility of biomolecules. *Biophysical Journal,* 65, 992–997.
39. Merkus, H. G. (ed.). 2009. *Particle Size Measurements: Fundamentals, Practice, Quality.* Springer Particle Technology Series, Springer Adis US, LLC., New York, NY, Vol. 17, ISBN: 978-1-4020-9015-8
40. Hinterdorfer, P., and Dufrêne, Y. F. 2006. Detection and localization of single molecular recognition events using atomic force microscopy. *Nature Methods,* 3(5), 347–355.
41. Ferre,D., Amare, A. and Burley, S. 1994. Use of dynamic light scattering to assess crystallizability of macromolecules and macromolecular assemblies. *Structure,* 2, 357–359.
42. William, E., and Swartz, B.K. Jr. 1973. X-ray photoelectron spectroscopy. *Analytical Chemistry,* 45(9), 788A–800.
43. Sweeney, S., Woehrle, G. H., and Hutchison, J. E. 2006. Rapid purification and size separation of gold nanoparticles via diafiltration. *Journal of American Chemical Society,* 128, 3190–3197; Lyon, L. A., Keating, C. D., Fox, A. P., Baker, B. E., He, L., Nicewarner, S. R., Mulvaney, S. P., and Natan, M. J. 1998. Raman spectroscopy. *Analytical Chemistry,* 70, 341R–361R.
44. Dutrow, B. 1997. Better living through minerals x-ray diffraction of household products. In: Brady, J., Mogk, D., and Perkins, D. (eds.) *Teaching Mineralogy,* Mineralogical Society of America, Chantilly, VA, pp. 349–359.
45. Whitfield, P., and Mitchell, L. 2004. X-ray diffraction analysis of nanoparticles: Recent developments, potential problems and some solutions. *International Journal of Nano Science,* 3(6), 757–763.
46. Skoog, D. A., Holler, F. J., and Crouch, S. R. 2007. *Principles of Instrumental Analysis,* 6th ed., Thomson Brooks-Cole, California.
47. Blake, C. C., Geisow, M. J., Oatley, S. J., Rerat, B., and Rerat, C. 1978. Structure of prealbumin: Secondary, tertiary and quaternary interactions determined by Fourier refinement at 1.8 Å. *Journal of Molecular Biology,* 121, 339–356.
48. Griffiths, P. R., Hirsche, B. L., and Manning, C. J. 1999. Ultra-rapid-scanning Fourier transform infrared spectrometry. *Vibrational Spectroscopy,* 19, 165–176.
49. Marvina, L. F., Robertsb, M. A., and Faya, L. B. 2003. Matrix-assisted laser desorption/ionization time-of-flight mass spectrometry in clinical chemistry. *Clinica Chimica Acta,* 337, 11–21.
50. Binnig, G., Quate, C. F., and Gerber, C.H. 1986. Atomic force microscope. *Physics Review Letters,* 56, 930–933.

51. Sooväli, E.-I., Rõõm, A., Kütt, I., and Kaljurand, I. 2006. Leito. Uncertainty sources in UV–Vis spectrophotometric measurement. *Accreditation Quality Assurance*, 11, 246–255.
52. Boudjemline, A., Saridakis, E., and Swann, M. 2011. Use of dual polarization interferometry as a diagnostic tool for protein crystallization. *American Chemical Society*, 83(20), 7881–7887.
53. Boudjemline, A., Saridakis, E., Swann, M. J., Govada, L., Mavridis, I. M., and Chayen, N. E. 2011. Use of dual polarization interferometry as a diagnostic tool for protein crystallization. *Analysis Chemistry*, 83, 7881–7887.
54. Judd, C. S. 1995. Proton NMR basics. *Chemical Education* 72(8), 706.
55. Vartanyants I. A. and Robinson, I. K. 2001. Partial coherence effects on the imaging of small crystals using coherent x-ray diffraction. *Journal of Physics Condensed Matter*, 13, 10593–10611.
56. Filipe, V., Hawe, A., and Jiskoot, W. 2010. Critical evaluation of Nanoparticle Tracking Analysis (NTA) by NanoSight for the measurement of nanoparticles and protein aggregates. *Pharmaceutical Research* 27(5), 796–810.

3

Nanoparticle Lung Delivery and Inhalation Aerosols for Targeted Pulmonary Nanomedicine

Heidi M. Mansour, Chun-Woong Park, and Don Hayes, Jr.

CONTENTS

3.1 Introduction 43
3.2 Anatomy of the Human Respiratory Tract and Inhalation
    Aerosol Particle Deposition 45
3.3 Respiratory Diseases and Targeted Pulmonary Nanomedicine 48
    3.3.1 Chronic Obstructive Pulmonary Disease and Asthma 48
    3.3.2 Cystic Fibrosis 48
    3.3.3 Tuberculosis 49
    3.3.4 Infectious Diseases 50
    3.3.5 Vaccination 51
3.4 Nanoparticle Lung Delivery Systems 51
    3.4.1 Polymer-Based Nanocarriers 51
        3.4.1.1 Polymeric Micelles 51
        3.4.1.2 Polymeric Nanoparticles 53
    3.4.2 Lipid-Based Nanocarriers 54
        3.4.2.1 Solid-Lipid Nanoparticles 54
        3.4.2.2 Liposomes 55
3.5 In Vitro and In Vivo Characterization of Targeted Pulmonary
    Nanomedicine Delivery Systems 57
3.6 Conclusion and Future Direction 60
References 60

3.1 Introduction

Nanomedicine drug-delivery systems have a number of advantages[1-3]: (1) to achieve relatively uniform distribution of drug dose; (2) to enhance the apparent solubility of a poorly water-soluble drug; (3) to control drug release that can consequently reduce the dosing frequency; (4) to achieve macromolecule delivery of therapeutic proteins and polypeptides; (5) to reduce side effects and toxicity; (6) to improve patient compliance; and (7) to provide strategies for intracellular targeted delivery. In addition, targeted pulmonary delivery systems can have several therapeutic advantages for the treatment of respiratory diseases as well as systemic delivery via the lung. The respiratory system has anatomical and physiological advantages: (1) a large surface area; (2) a thin physical barrier of alveolar epithelium; (3) the absence of extreme pH and low metabolism relative to other organ systems; (4) no hepatic first-pass effect; (5) rich blood supply; and (6) rapid systemic delivery from the alveolar region to the lung.[4] There has been an increasing interest in the therapeutic application of targeted pulmonary nanomedicine for the respiratory diseases and some examples are listed in Table 3.1.

The size range of 1–1000 nm has frequently been used as the scientific definition in both nanotechnology and pharmaceutical sciences.[46–49] The European Science Foundation (ESF) defines nanomedicine as "the science and technology of diagnosing, treating, and preventing disease and traumatic injury, of relieving pain, and of preserving and improving human health, using molecular tools and molecular knowledge of the human body."[50] There are five main categories by the ESF which are "analytical tools," "nanoimaging," "nanomaterials and nanodevices," "novel therapeutics and drug-delivery systems," and

TABLE 3.1

Respiratory Diseases and Targeted Pulmonary Nanomedicine Delivery Systems

Lung Disease	Drugs	Nanoparticle Delivery Systems
COPD and asthma	Budesonide	Liposomes,[5] polymer-base,[6] drug-base,[7–9] lipid-base[10]
	Fluticasone	liposome,[11] drug-base,[12] lipid-base[13]
	Beclomethasone	Liposomes,[14] drug-base,[15] polymer-base,[16] lipid-base[17]
	Salbutamol	Drug-base,[18] polymer-base,[11] lipid-base[19]
Cystic fibrosis (CF)	DNA	Polymer-base,[20] lipid-base[21]
Tuberculosis (TB)	Rifampicin	Liposomes,[22] polymer-base[23]
	Isoniazid/Pyrazinamide	Polymer-base[24]
Infectious disease (ID)	Amphotericin B	Liposomes[25,26]
	Itraconazole	Liposomes, drug-base,[27] polymer-base[28]
	Tobramycin	Liposomes,[29] drug-base[30]
	Ciprofloxacin	Liposomes,[31–33] drug-base[34,35]
Vaccination	Tetanus toxoid	Polymer-base[36]
	RSV antigens	Polymer-base[37]
Lung cancer	Paclitaxel	Liposomes,[38] lipid-base[39]
	Doxorubicin	Polymer-base[40]
Immunosuppression	Cyclosporine A	Liposomes,[41,42] polymer-base[43]
	Tacrolimus	Liposomes,[44] drug-base[45]

"clinical, regulatory, and toxicological issues."[51] With the National Institutes of Health (NIH) Roadmap for Medical Research in Nanomedicine, it had also been defined as "an offshoot of nanotechnology, refers to highly specific medical interventions at the molecular scale for curing disease or repairing damaged tissues, such as bone, muscle, or nerve."[52] In summary, nanomedicine delivery has focused on alternative technology to achieve unmet medical needs in novel drug-delivery systems such as achieving high local drug accumulation at the target site, protection of biologically unstable drugs against potential enzymatic or hydrolytic degradation in the body, increased drug-loading capacity, a longer circulation time *in vivo*, and controlled drug-release profiles.[53] There are two classifications of nanocarrier types[54]: (1) "hard type" (i.e., polymeric nanoparticles,[55–58] lipid nanoparticles[48,59–66]) with low flexibility and elasticity; and (2) "soft type" (i.e., liposomes,[67–71] nanoemulsions,[72–74] submicron lipid emulsions,[75–80] nanogels,[81–83] and polymeric micelles[84–86]), which can be reformed and deformed easily. Another classification scheme is as a "polymer-based nanocarriers" and "lipid-based nanocarriers."[54] There are examples of sugar, polymer, lipid, and phospholipid carriers for pulmonary nanomedicine delivery in Figure 3.1.

3.2 Anatomy of the Human Respiratory Tract and Inhalation Aerosol Particle Deposition

The respiratory tract is the organ of gas exchange with the nickname "the organ of life" due to its vital role of respiration. There are several types of cells to scavenge foreign matter, to sweep the mucous membranes with cilia for the lining of the smallest air passages, and to control the blood pressure.[87] Specifically, the physiological roles of the pulmonary system are: (1) to supply oxygen, (2) to remove endogenous wastes and toxins, and (3) to defend against hostile intruders. The respiratory tract can be divided into two main parts: (1) the upper respiratory tract (i.e., nose, nasal cavity, and the pharynx) and (2) the lower respiratory tract (i.e., larynx, trachea, bronchi, and the lung).[88] Anatomically, the lung can be defined as a series of bifurcating tubes from the trachea to the alveoli.[89] The trachea divides into two main bronchi, which divide into smaller bronchioles with several branches leading to the respiratory bronchioles followed by the alveolar ducts and alveoli. There exists anatomical models of the human lung by the construction of symmetrical[90] and asymmetrical[91] branching. The Weibel symmetrical branching model has been a significant model, which comprises 24 generations.[90] The airway from the trachea to the terminal bronchioles is ranged as a generation index 0–16, which is called the conducting zone, and the airways from the respiratory bronchioles to the alveolar sacs (generation index 17–23) are called the transitional and respiratory zone.

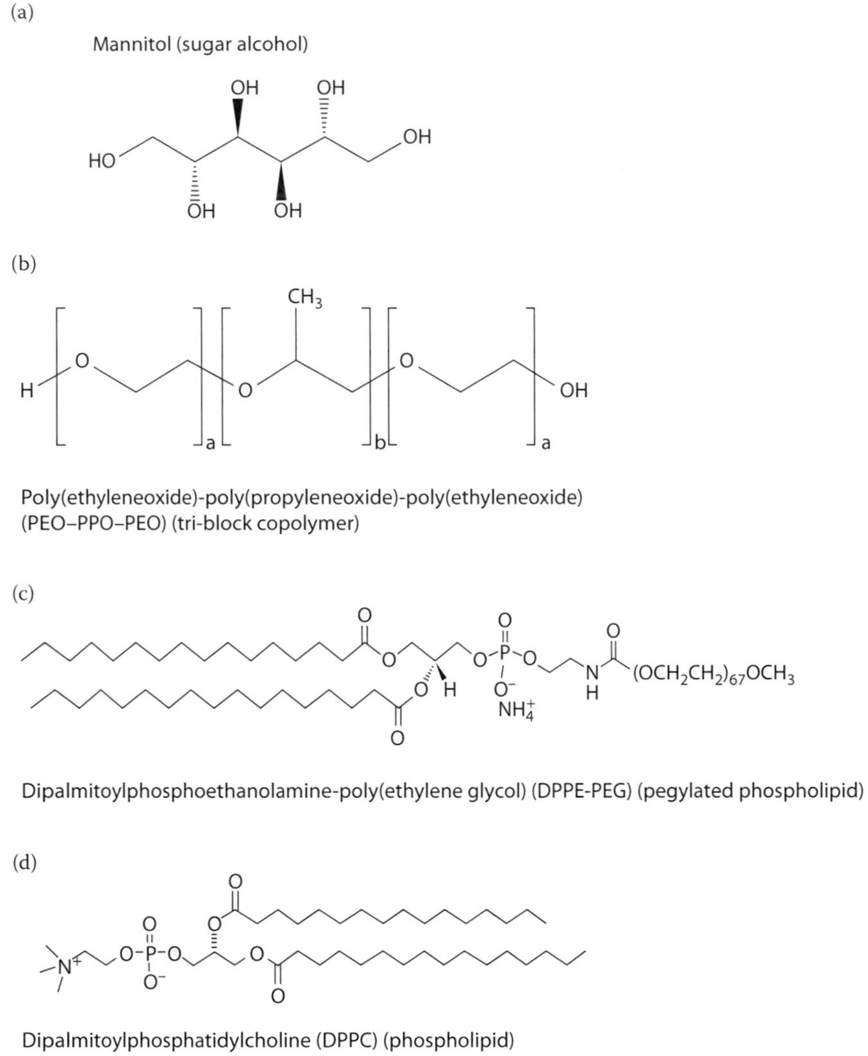

(a)

Mannitol (sugar alcohol)

(b)

Poly(ethyleneoxide)-poly(propyleneoxide)-poly(ethyleneoxide)
(PEO–PPO–PEO) (tri-block copolymer)

(c)

Dipalmitoylphosphoethanolamine-poly(ethylene glycol) (DPPE-PEG) (pegylated phospholipid)

(d)

Dipalmitoylphosphatidylcholine (DPPC) (phospholipid)

FIGURE 3.1
Examples of sugar, polymer, lipid, and phospholipid for the targeted pulmonary nanomedicines: (a) Mannitol, (b) PEO–PPO–PEO (tri-block copolymer), (c) DPPE-PEG (pegylated phospholipid), (d) DPPC (phospholipid). (ChemDraw Ultra 10.0, ChemOffice 2006, Cambridgesoft, Cambridge, MA.)

Examples of active agents for targeted pulmonary nanomedicine delivery are listed in Figure 3.2. The clinical efficacy of these active agents is proportional to the amount of active agent reaching the airways.[92] This means that a higher lung deposition of the active agent can achieve a higher clinical efficacy with a smaller dose amount of active agents. The deposition of inhaled particles in the different regions of the respiratory system is very complex

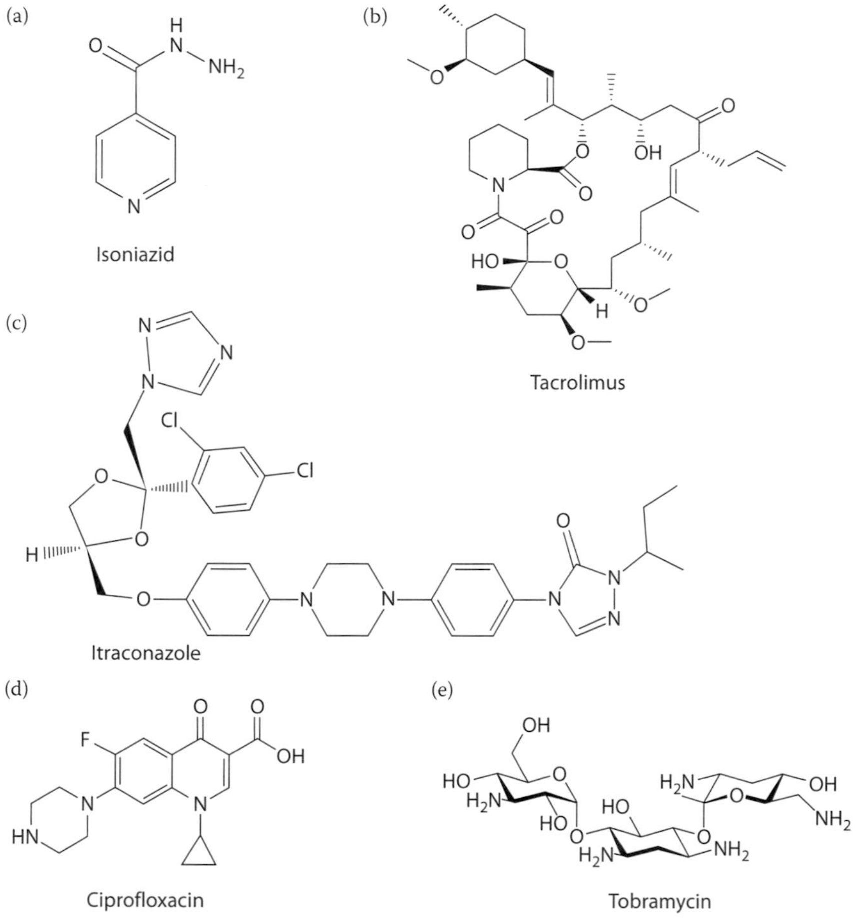

FIGURE 3.2
Examples of active agent for the targeted pulmonary nanomedicines: (a) Isoniazid, (b) Tacrolimus, (c) Itraconazole, (d) Ciprofloxacin, and (e) tobramycin. (ChemDraw Ultra 10.0, ChemOffice 2006, Cambridgesoft, Cambridge, MA.)

with individual variation due to differences in breathing rates and respiratory volume due to lung volume, and health status of individuals.

Depending on particle size, airflow, and location in the respiratory system along with the physicochemical properties of inhaled drug aerosol particles, deposition in the airways are by the following three main deposition mechanisms[89]: (1) inertial impaction by inertial forces,[93] (2) sedimentation by gravitational forces (also known as gravitational settling),[94] and (3) diffusion due to Brownian motion.[95,96] The respiratory deposition by the "impaction" mechanism is mainly based on the ratio of particle stopping distance to airway dimensions,[97] which means that large particles (10 μm and larger in aerodynamic size) impact on bronchial bifurcations due to inertial impaction as a result of high momentum, high air velocity, and sharp airflow directional change in the oro-pharyngeal bifurcation. "Sedimentation" by gravitational forces acts on smaller particles (e.g., 1–5 μm in aerodynamic size) which have lower momentum in the bronchiolar region where the directional change decreases and the air veloc-ity has slowed down.[98] "Diffusion" in the terminal and respiratory bronchioles and alveolar region, where particles below 1 μm in aerodynamic size deposit as a function of Brownian motion[89] rather than gravitational forces.

3.3 Respiratory Diseases and Targeted Pulmonary Nanomedicine

3.3.1 Chronic Obstructive Pulmonary Disease and Asthma

Chronic obstructive pulmonary disease (COPD) and asthma are among the major pulmonary diseases worldwide where COPD is predicted to be the third most common cause of death by 2020.[99] Similarities between COPD and bron-chial asthma exist, such as airway wall thickening visible upon imaging by computed tomography (CT) or reversibility and airway hyper-responsiveness in pulmonary function testing.[100] However, there are some differences in air-way inflammation between the two diseases. In the case of bronchial asthma, airway inflammation is through activated T-lymphocytes (i.e., CD4+ Th2 cells), eosinophils and mast cells. In contrast, stable COPD involves an increased number of T-lymphocytes (i.e., CD8+ T cells), macrophages, and neutrophils.

Potent nanoparticles of a P-selectin antagonist were investigated with strong anti-inflammatory effects in a murine model of allergic asthma.[101] Because selective P-selectin inhibitors may lead to an inhibition of the ongo-ing inflammatory processes present in allergic bronchial asthma, P-selectin inhibitors were synthesized using polyvalent polymer nanoparticles. Nanoparticle formulations were tested in which the ratio of fucose, sulfate, and polyethylene glycol were varied. The efficacy of formulation changes were evaluated in an *in vitro* recirculating loop assay. In the absence of polym-erized lipid nanoparticle (PLNP), the number of U-937 cells interacting with the coated capillary tubes gradually increased with time. In summary, these studies demonstrated the discovery of a P-selectin inhibitor with potent *in vivo* activity by using a physiologically relevant *in vitro* shear assay system.

3.3.2 Cystic Fibrosis

Cystic fibrosis (CF), an autosomal recessive genetic disorder, is caused by a dysfunction of the epithelial chloride channel CFTR (cystic fibrosis trans-membrane regulator),[102] which has more than 900 mutations of the CFTR gene known.[103] The hypersecretory-induced airway changes in CF are characterized by submucosal gland and goblet cell hyper- and metaplasia, leading to mucus overproduction, increased mucus viscocity, and inhibition of the mucociliary clearance.[102] As a result, chronic inflammatory changes and bacterial colonization result.[104,105] Gel-forming mucin glycoproteins between 10 and 40 million Da are the major components of airway mucus.[106–109] The mucins can be mainly produced by two kinds of airway cell types: goblet cells (i.e., MUC2 and MUC5AC mucins expression) and glandular cells (i.e., MUC5B and MUC7 mucins expression).[104,110,111] Mucus hypersecretion as well as the deficient channel protein CFTR can be targeted by pulmonary nanomedicine delivery systems. In a recent study, Truong-Le and coworkers[20] reported that the DNA and gelatin nanoparticle coacervate containing chloroquine and calcium, and with the cell ligand transferrin covalently bound to the gelatin, had been prepared as a gene delivery vehicle. Nanospheres with the DNA achieved incorporation over 98% of the DNA in the reaction. DNA into the nanosphere was partially resistant to digestion with concentrations of DNase I that resulted in extensive degradation of free DNA but was completely degraded by high concentrations of DNase. In transfection studies of cultured human tracheal epithelial cells (9HTEo) with nanospheres containing the DNA, a CFTR expression in over 50% of the cells was found, and resulted that human bronchial epithelial cells (IB-3-1) defective in CFTR-mediated chloride transport regained an effective transport activity when transfected with nanospheres containing the CFTR transgene. In summary, the biological integrity of the optimized nanospheres with the DNA was demonstrated with a nanomedicine pulmonary delivery system utilizing DNA encoding the CFTR. To further understand how to effectively deliver genes to the airways of CF patients, Sanders et al.[21] explained that the extent of CF sputum presents a physical barrier to the transport of nanospheres of a size comparable to that of lipoplexes and other transfection systems currently being clinically evaluated for CF gene therapy. It was also observed that an extremely low percentage of nanospheres (0.3%) moved through a 220 mm thick CF sputum layer after 150 min, and the largest nanospheres studied (560 nm) were almost completely blocked by the sputum, whereas the smaller nanospheres (124 nm) were retarded only by a factor of 1.3 as compared with buffer. Surprisingly, the nanospheres diffused significantly more easily through the more viscoelastic sputum samples. These phenomena could be explained by the structure of the network in sputum becomes more macroporous as the sputum becomes more viscoelastic. Recombinant human DNase (dornase alfa) was also developed as a food and drug administration (FDA)-approved marketed product (Pulmozyme®, Genentech, USA) to degrade the large amount of free DNA that accumulates within CF mucus, leading to an improvement in the viscoelastic properties of airway secretions and promoting airway clearance.[112,113]

3.3.3 Tuberculosis

Tuberculosis (TB) has been another therapeutic area of focus in targeted pulmonary nanomedicine delivery. Pandey et al.[24] reported on the formulation of three antituberculosis drugs (i.e., rifampicin, isoniazid, and pyrazin-amide) encapsulated in poly(DL-lactide-*co*-glycolide) as nanoparticles suit-able for nebulization. This nanomedicine formulation was evaluated with the pharmacokinetics of each drug and its chemotherapeutic potential in *Mycobacterium tuberculosis*-infected guinea pigs. Sustained therapeutic drug levels in the plasma for 6–8 days and in the lungs for up to 11 days with a single nebulization to guinea pigs was achieved. The elimination half-life and the mean residence time of the drugs in these nanomedicine pulmonary formulations were significantly prolonged compared to oral administration (12.7-, 32.8-, and 14.7-fold for rifampicin, isoniazid, and pyrazinamide, respectively). It demonstrated that pulmonary administration of antituberculosis drug nanoparticles can be used experimentally to improve pharmacological management of pulmonary tuberculosis.

Ohashi et al.[23] also reported on rifampicin (RIF)/poly(lactic-*co*-glycolic acid) (PLGA) nanoparticle-containing mannitol (MAN) microspheres for inhala-tion therapy of tuberculosis using a four-fluid nozzle spray drier in one step, such that the RIF and PLGA acetone/methanol (2/1) solution and MAN aque-ous solution were supplied through different liquid passages of the four-fluid nozzle spray drier to obtain MAN microspheres including RIP/PLGA nanoparticles. These had a mean diameter of 213 nm, and showed good *in vitro* aerosol performance evaluated by an inertial cascade impactor. *In vivo* cell uptake of RIF from the (RIF/PLGA)/MAN formulations was about 4% at 1 h after administration increasing to 9.3% at 4 h. *In vivo* imaging study suggested that the micron-sized (RIF/PLGA)/MAN formulations were rapidly excreted from the lungs, but that it may be difficult to clear the nano-sized RIF/PLGA particles, resulting in their retention. Thus, the RIF/PLGA nanoparticles were recognized by alveolar macrophages and the uptake of RIF increased.

3.3.4 Infectious Diseases

Bacterial and viral infections have important therapeutic considerations because the progression of COPD, asthma, and CF along with secondary lung infections can lead to a progressive destruction of lung tissue resulting in respiratory failure.[114] Targeted delivery of anti-infective drugs (i.e., antimicro-bial agents) to the lung has been highly desirable with major advantages in the reduced systemic side effects and higher dose levels of the applicable medica-tion at the site of drug action (i.e., deposition to the alveolar site of the infection can reach high local concentration and therefore inhaled drugs can reduce the occurrence of serious systemic adverse effects by dose reduction).[100,115] The alveolar and bronchial epithelium is a site with major opportunity for drug delivery and therapy.[105] The slow development of new classes of antimicrobi-als for the treatment of resistant bacterial infections has increased the need for targeted delivery of antimicrobials directly to the site of lung infection. Targeted pulmonary nanomedicine delivery of antibiotics has focused on the treatment of pulmonary infections particularly chronic pulmonary infections in CF patients.[116–120] Yang et al.[121] recently reported that inhalable dry powders containing DNase and/or ciprofloxacin were produced by spray drying with dipalmitylphosphatidylcholine, albumin, and lactose as excipients, with the mass median aerodynamic diameters below 5 μm. With the study in an artificial sputum containing *Pseudomonas aeruginosa*, Cipro/DNase formulation showed better antibacterial activity than Cipro powder. Therefore, inhalational delivery of antibiotics to the CF airway could be optimized when the sputum barrier could be concomitantly addressed. Cheow et al.[122] reported that inhaled antibiotic-loaded PLGA and PCL polymeric drug nanoparticles had sustained release capability as promising antibiofilm formulations in the fight against respiratory biofilm infections which was attributed to their ability to penetrate the biofilm sputum. The antibacterial efficacy and physical characteristics of antibiotic-loaded polymeric nanoparticles were also evaluated.

3.3.5 Vaccination

Targeted pulmonary nanomedicine delivery can include vaccination formulations for long-lasting, noninvasive, and protective immunization to respiratory viral infections. Vila and coworkers[36] reported on polylactic acid (PLA) nanoparticles coated with a hydrophilic PEG-coating and tetanus toxoid. PLA nanoparticles suffered from immediate aggregation upon incubation with lysozyme, whereas the PEG-coated nanoparticles remained stable and deaggregated. The antibody levels elicited following intranasal administration of PEG-coated nanoparticles were significantly higher than those corresponding to PLA nanoparticles. Furthermore, PEG–PLA nanoparticles generated an increasing and a long-lasting response. Chitosan–DNA nanospheres containing a cocktail of plasmid DNAs encoding respiratory syncytial virus (RSV) antigens were prepared by Kumar and coworkers.[37] Following *in vivo* and *in vitro* studies of these nanospheres, there was a significant reduction of viral antigen load and viral titers after an acute RSV infection in mice animal model, and the induction of RSV-specific nasal IgA antibodies, cytotoxic T lymphocytes, IgG antibodies, and interferon-gamma production.

3.4 Nanoparticle Lung Delivery Systems

3.4.1 Polymer-Based Nanocarriers

3.4.1.1 Polymeric Micelles

As the colloidal nanocarrier systems, polymeric micelles, which are amphiphilic macromolecules that self-assemble in an aqueous environment, have promising applications in pulmonary targeted nanomedicine delivery. Poorly water-soluble drugs can be entrapped in the core of micelles, which can possibly make them to have high level of apparent water solubility. The hydrophilic outer shell can effectively protect the active agents. In addition, the outer surface of the shell can be modified to prevent recognition by the reticuloendothelial system (RES), and therefore increase the circulation time in the body. Another remarkable property of polymeric micelles is the flexibility in their size and shape *in vivo*. Polymeric micelles can also be selectively targeted in a broad range of disease sites with these attractive features. Polymeric micelles can be applied in the solubilization of water-insoluble drugs,[123] gene delivery[124] (e.g., siRNA) as well as macromolecule delivery[85] (e.g., therapeutic proteins and polypeptides).

Jones and Leroux[125] investigated beclomethasone dipropionate (BDP)-loaded polymeric micelles as an inhalation aerosol dosage form to treat asthma and COPD. These results showed that the polymeric micelles can evade the mononuclear phagocytic system by the bulky hydrophilic outer shell and also sustain the release of the drug.[126] In addition, polymeric micelles may be promising to pass through the mucus layer associated with bronchial inflammatory diseases directly to their receptors in the epithelial cells. Gaber et al.[127] reported on the potential of using poly-(ethylene oxide)-block-distearoyl phosphatidyl-ethanolamine (mPEG-DSPE) polymer to prepare BDP-loaded polymeric micelles with high entrapment efficiency and mass median aerodynamic diameter of less than 5 µm demonstrating sustained release properties. Lyophilized BDP-loaded micelles with entrapment efficiency of more than 96% were achieved and the particle size of the BDP-loaded micelles was about 22 nm. *In vitro* drug release showed a promising sustained release profile over six days following the Higuchi model. The high encapsulation efficiency, comparable inhalation properties, sustained release behavior together with biocompatibility nature of the polymer support the potential of BDP-loaded polymeric micelles as a versatile delivery system to be used in the treatment of asthma and COPD.

Chao et al.[128] reported on the efficient inhalation gene delivery to the lung using a biocompatible, nonionic poly(ethyleneoxide)-poly(propyleneoxide)-poly(ethyleneoxide) (PEO–PPO–PEO) polymeric micelles as a carrier and combined it with ethanol as a penetration enhancer to enhance membrane penetration of delivered DNA. The results showed that β-gal activity was significantly increased by 38% in the lung around the bronchioles when inhalation of polymeric micelles and 10% ethanol were given. The 10% ethanol also increased the intracellular apparent permeability by 42% in the stomach and by 141% in the intestine at 48 h after the first dose. Also delivery of DNA encoding a functional human CFTR using the same inhalation delivery method coformulated with 10% ethanol, an increased expression of CFTR in the lung was detected by immunostaining. Yang et al.[129] recently investigated a novel pulmonary delivery platform of microparticles containing micelles in which a therapeutic photosensitizing drug, hematoporphyrin (Hp), was encapsulated. For these microparticle formulations with micelles, different poloxamers were used to form micellar Hp, and one of these, Pluronic

L122-Hp, was subsequently incorporated into lactose microparticles by spray drying. Photodynamic activity of the various Hp samples were evaluated in human lung epithelial carcinoma A549 cells using a light-emitting diode (LED) device at a wavelength of 630 ± 5 nm. The cellular uptake of micellar Hp and lactose-micellar Hp measured on A549 cells was at least two-fold higher than those obtained with the Hp at equivalent concentrations. Micellar Hp exhibited higher cytotoxicity than Hp due to reduced formation of Hp aggregates and increased cellular uptake. With these promising results, microparticles containing micelles have the potential for delivering micelle-encapsulated hydrophobic drugs for targeted therapy of pulmonary diseases.

3.4.1.2 Polymeric Nanoparticles

The main roles of polymeric nanoparticles in drug-delivery system are to carry the drug molecules, to protect drugs from degradation, and to provide controlled drug release.[3] In pharmaceutical and medical applications, polymers should have both biodegradability and biocompatibility[130] *in vivo*. The process of biodegradation can be described as two main steps: (1) water penetration into polymeric matrix for the breakdown of the chemical bonds by hydrolysis; and (2) surface erosion of the polymer with increasing conversion rate of the polymer into water-soluble structures.

Polyester-based polymers are commonly used in pulmonary targeted nanomedicine delivery systems, such as polycaprolactone (PCL), polylactide acid (PLA), and polylactic-*co*-glycolic acid (PLGA), which are FDA-approved[130] inactive ingredients with biodegradability and biocompatibility. PLGA have been the most studied diblock copolymer for drug delivery offering enhanced drug encapsulation, sustained release property, nontoxicity, and is present in several commercially available pharmaceutical products.[130] Degradation and release rates of PLGA-based systems can mainly be affected by molecular weight and the lactide/glycolide ratio of PLGA.[131–133]

Naturally derived polymers[130] such as chitosan,[134–136] alginate,[137] hyaluronic acid,[138,139] and collagen (e.g., gelatin),[140–143] have also been investigated. There have been a number of targeted pulmonary drug-delivery systems using polymeric nanoparticles. These reported investigations have included targeted pulmonary nanomedicines such as antiasthmatic drugs,[144,145] antituberculosis drugs,[24,146] pulmonary hypertension drugs,[147] and anticancer drugs.[143,148] In addition, polymer-based gene carriers as cationic polymer-based nanoparticles have been studied for gene delivery to the lungs.[149,150] In particular, PEI with liposomes/PEGs or conjugations of PEI with ligands such as transferrin have been investigated intensively.[151–155]

Ungaro et al.[156] reported that PLGA containing insulin with optimal aerodynamic properties were fabricated by a double emulsion method by aid of hydroxypropyl-β-cyclodextrin (HPβCD). The aerosolization properties and the release features of PLGA/HPβCD/insulin large porous particles (LPP) were investigated in depth. Confocal microscopy studies, performed after administration of labeled PLGA/HPβCD/insulin LPP to the rat lung by means of a low-scale dry powder inhaler (DPI), suggest that particles reach the alveoli and remain *in situ* after delivery. *In vivo* data showed that PLGA/HPβCD/insulin LPP could reach the alveoli and release insulin, which was absorbed in its bioactive form.

Dailey et al.[157] investigated surfactant-free, biodegradable nanoparticle systems with the branched polyester, diethylaminopropyl amine-poly(vinyl alcohol)-grafted-poly(lactide-*co*-glycolide) (DEAPA-PVAL-g-PLGA) alone, as well as with increasing amounts of carboxymethyl cellulose (CMC). In detail, three formulations were studied: cationic nanoparticles without CMC, cationic nanoparticles with CMC, and anionic nanoparticles with an excess of CMC. Surfactant-free nanoparticles from DEAPA-PVAL-g-PLGA could be versatile drug-delivery systems; however, only the anionic formulations investigated were proven suitable for aerosol therapy.

Yamamoto et al.[158] reported that peptide-loaded PLGA nanospheres could be granulated with the sugar alcohol, mannitol. A spray drying fluidized-bed granulator was used to form soft matrix composite granules. Nanosphere suspension could be easily obtained by dispersing the composite granules in distilled water. More than 50% of the composite granules were delivered to the bronchioles and the alveoli of rat, and it had strong and prolonged pharmacological effects compared to the inhalation of insulin solution.

3.4.2 Lipid-Based Nanocarriers

3.4.2.1 Solid-Lipid Nanoparticles

Solid-lipid nanoparticles (SLNs) are nano-sized colloidal nanocarrier systems developed at the beginning of the 1990s.[159,160] SLNs based on solid lipids at room temperature, surfactant(s), and an aqueous medium.[161–163] There are various advantages of SLNs: (1) bioavailability enhancement of poorly water-soluble drugs; (2) decrease of toxicity *in vivo* following a high biocompatibility and biodegradability; (3) physicochemical stabilization of unstable drugs in biological and storage conditions; (4) modulation of drug release profiles *in vitro* and *in vivo*; (5) low manufacturing cost; and (6) use of various administration routes such as parenteral, oral, ocular, and dermal.[62,164] The nanostructure lipid carriers (NLCs) are highly similar to SLNs, but the NLCs contain a solid matrix that entraps liquid lipid nano-compartments, which have advantages over SLNs such as a higher solubility for drugs than solid lipids, a higher drug-loading capacity, lower drug expulsion during storage, and higher level of sustained release effects.[63] Although SLNs and NLCs as nanocarriers used in drug delivery systems have remarkable advantages, toxicological profiles of SLNs and NLCs should be confirmed. In this case, physiological endogenous lipids can be used for SLNs and NLCs because physiological lipids have little or no cytotoxicity.[165,166] Several preparation methods for SLNs have been used, which are based on the basic principles of cold high-pressure homogenization, hot high-pressure homogenization, multiple emulsion technique, and hot homogenization methods followed by ultrasonication.

Pulmonary targeted delivery of SLNs have been studied for antituberculosis drugs,[167] cancer chemotherapeutic drugs,[168,169] and macromolecules (i.e., insulin, HIV 1 TAT-peptide109).[170,171] Pandey and Khuller[167] evaluated the chemotherapeutic potential of nebulized SLNs incorporating rifampicin, isoniazid, and pyrazinamide against experimental tuberculosis. The SLNs prepared by the "emulsion solvent diffusion" technique possessed a favorable mass median aerodynamic diameter suitable for bronchoalveolar drug delivery. On nebulization of drug-loaded SLNs to infected guinea pigs at every 7th day, no tubercle bacilli could be detected in the lungs/spleen after 7 doses of treatment whereas 46 daily doses of orally administered drugs were required to obtain an equivalent therapeutic benefit. Further, there was no evidence of any biochemical hepatotoxicity.

Lung cancer-targeted nanomedicine was investigated using camptothecins,[168] inhibitors of topoisomerase I which is one of the key enzymes for DNA replication and subsequent cell proliferation. Preclinical and clinical evaluations in this study had shown that the camptothecins were active against lung cancer and other solid malignancies with novel aerosol routes of drug administration, and their application in combination therapy. Epirubicin-loaded SLNs as an inhalable formulation for treatment of lung cancer was studied.[169] The drug concentrations in lungs and in plasma after inhalation of epirubicin-SLNs were much higher than those after administration of epirubicin solution.

Lymphatic uptake of pulmonary administered SLNs after aerosolization and clearance from the lungs has been reported.[172,173] SLNs with griceryl behenate were radiolabeled by D,L-hexamethylpropylene amine oxime (HMPAO) coupled with [99m]Tc. Wistar rats were treated by endotracheal administration and lymphatic uptake was determined upon organ sampling. Delivered SLNs were rapidly eliminated from rat lungs. In summary, translocation of SLNs across the lung mucosa and their uptake into the lymphatics could demonstrate their usefulness as potential drug carriers for pulmonary lymphatic delivery which may have novel application in the treatment of lung cancer metastases which are known to circulate in the lymphatic system.

3.4.2.2 Liposomes

Liposomes have been extensively investigated for controlled delivery to the lung, which are commonly defined as the phospholipid self-assemblies with a size range of 50–1000 nm.[174] Liposomal formulations can be formed by one bilayer (unilamellar) or several lipid bilayers (multilamellar) with an aqueous phase associated with the polar headgroups both inside and between the multiple bilayers. Liposomal nanomedicine delivery systems[164] can entrap hydrophilic drugs in the aqueous core or lipophilic drugs in the phospholipid bilayers. Since they are compromised of biomembrane phospholipids, they are nontoxic, nonimmunogenic, and biodegradable.[164] The amphiphilic nature of liposomes provide versatility as drug-delivery systems.[175] Phospholipid bilayers have unique nanomaterial properties of characteristic hydration properties[176] and spreading functionality[177] on surfaces which provide versatility. They also serve as robust biomimetic lung surfactant models[178] for drug-delivery applications in the context of interfacial and spreading properties.

Conventional liposomes given by injection can have a relatively short blood circulation time due to rapid accumulation by the phagocytic cells of the mononuclear phagocyte system (MPS) and by the reticuloendothelial system (RES) uptake.[179,180] Long-circulating liposomes have a coating on the liposome surface comprised of an inert biocompatible polymer of polyethylene glycol (PEG) as a protective layer over the liposome surface to reduce opsonization.[181–184] Such PEG-coated liposomes are also known as "stealth" or "sterically stabilized" liposomes with their MPS-escaping capability and their steric hindrance stabilization mechanism providing long circulation times.[185] Immunoliposomes have been prepared with specific surface-attached antibodies, such as immunoglobulin G (IgG), for surface cell recognition and targeted.[181] Cationic liposomes are used in the development of advanced delivery of oligonucleotides and genetic material.[186] The cationic lipid component interacts electrostatically with the negatively charged DNA, thereby condensing the DNA into a more compact structure. The resulting lipid–DNA complexes (also known as "lipoplexes") provide protection and promote cellular internalization and expression of the condensed plasmid.[186] Compared with viral vector gene delivery, cationic liposomes are relatively easy to prepare, reasonably inexpensive, and nonimmunogenic.[187]

Proliposomes have been studied as dry, free-flowing particles, which have the ability to form liposomal dispersion when dispersed in aqueous phase.[188] Pulmonary drug delivery of therapeutic liposomal dry powder inhalation aerosols[189] offer many unique advantages and can enhance drug residence time in the lung, provide controlled release, and spreading on the lung fluid surface. Proliposomes can be prepared by various nanoparticulate preparation methods (i.e., freeze-drying, spray-drying, spray freeze-drying, and supercritical-fluid technology).[190,191]

Nebulization of rehydrated freeze-dried beclomethasone dipropionate (BDP) liposomal preparations[192] showed that the lipid with a low transition temperature (T_m) (i.e., dilauroyl phosphatidylcholine (DLPC)) incorporated a higher amount of BDP than lipid with a high T_m (i.e., dipalmitoyl phosphatidylcholine (DPPC)). The rehydrated BDP–DLPC liposomes showed a higher output (78.3%) and a higher fine particle fraction (FPF) (75.0%) and smaller mass median aerodynamic diameter (MMAD) than the other rehydrated liposome preparations. Changsan et al.[22] reported that RIF encapsulated liposomes could be an alternative formulation for delivery to the respiratory tract. Four liposome suspensions were prepared, containing different millimole ratios of cholesterol (CH) and soybean L-∞-phosphatidylcholine (SPC) by the chloroform film method, followed by freeze-drying. Higher CH content in the liposome formulation resulted in a smaller change in size distribution with time, and higher CH content was associated with an increase in the ^{2}H NMR splitting, indicative of an increase in order of the lipid acyl chains. SS-NMR results indicated that RIF was located between the acyl chains of the phospholipid bilayer and associated with CH molecules. RIF in dry powder formulations was considerably more stable when compared with RIF aqueous solutions and RIF liposomal suspensions.

Wijagkanalan et al.[193] investigated that inhalation of bacterial endotoxin with the selective targeting of mannosylated liposomes to alveolar macrophages could induce pulmonary inflammation by activation of nuclear factor κB (NFκB), production of cytokines and chemokines, and neutrophil activation. In this study, the anti-inflammatory effects of dexamethasone palmitate incorporated in mannosylated liposomes (DPML) significantly inhibited tumor necrosis factor α, interleukin-1β, and cytokine-induced neutrophil chemoattractant-1 levels, suppressed neutrophil infiltration and myeloperoxidase activity, and inhibited NFκB and p38 mitogen-activated protein kinase activation in the lung. These results prove the value of inhaled mannosylated liposomes as powerful targeting systems for the delivery of anti-inflammatory drugs to alveolar macrophages to improve their efficacy against lung inflammation. Bi et al.[194] reported that dry powder inhalation of insulin-loaded liposomes could be prepared by novel spray-freeze-drying method, and influence of different kinds and amounts of lyoprotectants was also evaluated for the best preservation of the drug entrapped in the liposome bilayers after the dehydration–rehydration cycle. The *in vivo* study of intratracheal instillation of insulin-loaded liposomes to diabetic rats showed successful hypoglycemic effect with low blood glucose level and long-lasting period and a relative pharmacological bioavailability as high as 38.38% in the group of 8 IU/kg dosage. Behr et al.[195] studied a liposomal cyclosporine A (CsA) PARI nebulized formulation which was able to be deposited to the peripheral lung using the PARI eFlow® nebulizer with good tolerance and no drug-related side effects were observed. Once or twice daily dosing of 10 mg CsA resulted in a sufficient peripheral lung deposition of approximately 14 and 28 mg/week, respectively.

3.5 *In Vitro* and *In Vivo* Characterization of Targeted Pulmonary Nanomedicine Delivery Systems

There are various preparation methods[3,196] for targeted pulmonary nanomedicine delivery systems which are listed in Table 3.2. After preparation, an array of comprehensive physicochemical,[205] surface analytical,[206] and imaging techniques[207] can be employed for an in-depth understanding of the behavior of nanoparticulate pulmonary inhalation aerosols[205] *in vitro, in vivo,* and *ex vivo.* These are listed in Table 3.3.

TABLE 3.2

Preparation Methods Used in Design and Formulation of Targeted Pulmonary
Nanomedicine Delivery Systems

Method	Description
Nano-milling (e.g., wet-milling)	A rotating milling shaft, which is circulating through a milling chamber, presents both high shear rate and impaction for the production of a mechanical stress between the milling media and slurry containing raw drug particles and stabilizer. The milling media might be based on material science, and can be used with the beads of glass, zirconium oxide, or cross-linked polystyrene resin.[27,197,198]
High-pressure homogenization	A slurry feeding stream, usually composed of drug coarse particle and stabilizer, is pressurized with an intensifier pump to 100–2000 bar. The processing time depends on the homogenization pressure, which in turn determines the flow rate, number of cycles, solid loading, and amount of materials to be processed.[199]
Spray drying	Spray drying (SD) is a robust and effective method for designing and manufacturing aerosol formulations.[3,164,196,200] The feed solution is pumped to the nozzle where it is atomized by the nozzle gas. The atomized droplets are then dried by the preheated drying gas during primary drying followed by secondary drying thus forming dry particles that are collected via a cyclone and sample collector.
Spray freeze drying	Spray freeze drying (SFD)[3,164,196] is an combination of spray-drying and freeze-drying processing steps. This method has been proposed to evaporate solvents with cryogenic fluids and freeze drying at a wide range of cooling rates (102–106 K/s). The cooling rate is maintained at a sufficiently higher rate than those used in the conventional lyophilization (~1 K/s).[199] This technique involves the atomization of an aqueous drug solution into a spray chamber filled with a cryogenic liquid (liquid nitrogen) or halocarbon refrigerant such as chlorofluorocarbon or fluorocarbon.[201,202]
Supercritical fluid technology	The most common in pulmonary aerosols are supercritical antisolvent precipitation (SAS) and supercritical fluid extraction of emulsions (SFEE).[3,196] SAS is based on rapid precipitation when a drug solution is brought into contact with a supercritical CO_2. SFEE is based on extraction of the organic phase in oil-in-water or multiple emulsions using supercritical CO_2.[203,204]
Antisolvent	Mixing a solution with an antisolvent generating supersaturation that subsequently induces nucleation and simultaneous growth by condensation and coagulation. The drug must be soluble in the solvent but practically insoluble in the antisolvent. The solvent and antisolvent must also be miscible at the operating conditions.[3,199]

Aerosol inhalation deposition behavior[89] can be affected by air flow, directional change, passage of an obstacle, and curvilinear motion. Inertial impaction is the aerosol characterization method based on curvilinear motion of suspended particles that is extensively applied for collection, measurement, and aerosol separation.[97] Inertial impaction[89] is based on the theory of Stokes' law.[3]

TABLE 3.3

Characterization Methods for Targeted Pulmonary Nanomedicine
Delivery Systems

Type	Method	Measurement
In vitro	*In vitro* release test	Drug release rate and release mechanism
	Inertial impaction[89]	Aerodynamic size and aerodynamic size distribution of aerosolized particles
	Karl Fischer titration[205,200]	Water content quantification
	Laser size diffraction[200]	Particle size and size distribution
	SEM[205,200]	Electron imaging of particles and surfaces
	XRPD[205,200]	Molecular order assessment
	DSC[205,200]	Thermal analysis of phase behavior
	AFM[205,206]	Nanotopographical imaging, adhesive/cohesive forces
In vivo	Gamma-scintigraphy[196,207]	Imaging of aerosol deposition in the respiratory tract
	Pharmacokinetics/ Pharmacodynamics	Pharmacokinetic parameters and biodistribution
Ex vivo	Isolated perfused lung[196]	Characterization of drug transport, disposition, and its mechanism *ex vivo*

Abbreviations: AFM, atomic force microscopy; DSC, differential scanning calorimetry; SEM, scanning electron microscopy; XRPD, x-ray powder diffraction.

Cascade impactors are based on curvilinear motion of particles in the aerosol stream.[89] The Andersen cascade impactor (ACI) and next-generation impactor (NGI) are common cascade impactors[89] with the former having a historical precedence in environmental inhalation toxicology and the latter being recently developed by pharmaceutical inhalation aerosol scientists. The twin-stage liquid impinger (TSLI) and multi-stage liquid impingers (MSLI) are also based on the principles of inertial impaction. A single jet per impactor stage is located above the flat collection plate. Particles over a certain value (i.e., cut-off size) cannot be retained in the streamlines and will impact on the collection plate and be deposited on it.[208,209] The Nano-MOUDI™ impactor has been recently developed for purpose of measuring ultra-fine aerosol particles.[210–213]

Physiochemical and surface analytical techniques used in characterization of inhalation aerosols have been previously described in-depth.[205,206] Scanning electron microscopy (SEM)[200,205] is a unique electron imaging method for imaging particle morphology and surface morphology which influence aerosol dispersion of dry powders. With its high resolution (magnifications in the range 20–100,000 times), a gold-palladium-coated sample can be scanned by a fine beam of electrons of medium energy (5–50 keV), which is routinely used for imaging particles in the micron and smaller size range and for examining the surfaces of larger particles.[205] Atomic force microscopy (AFM)[205,206] enables imaging of surface nanotopography and measurement of surface energy and adhesive/cohesive forces on the order of 10^{-6}–10^{-9} m.[214] There are several experimental factors including: (1) the cantilever tip consistency; (2) the physical and chemical properties of colloid probe and substrate surfaces; (3) environmental issues, such as temperature and relative humidity; and (4) the contact area determination or normalization.[205] X-ray powder diffraction (XRPD)[200,205] directly measures the degree of molecular order.[3,215,216] Differential scanning calorimetry (DSC)[200,205] is also a robust thermal analytical method for phase behavior and phase transitions of pharmaceutical materials including nanoparticles.[217]

Many *in vitro* pulmonary cell culture models[196] have been developed for various pulmonary cell types representing different lung regions.[218–223] *In vivo* and *ex vivo* evaluation[196,207] can be performed via aerosolization by nebulization (liquid aerosols), microspraying (liquid aerosols), or insufflation (dry powder aerosols). Restraint-free small animal inhalation dosing chambers for *in vivo* aerosolization has been reported with itraconazole aerosols,[28,224,225] microspraying by the microsprayer rodent device, or insufflation by the dry powder insufflators rodent device.

3.6 Conclusion and Future Direction

Interest in inhalation nanomedicine delivery continues to increase due to its demonstrated successful application to address medical needs and the significant fundamental advances in nanotechnology, material science, and particle engineering design. Recent advances in therapeutic macromolecules and biotherapeutics have also increased the growth of inhalation pulmonary nanomedicine delivery. Through basic and applied research combined with *in vivo* efficacy and safety studies, targeted pulmonary nanomedicine delivery as inhalation aerosols provides great potential as a novel therapeutic paradigm.

References

1. Sung, J. C., Pulliam, B. L., and Edwards, D. A., Nanoparticles for drug delivery to the lungs, *TRENDS in Biotechnology* 25 (12), 563–570, 2007.

2. Bailey, M. M. and Berkland, C. J., Nanoparticle formulations in pulmonary drug delivery, *Medicinal Research Reviews* 29 (1), 196–212, 2009.
3. Mansour, H. M., Rhee, Y. S., and Wu, X., Nanomedicine in pulmonary delivery, *International Journal of Nanomedicine* 4, 299, 2009.
4. Kulkarni, V. S., *Handbook of Non-Invasive Drug Delivery Systems: Science & Technology* (Personal care & cosmetic technology series), Elsevier Inc, Burlington, MA, 2009.
5. Joshi, M. R. and Misra, A., Liposomal budesonide for dry powder inhaler: Preparation and stabilization, *AAPS PharmSciTech* 2 (4), 44, 2001.
6. Martin, T. M., Bandi, N., Shulz, R., Roberts, C. B., and Kompella, U. B., Preparation of budesonide and budesonide-PLA microparticles using super-critical fluid precipitation technology, *AAPS PharmSciTech* 3 (3), 16–26, 2002.
7. El Gendy, N., Gorman, E. M., Munson, E. J., and Berkland, C., Budesonide nanoparticle agglomerates as dry powder aerosols with rapid dissolution, *Journal of Pharmaceutical Sciences* 98 (8), 2731–2746, 2009.
8. Jacobs, C. and Muller, R. H., Production and characterization of a budesonide nanosuspension for pulmonary administration, *Pharmaceutical Research* 19 (2), 189–194, 2002.
9. Shrewsbury, S. B., Bosco, A. P., and Uster, P. S., Pharmacokinetics of a novel sub-micron budesonide dispersion for nebulized delivery in asthma, *International Journal of Pharmaceutics* 365 (1–2), 12–17, 2009.
10. Mezzena, M., Scalia, S., Young, P. M., and Traini, D., Solid lipid budesonide mic-roparticles for controlled release inhalation therapy, *The AAPS Journal* 11 (4), 771–778, 2009.
11. Beck-Broichsitter, M., Gauss, J., Gessler, T., Seeger, W., Kissel, T., and Schmehl, T., Pulmonary targeting with biodegradable salbutamol-loaded nanoparticles, *Journal of Aerosol Medicine and Pulmonary Drug Delivery* 23 (1), 47–57, 2010.
12. Kubavat, H., Shur, J., and Price, R., The influence of crystallization processes on the nano-mechanical properties of fluticasone propionate, *Drug Delivery to the Lungs 22th Conference*, Edinburgh, Scotland, UK. 10–12 December, 2011.
13. Doktorovova, S., Araujo, J., Garcia, M. L., Rakovsk ¥, E., and Souto, E. B., Formulating fluticasone propionate in novel PEG-containing nanostructured lipid carriers (PEG-NLC), *Colloids and Surfaces B: Biointerfaces* 75 (2), 538–542, 2010.
14. Saari, S. M., Vidgren, M. T., Koskinen, M. O., Turjanmaa, V. M. H., Waldrep, J. C., and Nieminen, M. M., Regional lung deposition and clearance of 99mTc-labeled beclomethasone-DLPC liposomes in mild and severe asthma, *Chest* 113 (6), 1573, 1998.
15. Wang, Z., Chen, J. F., Le, Y., Shen, Z. G., and Yun, J., Preparation of ultrafine beclomethasone dipropionate drug powder by antisolvent precipitation, *Industrial & Engineering Chemistry Research* 46 (14), 4839–4845, 2007.
16. Hyvonen, S., Peltonen, L., Karjalainen, M., and Hirvonen, J., Effect of nano-precipitation on the physicochemical properties of low molecular weight poly (L-lactic acid) nanoparticles loaded with salbutamol sulphate and beclometha-sone dipropionate, *International Journal of Pharmaceutics* 295 (1–2), 269–281, 2005.
17. Jaafar-Maalej, C., Andrieu, V., Elaissari, A., and Fessi, H., Beclomethasone-loaded lipidic nanocarriers for pulmonary drug delivery: Preparation, charac-terization and *in vitro* drug release, *Journal of Nanoscience and Nanotechnology* 11 (3), 1841–1851, 2011.

18. Ahmad, F. J., Mittal, G., Jain, G. K., Malhotra, G., Khar, R. K., and Bhatnagar, A., Nano-salbutamol dry powder inhalation: A new approach for treating broncho-constrictive conditions, *European Journal of Pharmaceutics and Biopharmaceutics* 71 (2), 282–291, 2009.

19. Hong, Y., Hu, F., and Yuan, H., Effect of PEG2000 on drug delivery characterization from solid lipid nanoparticles, *Pharmazie* 61 (4), 312–315, 2006.

20. Truong-Le, V. L., Walsh, S. M., Schweibert, E., Mao, H. Q., Guggino, W. B., August, J. T., and Leong, K. W., Gene transfer by DNA-gelatin nanospheres* 1, *Archives of Biochemistry and Biophysics* 361 (1), 47–56, 1999.

21. Sanders, N. N., De Smedt, S. C., Van Rompaey, E., Simoens, P., De Baets, F., and Demeester, J., Cystic fibrosis sputum. A barrier to the transport of nanospheres, *American Journal of Respiratory and Critical Care Medicine* 162 (5), 1905, 2000.

22. Changsan, N., Chan, H. K., Separovic, F., and Srichana, T., Physicochemical characterization and stability of rifampicin liposome dry powder formulations for inhalation, *Journal of Pharmaceutical Sciences* 98 (2), 628–639, 2009.

23. Ohashi, K., Kabasawa, T., Ozeki, T., and Okada, H., One-step preparation of rifampicin/poly (lactic-*co*-glycolic acid) nanoparticle-containing mannitol microspheres using a four-fluid nozzle spray drier for inhalation therapy of tuberculosis, *Journal of Controlled Release* 135 (1), 19–24, 2009.

24. Pandey, R., Sharma, A., Zahoor, A., Sharma, S., Khuller, G., and Prasad, B., Poly (DL-lactide-co-glycolide) nanoparticle-based inhalable sustained drug delivery system for experimental tuberculosis, *Journal of Antimicrobial Chemotherapy* 52 (6), 981, 2003.

25. Shah, S. and Misra, A., Development of liposomal amphotericin B dry powder inhaler formulation, *Drug Delivery* 11 (4), 247–253, 2004.

26. Vyas, S. P., Quraishi, S., Gupta, S., and Jaganathan, K., Aerosolized liposome-based delivery of amphotericin B to alveolar macrophages, *International Journal of Pharmaceutics* 296 (1–2), 12–25, 2005.

27. Yang, W., Johnston, K. P., and Williams III, R. O., Comparison of bioavailability of amorphous versus crystalline itraconazole nanoparticles via pulmonary administration in rats, *European Journal of Pharmaceutics and Biopharmaceutics* 75 (1), 33–41, 2010.

28. Yang, W., Tam, J., Miller, D. A., Zhou, J., McConville, J. T., Johnston, K. P., and Williams III, R. O., High bioavailability from nebulized itraconazole nanoparticle dispersions with biocompatible stabilizers, *International Journal of Pharmaceutics* 361 (1–2), 177–188, 2008.

29. Omri, A., Beaulac, C., Bouhajib, M., Montplaisir, S., Sharkawi, M., and Lagace, J., Pulmonary retention of free and liposome-encapsulated tobramycin after intra-tracheal administration in uninfected rats and rats infected with Pseudomonas aeruginosa, *Antimicrobial Agents and Chemotherapy* 38 (5), 1090, 1994.

30. Pilcer, G., Vanderbist, F., and Amighi, K., Preparation and characterization of spray-dried tobramycin powders containing nanoparticles for pulmonary delivery, *International Journal of Pharmaceutics* 365 (1–2), 162–169, 2009.

31. Finlay, W. and Wong, J., Regional lung deposition of nebulized liposome-encap-sulated ciprofloxacin, *International Journal of Pharmaceutics* 167 (1–2), 121–127, 1998.

32. Sweeney, L. G., Wang, Z., Loebenberg, R., Wong, J. P., Lange, C. F., and Finlay, W. H., Spray-freeze-dried liposomal ciprofloxacin powder for inhaled aerosol drug delivery, *International Journal of Pharmaceutics* 305 (1–2), 180–185, 2005.

33. Conley, J., Yang, H., Wilson, T., Blasetti, K., Di Ninno, V., Schnell, G., and Wong, J. P., Aerosol delivery of liposome-encapsulated ciprofloxacin: Aerosol characterization and efficacy against Francisella tularensis infection in mice, *Antimicrobial Agents and Chemotherapy* 41 (6), 1288, 1997.
34. Zhao, H., Le, Y., Liu, H., Hu, T., Shen, Z., Yun, J., and Chen, J. F., Preparation of microsized spherical aggregates of ultrafine ciprofloxacin particles for dry powder inhalation (DPI), *Powder Technology* 194 (1–2), 81–86, 2009.
35. El-Gendy, N., Desai, V., and Berkland, C., Agglomerates of ciprofloxacin nanoparticles yield fine dry powder aerosols, *Journal of Pharmaceutical Innovation* 5 (3), 79–87, 2010.
36. Vila, A., Sanchez, A., Evora, C., Soriano, I., Vila Jato, J., and Alonso, M., PEG-PLA nanoparticles as carriers for nasal vaccine delivery, *Journal of Aerosol Medicine* 17 (2), 174–185, 2004.
37. Kumar, M., Kong, X., Behera, A. K., Hellermann, G. R., Lockey, R. F., and Mohapatra, S. S., Chitosan IFN-gamma-pDNA nanoparticle (CIN) therapy for allergic asthma, *Genetic Vaccines and Therapy* 1 (3), 1–10, 2003.
38. Koshkina, N. V., Waldrep, J. C., Roberts, L. E., Golunski, E., Melton, S., and Knight, V., Paclitaxel liposome aerosol treatment induces inhibition of pulmonary metastases in murine renal carcinoma model, *Clinical Cancer Research* 7 (10), 3258, 2001.
39. Hureaux, J., Lagarce, F., Gagnadoux, F., Vecellio, L., Clavreul, A., Roger, E., Kempf, M., Racineux, J. L., Diot, P., and Benoit, J. P., Lipid nanocapsules: Ready-to-use nanovectors for the aerosol delivery of paclitaxel, *European Journal of Pharmaceutics and Biopharmaceutics* 73 (2), 239–246, 2009.
40. Azarmi, S., Tao, X., Chen, H., Wang, Z., Finlay, W. H., Lobenberg, R., and Roa, W. H., Formulation and cytotoxicity of doxorubicin nanoparticles carried by dry powder aerosol particles, *International Journal of Pharmaceutics* 319 (1–2), 155–161, 2006.
41. Gilbert, B. E., Knight, C., Alvarez, F. G., Waldrep, J. C., Rodarte, J. R., Knight, V., and Eschenbacher, W. L., Tolerance of volunteers to cyclosporine A-dilauroylphosphatidylcholine liposome aerosol, *American Journal of Respiratory and Critical Care Medicine* 156 (6), 1789, 1997.
42. Letsou, G. V., Safi, H. J., Reardon, M. J., Ergenoglu, M., Li, Z., Klonaris, C. N., Baldwin, J. C., Gilbert, B. E., and Waldrep, J. C., Pharmacokinetics of liposomal aerosolized cyclosporine A for pulmonary immunosuppression, *The Annals of Thoracic Surgery* 68 (6), 2044, 1999.
43. Zijlstra, G. S., Rijkeboer, M., Van Drooge, D. J., Sutter, M., Jiskoot, W., Van De Weert, M., Hinrichs, W. L. J., and Frijlink, H. W., Characterization of a cyclosporine solid dispersion for inhalation, *The AAPS Journal* 9 (2), 190–199, 2007.
44. Chougule, M., Padhi, B., and Misra, A., Nano-liposomal dry powder inhaler of tacrolimus: Preparation, characterization, and pulmonary pharmacokinetics, *International Journal of Nanomedicine* 2 (4), 675, 2007.
45. Sinswat, P., Overhoff, K. A., McConville, J. T., Johnston, K. P., and Williams III, R. O., Nebulization of nanoparticulate amorphous or crystalline tacrolimus-Single-dose pharmacokinetics study in mice, *European Journal of Pharmaceutics and Biopharmaceutics* 69 (3), 1057–1066, 2008.
46. Brigger, I., Dubernet, C., and Couvreur, P., Nanoparticles in cancer therapy and diagnosis, *Advanced Drug Delivery Reviews* 54 (5), 631–651, 2002.
47. Tiwari, S. B. and Amiji, M. M., A review of nanocarrier-based CNS delivery systems, *Current Drug Delivery* 3 (2), 219–232, 2006.

48. Kaur, I. P., Bhandari, R., Bhandari, S., and Kakkar, V., Potential of solid lipid nanoparticles in brain targeting, *Journal of Controlled Release* 127 (2), 97–109, 2008.
49. Davis, M. E., Nanoparticle therapeutics: An emerging treatment modality for cancer, *Nature Reviews Drug Discovery* 7 (9), 771–782, 2008.
50. ESF, Nanomedicine—An ESF–European Medical Research Councils (EMRC) Forward Look Report. Strasbourg cedex, France, 2004.
51. Webster, T. J., Nanomedicine: What's in a definition?, *International Journal of Nanomedicine* 1 (2), 115, 2006.
52. NIH, N. I. o. H., National Institute of Health Roadmap for Medical Research: Nanomedicine, USA, 2006.
53. Torchilin, V. P., Lipid-core micelles for targeted drug delivery, *Current Drug Delivery* 2 (4), 319–327, 2005.
54. Florence, A. T., Pharmaceutical aspects of nanotechnology, in *Chapter 12 in Modern Pharmaceutics, Volume 2: Applications and Advances*, Florence, A. T. and Siepmann, J. (eds.), Informa Healthcare, New York, 2009.
55. Von Werne, T. and Patten, T. E., Preparation of structurally well-defined polymer-nanoparticle hybrids with controlled/living radical polymerizations, *Journal of the American Chemical Society* 121 (32), 7409–7410, 1999.
56. Pridgen, E. M., Langer, R., and Farokhzad, O. C., Biodegradable, polymeric nanoparticle delivery systems for cancer therapy, *Nanomedicine* 2 (5), 669–680, 2007.
57. Hussain, F., Hojjati, M., Okamoto, M., and Gorga, R. E., Review article: Polymer-matrix nanocomposites, processing, manufacturing, and application: An overview, *Journal of Composite Materials* 40 (17), 1511, 2006.
58. van Vlerken, L. E. and Amiji, M. M., Multi-functional polymeric nanoparticles for tumour-targeted drug delivery, 2006.
59. Almeida, A. J. and Souto, E., Solid lipid nanoparticles as a drug delivery system for peptides and proteins, *Advanced Drug Delivery Reviews* 59 (6), 478–490, 2007.
60. Joshi, M. D. and Muller, R. H., Lipid nanoparticles for parenteral delivery of actives, *European Journal of Pharmaceutics and Biopharmaceutics* 71 (2), 161–172, 2009.
61. Muchow, M., Maincent, P., and Muller, R. H., Lipid nanoparticles with a solid matrix (SLN¢ç, NLC¢ç, LDC¢ç) for oral drug delivery, *Drug Development and Industrial Pharmacy* 34 (12), 1394–1405, 2008.
62. MuEller, R. H., MaEder, K., and Gohla, S., Solid lipid nanoparticles (SLN) for controlled drug delivery-a review of the state of the art, *European Journal of Pharmaceutics and Biopharmaceutics* 50 (1), 161–177, 2000.
63. Muller, R., Radtke, M., and Wissing, S., Solid lipid nanoparticles (SLN) and nanostructured lipid carriers (NLC) in cosmetic and dermatological preparations, *Advanced Drug Delivery Reviews* 54, S131–S155, 2002.
64. Pardeike, J., Hommoss, A., and Muller, R. H., Lipid nanoparticles (SLN, NLC) in cosmetic and pharmaceutical dermal products, *International Journal of Pharmaceutics* 366 (1–2), 170–184, 2009.
65. Schafer-Korting, M., Mehnert, W., and Korting, H. C., Lipid nanoparticles for improved topical application of drugs for skin diseases, *Advanced drug Delivery Reviews* 59 (6), 427–443, 2007.
66. Wissing, S., Kayser, O., and Muller, R., Solid lipid nanoparticles for parenteral drug delivery, *Advanced Drug Delivery Reviews* 56 (9), 1257–1272, 2004.

67. Crommelin, D. J. A. and Storm, G., Liposomes: From the bench to the bed, *Journal of Liposome Research* 13 (1), 33–36, 2003.
68. Metselaar, J. M., Mastrobattista, E., and Storm, G., Liposomes for intravenous drug targeting: Design and applications, *Mini Reviews in Medicinal Chemistry* 2 (4), 319–329, 2002.
69. Brandl, M., Liposomes as drug carriers: A technological approach, *Biotechnology Annual Review* 7, 59–85, 2001.
70. Lasic, D. D. and Martin, F., *Stealth Liposomes*, CRC Press, Boca Raton, FL, 1995.
71. Gregoriadis, G. and Florence, A. T., *Liposomes in drug delivery*, CRC Press, Boca Raton, FL, 1993.
72. Lawrence, M. J. and Rees, G. D., Microemulsion-based media as novel drug delivery systems, *Advanced Drug Delivery Reviews* 45 (1), 89–121, 2000.
73. Wu, W., Wang, Y., and Que, L., Enhanced bioavailability of silymarin by self-microemulsifying drug delivery system, *European Journal of Pharmaceutics and Biopharmaceutics* 63 (3), 288–294, 2006.
74. Jadhav, K., Shaikh, I., Ambade, K., and Kadam, V., Applications of microemulsion based drug delivery system, *Current Drug Delivery* 3 (3), 267–273, 2006.
75. Hashida, M., Kawakami, S., and Yamashita, F., Lipid carrier systems for targeted drug and gene delivery, *Chemical & Pharmaceutical Bulletin* 53 (8), 871–880, 2005.
76. Davis, S. S., Washington, C., West, P., Illum, L., Liversidge, G., Sternson, L., and Kirsh, R., Lipid emulsions as drug delivery systems, *Annals of the New York Academy of Sciences* 507 (1), 75–88, 1987.
77. Collins-Gold, L., Lyons, R., and Bartholow, L., Parenteral emulsions for drug delivery, *Advanced Drug Delivery Reviews* 5 (3), 189–208, 1990.
78. Charman, W. N., Lipids, lipophilic drugs, and oral drug delivery—Some emerging concepts, *Journal of Pharmaceutical Sciences* 89 (8), 967–978, 2000.
79. Jamaty, C., Bailey, B., Larocque, A., Notebaert, E., Sanogo, K., and Chauny, J. M., Lipid emulsions in the treatment of acute poisoning: A systematic review of human and animal studies, *Clinical Toxicology* 48 (1), 1–27, 2010.
80. Pouton, C. W., Lipid formulations for oral administration of drugs: Non-emulsifying, self-emulsifying and "self-microemulsifying" drug delivery systems, *European Journal of Pharmaceutical Sciences* 11, S93–S98, 2000.
81. Vinogradov, S. V., Colloidal microgels in drug delivery applications, *Current Pharmaceutical Design* 12 (36), 4703, 2006.
82. Vinogradov, S. V., Zeman, A. D., Batrakova, E. V., and Kabanov, A. V., Polyplex nanogel formulations for drug delivery of cytotoxic nucleoside analogs, *Journal of Controlled Release* 107 (1), 143–157, 2005.
83. Raemdonck, K., Demeester, J., and De Smedt, S., Advanced nanogel engineering for drug delivery, *Soft Matter* 5 (4), 707–715, 2008.
84. Kataoka, K., Harada, A., and Nagasaki, Y., Block copolymer micelles for drug delivery: Design, characterization and biological significance, *Advanced Drug Delivery Reviews* 47 (1), 113–131, 2001.
85. Nasongkla, N., Bey, E., Ren, J., Ai, H., Khemtong, C., Guthi, J. S., Chin, S. F., Sherry, A. D., Boothman, D. A., and Gao, J., Multifunctional polymeric micelles as cancer-targeted, MRI-ultrasensitive drug delivery systems, *Nano Letters* 6 (11), 2427–2430, 2006.
86. Maeda, H., Bharate, G., and Daruwalla, J., Polymeric drugs for efficient tumor-targeted drug delivery based on EPR-effect, *European Journal of Pharmaceutics and Biopharmaceutics* 71 (3), 409–419, 2009.

87. Cotes, J. E. and Leathart, G. L., *Lung Function*. Wiley Online Library, 1993.
88. Haverich, A., Scott, W., and Jamieson, S., Twenty years of lung preservation—A review, *The Journal of Heart Transplantation* 4 (2), 234, 1985.
89. Hickey, A. J. and Mansour, H. M., Delivery of drugs by the pulmonary route, in *Modern Pharmaceutics*, 5th ed., Florence, A. T. and Siepmann, J. (eds), Taylor & Francis, Inc., New York, 2009, pp. 191–219.
90. Weibel, E. R., Morphometry of the human lung, *Anesthesiology* 26 (3), 367, 1965.
91. Horsfield, K. and Woldenberg, M. J., Branching ratio and growth of tree-like structures, *Respiration Physiology* 63 (1), 97–107, 1986.
92. Pauwels, R., Newman, S., and Borgstrom, L., Airway deposition and airway effects of antiasthma drugs delivered from metered-dose inhalers, *European Respiratory Journal* 10 (9), 2127, 1997.
93. Yu, C. and Diu, C., A comparative study of aerosol deposition in different lung models, *American Industrial Hygiene Association Journal* 43 (1), 54–65, 1982.
94. Pich, J., Theory of gravitational deposition of particles from laminar flows in channels, *Journal of Aerosol Science* 3 (5), 351–361, 1972.
95. Ingham, D., Diffusion of aerosols from a stream flowing through a cylindrical tube, *Journal of Aerosol Science* 6 (2), 125–132, 1975.
96. Landahl, H., Particle removal by the respiratory system note on the removal of airborne particulates by the human respiratory tract with particular reference to the role of diffusion, *Bulletin of Mathematical Biology* 25 (1), 29–39, 1963.
97. Hinds, W. C., *Aerosol technology: Properties, behavior, and measurement of airborne particles*, Wiley-Interscience, New York, 1982.
98. Smola, M., Vandamme, T., and Sokolowski, A., Nanocarriers as pulmonary drug delivery systems to treat and to diagnose respiratory and non respiratory diseases, *International Journal of Nanomedicine* 3 (1), 1, 2008.
99. Halbert, R., Natoli, J., Gano, A., Badamgarav, E., Buist, A., and Mannino, D., Global burden of COPD: Systematic review and meta-analysis, *European Respiratory Journal* 28 (3), 523, 2006.
100. Pison, U., Welte, T., Giersig, M., and Groneberg, D. A., Nanomedicine for respiratory diseases, *European Journal of Pharmacology* 533 (1–3), 341–350, 2006.
101. John, A. E., Lukacs, N. W., Berlin, A. A., Palecanda, A., Bargatze, R. F., Stoolman, L. M., and Nagy, J. O., Discovery of a potent nanoparticle P-selectin antagonist with anti-inflammatory effects in allergic airway disease, *The FASEB Journal* 17 (15), 2296, 2003.
102. Rosenstein, B. J. and Zeitlin, P. L., Prognosis in cystic fibrosis, *Current Opinion in Pulmonary Medicine* 1 (6), 444, 1995.
103. Stern, R. C., The diagnosis of cystic fibrosis, *The New England Journal of Medicine* 336 (7), 487, 1997.
104. Groneberg, D., Eynott, P., Lim, S., Oates, T., Wu, R., Carlstedt, I., Roberts, P., McCann, B., Nicholson, A., and Harrison, B., Expression of respiratory mucins in fatal status asthmaticus and mild asthma, *Histopathology* 40 (4), 367–373, 2002.
105. Ramsey, B. W., Management of pulmonary disease in patients with cystic fibrosis, *The New England Journal of Medicine* 335 (3), 179, 1996.
106. Davies, J., Hovenberg, H., Linden, C., Howard, R., Richardson, P., Sheehan, J., and Carlstedt, I., Mucins in airway secretions from healthy and chronic bronchitic subjects, *Biochemical Journal* 313 (Pt 2), 431, 1996.
107. Gupta, R. and Jentoft, N., The structure of tracheobronchial mucins from cystic fibrosis and control patients, *Journal of Biological Chemistry* 267 (5), 3160, 1992.

108. Thornton, D. J., Sheehan, J. K., Lindgren, H., and Carlstedt, I., Mucus glyco-proteins from cystic fibrotic sputum. Macromolecular properties and structural architecture, *Biochemical Journal* 276 (Pt 3), 667, 1991.
109. Thornton, D., Davies, J., Kraayenbrink, M., Richardson, P., Sheehan, J., and Carlstedt, I., Mucus glycoproteins from normal human tracheobronchial secre-tion, *Biochemical Journal* 265 (1), 179, 1990.
110. Sharma, P., Dudus, L., Nielsen, P. A., Clausen, H., Yankaskas, J. R., Hollingsworth, M. A., and Engelhardt, J. F., MUC5B and MUC7 are differentially expressed in mucous and serous cells of submucosal glands in human bronchial airways, *American Journal of Respiratory Cell and Molecular Biology* 19 (1), 30–37, 1998.
111. Wickstrom, C., Davies, J., Eriksen, G., Veerman, E., and Carlstedt, I., MUC5B is a major gel-forming, oligomeric mucin from human salivary gland, respira-tory tract and endocervix: Identification of glycoforms and C-terminal cleavage, *Biochemical Journal* 334 (Pt 3), 685, 1998.
112. Flume, P. A., O'Sullivan, B. P., Robinson, K. A., Goss, C. H., Mogayzel Jr, P. J., Willey-Courand, D. B., Bujan, J., Finder, J., Lester, M., and Quittell, L., Cystic fibro-sis pulmonary guidelines: Chronic medications for maintenance of lung health, *American Journal of Respiratory and Critical Care Medicine* 176 (10), 957, 2007.
113. Cimmino, M., Nardone, M., Cavaliere, M., Plantulli, A., Sepe, A., Esposito, V., Mazzarella, G., and Raia, V., Dornase alfa as postoperative therapy in cystic fibrosis sinonasal disease, *Archives of Otolaryngology Head and Neck Surgery* 131 (12), 1097, 2005.
114. Koch, C. and Hiby, N., Pathogenesis of cystic fibrosis, *Lancet* 341 (8852), 1065, 1993.
115. Park, C. W., Hayes, D. J., and Mansour, H. M., Pulmonary inhalation aerosols for targeted antibiotics delivery, *European Pharmaceutical Review* 16 (1), 32–36, 2011.
116. Flume, P. and Klepser, M. E., The rationale for aerosolized antibiotics, *Pharmacotherapy* 22 (3 Part 2), 71–79, 2002.
117. Craig, W. A., Pharmacokinetic/pharmacodynamic parameters: Rationale for antibacterial dosing of mice and men, *Clinical Infectious Diseases* 26 (1), 1–10, 1998.
118. FitzSimmons, S. C., The changing epidemiology of cystic fibrosis, *The Journal of Pediatrics* 122 (1), 1–9, 1993.
119. Beringer, P. M., New approaches to optimizing antimicrobial therapy in patients with cystic fibrosis, *Current Opinion in Pulmonary Medicine* 5 (6), 371, 1999.
120. Geller, D. E., Aerosol antibiotics in cystic fibrosis, *Respiratory Care* 54 (5), 658–670, 2009.
121. Yang, Y., Tsifansky, M. D., Wu, C. J., Yang, H. I., Schmidt, G., and Yeo, Y., Inhalable antibiotic delivery using a dry powder co-delivering recombinant deoxyribonu-clease and ciprofloxacin for treatment of cystic fibrosis, *Pharmaceutical Research* 27 (1), 151–160, 2010.
122. Cheow, W. S., Chang, M. W., and Hadinoto, K., Antibacterial efficacy of inhal-able antibiotic-encapsulated biodegradable polymeric nanoparticles against E. coli biofilm cells, *Journal of Biomedical Nanotechnology* 6 (4), 391–403, 2010.
123. Kwon, G. S., Polymeric micelles for delivery of poorly water-soluble com-pounds, *Critical Reviews in Therapeutic Drug Carrier Systems* 20 (5), 357–403, 2003.
124. Nishiyama, N. and Kataoka, K., Current state, achievements, and future prospects of polymeric micelles as nanocarriers for drug and gene delivery, *Pharmacology & Therapeutics* 112 (3), 630–648, 2006.

125. Jones, M. C. and Leroux, J. C., Polymeric micelles-a new generation of colloidal drug carriers, *European Journal of Pharmaceutics and Biopharmaceutics* 48 (2), 101–111, 1999.
126. Marsh, D., Bartucci, R., and Sportelli, L., Lipid membranes with grafted polymers: Physicochemical aspects, *Biochimica et Biophysica Acta (BBA)-Biomembranes* 1615 (1–2), 33–59, 2003.
127. Gaber, N. N., Darwis, Y., Peh, K. K., and Tan, Y. T. F., Characterization of polymeric micelles for pulmonary delivery of beclomethasone dipropionate, *Journal of Nanoscience and Nanotechnology*, 6 9 (10), 3095–3101, 2006.
128. Chao, Y. C., Chang, S. F., Lu, S. C., Hwang, T. C., Hsieh, W. H., and Liaw, J., Ethanol enhanced *in vivo* gene delivery with non-ionic polymeric micelles inhalation, *Journal of Controlled Release* 118 (1), 105–117, 2007.
129. Yang, Y. T., Chen, C. T., Yang, J. C., and Tsai, T., Spray-dried microparticles containing polymeric micelles encapsulating hematoporphyrin, *The AAPS Journal* 12 (2), 138–146, 2010.
130. Mansour, H. M., Sohn, M., Al-Ghananeem, A., and DeLuca, P. P., Materials for pharmaceutical dosage forms: Molecular pharmaceutics and controlled release drug delivery aspects. Invited Paper. *International Journal of Molecular Sciences: Special Issue-Material Sciences and Nanotechnology Section—Biodegradability of Materials*, 11, 3298–3322, 2010.
131. Houchin, M. and Topp, E., Chemical degradation of peptides and proteins in PLGA: A review of reactions and mechanisms, *Journal of Pharmaceutical Sciences* 97 (7), 2395–2404, 2008.
132. Na, D. H. and DeLuca, P. P., PEGylation of octreotide: I. Separation of positional isomers and stability against acylation by poly (D, L-lactide-co-glycolide), *Pharmaceutical Research* 22 (5), 736–742, 2005.
133. Na, D. H., Lee, K. C., and DeLuca, P. P., PEGylation of octreotide: II. Effect of N-terminal mono-PEGylation on biological activity and pharmacokinetics, *Pharmaceutical Research* 22 (5), 743–749, 2005.
134. Kumar, R. and Majeti, N., A review of chitin and chitosan applications, *Reactive and Functional Polymers* 46 (1), 1–27, 2000.
135. Wei, L., Cai, C., Lin, J., and Chen, T., Dual-drug delivery system based on hydrogel/micelle composites, *Biomaterials* 30 (13), 2606–2613, 2009.
136. Smidsrd, O. and Skjaok-Brk, G., Alginate as immobilization matrix for cells, *Trends in Biotechnology* 8, 71–78, 1990.
137. Rowley, J. A., Madlambayan, G., and Mooney, D. J., Alginate hydrogels as synthetic extracellular matrix materials, *Biomaterials* 20 (1), 45–53, 1999.
138. Liao, Y. H., Jones, S. A., Forbes, B., Martin, G. P., and Brown, M. B., Hyaluronan: Pharmaceutical characterization and drug delivery, *Drug Delivery* 12 (6), 327–342, 2005.
139. Malafaya, P. B., Silva, G. A., and Reis, R. L., Natural-origin polymers as carriers and scaffolds for biomolecules and cell delivery in tissue engineering applications, *Advanced Drug Delivery Reviews* 59 (4–5), 207–233, 2007.
140. Friess, W., Collagen-biomaterial for drug delivery1, *European Journal of Pharmaceutics and Biopharmaceutics* 45 (2), 113–136, 1998.
141. Schoof, H., Apel, J., Heschel, I., and Rau, G., Control of pore structure and size in freeze dried collagen sponges, *Journal of Biomedical Materials Research* 58 (4), 352–357, 2001.

142. Kojima, C., Tsumura, S., Harada, A., and Kono, K., A collagen-mimic dendrimer capable of controlled release, *Journal of the American Chemical Society* 131 (17), 6052–6053, 2009.

143. Tseng, C. L., Su, W. Y., Yen, K. C., Yang, K. C., and Lin, F. H., The use of biotinyl-ated-EGF-modified gelatin nanoparticle carrier to enhance cisplatin accumulation in cancerous lungs via inhalation, *Biomaterials* 30 (20), 3476–3485, 2009.

144. Seong, J. H., Lee, K. M., Kim, S. T., Jin, S. E., and Kim, C. K., Polyethylenimine based antisense oligodeoxynucleotides of IL 4 suppress the production of IL 4 in a murine model of airway inflammation, *The Journal of Gene Medicine* 8 (3), 314–323, 2006.

145. Wernig, K., Griesbacher, M., Andreae, F., Hajos, F., Wagner, J., Mosgoeller, W., and Zimmer, A., Depot formulation of vasoactive intestinal peptide by protamine-based biodegradable nanoparticles, *Journal of Controlled Release* 130 (2), 192–198, 2008.

146. Zahoor, A., Sharma, S., and Khuller, G., Inhalable alginate nanoparticles as anti-tubercular drug carriers against experimental tuberculosis, *International Journal of Antimicrobial Agents* 26 (4), 298–303, 2005.

147. Kimura, S., Egashira, K., Chen, L., Nakano, K., Iwata, E., Miyagawa, M., Tsujimoto, H., Hara, K., Morishita, R., and Sueishi, K., Nanoparticle-mediated delivery of nuclear factor {kappa} B decoy into lungs ameliorates monocrotaline-induced pulmonary arterial hypertension, *Hypertension* 53 (5), 877, 2009.

148. Beck-Broichsitter, M., Schmehl, T., Seeger, W., and Gessler, T., Evaluating the controlled release properties of inhaled nanoparticles using isolated, perfused, and ventilated lung models, *Journal of Nanomaterials* 2011, 1–16, 2011.

149. Densmore, C. L., Advances in noninvasive pulmonary gene therapy, *Current Drug Delivery* 3 (1), 55–63, 2006.

150. De Smedt, S. C., Demeester, J., and Hennink, W. E., Cationic polymer based gene delivery systems, *Pharmaceutical Research* 17 (2), 113–126, 2000.

151. Ogris, M. and Wagner, E., Tumor-targeted gene transfer with DNA polyplexes, *Somatic Cell and Molecular Genetics* 27 (1), 85–95, 2002.

152. Rudolph, C., Schillinger, U., Plank, C., Gessner, A., Nicklaus, P., Muller, R., and Rosenecker, J., Nonviral gene delivery to the lung with copolymer-protected and transferrin-modified polyethylenimine, *Biochimica et Biophysica Acta (BBA)-General Subjects* 1573 (1), 75–83, 2002.

153. Eliyahu, H., Joseph, A., Schillemans, J., Azzam, T., Domb, A., and Barenholz, Y., Characterization and *in vivo* performance of dextran-spermine polyplexes and DOTAP/cholesterol lipoplexes administered locally and systemically, *Biomaterials* 28 (14), 2339–2349, 2007.

154. Chono, S., Li, S. D., Conwell, C. C., and Huang, L., An efficient and low immu-nostimulatory nanoparticle formulation for systemic siRNA delivery to the tumor, *Journal of Controlled Release* 131 (1), 64–69, 2008.

155. Ko, Y. T., Kale, A., Hartner, W. C., Papahadjopoulos-Sternberg, B., and Torchilin, V. P., Self-assembling micelle-like nanoparticles based on phospholipid-poly-ethyleneimine conjugates for systemic gene delivery, *Journal of Controlled Release* 133 (2), 132–138, 2009.

156. Ungaro, F., d'Emmanuele di Villa Bianca, R., Giovino, C., Miro, A., Sorrentino, R., Quaglia, F., and La Rotonda, M. I., Insulin-loaded PLGA/cyclodextrin large porous particles with improved aerosolization properties: *In vivo* deposition and hypoglycaemic activity after delivery to rat lungs, *Journal of Controlled Release* 135 (1), 25–34, 2009.

157. Dailey, L., Kleemann, E., Wittmar, M., Gessler, T., Schmehl, T., Roberts, C., Seeger, W., and Kissel, T., Surfactant-free, biodegradable nanoparticles for aerosol therapy based on the branched polyesters, DEAPA-PVAL-g-PLGA, *Pharmaceutical Research* 20 (12), 2011–2020, 2003.

158. Yamamoto, H., Hoshina, W., Kurashima, H., Takeuchi, H., Kawashima, Y., Yokoyama, T., and Tsujimoto, H., Engineering of poly (DL-lactic-co-glycolic acid) nano-composite particle for dry powder inhalation dosage forms of insulin with spray fluidized bed Granulating system, *Journal of the Society of Powder Technology, Japan* 41, 514–521, 2004.

159. Muller, R. H., Mader, K., and Gohla, S., Solid lipid nanoparticles (SLN) for controlled drug delivery—A review of the state of the art, *European Journal of Pharmaceutics and Biopharmaceutics* 50 (1), 161–177, 2000.

160. Siekmann, B. and Westesen, K., Sub-micron sized parenteral carrier systems based on solid lipids, *Pharmaceutical and Pharmacological Letters* 1, 123–126, 1992.

161. Muchow, M., Maincent, P., and Muller, R. H., Lipid nanoparticles with a solid matrix (SLN, NLC, LDC) for oral drug delivery, *Drug Development and Industrial Pharmacy* 34 (12), 1394–1405, 2008.

162. Joshi, M. D. and Muller, R. H., Lipid nanoparticles for parenteral delivery of actives, *European Journal of Pharmaceutics and Biopharmaceutics* 71 (2), 161–172, 2009.

163. Mehnert, W. and Mader, K., Solid lipid nanoparticles: Production, characterization and applications, *Advanced Drug Delivery Reviews* 47 (2–3), 165–196, 2001.

164. Mansour, H. M., Rhee, Y. S., Park, C. W., and DeLuca, P. P., Lipid nanoparticulate drug delivery and nanomedicine, in *Lipids in Nanotechnology*, First ed., Moghis, A. American Oil Chemists Society (AOCS) Press, Urbana, Illinois, 2011, pp. 221–268.

165. Muller, R. H., Ruhl, D., Runge, S., Schulze-Forster, K., and Mehnert, W., Cytotoxicity of solid lipid nanoparticles as a function of the lipid matrix and the surfactant, *Pharmaceutical Research* 14 (4), 458–462, 1997.

166. Heydenreich, A., Westmeier, R., Pedersen, N., Poulsen, H., and Kristensen, H., Preparation and purification of cationic solid lipid nanospheres—Effects on particle size, physical stability and cell toxicity, *International Journal of Pharmaceutics* 254 (1), 83–87, 2003.

167. Pandey, R. and Khuller, G., Solid lipid particle-based inhalable sustained drug delivery system against experimental tuberculosis, *Tuberculosis* 85 (4), 227–234, 2005.

168. Koshkina, N., Waldrep, J., and Knight, V., Camptothecins and lung cancer: Improved delivery systems by aerosol, *Current Cancer Drug Targets* 3 (4), 251–264, 2003.

169. Hu, L., Jia, Y., and WenDing, Preparation and characterization of solid lipid nanoparticles loaded with epirubicin for pulmonary delivery, *Pharmazie* 65 (8), 585–587, 2010.

170. Liu, J., Gong, T., Fu, H., Wang, C., Wang, X., Chen, Q., Zhang, Q., He, Q., and Zhang, Z., Solid lipid nanoparticles for pulmonary delivery of insulin, *International Journal of Pharmaceutics* 356 (1–2), 333–344, 2008.

171. Rudolph, C., Schillinger, U., Ortiz, A., Tabatt, K., Plank, C., Muller, R. H., and Rosenecker, J., Application of novel solid lipid nanoparticle (SLN)-gene vector formulations based on a dimeric HIV-1 TAT-peptide *in vitro* and *in vivo*, *Pharmaceutical Research* 21 (9), 1662–1669, 2004.

172. Videira, M., Gano, L., Santos, C., Neves, M., and Almeida, A., Lymphatic uptake of lipid nanoparticles following endotracheal administration, *Journal of Microencapsulation* 23 (8), 855–862, 2006.

173. Videira, M. A., Botelho, M., Santos, A. C., Gouveia, L. F., Pedroso de Lima, J., and Almeida, A. J., Lymphatic uptake of pulmonary delivered radiolabelled solid lipid nanoparticles, *Journal of Drug Targeting* 10 (8), 607–613, 2002.

174. Gershkovich, P., Wasan, K. M., and Barta, C. A., A review of the application of lipid-based systems in systemic, dermal/transdermal, and ocular drug delivery, *Critical Reviews in Therapeutic Drug Carrier Systems* 25 (6), 545, 2008.

175. El Maghraby, G., Barry, B., and Williams, A., Liposomes and skin: From drug delivery to model membranes, *European Journal of Pharmaceutical Sciences* 34 (4–5), 203–222, 2008.

176. Mansour, H. M. and Zografi, G., The relationship between water vapor absorption and desorption by phospholipids and bilayer phase transitions, *Journal of Pharmaceutical Sciences* 96 (2), 377–396, 2007.

177. Mansour, H. M. and Zografi, G., Relationships between equilibrium spreading pressure and phase equilibria of phospholipid bilayers and monolayers at the air-water interface, *Langmuir: The ACS Journal of Surfaces and Colloids* 23 (7), 3809–3819, 2007.

178. Mansour, H. M., Damodaran, S., and Zografi, G., Characterization of the *in situ* structural and interfacial properties of the cationic hydrophobic heteropolypeptide, KL_4, in lung surfactant bilayer and monolayer models at the air-water interface: Implications for pulmonary surfactant delivery, *Molecular Pharmaceutics* 5 (5), 681–695, 2008.

179. Gabizon, A., Catane, R., Uziely, B., Kaufman, B., Safra, T., Cohen, R., Martin, F., Huang, A., and Barenholz, Y., Prolonged circulation time and enhanced accumulation in malignant exudates of doxorubicin encapsulated in polyethylene-glycol coated liposomes, *Cancer Research* 54 (4), 987, 1994.

180. Martin, F. J. and Papahadjopoulos, D., Irreversible coupling of immunoglobulin fragments to preformed vesicles. An improved method for liposome targeting, *Journal of Biological Chemistry* 257 (1), 286, 1982.

181. Torchilin, V. P., Recent advances with liposomes as pharmaceutical carriers, *Nature Reviews Drug Discovery* 4 (2), 145–160, 2005.

182. Klibanov, A. L., Maruyama, K., Torchilin, V. P., and Huang, L., Amphipathic polyethyleneglycols effectively prolong the circulation time of liposomes, *FEBS Letters* 268 (1), 235–237, 1990.

183. Blume, G. and Cevc, G., Molecular mechanism of the lipid vesicle longevity *in vivo*, *Biochimica et Biophysica Acta (BBA)-Biomembranes* 1146 (2), 157–168, 1993.

184. Wu, X. and Mansour, H. M., Nanopharmaceuticals II: Application of nanoparticles and nanocarrier systems in pharmaceutics and nanomedicine, *International Journal of Nanotechnology* 8 (1), 115–145, 2011.

185. Storm, G., Belliot, S. O., Daemen, T., and Lasic, D. D., Surface modification of nanoparticles to oppose uptake by the mononuclear phagocyte system, *Advanced Drug Delivery Reviews* 17 (1), 31–48, 1995.

186. Storm, G. and Crommelin, D. J. A., Liposomes: Quo vadis?, *Pharmaceutical Science & Technology Today* 1 (1), 19–31, 1998.

187. Felgner, P. L. and Ringold, G., Cationic liposome-mediated transfection, *Nature* 337 (6205), 387–388, 1989.

188. Rhee, Y. S. and Mansour, H. M., Nanopharmaceuticals I: Nanocarrier systems in drug delivery, *International Journal of Nanotechnology* 8 (1), 84–114, 2011.

189. Willis, L., Hayes, D. J., and Mansour, H. M., Therapeutic liposomal dry powder inhalation aerosols for targeted lung delivery, *Lung* 190 (3), 251–262, 2012.

190. Courrier, H., Butz, N., and Vandamme, T. F., Pulmonary drug delivery systems: Recent developments and prospects, *Critical Reviews in Therapeutic Drug Carrier Systems* 19 (4–5), 425–498, 2002.
191. Niven, R. W., Delivery of biotherapeutics by inhalation aerosol, *Critical Reviews in Therapeutic Drug Carrier Systems* 12 (2–3), 151, 1995.
192. Darwis, Y. and Kellaway, I., Nebulisation of rehydrated freeze-dried beclometh-asone dipropionate liposomes, *International Journal of Pharmaceutics* 215 (1–2), 113–121, 2001.
193. Wijagkanalan, W., Higuchi, Y., Kawakami, S., Teshima, M., Sasaki, H., and Hashida, M., Enhanced anti-inflammation of inhaled dexamethasone palmitate using mannosylated liposomes in an endotoxin-induced lung inflammation model, *Molecular Pharmacology* 74 (5), 1183, 2008.
194. Bi, R., Shao, W., Wang, Q., and Zhang, N., Spray-freeze-dried dry powder inhalation of insulin-loaded liposomes for enhanced pulmonary delivery, *Journal of Drug Targeting* 16 (9), 639–648, 2008.
195. Behr, J., Zimmermann, G., Baumgartner, R., Leuchte, H., Neurohr, C., Brand, P., Herpich, C., Sommerer, K., Seitz, J., and Menges, G., Lung deposition of a liposomal cyclosporine A inhalation solution in patients after lung transplantation, *Journal of Aerosol Medicine and Pulmonary Drug Delivery* 22 (2), 121–130, 2009.
196. Hickey, A. J. and Mansour, H. M., Volume 2: Formulation challenges of powders for the delivery of small molecular weight molecules as aerosols., in *Modified-Release Drug Delivery Technology* 2nd ed., Rathbone, M. J., Hadgraft, J., Roberts, M. S., and Lane, M. E. Informa Healthcare, New York, 2008, pp. 573–602.
197. Bilgili, E., Hamey, R., and Scarlett, B., Nano-milling of pigment agglomerates using a wet stirred media mill: Elucidation of the kinetics and breakage mechanisms, *Chemical Engineering Science* 61 (1), 149–157, 2006.
198. Robinson, G. M., Jackson, M. J., and Whitfield, M. D., A review of machining theory and tool wear with a view to developing micro and nano machining processes, *Journal of Materials Science* 42 (6), 2002–2015, 2007.
199. Zhang, J., Wu, L., Chan, H. K., and Watanabe, W., Formation, characterization, and fate of inhaled drug nanoparticles, *Advanced Drug Delivery Reviews*, 63 (6), 441–455, 2011.
200. Li, X. and Mansour, H. M., Physicochemical characterization and water vapor absorption of organic solution advanced spray dried trehalose microparticles and nanoparticles for targeted dry powder pulmonary inhalation delivery, *AAPS PharmSciTech: Special Theme: Advances in Pharmaceutical Excipients Research and Use: Novel Materials, Functionalities and Testing* 12 (4), 1420–1430, 2011.
201. Rogers, T. L., Johnston, K. P., and Williams III, R. O., Solution-based particle formation of pharmaceutical powders by supercritical or compressed fluid CO2 and cryogenic spray-freezing technologies, *Drug Development and Industrial Pharmacy* 27 (10), 1003–1015, 2001.
202. Subramaniam, B., Rajewski, R. A., and Snavely, K., Pharmaceutical processing with supercritical carbon dioxide, *Journal of Pharmaceutical Sciences* 86 (8), 885–890, 1997.
203. Shekunov, B. Y., Chattopadhyay, P., Seitzinger, J., and Huff, R., Nanoparticles of poorly water-soluble drugs prepared by supercritical fluid extraction of emulsions, *Pharmaceutical Research* 23 (1), 196–204, 2006.

204. Chattopadhyay, P., Huff, R., and Shekunov, B., Drug encapsulation using supercritical fluid extraction of emulsions, *Journal of Pharmaceutical Sciences* 95 (3), 667–679, 2006.

205. Hickey, A. J., Mansour, H. M., Telko, M. J., Xu, Z., Smyth, H. D. C., Mulder, T., McLean, R., Langridge, J., and Papadopoulos, D., Physical characterization of component particles included in dry powder inhalers. I. Strategy review and static characteristics, *Journal of Pharmaceutical Sciences* 96 (5), 1282–1301, 2007.

206. Wu, X., Li, X., and Mansour, H. M., Surface analytical techniques in solid-state particle characterization: Implications for predicting performance in dry powder inhalers. Invited Paper, *KONA Powder & Particle Journal* 28, 3–19, 2010.

207. Park, C. W., Rhee, Y. S., Vogt, F., Hayes, D. J., Zwischenberger, J. B., DeLuca, P. P., and Mansour, H. M., Advances in microscopy and complementary imaging techniques to assess the fate of drugs *ex-vivo* in respiratory drug delivery. Invited Paper., *Advanced Drug Delivery Reviews* 64 ((4) Special Theme Issue-Computational and Visualization Approaches in Respiratory Delivery.), 344–356, 2012.

208. Kwong, W. T. J., Ho, S. L., and Coates, A. L., Comparison of nebulized particle size distribution with Malvern laser diffraction analyzer versus Andersen cascade impactor and low-flow Marple personal cascade impactor, *Journal of Aerosol Medicine* 13 (4), 303–314, 2000.

209. Thompson, P. J., Drug delivery to the small airways, *American Journal of Respiratory and Critical Care Medicine* 157 (5), S199, 1998.

210. Sardar, S. B., Philip, M., Mayo, P. R., and Sioutas, C., Size-fractionated measurements of ambient ultrafine particle chemical composition in Los Angeles using the NanoMOUDI, *Environmental Science & Technology* 39 (4), 932–944, 2005.

211. Lin, C. C., Chen, S. J., Huang, K. L., Hwang, W. I., Chang-Chien, G. P., and Lin, W. Y., Characteristics of metals in nano/ultrafine/fine/coarse particles collected beside a heavily trafficked road, *Environmental Science & Technology* 39 (21), 8113–8122, 2005.

212. Venkatachari, P., Hopke, P. K., Brune, W. H., Ren, X., Lesher, R., Mao, J., and Mitchell, M., Characterization of wintertime reactive oxygen species concentrations in Flushing, New York, *Aerosol Science and Technology* 41 (2), 97–111, 2007.

213. Geller, M. D., Kim, S., Misra, C., Sioutas, C., Olson, B. A., and Marple, V. A., A methodology for measuring size-dependent chemical composition of ultrafine particles, *Aerosol Science and Technology* 36 (6), 748–762, 2002.

214. Bunker, M., Davies, M., and Roberts, C., Towards screening of inhalation formulations: Measuring interactions with atomic force microscopy, *Expert Opinion on Drug Delivery*, 2 (4), 613–624, 2005.

215. Zhu, X., Birringer, R., Herr, U., and Gleiter, H., X-ray diffraction studies of the structure of nanometer-sized crystalline materials, *Physical Review B* 35 (17), 9085, 1987.

216. Nagvekar, A. A., Trickler, W. J., and Dash, A. K., Current analytical methods used in the *in vitro* evaluation of nano-drug delivery systems, *Current Pharmaceutical Analysis* 5 (4), 358–366, 2009.

217. Saleki-Gerhardt, A., Ahlneck, C., and Zografi, G., Assessment of disorder in crystalline solids, *International Journal of Pharmaceutics* 101 (3), 237–247, 1994.

218. Steimer, A., Haltner, E., and Lehr, C. M., Cell culture models of the respiratory tract relevant to pulmonary drug delivery, *Journal of Aerosol Medicine* 18 (2), 137–182, 2005.

219. Borchard, G., Cassara, M. L., Roemele, P. E. H., Florea, B. I., and Junginger, H. E., Transport and local metabolism of budesonide and fluticasone propionate in a human bronchial epithelial cell line (Calu 3), *Journal of Pharmaceutical Sciences* 91 (6), 1561–1567, 2002.
220. Ehrhardt, C., Fiegel, J., Fuchs, S., Abu-Dahab, R., Schaefer, U., Hanes, J., and Lehr, C. M., Drug absorption by the respiratory mucosa: Cell culture models and particulate drug carriers, *Journal of Aerosol Medicine* 15 (2), 131–139, 2002.
221. Foster, K. A., Avery, M. L., Yazdanian, M., and Audus, K. L., Characterization of the Calu-3 cell line as a tool to screen pulmonary drug delivery, *International Journal of Pharmaceutics* 208 (1–2), 1–11, 2000.
222. Foster, K. A., Oster, C. G., Mayer, M. M., Avery, M. L., and Audus, K. L., Characterization of the A549 cell line as a type II pulmonary epithelial cell model for drug metabolism, *Experimental Cell Research* 243 (2), 359–366, 1998.
223. Manford, F., Tronde, A., Jeppsson, A. B., Patel, N., Johansson, F., and Forbes, B., Drug permeability in 16HBE14o-airway cell layers correlates with absorption from the isolated perfused rat lung, *European Journal of Pharmaceutical Sciences* 26 (5), 414–420, 2005.
224. Vaughn, J. M., McConville, J. T., Burgess, D., Peters, J. I., Johnston, K. P., Talbert, R. L., and Williams III, R. O., Single dose and multiple dose studies of itraconazole nanoparticles, *European Journal of Pharmaceutics and Biopharmaceutics* 63 (2), 95–102, 2006.
225. McConville, J. T., Overhoff, K. A., Sinswat, P., Vaughn, J. M., Frei, B. L., Burgess, D. S., Talbert, R. L., Peters, J. I., Johnston, K. P., and Williams, R. O., Targeted high lung concentrations of itraconazole using nebulized dispersions in a murine model, *Pharmaceutical Research* 23 (5), 901–911, 2006.

4

Biological Systems for the Delivery of Nanoparticles

Niketa Dixit, Mark Glaum, Arun Kumar, and Don F. Cameron

CONTENTS

4.1 Introduction 75
4.2 Bacteria as a Carrier to Deliver Nanoparticles 76
    4.2.1 Bacterial Magnetic Nanoparticles 77
4.3 Cells as a Carrier to Deliver Nanoparticles 78
4.4 Virus as a Carrier to Deliver Nanoparticles 80
    4.4.1 Challenges in Viral Nanoparticle-Based Drug-Delivery
        Systems 81
    4.4.2 Future Possibilities 82
    4.4.3 Plant Virus for Nanoparticle Delivery 82
    4.4.4 Oncolytic Viruses for Nanoparticle Delivery 83
    4.4.5 Virus-Like Particles for Drug Delivery 83
References 84

4.1 Introduction

There is increasing optimism that nanotechnology, as applied to medicine, will bring significant advances in the diagnosis and treatment of disease. The advent of nanotechnology has enabled the precise manufacture of materials with desirable properties and the removal of undesirable features. Anticipated applications in medicine include drug delivery, both *in vitro* and *in vivo* diagnostics, nutraceuticals and production of improved biocompatible materials. One of the most significant challenges facing the treatment of diseases is early intervention to deliver specific therapeutic cargo efficiently into cells to alter gene expression and subsequent protein production. Recent advances in nanotechnology have been used to deliver such cargoes into single cells through the use of nanoparticles for imaging, diagnostics, and therapeutics. For example, the gold and silver nanoparticles coated with antibodies can regulate the process of membrane receptor internalization. This binding and activation of membrane receptors, and the subsequent protein expression, is strongly dependent on nanoparticle size [1].

Although significant advances have been made in nanoparticle–cell interaction, many difficulties remain in delivering the nanoparticles to tumor sites, mainly because of the physical barriers encountered in solid tumors, such as malformed blood supplies, elevated interstitial pressure, and large transport distances in the tumor interstitium [2]. Researchers have over time been able to show that medicine designed at the nanoscale offers unprecedented opportunities for targeted treatment of serious diseases such as cancer. Clearly, nanostructures of different sizes, shapes, and material properties have many applications in biomedical imaging, clinical diagnostics, and therapeutics.

In spite of what has been achieved so far, a complete understanding of how cells interact with nanostructures, at the molecular level remains poorly understood; and how, for example, the body's immune system plays a part in the drug-delivery process [3].

Biological systems used as a carrier to deliver nanoparticle/biomolecule are

a. Bacteria

b. Cells

c. Viruses

d. Virus-like particles (VLPs)

4.2 Bacteria as a Carrier to Deliver Nanoparticles

Nanoparticles and bacteria can be used to deliver genes and proteins into mammalian cells for monitoring or altering gene expression and protein production. It is possible to use nanoparticles and bacteria to deliver DNA-based model drug molecules *in vivo* and *in vitro*. Researchers have demonstrated that bacteria can be loaded with nanoparticles, which are carried on the bacteria surface and can be delivered into tissues and cells. Following nanoparticle incubation with loaded bacteria, the cargo-carrying bacteria ("microbots") were internalized by the cells, and the genes released from the nanoparticles were expressed in the cells. Mice injected with microbots also successfully expressed the genes as seen by luminescence in different organs [4]. This approach may be used to deliver different types of cargo into live animals and a variety of cells in culture without the need for complicated genetic manipulations. Cells control their function and state through numerous processes of intracellular signaling events that are normally triggered by the binding of a ligand molecule with cell surface receptors. The extent of receptor–ligand binding and receptor crosslinking affects the intensity and duration of intracellular signaling and other downstream events, such as those seen with the trans-membrane receptor tyrosine kinases [5]. Ligands with multiple receptor binding sites, known as multivalent ligands, can crosslink the membrane receptors more efficiently to regulate signaling processes [6]. Nanoparticles coated with antibodies could potentially function as multivalent ligands that are capable of crosslinking surface receptors. By changing the size, shape, and material properties of the engineered nanoparticles, the degree of receptor crosslinking and subsequent cell responses can be precisely controlled. Recent observations in biological systems suggest that the physical parameters of nanoparticles can affect their nonspecific uptake in cells, with potential to induce cellular responses [7]. However, these studies provide limited information regarding the cellular processes involved in nanoparticle trafficking and their ensuing functional impact.

Bacteria also have been used as a nonviral means to transfer plasmid DNA into mammalian cells through a process called "bactofection." Several intracellular bacteria, including *Listeria monocytogenes*, which is responsible for foodborne infections in humans and animals [8], can penetrate mammalian cells that are normally nonphagocytic. These bacteria need specific surface molecules that interact with host cell receptors and once it is inside the cells, the bacteria carriers are disrupted by treatment with antibiotics and the DNA is released. *L. monocytogenes*-based bactofection systems have shown efficient transfer of genetic material inside the cells [9].

Other earlier reports include use of attenuated (reduced infectivity) bacteria such as *Shigella* [10] and *Salmonella typhimurium* [11] for the delivery of DNA-based vaccines. Bacteria themselves have additional advantages as delivery systems. For example, attenuated strains of *Escherichia coli*, *S. typhimurium*, *Vibrio cholerae*, and *L. monocytogenes* have been shown to be capable of multiplying selectively in tumors and in the case of *Clostridium* and *Bifidobacterium* spp. they even inhibit tumor growth [12]. Some of the unique properties of attenuated *Listeria* strains make them an ideal nonviral gene-delivery vehicle [13]. It should also be noted that antibiotics can control bacterial replication in the body or activate gene-based therapeutic molecules, as in the case with tetracycline-regulated control of gene expression.

4.2.1 Bacterial Magnetic Nanoparticles

Bacterial magnetic nanoparticles (BMPs), which are produced from magnetotactic bacteria, *Magnetospirillum* [14], are composed of Fe_3O_4 nanocrystals and a membrane coating that consists of phosphatidylethanolamine, phosphatidylglycerol, and other biological species containing abundant amino groups [15]. BMPs have been used successfully in numerous applications, including the immobilization of enzymes [16], the extraction of DNA and RNA [17], the sensitive detection and concentration of toxic substances [18], and the fabrication of magnetic nanotubes [19] and nanocrystalline magnetite [20]. Recently, BMPs have been shown to be a drug carrier with a higher drug-loading ratio than some artificial magnetic particles [21]. By using the abundant amino groups on their surface membranes, large quantities of chemotherapeutic agents can be attached efficiently. Besides the amino groups, there also exists an abundance of other functional groups, such as glycerol on the surface coating of the BMPs, and this offers a convenient approach to couple another ligand to the BMPs. The researchers have designed the system that combines two kinds of interactions: a magnetic dipole interaction and a ligand–receptor interaction for tumor targeting. In this system, the galactosyl-terminating ligand, which can selectively enter hepatocytes and hepatocellular carcinoma cells via the asialoglycoprotein receptor (ASGP-R) [22], is used as a hepatotropic ligand. Doxorubicin (DOX) was used as an anticancer agent and was bound to the surface of the BMPs. By chemically coupling both doxorubicin and the galactosyl ligand to the membrane surface of the BMPs, they have developed an efficient approach for generating bifunctional bacterial magnetic nanoparticles (BBMPs) with a high drug load ratio for tumor targeting [23].

The understanding of how engineered nanoparticles of different geometries interact with bacteria requires the study of the molecular events involved in nanoparticle and bacterial membrane receptor binding, endocytosis, and subsequent signaling activation vide insights into nanotoxicity.

4.3 Cells as a Carrier to Deliver Nanoparticles

Although significant efforts have been devoted to bridging the gap between synthetic nanomaterials and biological entities, an RBC-mimicking delivery vehicle has remained elusive to biomedical researchers. One major challenge lies in the difficulty in functionalizing nanoparticles with the complex surface chemistry of a biological cell. Despite the recent progress in reducing macrophage engulfment of polystyrene beads following their conjugation with an immunosuppressive RBC–membrane protein, CD47 [24], current chemistry-based bioconjugation techniques often lead to protein denaturation. Particularly difficult to treat by any drug-delivery system is the deep lung, the site of serious and urgent lung diseases such as acute respiratory distress syndrome (ARDS), post-lung transplantation complications, and lung cancers. This is due to methodological limitations in targeting the deep-lung pathologies with high efficiency drug distribution. The primary methodological approach to treating the lung is by inhalation therapy which is most effective in upper airway diseases. However, meeting the efficient delivery of most macromolecules to the deep lung is difficult because a sustained drug release goal can be somewhat problematic due to their low system efficiency and low drug mass per puff. Also, the lungs tend to expel materials that poor formulation stability for macromolecules, and poor are introduced via the airway and it is, therefore, difficult to do dosing reproducibility [25–26].

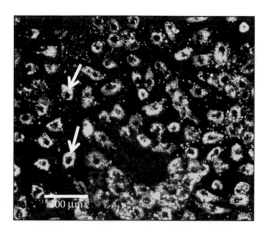

FIGURE 4.1
Isolated rat Sertoli cells *in vitro* are preloaded with FITC-labeled nanoparticles (arrows).

Arun Kumar and Don F. Cameron et al. [25] showed that Sertoli cells can be used as a vehicle for the delivery of nanoencapsulated drugs into deep lung tissue (Figure 4.1). To overcome drug-delivery limitations inhibiting the optimization of deep-lung therapy, isolated rat Sertoli cells preloaded with chitosan nanoparticles were used to obtain a high-density distribution and concentration (92%) of the nanoparticles in the lungs of mice by way of the peripheral venous vasculature rather than the more commonly used pulmonary route (Figure 4.2).

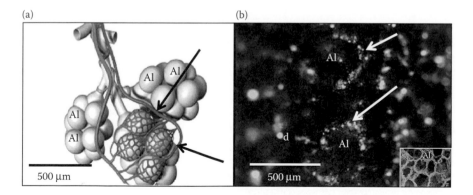

FIGURE 4.2
Pre-loaded rat Sertoli cell were injected into the peripheral venous vasculature of the mouse and, by way of the pulmonary arterial vasculature, distributed into the deep lung via the small peri-alveolar arterioles (graphically illustrated in a, arrows) where the FITC label (b, arrows) is seen in these vessels (b, arrows) and the pulmonary interstitial tissue (b). Individual alveoli (Al), which comprise an alveolar sac, are illustrated by scanning electron microscopy (b, insert) and graphically (a).

Sertoli cells were preloaded with chitosan nanoparticles coupled with the anti-inflammatory compound curcumin and then injected intravenously into control or experimental mice with deep-lung inflammation. By 24 h postinjection, most of the curcumin load (~90%) delivered in the injected Sertoli cells was present and distributed throughout the lungs, including the perialveolar sac area in the lower lungs. This was based on the high-density, positive quantification of both nanoparticles and curcumin in the lungs. There was a marked positive therapeutic effect achieved 24 h following curcumin treatment delivered by this Sertoli cell nanoparticle protocol (SNAP). Results identify a novel and efficient protocol for targeted delivery of drugs to the deep lung mediated by extratesticular Sertoli cells [25]. Utilization of SNAP cell-mediated delivery may optimize drug therapy for conditions such as ARDS, status asthmaticus, pulmonary hypertension, lung cancer, and complications following lung transplantation where the use of high concentrations of anti-inflammatory drugs is desirable, but often limited by risks of systemic drug toxicity.

Although this novel cell-mediated drug-delivery protocol to the deep lung offers the potential to treat lung pathologies far more effectively than current protocols and may constitute a significant advancement in lung therapy, drug delivery to other tissues and cells remains in its infancy.

4.4 Virus as a Carrier to Deliver Nanoparticles

Viral nanoparticles (VNPs) are emptied virus cells that can carry drugs directly to cancer cells to kill them. Scientists have engineered VNPs from plant viruses, insect viruses, and animal viruses [27]. It is recommended that to avoid using human viruses in order to minimize the chance of the virus interacting with human proteins and causing toxic side effects, infection, and immune response. Mostly, the scientists work with plant viruses, because they are easiest to produce in large quantities [28]. Plant viruses are also ideal, because they can self-assemble around a nanoparticle *in vitro* and hold approximately 10 cubic nanometers of particles [29]. Therefore, many molecules of cancer drugs can fit in plant VNPs. Many researchers have worked with the Cowpea mosaic virus (CPMV), a VNP about 30 nm in diameter created from a plant virus. The researchers from John Innes Center reported the first CPMV generated through proteolytic processing. They have used plant cells to create CPMV nanoparticles that were empty of RNA, meaning that the particles would be unable to infect organisms. They also found that by creating the virus particles in plant cells, there was no danger to the structure of the capsid. This would provide more opportunities to create mutations that allow for changes in the protein coating, which would in turn expand the possible uses of nanoparticles [30]. One of the major benefits of using VNPs in a drug-delivery system is that molecules can easily be attached to the nanoparticles' surfaces to enable the virus cells to bond only to the cancer cells, rather than the surrounding cells. VNPs based on plant viruses such as CPMV can be used for a broad range of biomedical applications because they present a robust scaffold that allows functionalization by chemical conjugation and genetic modification, thereby offering an efficient drug-delivery platform that can target specific cells and tissues. VNPs such as CPMV show natural affinity to cells; however, cellular uptake is inefficient [31]. The chemical modification of the CPMV surface with a highly reactive, specific, and UV-traceable hydrazone linker allows bioconjugation of polyarginine (R5) cell-penetrating peptides (CPPs), which can overcome these limitations [32]. Research shows that the resulting CPMV–R5 particles can be taken up by a human cervical cancer cell line (HeLa) more efficiently than native particles. The nanoparticles uptake efficiency is dependent on the density or concentration of R5 peptides on the surface of the VNP particles. The plasma membranes are taken up by VNPs into the cells via an energy-dependent mechanism whereas particles with low concentration of peptide are slowly taken up by the cells. This research has provided the groundwork for the development of efficient drug-delivery formulations based on CPMV–R5.

The researcher at The Scripps Research Institute studied the canine parvovirus and tumor specificity in VNPs. They found that the transferrin receptor on the canine parvovirus responded to transferrin released in human bodies, even though it is a canine virus [33]. In humans, transferrin is released during cell growth, so tumor cells have a lot of transferrin receptor expression. The increased expression in tumor cells attracts the canine parvovirus. If the canine parvovirus is filled with a drug to kill cancer cells, it would become a tumor-specific drug-delivery system [34]. Tumor cells express increased levels of other substances too, such as integrins. If VNPs are coated in a substance that bonds with integrins, they would be as tumor specific as the canine parvovirus [35]. Once the nanoparticles attach to the tumor cells, they can release whatever drug they contained and kill only the tumor cell. Alternatively, an imaging agent attached to or encased within the nanoparticles would allow scientists and doctors to image the tumor after the nanoparticle has attached to it [36]. Another way to draw the nanoparticles to the cancer cells is through attaching iron oxide to the viruses and using magnets to attract them to the tumors. Research has shown that it is possible to attach iron oxide nanoparticles to the CPMV and found that the groupings of iron oxide nanoparticles had large magnetic dipoles and increased magnetic field strength [37]. These characteristics would allow the CPMV to be drawn to the tumors by an external magnetic device, thus facilitating imaging and targeted drug delivery.

4.4.1 Challenges in Viral Nanoparticle-Based Drug-Delivery Systems

While VNPs are useful in their specificity, there are some problems by using them for drug delivery. As viruses are made of proteins, the human immune system will attack the VNPs, even though the viruses that scientists are experimenting with now are nonhuman viruses. Thus, the VNPs cannot have repeated use. Researchers at The Scripps Research Institute are currently looking into ways around the immune system's response by coating the VNPs in a special polymer substance to mask their protein composition [38]. Another problem, which has not been as extensively researched, is the toxicity of the VNPs once they are in the body. Most human viruses have been found to be highly toxic when used as VNPs. However, many experiments have demonstrated that the toxicity of the virus-based drug delivery in mice to be safe and nontoxic. Nonhuman viruses tend to have lower toxicity when used as nanoparticles in cancer treatment [39]. However, VNPs of either type that have iron oxide connected to them have a much higher chance of being toxic to the body. More research is needed on how to break up the nanoparticles that might be attached to a plant virus so that the particles can leave the body.

4.4.2 Future Possibilities

VNPs could revolutionize cancer treatment, acting not only as a safer, more specific form of cancer treatment, but also as a new imaging tool. The nanoparticles could create a type of drug delivery that is extremely tumor-specific with greatly reduced side effects. The VNPs would be more soluble and have higher drug efficacy than current treatments. The ease with which molecules can be attached to the VNPs and in turn fuse the nanoparticles to cancer cells is one factor that makes the nanoparticles tumor-specific. In the future, VNPs used in this form of cancer treatment could allow cancer patients to continue to lead relatively normal lives. The VNPs would take medication straight to the tumors and kill only the cancer cells, leaving the surrounding cells healthy.

4.4.3 Plant Virus for Nanoparticle Delivery

The most important property of the virus is its built-in sensor-actuator system. When the virus carrying the therapeutic agent enters a cell, it senses a change in chemical environment and automatically unloads its cargo. Therefore, the highly toxic therapeutic agent is released only in a cell, never in the blood stream as with manmade particles that depend upon capsule degradation or require an external trigger to open the particles for the release of their content. The benefit derived from this feature of the NanoVector nanoparticle is the minimization of the toxic side effects associated with free anticancer drugs in the blood stream that attack healthy cells. A second feature of the plant virus is that its automatic release of cargo is not instantaneous once the virus enters a cell [40]. This allows time for the licensed two-stage targeting in which nuclear importins attached to the nanoparticle guide it into the cell nucleus where it unloads its therapeutic agent, thereby maximizing efficacy and evading the cancer cell defenses. Delivery to the nucleus overcomes multidrug resistance that occurs with current drug therapies.

4.4.4 Oncolytic Viruses for Nanoparticle Delivery

Viruses have long been envisaged as nanoparticle vectors suitable for drug delivery, vaccines, and gene therapy, by harnessing their fusogenic cell receptor-binding properties and unsurpassed transfection efficiency [41]. A major thrust in cancer therapy involves the development of viruses for oncolytic activity. Oncolytic viruses are engineered to replicate selectively within cancer cells and induce toxic effects such as cell lysis and apoptosis, by mechanisms that exploit tumor selectivity, by use of intrinsically tumor selective viruses, gene deletion, replication-selective gene insertion, and modification of the virus coat [42]. Adenoviruses are the most commonly used virotherapeutic models, where mechanisms for initial fiber protein binding with CAR cell surface receptors have been actively investigated for tissue and organ targeting in human gene therapy [43]. For example, a phase II clinical study using DNA deleted adenovirus Onyx 015 demonstrated a selective response in most patients with p53 mutant cancers [44]. Other viruses, for example, oncolytic herpes simplex virus strain containing an inactivated insertion of ICP6 protein, responsible for viral DNA synthesis in nondividing cells, was used to selectively target rapidly dividing tumor cells with greater expression of the protein [45]. Recently researchers have [46] reported how a novel human telomerase (enzyme involved in cancer cell proliferation) reverse transcriptase (m-hTERT) promoter was engineered to enable oncolytic adenoviruses to conditionally replicate selectively in tumor cells by incorporating an adenoviral gene necessary for viral replication under the control of the m-hTERT promoter. These researches have shown that a cytopathic effect in only cancer cells, and demonstrate how the usage of telomerase-based viral strategies can achieve universal treatment of human malignancies. A variety of nanoassembled structures have been proposed by the researchers in which viruses are used for their regular geometries, with well-characterized surface properties and nanoscale dimensions for various applications.

4.4.5 Virus-Like Particles for Drug Delivery

The self-assembly of VLPs is composed of an icosahedral virus protein coat encapsulating a functionalized spherical nanoparticle core. The recent development of efficient VLPs provides an example of how biomimetic self-organization can combine the natural characteristics of virus capsids with the exquisite physical properties of nanoparticles [47]. Interactions between the artificial cargo and the protein carrier affects both the self-assembly and the stability of the resulting structure, yet very little is known about them. Progress toward the basic development and the practical use of

VLPs requires an understanding of how relevant parameters contribute to complex formation. Symmetric VLPs may provide a technology for therapeutic or diagnostic agent delivery that is improved over amorphous shell nanoparticles that are already known to be efficient in similar applications [34,35]. The advantage of a regular surface protein structure provides the binding domains for multifunctional nanoparticles. It has been shown in several situations that receptor-mediated targeting can be achieved even when using amorphous coatings [48].

The principle challenges for nanoparticle delivery currently include: effective nanoparticle carrier systems, limited life time in body fluids, nanoparticle transduction across the cellular membrane, avoidance of the exocytotic pathways, and target specificity. These new approaches of drug delivery will open the way to treat the diseases which are hard to treat by the current approach.

References

1. Sperling, R. A., Gil, P. R., Zhang, F., Zanella, M., and Parak, W. J. 2008. Biological applications of gold nanoparticles. *Chem. Soc. Rev.*, 37, 1896.
2. Rakesh, K. 1987. Transport of molecules in the tumor interstitium: A review. *Jain Cancer Res*, 47, 3039–3051.
3. Nishihira, J. 2012. Molecular function of macrophage migration inhibitory factor and a novel therapy for inflammatory bowel disease. *Ann New York Acad Sci*, 1271, 53–57.
4. Akin, D., Sturgis, J., Ragheb, K., Sherman, D., Burkholder, K., Paul, J., Arun, R., Bhunia, K. Mohammed, S., and Bashir, R. 2007. Bacteria-mediated delivery of nanoparticles and cargo into cells. *Nat Nanotechnol*, 2, 441–449.
5. Cadena, D. L. and Gill, G. N. 1992. Receptor tyrosine kinases. *FASEB J*, 6, 2332–2337.
6. Gestwicki, J. E., Cairo, C. W., Strong, L. E., Oetjen, K. A., and Kiessling, L. L. 2002. Influencing receptor–ligand binding mechanisms with multivalent ligand architecture. *J Am Chem Soc.* 18, 124(50), 14922–14933.
7. Sen, K. D., Desai, D., Senthilkumar, R., Johansson, E. M, Råtts, N., Odén, M., Eriksson, J. E, Sahlgren, C., Toivola, D. M., and Rosenholm, J. M. Shape engineering vs organic modification of inorganic nanoparticles as a tool for enhancing cellular internalization. *Nanoscale Res Lett.* 7(1), 358.
8. Larsen, M. D., Griesenbach, U., Goussard, S., Gruenert, D. C., Geddes, D. M., Scheule, R. K, Cheng, S. H., Courvalin, P., Grillot-Courvalin, C., and Alton, E. W. 2008. Bactofection of lung epithelial cells *in vitro* and *in vivo* using a genetically modified *Escherichia coli*. *Gene Ther.* 15(6), 434–442.
9. Tangney, M. and Gahan, C. G. 2010. Listeria monocytogenes as a vector for anticancer therapies. *Curr Gene Ther.* 10(1), 46–55.
10. Ogawa, M. and Sasakawa, C. 2006. Shigella and autophagy. *Autophagy*, 2(3), 171–174.

11. Mohler, V. L., Heithoff, D. M, Mahan, M. J., Hornitzky, M. A., Thomson, P. C., and House, J. K. 2012. Development of a novel in-water vaccination protocol for DNA adenine methylase deficient *Salmonella enterica* serovar *Typhimurium* vaccine in adult sheep. *Vaccine*. 30(8), 1481–1491.

12. Hara, N., Alkanani, A. K., Ir, D., Robertson, C. E., Wagner, B. D., Frank, D. N., and Zipris, D. 2012. Prevention of virus-induced type 1 diabetes with antibiotic therapy. *J Immunol* 189(8), 3805–3814.

13. Bolhassani, A. and Zahedifard, F. 2012. Therapeutic live vaccines as a potential anticancer strategy. *Int J Cancer* 131(8), 1733–1743.

14. Ruder, W. C., Hsu, C.P., Edelman, B. D Jr, Schwartz, R., and Leduc, P. R. 2012. Biological colloid engineering: Self-assembly of dipolar ferromagnetic chains in a functionalized biogenic ferrofluid. *Appl Phys Lett* 101(6), 63701.

15. Sonkaria, S., Fuentes, G., Verma, C., Narang, R., Khare, V., Fischer, A., and Faivre, D. 2012. Insight into the assembly properties and functional organisation of the magnetotactic bacterial actin-like homolog, MamK. *PLoS One* 7(5), e34189.

16. Rong, C., Zhang, C., Zhang, Y., Qi, L., Yang, J., Guan, G., Li, Y., and Li, J. 2012. FeoB2 Functions in magnetosome formation and oxidative stress protection in *Magnetospirillum gryphiswaldense* strain MSR-1. *J Bacteriol* 194(15), 3972–3976.

17. Bo, T., Wang, K., Ge, X., Chen, G., and Liu, W. 2012. Compromised DNA damage repair promotes genetic instability of the genomic magnetosome island in *Magnetospirillum magneticum* AMB-1. *Curr Microbiol* 65(1), 98–107.

18. Shin, J., Yoo, C. H., Lee, J., and Cha, M. 2012. Cell response induced by internalized bacterial magnetic nanoparticles under an external static magnetic field. *Biomaterials* 33(22), 5650–5657.

19. Alphandéry, E., Guyot, F., and Chebbi, I. 2012. Preparation of chains of magnetosomes, isolated from *Magnetospirillum magneticum* strain AMB-1 magnetotactic bacteria, yielding efficient treatment of tumors using magnetic hyperthermia. *Int J Pharm* 434(1–2), 444–452.

20. Kang, H. J., Kim, J. Y., Lee, H. J., Kim, K. H., Kim, T. Y., Lee, C. S., Lee, H. C., Park, T. H., Kim, H. S., and Park, Y. B. 2012. Magnetic bionanoparticle enhances homing of endothelial progenitor cells in mouse hindlimb ischemia. *Korean Circ J* 42(6), 390–396.

21. Guo, L., Huang, J., and Zheng, L. M. 2011. Control generating of bacterial magnetic nanoparticle – doxorubicin conjugates by poly-L-glutamic acid surface modification. *Nanotechnology* 22(17), 175102.

22. Zhao, X., Yu, Z., Dai, W., Yao, Z., Zhou, W., Zhou, J., Yang, Y. et al. 2011. Construction and characterization of an anti-asialoglycoprotein receptor single-chain variable-fragment-targeted melittin. *Biotechnol Appl Biochem* 58(6), 405–411.

23. Sun, J. B., Duan, J. H., Dai, S. L., Ren, J., Guo, L., Jiang, W., and Li, Y. 2008. Preparation and anti-tumor efficiency evaluation of doxorubicin-loaded bacterial magnetosomes: Magnetic nanoparticles as drug carriers isolated from *Magnetospirillum gryphiswaldense*. *Biotechnol Bioeng* 101(6), 1313–1320.

24. Tibbe, A. G., de Grooth, B. G., Greve, J., Rao, C., Dolan, G. J., and Terstappen, L. W. 2002. Cell analysis system based on compact disk technology. *Cytometry* 47(3), 173–182.

25. Kumar, A., Glaum, M., El-Badri, N., Mohapatra, S., Haller, E., Park, S., Patrick, L., Nattkemper, L., Vo, D., and Cameron, D. F. 2011. Initial observations of cell-mediated drug delivery to the deep lung. *Cell Transplant* 20(5), 609–618.

26. Shur, J., Lee, S., Adams, W., Lionberger, R., Tibbatts, J., and Price, R. 2012. Effect of device design on the *in vitro* performance and comparability for capsule-based dry powder inhalers. *AAPS J* 14(4), 667–676.

27. Shukla, S., Ablack, A. L., Wen, A. M., Lee, K. L., Lewis, J. D., and Steinmetz, N. F. 2013. Increased tumor homing and tissue penetration of the filamentous plant viral nanoparticle potato virus X. *Mol Pharm* 10(1), 33–42.

28. Wu, Z., Chen, K., Yildiz, I., Dirksen, A., Fischer, R., Dawson, P. E., and Steinmetz, N. F. Development of viral nanoparticles for efficient intracellular delivery. *Nanoscale* 4(11), 3567–3576.

29. Ahmed, M. and Narain, R. 2012. The effect of molecular weight, compositions and lectin type on the properties of hyperbranched glycopolymers as non-viral gene delivery systems. *Biomaterials* 33(15), 3990–4001.

30. Agrawal, A. and Manchester, M. 2012. Differential uptake of chemically modified cowpea mosaic virus nanoparticles in macrophage subpopulations present in inflammatory and tumor microenvironments. *Biomacromolecules* 13(10), 3320–336.

31. Lewis, J. D., Destito, G., Zijlstra, A., Gonzalez, M. J., Quigley, J. P., Manchester, M., and Stuhlmann, H. 2006. Viral nanoparticles as tools for intravital vascular imaging. *Nat Med* 12(3), 354–360.

32. Muldoon, L. L., Nilaver, G., Kroll, R. A., Pagel, M. A., Breakefield, X. O., Chiocca, E. A., Davidson, B. L., Weissleder, R., and Neuwelt, E. A. 1995. Comparison of intracerebral inoculation and osmotic blood–brain barrier disruption for delivery of adenovirus, herpesvirus, and iron oxide particles to normal rat brain. *Am J Pathol* 147(6), 1840–1851.

33. Raty, J. K., Liimatainen, T., Wirth, T., Airenne, K. J., Ihalainen, T. O., Huhtala, T., Hamerlynck, E. et al. 2006. Magnetic resonance imaging of viral particle biodistribution in vivo. *Gene Ther* 13(20), 1440–1446.

34. Niikura, K., Sugimura, N., Musashi, Y., Mikuni, S., Matsuo, Y., Kobayashi, S., Nagakawa, K. et al. 2013. Virus-like particles with removable cyclodextrins enable glutathione-triggered drug release in cells. *Mol Biosyst* 9(3), 501–507.

35. Schneemann, A., Speir, J. A., Tan, G. S., Khayat, R., Ekiert, D. C., Matsuoka, Y., and Wilson, I. A. 2012. A virus-like particle that elicits cross-reactive antibodies to the conserved stem of influenza virus hemagglutinin. *J Virol* 86(21), 11686–11697.

36. Singh, P., Prasuhn, D., Yeh, R. M., Destito, G., Rae, C. S., Osborn, K., Finn, M. G., and Manchester, M. 2007. Bio-distribution, toxicity and pathology of cowpea mosaic virus nanoparticles in vivo. *J Controlled Release* 120(1–2), 41–50.

37. Koudelka, K. J., Destito, G., Plummer, E. M., Trauger, S. A., Siuzdak, G., and Manchester, M. 2009. Endothelial targeting of cowpea mosaic virus (CPMV) via surface vimentin. *PLoS Pathog* 5(5), 38.

38. Nycholat, C. M., Rademacher, C., Kawasaki, N., and Paulson, J. C. 2012. In silico-aided design of a glycan ligand of sialoadhesin for in vivo targeting of macrophages. *J Am Chem Soc* 134(38), 15696–15699.

39. Zahid, M. and Robbins, P. D. 2012. Protein transduction domains: Applications for molecular medicine. *Curr Gene Ther* 12(5), 374–380.

40. Sharma, P., Chawla, A., Arora, S., and Pawar, P. 2012. Novel drug delivery approaches on antiviral and antiretroviral agents. *J Adv Pharm Technol Res* 3(3), 147–59.

41. Thorne, S. H. 2007. Strategies to achieve systemic delivery of therapeutic cells and microbes to tumors. *Expert Opin Biol Ther* 7(1), 41–51.

42. Miranda, E., Maya, P. H., Oberg, D., Cherubini, G., Garate, Z., Lemoine, N. R., and Halldén, G. 2012. Adenovirus-mediated sensitization to the cytotoxic drugs docetaxel and mitoxantrone is dependent on regulatory domains in the E1ACR1 gene-region. *PLoS One* 7(10), e46617.
43. Zhang, H., Wang, H., Zhang, J., Qian, G., Niu, B., Fan, X., Lu, J., Hoffman, A. R., Hu, J. F., and Ge, S. 2009. Enhanced therapeutic efficacy by simultaneously targeting two genetic defects in tumors. *Mol Ther* 17(1), 57–64.
44. Fields, R. J., Cheng, C. J, Quijano, E., Weller, C., Kristofik, N., Duong, N., Hoimes, C., Egan, M. E., and Saltzman, W. M. 2012. Surface modified poly(β amino ester)-containing nanoparticles for plasmid DNA delivery. *J Control Release* 164(1):41–48.
45. Alemany, R. 2012. Design of improved oncolytic adenoviruses. *Adv Cancer Res* 115, 93–114.
46. Oh, W., Ghim, J., Lee, E. W., Yang, M. R., Kim, E. T., Ahn, J. H., and Song, J. 2009. PML-IV functions as a negative regulator of telomerase by interacting with TERT. *J Cell Sci* 122(Pt 15), 2613–2622.
47. Blokhina, E. A., Kuprianov, V. V., Stepanova, L. A., Tsybalova, L. M., Kiselev, O. I., Ravin, N. V., and Skryabin, K. G. 2012. A molecular assembly system for presentation of antigens on the surface of HBc virus-like particles. *Virology* pii: S0042–6822(12)00455–2.
48. Hadiji-Abbes, N., Martin, M., Benzina, W., Karray-Hakim, H., Gergely, C., Gargouri, A., and Mokdad-Gargouri, R. 2012. Extraction and purification of hepatitis B virus-like M particles from a recombinant *Saccharomyces cerevisiae* strain using alumina powder. *J Virol Methods* pii: S0166–0934(12)00353–9.

5

Nanodermatology: The Giant Role of Nanotechnology in Diagnosis and Treatment of Skin Disease

Adam Friedman

CONTENTS

5.1 Introduction 90
5.2 Structure and Function of the Skin 90
5.3 Topical Drug Delivery 92
5.4 Challenges in Topical Drug Delivery 94
5.5 Nanotechnology for the Diagnosis and Treatment of Skin Disease 95
    5.5.1 Acne Vulgaris 96
    5.5.2 Atopic Dermatitis 98
    5.5.3 Skin Cancer 101
    5.5.4 Dermatophytosis 103
        5.5.4.1 Nano-Silver 104
        5.5.4.2 Chitosan 104
        5.5.4.3 Titanium Dioxide 105
        5.5.4.4 Soybean Oil-Derived Nanoemulsions 105
        5.5.4.5 Antifungal Encapsulated Nanomaterials 106
    5.5.5 Psoriasis 106
        5.5.5.1 Diagnosis 107
        5.5.5.2 Treatment 108
5.6 Nanotechnology and Cosmeceuticals 109
    5.6.1 Introduction 109
    5.6.2 Nanocosmetics 109
    5.6.3 Nanoemollients 111
    5.6.4 Nanocleansers 111
    5.6.5 Nanosunscreens 112
5.7 Conclusions 113
References 113

5.1 Introduction

Cutaneous drug delivery offers many advantages over alternative routes of administration with regard to target-specific impact, decreased systemic toxicity, avoidance of first-pass metabolism, variable dosing schedules, and broadened utility to diverse patient populations. A complicating factor is that the skin has evolved mechanisms to impede exogenous molecules, especially hydrophilic ones, from safe passage. The horny layer of the stratum corneum (the topmost layer of the skin) is tightly bonded to an intercellular lipid matrix, making the passage of therapeutics a serious challenge.[1] This strong barrier to molecular activity is quite effective at blocking large molecules, which of course make up the majority of active therapeutics.[2] Many substances that could, in theory, be used as topical therapeutics have several disadvantages in that they are (i) weakly or not soluble in water; (ii) degraded or inactivated prior to reaching the appropriate target; and (iii) nonspecifically distributed to tissues and organs, resulting in undue adverse side effects and limited efficacy at the target site.

There is currently a great need for new topical therapies that both improve upon the limitations of currently available medications such as irritation and repeated application as well as offer enhanced efficacy. In addition to generating entirely new compounds, reformulation of well-established, FDA-approved products in superior vehicles is also a useful and cost-effective approach. Novel delivery vehicles generated through nanotechnology are raising the exciting prospect for controlled and sustained drug delivery across the impenetrable skin barrier. Particles of 500 nm and smaller exhibit a host of unique properties that are superior to their bulk material counterparts.[3–5] Small size is a necessary feature but other properties are needed for nanomaterials to achieve efficacy as a topical delivery vehicle. Optimally, these nanoparticles should (i) carry drugs through the primary skin barrier; (ii) release the transported drug spontaneously once penetration is achieved; and (iii) exhibit low rates of cutaneous drug clearance allowing for deep/targeted deposition and prolonged action of the transported drugs. Additionally, these products should be able to adjust to relevant physiologic variations as part of their design and targeting.

In this chapter, cutaneous physiology and pharmacology will be reviewed as a means to highlight the utility and potential of nanotechnology as a versatile approach to both the diagnosis and treatment of skin disease.

5.2 Structure and Function of the Skin

The skin is a complex multilayered organ consisting of three major components, including the epidermis, dermis, and underlying subcutaneous tissue,

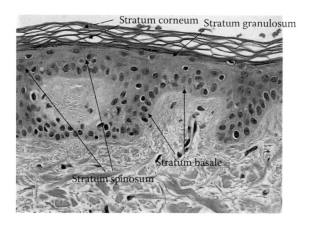

FIGURE 5.1
(See color insert.) Histology of human skin.

with the barrier functions largely owing to the upper layers of the epidermis. Keratinocytes, the key cell type of the epidermis, are arranged in several strata and both their shape and function are associated with this placement. The following order of levels or strata follows from deepest to most super-ficial: stratum basale (basal cell layer), stratum spinosum, stratum granulo-sum, and stratum corneum (Figure 5.1).

Keratinocytes are protein-rich cells composed mostly of keratin and kera-tohyalin. Keratin provides structure and tensile strength by forming bun-dles that stretch across the cell. In the stratum basale, keratin filaments are arranged perpendicularly, attaching the basal keratinocyte, specifically the hemidesmosomal plaque, within the basal cells, to the overlying epidermis as a means of providing adhesion to the basement membrane. In the stratum spinosum, keratin filaments are displayed in a concentric pattern around the nucleus and inserting into peripheral keratinocytes via desmosomal proteins, forming "spines" histologically (especially apparent in the setting of spongiosis or epidermal edema, a hallmark of eczematous processes). Keratohyalin granules, which become more apparent in the "granular" layer or stratum granulosum, are composed of several proteins such as profilag-grin, which is eventually cleaved into filaggrin peptides, and loricrin, both of which are important components of the cornified envelope. This envelope is the major structure providing protection to the epidermis and to which both intracellular keratins and extracellular lipids attach. The lipid "cement" comes from lamellar granules, which first appear in the spinous layer, but serve a very important role higher up in the epidermis. These lysosomal structures contain lipid precursors such as glycoproteins, phospholipids, and free sterols, which are discharged into the extracellular space at the junc-tion of the granular and horny layers to solidify the barrier and mediate stra-tum corneum adhesion with fillagrin. The stratum corneum is in essence the impeding brick wall preventing safe passage of topical therapies. Looking a bit closer, corneocytes (i.e., differentiated keratinocytes) are interconnected via corneodesmosomes, specialized adhesion molecules, which provide the stratum corneum the ability to resist shearing forces. Corneodesmosomes have been likened to "iron rods" that extend through this "brick wall," further supporting its tensile strength. The stratum corneum therefore provides physical and mechanical protection, barrier to water loss, and importantly barrier to preventing permeation of exogenous substances.[6–9]

At the intersection of the epidermis and dermis exists the basement membrane zone, which is composed of transmembrane proteins spanning between the epidermis and dermis allowing for proper adhesion and communication.[10] The dermis is a 1–2-mm-thick layer, composed of collagen (contributing at least 70% of the dry weight of the skin) and elastic fibers in a jelly-like material composed of highly hydrophilic glycosaminoglycans.[11,12] In addition to containing capillary and lymphatic vessels, important targets in drug delivery, the dermis contains appendageal structures that include apocrine, eccrine, and sebaceous glands, nerve endings, and hair follicles. Below the dermis is the subcutaneous layer composed of adipocytes, which provide insulation, protective padding, and energy storage.

5.3 Topical Drug Delivery

When considering topical drug delivery, certain concepts must be delineated and defined. Penetration of a topical drug refers to the entrance of the drug into a particular skin layer, whereas permeation is the passage of the drug from one skin layer to a structurally different layer. Furthermore, absorption of topical agents indicates that it is taken up by the vasculature within the skin for systemic distribution.[13–15]

The topical application of drugs for the purpose of treating skin disease has many advantages, particularly the ability to target the disease site without significant risk of systemic absorption and importantly side effects. Transdermal drug delivery has several key advantages, including access to the circulation without undergoing significant first-pass metabolism, since the skin has a relatively low capacity to enzymatically alter drugs as compared with the gastrointestinal tract. There is also significant ease of administration due to its noninvasive, painless, and readily accessible nature (particularly compared to the oral route, which can often be compromised due to access or nausea).[8,13,16,17]

With respect to penetration, the transport of topically applied materials occurring across the stratum corneum is largely passive diffusion and is reliant on the physiochemical properties of the permeating agent. There are two major routes through which this diffusion across the skin can occur. The first is transappendageal, relying on the natural imperfections in skin integrity

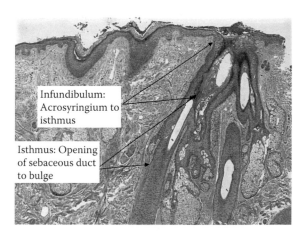

Infundibulum:
Acrosyringium to
isthmus

Isthmus: Opening
of sebaceous duct
to bulge

FIGURE 5.2
(**See color insert.**) Histology of the pilosebaceous unit.

associated with hair follicles (Figure 5.2) and sweat glands. These openings can potentially allow the topical drug to bypass the low diffusivity of the stratum corneum.[6] Furthermore, this route may aid in the delivery of charged ions, and large polar molecules, which are generally slow, permeate through the stratum corneum. Ultimately, the choice of the vehicle will affect its ability to utilize transfollicular penetration. The second pathway is through the epidermis itself, and is subdivided into two potential avenues, transcellular and intercellular. Hydrophilic compounds are likely to flow through the transcellular route, while lipophilic materials are preferential for the more roundabout intercellular route. It is believed that the latter pathway is the predominant route of entry for most topical therapies. Unfortunately, this pathway also serves as an impressive impediment for therapeutic intended for topical delivery.[18]

Transappendageal penetration of drugs occurs through natural imperfections in the skin due to the presence of sweat glands, sebaceous glands, and hair follicles. These pathways are unlikely to play a significant role in drug diffusion as they only make up a small percentage of the cutaneous surface area. Of the possible appendageal routes, passage through hair follicles is likely to play the greatest role, as the opening of the hair follicle is relatively large, and the presence of sebum in the duct of the pilosebaceous gland may allow for an easy route for lipophilic drugs to diffuse.[19,20]

Upon overcoming and passing through the stratum corneum, drug molecules reach the moist, live component of the epidermis, which, unlike the stratum corneum, provide little resistance to diffusing compounds. Owing to the tight adhesion between cells resulting from the desmosomal connections, agents must diffuse directly through the cell membranes and cytosol, and therefore, agents that are extremely hydrophilic or lipophilic may have difficulty passing through the remainder of the epidermis.

To reach the systemic circulation, drugs must continue through the epidermis and into the upper or papillary dermis, where small capillaries reside.

Importantly, the release of drug from its delivery vehicle, beyond the skin barrier, and into the underlying skin layers, is characterized by its pharmacokinetics. A topical delivery system/vehicle is a substance that carries a drug with and through the skin. The vehicle itself can have therapeutic properties, even serving as an effective emollient, often evidenced by the substantial vehicle responses when being used as the control arm in clinical investigations. The make-up and components of a vehicle must often meet certain standards to be considered cosmetically acceptable by users, such as being nonallergenic, nonirritating, and invisible. Equally important, a vehicle should appropriately release the payload, ensuring that the amount of active drug formulated into the delivery system is facilitated through the stratum corneum and not retained within the vehicle itself. The kinetics and degree of percutaneous absorption are determined by the formulation. The physiochemical properties of the formulation influence the properties of the release and absorption of the drug.

5.4 Challenges in Topical Drug Delivery

There are various factors that contribute to the difficulty of percutaneous penetration of drugs. Most important is the stratum corneum, whose interwoven kevlar keratin-rich corneocytes amidst a sea of thick lipid provides an almost impenetrable fortress through which drug molecules must travel. Since the movement of drugs through the skin occurs by diffusion, molecular size is an important limiting factor. For drugs to passively traverse the stratum corneum efficiently, a molecular mass of 500 Da generally appears to be the upper limit.[2] Once drug molecules are able to pass through the stratum corneum, the rest of the epidermis provides little resistance. Chemical and physical factors of drugs that favor passive percutaneous drug absorption include low melting point and solubility in oil and water.[14]

To overcome size limitations, various mechanisms that disrupt the barrier have been employed. Mechanical abraders and microneedles can open a limited number of relatively wide ($\geq 10^3$ nm) pores in the skin barrier that can allow for transient passage of small and even large molecules (or even bacteria).[21] Disruption with either ultrasound (phonopheresis) or high-voltage electrical pulsing (electroporation) has been used to force larger materials through this complex barrier. Chemical penetration enhancers are also utilized to perturb the epidermal barrier, although safety concerns have limited their efficacy[22-24]—there is potential for these drugs and/or delivery vehicles to cause irritant and allergic reactions.

An important point to note is that effective topical drug therapy is not only dependent on the agent itself but also on the vehicle in which this material is delivered. Poor drug–vehicle interaction could potentially lead to inactivation of the drug due to, for example, instability in the formulation. Binding of the drug to vehicle ingredients may also inhibit adequate delivery to the affected layer of the skin. A formulation needs to be carefully constructed to account for specific drug and biological parameters to prevent delivery and therefore treatment failure.

5.5 Nanotechnology for the Diagnosis and Treatment of Skin Disease

The development of nanoparticulate carriers for drugs is a novel area in science that provides the technology to work at the molecular level, leading to devices or delivery systems with unique properties and functions. These carriers offer numerous advantages such as overcoming a healthy intact skin barrier to allow either intradermal or transdermal drug delivery to relatively impermeable sites of the target tissue, accumulation in action sites, and reduction of side effects.[3,25–27] One approach to reduce these side effecta is to use conventional formulations containing lower concentrations of active ingredients, which often fall short and result in poor clinical outcomes. Novel delivery systems, on the other hand, present the potential to reduce the side effects without compromising efficacy. Vesicular and particulate drug delivery systems such as liposomes, niosomes, micro/nanospheres or sponges, solid lipid nanoparticles (SLNs), and nanoemulsions all have the potential for improved penetration and controlled release of active substances.[14,28–34] The application of these systems to the skin distributes the topical agents gradually and, in some cases, has demonstrated the ability to reduce the irritancy of some drugs while maintaining a similar efficacy when compared with conventional formulations.

In addition to the controlled release of the drug into the epidermis, these systems can also promote follicular targeting, creating high local concentrations of the active compounds in the pilosebaceous unit.[35–38] As discussed earlier, a topically applied material has basically three possibilities to penetrate into the skin: transcellular, intercellular, and follicular. The hair follicle is a skin appendage with a complex structure containing many cell types that produce highly specialized proteins. The hair follicle is in a continuous cycle of growth: anagen is the hair growth phase, catagen the involution phase, and telogen is the resting phase. When considering targeted therapy, the hair follicle represents a great site for skin treatment, owing to its deep extension into the dermis and thus provides much deeper penetration and absorption of compounds beneath the skin than seen with the transdermal route (Figure 5.2). In the case of skin diseases and of cosmetic products, delivery to sweat glands or to the pilosebaceous unit is essential for the effectiveness of certain drugs, specifically in acne vulgaris. Increased accumulation in the pilosebaceous unit could result in improved outcomes related to topical therapy. The vesicular and particulate drug delivery systems have the advantage of penetrating more efficiently into the hair follicles than do nonparticulate systems, such as conventional formulations, so long as the size is selected in an appropriate manner.[37] This provides a high local concentration over a prolonged period of time allowing for increased efficacy.

To fully capture the potential of nanotechnology in dermatology, examples of currently utilized and investigated nanomaterials will be reviewed pertaining to several common dermatologic diseases.

5.5.1 Acne Vulgaris

Acne vulgaris is one of the most common dermatologic diseases. It affects between 40 and 50 million people each year (Figure 5.3).[39] Acne is most often an isolated problem; however, it may also be associated with underlying disease or exogenous influences such as polycystic ovarian syndrome, hyperandrogenism, hypercortisolism, precocious puberty, and corticosteroid therapy.[39]

Topical therapies for acne vulgaris, including benzoyl peroxide (BP), salicylic acid, topical antibiotics such as clindamycin, and retinoids all suffer from various related side effects, including irritation, erythema, xerosis, peeling and scaling, bacterial resistance, and resulting dyschromia from the associated irritation in patients of darker skin types. These adverse events often serve as major limiting factors influencing patient compliance and ultimately impacting efficacy.[40–44] The pursuit to improve the efficacy and safety profiles of our armament of acne therapeutics through nanoencapsulation has been rigorous and will be briefly reviewed.

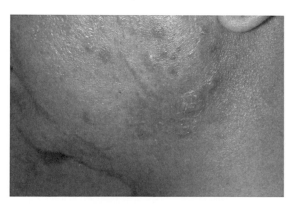

FIGURE 5.3
(See color insert.) Nodulocystic acne vulgaris.

BP has both a mild keratolytic and potent bactericidal effect to which *Propionibacterium acnes* has yet to demonstrate resistance.[45] Although an effective acne therapy, skin irritation is an expected adverse event, and is unfortunately appreciated at efficacious doses. Encapsulation in liposomes is one approach being used to improve the efficacy by reducing the side effects associated with topical application and ultimately improving patient compliance. In one small ($n = 30$) clinical trial, liposomal BP gels significantly improved therapeutic responses (about twofold) at all evaluation time points as compared with those of the commercially available BP gel.[46] Furthermore, liposomal BP gels demonstrated significantly less irritation in the first 2 weeks of treatment, with no reports of "burning" as per subjects. Conversely, the BP gel-treated group showed increased irritation through the eighth week of treatment. Stability evaluation of the BP liposomes demonstrated a good stability profile (almost 100% of drug retained, 90 days) at refrigeration temperature (2–8°C) compared with room temperature (25°C) and body temperature (37°C).

Several extensive investigations on cutaneous irritation, percutaneous absorption *in vitro* and *in vivo*, and the efficacy of the encapsulated BP in microspheres have been pursued.[35,47–50] In one study, cumulative irritancy of BP microspheres versus BP lotion was evaluated over 21 days in rabbits and humans.[50] The lotion containing free BP at 2.5% and 5% produced significantly greater irritation than that observed in entrapped BP.

Antibiotics have been utilized in the management of inflammatory acne vulgaris for decades,[43,51,52] with clindamycin being one of the most commonly used options. In previous studies, lipid compositions have been evaluated in an attempt to improve the effectiveness of clindamycin-encapsulated liposomes in acne treatment.[53–55]

In one study, treatment of acne patients with liposomal clindamycin resulted in better efficacy than nonliposomal lotion forms.[55] Application of a conventional lotion solution, a nonliposomal emulsion lotion, and a liposomal emulsion lotion resulted in decreases of 42.9%, 48.3%, and 62.8%, respectively, in the total number of lesions after a 4-week treatment.

Salicylic acid, a keratolytic agent with both comedolytic and antimicrobial activity, is available over the counter as well as is incorporated into peeling agents. It has been efficiently used in the treatment of acne as well as cosmetic repair of postinflammatory pigment alteration and pitted scars.[40,42,43] The majority of work to date on salicylic acid liposomes has been primarily preclinical.[56,57] In one investigation, when compared with free salicylic acid dispersion, salicylic liposomes not only prolonged the release of salicylic acid across the porcine skin but also enhanced its retention in the skin by a factor of 10.[56] Furthermore, the stability of the liposomal preparation was demonstrated after 12 weeks of storage at refrigeration temperature (4–5°C).

Retinoids regulate several critical physiological and pathological processes. These biological response modifiers exert their pleiotropic effects through the interaction with nuclear receptors.[28,58] In acne treatment, topical retinoids are very important because they reverse the abnormal desquamation by affecting follicular epithelial turnover and maturation of cells. In addition, some topical retinoids have an effect on inflammation by modulating the immune response, inflammatory mediators, and migration of inflammatory cells.[59] Tretinoin or all-*trans* retinoic acid, is a polymechanistic, effective drug that is frequently used in the topical treatment of mild-to-moderate acne. Retinoic acid both enables comedolysis and normalizes the maturation of the follicular epithelium so as to cease comedone formation, as well as has been shown to have anti-inflammatory and possibly even antimicrobial activity.[28] Unfortunately, topical application of retinoic acid and its derivatives generally results in local irritation, mild-to-severe erythema, dryness, peeling, and scaling.[28,58]

With respect to preclinical animal studies, there have been a number of investigations suggesting increased skin penetration, yet decreased percutaneous absorption of retinoic acid encapsulated in liposomes.[31,60–66] Even more importantly, the SLN have been used to enhance the photostability of retinoic acid in comparison to methanolic retinoic acid solution when both formulations were exposed to 180 min of natural sunlight.[67] Attempts to increase the efficacy and tolerability of retinoic acid have also been pursued using microspheres and microsponges.[68–77] In fact, there are currently commercially available formulation of Retin-A-loaded microspheres (Retin-A, Micro™, Ortho Dermatological). *Ex vivo* mouse skin cutaneous permeation studies demonstrated that the retinoic acid permeation from this microsponge technology was significantly less than that observed with the gel form of the native drug. A multicenter, double-blind, placebo-controlled, 12-week study was undertaken, revealing a statistically significant reduction in inflammatory and noninflammatory acne lesions treated using retinoic acid-loaded microsponges as compared to control.

In addition to the encapsulation of known drugs into nanodelivery vehicles, nanomaterials with inherent therapeutic properties have been used to combat acne. Nanoemulsions are currently being used to target the pilosebaceous unit for the treatment of acne. NB-003 is an antimicrobial oil-in-water emulsion in development for the topical treatment of acne. NB-003 has been shown to concentrate in the pilosebaceous unit and has potent *in vitro* bactericidal activity against multidrug-resistant clinical isolates of *P. acnes*.[78] NB-003 was evaluated in a pig skin model designed to mimic clinical studies that measures the reduction of *P. acnes* in human volunteers. It was found that NB-003 was more effective at reducing surface *P. acnes* on pig skin than commercial products containing BP.

5.5.2 Atopic Dermatitis

Atopic dermatitis (AD) is predominantly first seen in children,[79] with a prevalence of 6.8–17.2% of school-aged children being affected in the United States (Figure 5.4).[80] Only asthma and allergic rhinitis, components of the atopic spectrum, are seen in 30% and 35% of patients with AD, respectively.[81]

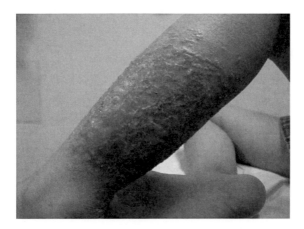

FIGURE 5.4
(**See color insert.**) Atopic dermatitis.

Childhood AD is financially and emotionally taxing on families.[82] Scratching and rubbing are common in both children and adults, which can disturb sleep and represents a significant cause of distress.[83]

Noninvasive or minimally invasive methods for the diagnosis of AD can offer significant advantages over predecessors.[84–86] Proteomic profiling is one method of assessing AD. In a pilot study of a small subset of patients with AD, the utility of proteomics was demonstrated.[87] Patients with a history of AD and eczema herpeticum and *Staphylococcus aureus* colonization were tape stripped on lesional and nonlesional skin. Proteins related to the skin barrier were assessed by mass spectrometry. Skin barrier proteins, including filaggrin-2, corneodesmosin, desmoglein-1, desmocollin-1, and transglutaminase-3, and proteins comprising natural moisturizing factor, such as arginase-1, caspase-14, and gamma-glutamyl cyclotransferase, were diminished in lesional skin when compared to nonlesional skin in patients with a history of AD and no history of eczema herpeticum. Epidermal fatty acid binding protein was expressed in higher levels in patients colonized with methicillin-resistant *S. aureus*. This study demonstrated that proteomic profiling might noninvasively give clues about the pathogenesis of AD. It may also be useful in personalized medicine, helping identify patients at risk for serious cutaneous bacterial and viral superinfections.

Therapy for AD can include topical therapies (baths, wraps, corticosteroids, immunomodulators, antihistamines, emollients, counter-irritants, barrier preparations); systemic therapies (antihistamines, anxiolytics, and immunosuppressive agents); phototherapy, and inpatient therapy.[88,89] Traditional therapies may lack specificity, may be inconvenient, and may be associated with systemic toxicity.

Tacrolimus, an immunomodulator originally used in the prevention of organ transplant rejection, has been formulated topically in a lipid nanoparticle.[90,91] The nanoparticulate form is more soluble than the unencapsulated counterpart. It has better delivery and retention kinetics in the epidermis. These characteristics predict greater efficacy, a longer duration of activity and reduced systemic release and toxicity.

AD is generally not associated with a higher incidence of allergic contact dermatitis, including nickel dermatitis. However, the most common cause of contact dermatitis is nickel, and nickel contact allergy can exacerbate AD. Nickel can be found on jewelry, and everyday items such as cabinet handles, cell phones, and coins. Nickel must penetrate the epidermis to induce contact allergy. Topical agents to reduce the penetration of nickel into skin have benefited from nanoformulation.[92,93] Calcium nanoparticles capture nickel ions by cation exchange, and cause nickel to remain on the skin surface. *In vitro*, and *in vivo*, this capture and ease of washing away nickel was demonstrated with nanoparticles of 500 nm and smaller containing calcium carbonate or calcium phosphate. About 90% fewer nanoparticles by mass are needed to match the efficacy of ethylene diamine tetra acetic acid.

One of the hallmarks of eczema is inflammation. Reactive oxygen species are generated during inflammation, and fullerenes have been shown to quench reactive oxygen species.[94–99] In an *in vivo* model of inflammation induced by phorbo 12-myristate 13-acetate, fullerene nanoparticles reduced inflammation and edema. Toxicity concerns regarding fullerenes and fullerols are being revised.

Clobetasol propionate is a potent topical corticosteroid used for the management of AD. A SLN containing clobetasol propionate has been developed and characterized.[100] Optimized nanoparticles have an average size of 177 nm and entrap 92% of the drug. The nanoparticulate form of clobetasol had a higher uptake in the epidermis and enhanced retention in the skin compared to unencapsulated clobetasol. In a double-blind pilot study of 16 patients with chronic eczema, both forms of clobetasol improved outcomes, but nanoparticulate clobetasol recipients had 1.9 times greater reduction in inflammation and 1.2-fold greater reduction in itching compared to native clobetasol recipients.

As one of the fundamental aspects of AD is impaired skin barrier function, the use of topical preparations that enhance the skin barrier can improve outcomes. Emollients have been shown to reduce the requirements for topical steroids. Replacement emollients that are optimized to correct the barrier defect typically contain physiologic lipids such as cholesterol, free fatty acids, and ceramide in appropriate proportions that mimic physiologic cutaneous conditions. Barrier creams containing ceramide-3 lipid nanoparticles in physiologic ratios showed improvement in disease severity and symptomatology for AD, irritant contact dermatitis, and allergic contact dermatitis.[88] Patients treated with balanced lipid barrier creams in combination with topical steroids had a more favorable response than patients treated with barrier cream alone.

5.5.3 Skin Cancer

The current incidence rates of melanoma have continued to increase since 1960, and are highest among the developed countries.[101] This may be the result of a change in behavior, increased screening, or a combination. It has long been known that melanoma occurs at the highest incidence in fair-skinned populations (Figure 5.5).[102] The USA SEER registries note that the rates are higher among non-Hispanic whites. The rates for white males are 19.4/100,000 and the rates for white females are 14.4/100,000.[101,103] Melanoma mortality has increased 157% in men of 65 years and older between 1969 and 1999.[104] When melanoma is identified in racial groups other than whites, it is more likely to be of more advanced stage.[101] Melanoma oncogenes that have been identified include neuroblastoma-RAS (NRAS), and other oncogenes from the RAS family. NRAS mutations have been found in approximately 15% of melanomas.[102] NRAS mutations have not been definitively associated with specific histopathological subtypes. In contrast, BRAF mutations have been reproducibly associated with specific clinical and histopathological subtypes. BRAF mutated melanomas are more likely to be found in younger patients with melanoma than in older patients. BRAF mutations are also more commonly of the superficial spreading melanoma (SSM) subtype, are more likely to be found on the trunk, and on intermittently rather than chronically sun-exposed skin.[105,106]

The goals of nanotechnology for the diagnosis of skin cancer are to be faster, more sensitive, more specific, less invasive, and require less tissue than traditional methods. Noninvasive methods of diagnosing skin cancer include near-infrared reflectance confocal microscopy, optical coherence tomography, and terahertz pulsed spectroscopy imaging.[85,86,107–134] The latter relies on changes in the nanomechanical properties of epidermal cells, the interstitium, and the extracellular matrix during the transition to malignancy. In the infrared spectrum (1060 nm), optical coherence tomography

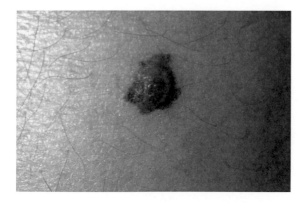

FIGURE 5.5
Melanoma.

has been used for the imaging of nonmelanoma skin cancer. Combining optical coherence tomography with photoacoustic scanning is being used for three-dimensional morphological imaging of the skin and may have applications for the delineation of tumors, vascular lesions, deeper soft tissue masses, wounds, and inflammatory diseases such as dermatitis and psoriasis.[86,134]

In some families at high risk for melanoma, mutations can be seen in the cyclin-dependent kinase inhibitor family (CDKN2A/CDK4). Lang and colleagues developed a high-throughput multiplexed bead-based PCR assay for detecting 39 different germline variants in kindreds prone to melanoma.[135] The assay was correctly able to identify 1540/1603 of susceptible individuals, and 1540/1545 individuals whose variants were included in the probe set. In addition, photoacoustic tomography using gold nanocages coupled to melanocyte stimulating hormone (MSH) allow for high-resolution real-time *in vivo* visualization of melanoma.[86,108] This can allow for early diagnosis, accurate staging, and image-guided resection of tumor.

Theranostics is the combination of simultaneous diagnosis and therapy of a target lesion.[141–145] Nanotechnology is particularly amenable to theranostics. A targeting ligand is coupled to a macromolecule that is visible by an imaging modality (e.g., near-infrared fluorescence). The same imaging modality can activate or deliver drug that leads to targeted therapy. An example would be a gold nanoshell tuned to a surface plasmon resonance frequency of 800 nm coupled to a targeting ligand such as melanocyte stimulating hormone.[146] These gold nanoparticles that can home to melanoma, are visible under NIR light, and can toxically heat up melanoma cells while leaving surrounding tissue unharmed. This type of selective photothermolysis of tumor has been demonstrated in murine models of melanoma. In addition, proteomics may allow for analysis of serologic markers for tumor presence, tumor burden, and for tracking tumor response to therapy.[147,148] Detection of small quantities of biomarkers accurately and rapidly using, for example, quantum dots, or nanocantilevers, may allow for more rapid characterization of tumor features.

Macromolecular antitumor drugs including photosensitizers such as protoporphyrin IX can be concentrated in tumors with the topical application of nitroglycerin.[149] Nitroglycerin enhances vascular drug delivery 2–3 fold. In murine models, nitroglycerin demonstrated enhanced therapeutic effect, yet no increased toxicity. Vehicles that enhance targeted delivery of nitroglycerin may be useful adjuncts in photodynamic therapy (PDT).

Topical delivery of therapeutic compounds may be enhanced by microneedle delivery. Examples include photosensitizers such as 5-aminolevulinic acid, vaccines, fluorescent dyes, and therapeutic antibodies.[150–155] Microneedles may be useful for the delivery of painless topical anesthesia prior to surgical intervention. Conversely, sampling of contents of suspicious neoplasms using a topically applied microneedle array may be

helpful in the diagnosis of malignant skin lesions.[156] Fiberoptic microneedles may be useful for the transdermal delivery of light for phototherapy or
photodynamic therapy.[157] Nanoscale optical fiber embedded light delivery
fabrics could be used to deliver phototherapy in a precise temporal and
spatial pattern.[158]

5.5.4 Dermatophytosis

The variety of lay terms used to describe dermatophyte infections under-
scores the ubiquity of this class of dermatologic disease. The nontrivial cost
of treatment for ring worm, athlete's foot, jock itch, thrush, and other cutaneous fungal infections, coupled with their pervasive nature, constitutes a
serious dermatologic concern (Figure 5.6).[159] Medicare expends 43 million
dollars annually on the treatment of onychomycosis (infection of the nail)
alone.[160] Dermatophyte infection extends across different age demographics
with adolescents and adults most often affected.[161] However, tinea capitis is
more common in children. Athletes who engage in contact sports are also at
increased risk of infection.[162]

Nanoparticles that consist of metals such as silver and metal oxides,
or biopolymers such as chitosan may be promising agents for antifungal
applications. These nanoparticles have the ability to bind to fungal cell
walls causing increased membrane permeability and disruption through
direct interactions, or generate damaging free radical. Mammalian cells are
able to phagocytose nanoparticles, and can subsequently degrade these
particles by lysosomal fusion, reducing toxicity, and free radical damage.
This may allow for the selectivity of the same nanoparticle to promote
tissue-forming cell functions, while also inhibiting bacterial functions that
lead to infection.

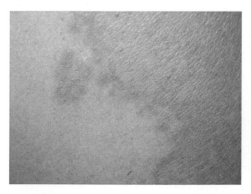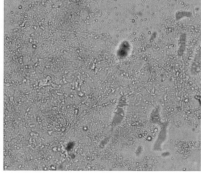

FIGURE 5.6
(**See color insert.**) Dermatophytosis—annular, scaly erythematous plaques (left); potassium
hydroxide wet prep demonstrating hyphae (right).

5.5.4.1 Nano-Silver

For centuries, silver (Ag) has been used for the treatment of burns and wounds to prevent infection.[163] Although the mechanism of its antimicrobial effects is not entirely known, it has been proposed that silver and silver ions (such as $AgNO_3$) penetrate bacterial cell walls and membranes via interaction with sulfur-containing proteins or thiol groups.[164] Once inside the cell, $AgNO_3$ targets and damages bacterial DNA and respiratory enzymes, leading to loss of the cell's replicating abilities and ultimately cell death.[163,165] The small size relative to the large surface area of silver nanoparticles (AgNps) makes them better able to penetrate bacterial cell walls and membranes, and as a result, the antimicrobial effect is directly dependent on nanoparticle size and shape.[163,166] Smaller nanoparticles (<10 nm) as well as triangular or truncated nanoparticles are more effective than larger particles that are round or rod-shaped.[164]

The stronger interaction of AgNps with microbial surfaces might also allow for lower Ag concentrations as compared to current silver agents, and may limit silver's toxicity, such as argyria. However, these benefits are largely theoretical, and the adverse effects of silver nanoparticles have yet to be fully characterized.[163] In one study, the antifungal activity of AgNps toward *Candida albicans* was demonstrated, and found to be similar to the antifungal activity in the minimal inhibitory concentration (MIC) values of amphotericin.[167] The mode of action of AgNps was shown to be its ability to dissipate the membrane potential of *C. albicans*. The results indicated AgNps have a similar mechanism of action to that of amphotericin b, which forms transmembrane pores causing leakage of cell constituents and eventually cell death. In addition, investigators showed that AgNps have either no effect or a weakly cytolytic effect on human erythrocytes, while amphotericin B incurred a higher hemolytic activity suggesting that AgNps may be a safer treatment. These data have been further corroborated by other investigators.[168–170]

5.5.4.2 Chitosan

Chitosan is a natural polysaccharide biopolymer derived from chitin, which is the principal structural component of the crustacean exoskeleton. The antimicrobial properties of chitosan result from its polycationic character in a weakly acidic pH, which favors interaction with negatively charged microbial cell walls and cytoplasmic membranes, resulting in decreased osmotic stability, membrane disruption, and eventual leakage of intracellular elements.[165,171,172] In addition, chitosan is able to enter the nuclei of bacteria and fungi and inhibit mRNA and protein synthesis by binding to microbial DNA.[172,173] When nanoscaled, chitosan has a higher surface-to-volume ratio, translating into higher surface charge density, increased affinity to bacteria and fungi, and greater antimicrobial activity.[173]

In one study, the *in vitro* antifungal activity of low-molecular-weight chitosan (LMWC) against 105 clinical *Candida* isolates were measured.[174] LMWC exhibited a significant antifungal activity, inhibiting over 89.9% of the clinical isolates examined (68.6% of which was completely inhibited). The species included several fluconazole-resistant strains and less susceptible species such as *Candida glabrata*, suggesting that chitosan may be a useful tool in the setting of antifungal drug resistance. Other studies have further supported the potential utility of chitosan as an antifungal agent,[175–177] though chitosan nanoparticles have yet to be fully explored as a topical antifungal agent.

5.5.4.3 Titanium Dioxide

Titanium dioxide (TiO_2) forms active oxygen species when exposed to ultraviolet light, a process called photocatalysis. These oxygen species, including hydrogen peroxide and hydroxyl radicals, damage bacterial cell membranes, resulting in cell death.[178,179] This antimicrobial property has been utilized in water and air purification, and recently has been investigated against pathogenic and opportunistic microorganisms.[180]

TiO_2 has also been combined with silver to create TiO_2–Ag nanoparticles (TiO_2–AgNPs) that were tested against Gram-negative bacteria, Gram-positive bacteria, and various fungi that are responsible for opportunistic infection and colonization of medical devices.[180] TiO_2–AgNPs demonstrated better antifungal activity against *C. albicans* and *Aspergillus fumigatus* when compared to AgNPs alone and conventional antifungals such as fluconazole.[180]

5.5.4.4 Soybean Oil-Derived Nanoemulsions

Antimicrobial nanoemulsions are stable oil-in-water emulsions composed of nanometer-sized, positively charged droplets that have broad-spectrum activity against enveloped viruses, fungi, and bacteria.[181–192] NB-002 is one such nanoemulsion that is currently being investigated as an antifungal agent. It contains the cationic quaternary ammonium compound cetylpyridinium chloride oriented at its oil–water interface, which stabilizes the nanoemulsion droplets, and contributes to the anti-infective activity. The NB-002 nanoemulsion was shown too exert broad, uniformly fungicidal activity against numerous dermatophyte species, including *T. rubrum*, *T. mentagrophytes*, and *E. floccosum* as well as the yeast *C. albicans*, the primary causes of human fungal hair, skin, and nail disease.[185,193,194] Its ability to serve as a topical treatment has been evaluated *ex vivo* with human cadaver skin samples, demonstrating that NB-002 can enter through a transfollicular route to enter the epidermal and dermal layers and that lateral diffusion occurs along tissue planes to sites distal from the application site.[189,195] Clinical studies of NB-002 for the treatment of onychomycosis have provided supporting results in its use as an effective topical treatment.[196]

5.5.4.5 Antifungal Encapsulated Nanomaterials

Liposomes have been employed to both enhance efficacy and improve delivery of antifungal agents. The best example and application of liposomal encapsulation is with amphotericin B. This is one of the mot effective antifungal agents, causing direct fungicidal activity by binding to ergosterol in fungal cell membranes and causing pore formation and ultimately cell death. However, the clinical use of this medication is limited due to severe, dose-limiting side effects. Amphotericin B, owing to its lipophilic nature, was an ideal candidate for liposomal encapsulation and was actually one of the first liposomal drugs to enter clinical trials in the late 1980s and continues to be a hot area of pursuit even today.[197–212] Several examples of products that have emerged from the initial studies include Abelcet®, Amphotec®, and Ambisome®.[205,206,213] However, the use of intravenous liposomal amphotericin b in the treatment of superficial dermatomycoses would be considered extreme, and no topical formulation is currently available. This example does set the template though for the use of liposomes to deliver topical antifungal agents, such as imidazoles (miconazole), triazoles (fluconazole and econazole), and polyenes (nystatin).

5.5.5 Psoriasis

Psoriasis is seen in 1.5–3% of individuals of European descent[214] and in 1.5% of the African American population (Figure 5.7).[215] In other populations, psoriasis is virtually nonexistent. China, for example, has a prevalence of psoriasis between 0% and 0.3%.[216] Although psoriasis can occur at any age, its peak age of onset is bimodal.[217] The first peak is at 16–22 years and the second is

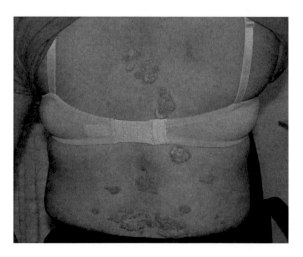

FIGURE 5.7
(See color insert.) Psoriasis.

at 57–60 years. The younger group tends to have a more severe disease and is more likely to have a family member with psoriasis. The older group has a milder, indolent course.

Genetic factors play a significant role in determining a patient's risk of developing psoriasis along with the age of onset, distribution, and severity.[218] Environmental factors such as trauma, infection, drugs, hormonal changes, alcohol, smoking, stress, and immune status also play a role in the development of psoriasis.[219]

5.5.5.1 Diagnosis

The diagnosis of psoriasis has traditionally been a clinical one with the recognition of characteristic skin lesions. Occasionally, when the diagnosis is in question, skin biopsies may be helpful. Recent attention in psoriasis has focused on genetic studies and the use of biomarkers both for the diagnosis of psoriasis and for monitoring therapy. Predicting susceptibility to psoriasis lies in the realm of bioinformatics. In one study of 451,724 single nucleotide polymorphisms (SNPs) in 2798 samples, it was determined that as few as 20 iteratively selected SNPs were able to predict psoriasis susceptibility with 68% accuracy.[220] Optical coherence tomography may also be useful in the diagnosis of psoriasis, the differentiation of nail psoriasis from onychomycosis, and for monitoring response to antipsoriatic therapy.[221]

The genes responsible for psoriasis map to a family of genes involved in chronic inflammation. These genes have also been implicated in AD, Crohn's disease, and rheumatoid arthritis. For example, genes involved in the IL-23 pathway have been implicated in psoriasis, ulcerative colitis, and Crohn's disease.[222-227] Genes in the endoplasmic reticulum aminopeptidase 1 (ERAP1) pathway are associated with Crohn's disease and with psoriasis. Other examples include IL-12 and TYK2.[228] Therapies that target IL-12 and IL-23 are demonstrating early success in the management of plaque-type psoriasis vulgaris. Hence, some of the therapies that have shown benefit in one condition have demonstrated crossover benefit in the others.

Currently, the diagnosis of psoriatic arthritis is challenging, based on history, examination, and rarely imaging techniques such as radiography and magnetic resonance. In psoriatic arthritis, surrogate markers of disease status such as soluble markers of cartilage and bone metabolism can be used to monitor the effects of treatment. For example, the soluble marker MMP-3 (matrix metalloprotease) and MIA (melanoma inhibitory activity, a marker for chondrocyte anabolism) have been used as a surrogate marker for efficacy of adalimumab in the treatment of psoriatic arthritis.[229] Early in adalimumab therapy, levels of MMP-3 fall, and MIA rise compared to placebo. Such screening can be helpful in the early phases of clinical trials to demonstrate efficacy. They can also be modified for an outpatient population to indirectly monitor response to therapy.

5.5.5.2 Treatment

Nanotechnology for the management of psoriasis involves enhancing drug delivery, promoting targeting of therapy, and reducing toxicity and side effects. Delivery of topical therapy can be mediated by encapsulation in SLNs. For topical steroids, this enhances deposition in the epidermis and papillary dermis, and minimizes systemic absorption, thus avoiding side effects such as atrophy and telangiectasia.[230–232] Topical preparations of cyclosporine also persist in the epidermis and dermal–epidermal junction, where they exert their action on psoriatic patches and plaques without systemic toxicity.[233] Methotrexate is typically given orally but suffers from side effects including hepatotoxicity. Topically administered methotrexate in SLNs may mitigate these concerns.[234–240]

Antibodies with biotherapeutic potential, the so-called biologics, such as adalimumab, efalizumab, infliximab, etanercept, and ustekinumab are essentially nanoparticles ($5 \times 5 \times 20$ nm) that have been specifically engineered to target certain receptors.[241] Biologics have proven effective in treating psoriasis with greater efficacy and fewer side effects than many other systemic agents.[242–246]

Because one component of psoriasis is keratinocyte hyperproliferation, some therapies involving siRNAs that favor apoptosis of keratinocytes may confer benefits in the management of psoriasis.[222,227,247–253]

Personalized medicine can play a role in psoriasis therapy.[254–256] Genetic variation can alter patient response to therapy and affect outcomes. The causes of this variability may include host factors such as psoriatic disease subset, specific disease genetic basis, concomitant illnesses, concomitant medications, as well as the patient's ability to metabolize and respond to medication. Furthermore, some patients may not tolerate therapies because of the vulnerability to medication toxicity. Identifying correct medications or combinations of medications suitable for a particular patient's psoriasis and general health profile will lead to tailored therapy that is less costly, more effective, and has fewer side effects. For example, methotrexate is a standard therapy for psoriasis. The benefits of methotrexate therapy include generally high efficacy, low cost, and convenient weekly dosing. The drawbacks of methotrexate include toxicity, and variable patient responsiveness.

While the mechanism of action of methotrexate action is still unclear, at least five key genes are believed to be involved in its metabolic pathway.[255,257] It is transported into cells via the folate carrier SLC19A1, and is actively transported out of the cell by ABCC1 and ABCG2, and its final activity is mediated by the adenosine receptors ADORA1 and ADORA2a. In one study, Warren et al. evaluated 374 patients with chronic plaque psoriasis and evaluated their methotrexate transmembrane transporters, and adenosine receptors. It was determined that SNPs within the efflux transporter genes ABC1 (ATP-binding cassette, subfamily C, member 1) and ABCG2 (ATP-binding cassette, subfamily G, member 2) are associated with a good response to methotrexate. One particular SNP in ABCC1, called rs246240, with two copies is associated with susceptibility to methotrexate toxicity.

5.6 Nanotechnology and Cosmeceuticals

5.6.1 Introduction

No discussion on nanotechnology in dermatology is complete without reviewing the long-standing role of nanomaterials in consumer and specifically cosmetic goods. Currently, nanotechnologies are being used in a broad range of commercial products soon to be or already available for consumers and patients—nanotechnologies are being employed predominantly as nanomaterials, as opposed to nanomachines or—computers, in sunscreens, emollients, soap, shampoo, lipstick, eye shadow, after shave products, deodorants, and antiaging products. The cosmetic industry leads in the number of patents for nanoparticles, which can be found in sunscreen, hair conditioner, shampoo, lipstick, eye shadow, after shave products, moisturizers, deodorants, and perfumes (Table 5.1).[3,25,258] Antiaging products are a big source of excitement for nanomaterials. Properly engineered, nanomaterials may be able to topically deliver retinoids, antioxidants, and drugs such as botulinum toxin or growth factors for collagen and elastin into the skin. A recent survey found that among the 270 or so nanotechnology products available, the majority are cosmetics. The following is a brief review on nanotechnology and cosmetics.

5.6.2 Nanocosmetics

Nanocosmetics are products that maintain or enhance the appearance of the skin, hair, and nails and capitalize on nanotechnology as their principal advantage. A broader definition would include products that help the appearance of the teeth and eyes. A broader definition would also include products that contain any nanomaterials on their ingredient list, rather than the active or key ingredient.

In the $200 billion global cosmetic industry, the current global market for nanotechnology is estimated to be $62 million and, barring curtailment through regulation, it was expected to grow annually at a rate of 16% and tech well over $150 million by 2012. Recently, in the "Nanotechnology Market Forecast to 2014," it was hypothesized that the global use of nanoparticles in cosmetic applications will grow at a CAGR of 17% during 2012–2014. Sunscreens are expected to account for the bulk of the growth, but other cosmetics, if they prove superior to current competitors, are likely to follow. The

TABLE 5.1

Dermatologic Consumer Products Containg Nanomaterials

Consumer Product	Manufacturer	Nanotechnology Contents
Sunscreens		
Soltan Facial Sun Defense Cream	Boots	Titanium dioxide
Blue Lizard Baby	Crown Laboratories, Inc	"Nanotechnological ingredients"
SPF 36 Lotion with Z-cote	Dermatome	Zinc oxide
Hawaiian Tropic sunscreen	Hawaiian Tropic	Zinc oxide
Cotz	Fallene	Titanium dioxide and zinc oxide
Daily Sun Defense	Skinceuticals	Zinc oxide
Physical UV Defense	Skinceuticals	Titanium dioxide and zinc oxide
Sport UV Defense	Skinceuticals	Zinc oxide
Ultimate UV Defense	Skinceuticals	Zinc oxide
Kids Tear Free	Banana Boat	Titanium dioxide and zinc oxide
Spectra3	Coppertone	Titanium dioxide and zinc oxide
Cosmetics		
Bionova Nano Skin Tech Range	Barney's New York	"Nanocomplexes"
Serge Lutens Blusher	Barney's New York	"Nanodispersion technology"
Coco Mademoiselle Fresh Moisturizer Mist	Chanel	Nanoemulsion
Defy: Age Management Exfoliator	Bellapelle Skin Studio	Fullerenes
After Glow Brush	ColoreScience	Nanovitamins A and E
Blush Colores	ColoreScience	Nanovitamins A and E
Sunforgettable Corrector Colores	ColoreScience	Titanium dioxide and zinc oxide
Moisturizing Dermatone Lips 'n Face Protection Crème	Dermatone	Zinc oxide
Dr Brandt New Lineless Cream	Dr Brandt	Fullerenes
Renutriv range	Este'e Lauder	Novasomes
Revitalift Double Lifting	L'Oreal Paris USA	Nanosomes
Hydra Flash Bronzer	Lancome	Nanocapsules
Renergie Microlift Eye	Lancome	Nanoparticles made of silicon and protein
Revlon Colorstay Stay Natural Powder	Revlon	Aluminum

growth of antiaging products may continue during a recession, especially as their cost is competitive when compared to procedures.

5.6.3 Nanoemollients

Emollients are substances that soften and soothe the skin by both preventing transepidermal water loss and in some cases serving as keratolytics to remove retained hyperkeratosis. Good emollients occlude the skin, contain humectants, and contain lubricants. Examples of moisturizers touting nanotechnology include Everyday Skin™ Penetrating Cream by Kara Vita that uses nanospheres to deliver emollients to dry skin along w/bioactive occlusive agents to strengthen the skin barrier. The manufacturer's goal is to have a single-application all-day-potent body moisturizer. The composition of the nanosphere and of the bioactive occlusant is proprietary. Another example is Arouge Deep NanoMoisture™ Care Set. The manufacturer's contents are proprietary. However, the company advertises the ability of its extremely small active ingredients to penetrate the skin deeply. "Arouge uses advanced technology to create extremely small moisture molecules. Because they are so small, they rapidly penetrate the deep layers of your skin. Arouge uses nanotechnology to make the molecules so small. Arouge has trademarked this solution, calling it NanoMoisture®. What this really means for your skin is that the moisture penetrates deeper, bringing the moisturizing and rejuvenating effects deeper into your skin than other skincare products." The company goes on to say, "Many people tell us that they are comfortable with their current facial care products, but they would like to extend their cleansing and moisturizing with the deeper and longer-lasting benefits of Arouge's NanoMoisture."

Lancome® makes HYDRA ZEN® cream that contains the proprietary ingredients Acticalm2™, Biolactone™, and nanoencapsulated triceramides. These are designed for long-lasting hydration, which, according to the manufacturer, protects the skin and keeps it fully hydrated and smooth all day long. Lancome also promotes Primordiale Nanolotion, which "melts into skin thanks to its ultra fine moisturizing texture (nano technology) combined with high tolerance sugar esters to bring intense hydration." Furthermore, Promordiale Nanolotion contains a Duplex System, which "combines two vegetal extracts with Vitamin E to ultra-smooth, refine your skin and improve its elasticity."

5.6.4 Nanocleansers

Cleansers debride, exfoliate, and decontaminate the skin. Some cleansers incorporate nano-silver as a disinfectant and skin decontaminant. They tout the importance of decreasing bacterial load on the skin gently. On example is Cosil Nano Beauty Soap (Natural Korea Company, Ltd). One company uses zinc oxide and nanomicelles to remove make-up and exfoliate the skin, giving the skin a "clean smooth" sensation after washing (Nano-Infinity Nano Tech Co., Ltd. Beautiful Face Series).

5.6.5 Nanosunscreens

A consensus exists that physical blockers like titanium dioxide (TiO_2) and zinc oxide (ZnO) can provide effective, comprehensive protection as sunscreens. For years, however, consumers did not favor products containing these ingredients because they formed an unattractive white coating on the skin. Today, owing to nanotechnology advances, titanium dioxide- and zinc oxide-based products have become far more desirable.

Sunscreens employing nanomaterials rely on the unique properties of metallic zinc and titanium at the nanoscale. Macro-sized zinc and titanium require oily vehicles for solubility. Their nano-sized counterparts are easily dispersed in water-based topical preparations. Hence, they are more cosmetically elegant when applied and less likely to be comedogenic. Furthermore, nano-sized zinc and titanium are much smaller than the wavelength of visible light (400–700 nm) and vanish on the skin without leaving a whitish film.[27,259,260] Also, because of their small size and ready solubility, nano-sized sunscreens are more easily dispersed on the skin and can provide better overall coverage of the skin. Finally, because they are physical blockers, they are more likely to block ultraviolet A and ultraviolet B light. Sunscreens containing these particles are widely available. Recently, manufacturers have shied away from mentioning them on their product lists, but independent laboratories working for Consumers Union have demonstrated nanoparticle content in several brands that specifically market themselves as nanoparticle free.[260–262]

Some concern has been raised that nanoparticles could be absorbed through the skin into the blood stream and create unintended health risks. From a common sense standpoint, they have raised a valid question, but little or no evidence exists to support fears that the nanoparticles used in sunscreens do penetrate into or through human skin. An underlying reason for this is that nanoparticles are naturally prone to tightly bonding together, causing them to act as larger aggregates rather than as separate, individual fine particles. The force required to break aggregates into component particles is far greater than any force applied during the sunscreen manufacturing or application process. Extensive safety testing has been conducted, and results have been independently reviewed by various organizations and regulatory bodies. Evidence from study after study has consistently shown that insoluble nanoparticles, such as those used in inorganic sunscreens, do not permeate human skin.[259,260,262–264] German and Australian health authorities have formally accepted these findings and acknowledged that UV attenuation forms of TiO_2 used in sunscreens do not pose any health risk. In a 2007 assessment, the European Union found no evidence of nanoscale particles absorbing through pig skin (the most appropriate substitute for human skin), healthy human skin, or the skin of patients suffering from skin disorders.

Recently, the Nanodermatology Society, a nonprofit physician-run organization founded in 2010, released a position statement on the use of nanomaterials in sunscreens detailing the available data regarding the safety of these ingredients and concluded based on all information available that they are safe and aid in the prevention of sun-related skin disease (http://www.nanodermsociety.org/documents/press/NDS_Sunscreen_Guidelines.pdf). This report was quickly followed by the release of the 2010 annual sunscreen report by the Environmental Working Group (EWG), a U.S.-based nonprofit organization that conducts independent research to protect human health and the environment, along with a corresponding report issued by the American Academy of Dermatology. Both concluded that the use of nanotechnology in sunscreen creams/lotions is safe, though the use of nanoparticles in aerosolized preparations such as sprays, may provide a means through which these particles can be inhaled and ultimately cause pulmonary inflammation and dysfunction. However, this risk is theoretical and has yet to be determined *in vivo*. In April 2012, the FDA released its preliminary guidelines for evaluating the safety of nanomaterials in cosmetics and commercial goods. The FDA is working with the White House, the National Nanotechnology Initiative, other U.S. government agencies, and international regulators to focus on generating data and coordinating policy approaches to ensure the safety and effectiveness of products using nanomaterials.

5.7 Conclusions

Nanotechnology is moving at a rapid pace in dermatology. A large array of products has already been developed for the health and beauty of the skin, eyes, nails, hair, and teeth. The delivery mechanisms of nanotechnology also allow for the topical application of drugs, which must currently be ingested or injected. It is likely that much progress will be made in nanotechnology and skin care in the future. It is likely that future advances will take place under the watchful eye of regulators with input from dermatologists, consumers, and scientists.

References

1. Elias PM. Stratum corneum defensive functions: An integrated view. *Journal of Investigative Dermatology.* Aug 2005;125(2):183–200.
2. Bos JD, Meinardi MM. The 500 Dalton rule for the skin penetration of chemical compounds and drugs. *Experimental Dermatology.* Jun 2000;9(3):165–169.

3. Nasir A. Nanotechnology and dermatology: Part I-potential of nanotechnology. *Clinics in Dermatology.* Jul-Aug 2010;28(4):458–466.

4. Cevc G, Vierl U. Nanotechnology and the transdermal route A state of the art review and critical appraisal. *Journal of Controlled Release.* Feb 2010;141(3): 277–299.

5. Farokhzad OC. Nanotechnology for drug delivery: The perfect partnership. *Expert Opinion on Drug Delivery.* Sep 2008;5(9):927–929.

6. Waller JM, Maibach HI. Age and skin structure and function, a quantitative approach (II): Protein, glycosaminoglycan, water, and lipid content and structure. *Skin Research and Technology: Official Journal of International Society for Bioengineering and the Skin.* Aug 2006;12(3):145–154.

7. Berardesca E, Maibach H. Racial differences in skin pathophysiology. *Journal of the American Academy of Dermatology.* Apr 1996;34(4):667–672.

8. Bauer EA, Cohen DE. Systems that enhance skin drug delivery. *Dermatologic Therapy.* Sep 2011;24(5):463.

9. Torin Huzil J, Sivaloganathan S, Kohandel M, Foldvari M. Drug delivery through the skin: Molecular simulations of barrier lipids to design more effective noninvasive dermal and transdermal delivery systems for small molecules, biologics, and cosmetics. *Wiley Interdisciplinary Reviews. Nanomedicine and Nanobiotechnology.* 2011;3(5):449–462.

10. Hashmi S, Marinkovich MP. Molecular organization of the basement membrane zone. *Clinics in Dermatology.* Jul-Aug 2011;29(4):398–411.

11. Divoux A, Clement K. Architecture and the extracellular matrix: The still unappreciated components of the adipose tissue. *Obesity Reviews.* May 2011;12(5):e494–e503.

12. Rock K, Fischer JW. [Role of the extracellular matrix in extrinsic skin aging]. *Der Hautarzt; Zeitschrift fur Dermatologie, Venerologie, und verwandte Gebiete.* Aug 2011;62(8):591–597.

13. Mak WC, Richter H, Patzelt A et al. Drug delivery into the skin by degradable particles. *European Journal of Pharmaceutics and Biopharmaceutics: Official Journal of Arbeitsgemeinschaft Fur Pharmazeutische Verfahrenstechnik e.V.* Sep 2011;79(1):23–27.

14. Korting HC, Schafer-Korting M. Carriers in the topical treatment of skin disease. *Handbook of Experimental Pharmacology.* 2010(197):435–468.

15. Kaur IP, Kakkar S. Topical delivery of antifungal agents. *Expert Opinion on Drug Delivery.* Nov 2010;7(11):1303–1327.

16. Prow TW, Grice JE, Lin LL et al. Nanoparticles and microparticles for skin drug delivery. *Advanced Drug Delivery Reviews.* May 30 2011;63(6):470–491.

17. Park K. Nanotechnology: What it can do for drug delivery. *Journal of Controlled Release.* Jul 2007;120(1–2):1–3.

18. Kircik L, Friedman A. Optimizing acne therapy with unique vehicles. *Journal of Drugs in Dermatology: JDD.* May 2010;9(5 Suppl ODAC Conf Pt 1):s53–57.

19. Ciotti S, Baker JR, Ma LF, Eisma R. Novel follicular-targeted nanoemulsion for acne. *Journal of the American Academy of Dermatology.* Mar 2010;62(3): AB24–AB24.

20. Lademann J, Otberg N, Jacobi U, Hoffman RM, Blume-Peytavi U. Follicular penetration and targeting. *The Journal of Investigative Dermatology. Symposium Proceedings/the Society for Investigative Dermatology, Inc. [and] European Society for Dermatological Research.* Dec 2005;10(3):301–303.

21. Staples M, Daniel K, Cima MJ, Langer R. Application of micro- and nano-electromechanical devices to drug delivery. *Pharmaceutical Research.* May 2006;23(5):847–863.

22. Kupper TS. Immune and inflammatory processes in cutaneous tissues. Mechanisms and speculations. *Journal of Clinical Investigation.* Dec 1990;86(6): 1783–1789.

23. Williams IR, Kupper TS. Immunity at the surface: Homeostatic mechanisms of the skin immune system. *Life Sciences.* 1996;58(18):1485–1507.

24. Cevc G. Transfersomes, liposomes and other lipid suspensions on the skin: Permeation enhancement, vesicle penetration, and transdermal drug delivery. *Critical Reviews in Therapeutic Drug Carrier Systems.* 1996;13(3–4):257–388.

25. Nasir A. NanoPresent and NanoFuture: The growing role of shrinking technology in dermatology. *Cosmetic Dermatology.* 2009;22(4):194–200.

26. Nasir A. Nanotechnology in vaccine development: A step forward. *Journal of Investigative Dermatology.* May 2009;129(5):1055–1059.

27. Hia J, Nasir A. Photonanodermatology: The interface of photobiology, dermatology and nanotechnology. *Photodermatology Photoimmunology & Photomedicine.* Feb 2011;27(1):2–9.

28. Trapasso E, Cosco D, Celia C, Fresta M, Paolino D. Retinoids: New use by innovative drug-delivery systems. *Expert Opinion on Drug Delivery.* May 2009;6(5): 465–483.

29. Kumar A, Agarwal SP, Ahuja A, Ali J, Choudhry R, Baboota S. Preparation, characterization, and *in vitro* antimicrobial assessment of nanocarrier based formulation of nadifloxacin for acne treatment. *Pharmazie.* Feb 2011;66(2):111–114.

30. Dominguez-Delgado CL, Rodriguez-Cruz IM, Escobar-Chavez JJ, Calderon-Lojero IO, Quintanar-Guerrero D, Ganem A. Preparation and characterization of triclosan nanoparticles intended to be used for the treatment of acne. *European Journal of Pharmaceutics and Biopharmaceutics.* 2011;79(1):102–107.

31. Castro GA, Oliveira CA, Mahecha GA, Ferreira LA. Comedolytic effect and reduced skin irritation of a new formulation of all-trans retinoic acid-loaded solid lipid nanoparticles for topical treatment of acne. *Archives of Dermatological Research.* September 2011;303(7):513–520.

32. Inui S, Aoshima H, Nishiyama A, Itami S. Improvement of acne vulgaris by topical fullerene application: Unique impact on skin care. *Nanomedicine.* Apr 2011;7(2):238–241.

33. Czermak P, Steinle T, Ebrahimi M, Schmidts T, Runkel F. Membrane-assisted production of S1P loaded SLNs for the treatment of acne vulgaris. *Desalination.* Jan 2010;250(3):1132–1135.

34. Chanda N, Kattumuri V, Shukla R et al. Bombesin functionalized gold nanoparticles show *in vitro* and *in vivo* cancer receptor specificity. *Proceedings of the National Academy of Sciences of United States of America.* May 2010;107(19):8760–8765.

35. Chourasia R, Jain SK. Drug targeting through pilosebaceous route. *Current Drug Targets.* Oct 2009;10(10):950–967.

36. de Leeuw J, de Vijlder HC, Bjerring P, Neumann HAM. Liposomes in dermatology today. *Journal of the European Academy of Dermatology and Venereology.* May 2009;23(5):505–516.

37. Castro GA, Ferreira LA. Novel vesicular and particulate drug delivery systems for topical treatment of acne. *Expert Opinion on Drug Delivery.* Jun 2008;5(6):665–679.

38. Bernard E, Dubois JL, Wepierre J. Importance of sebaceous glands in cutaneous penetration of an antiandrogen: Target effect of liposomes. *Journal of Pharmaceutical Sciences.* May 1997;86(5):573–578.
39. Zaenglein AL, Thiboutot DM. Chapter 37–Acne Vulgaris. In: Bolognia J, Jorizzo JL, Rapini RP, eds. *Dermatology.* London; New York: Mosby; 2003.
40. Smith EV, Grindlay DJ, Williams HC. What's new in acne? An analysis of systematic reviews published in 2009–2010. *Clinical and Experimental Dermatology.* Mar 2011;36(2):119–122; quiz 123.
41. Shah SK, Alexis AF. Acne in skin of color: Practical approaches to treatment. *Journal of Dermatological Treatment.* May 2010;21(3):206–211.
42. Merkviladze N, Gaidamashvili T, Tushurashvili P, Ekaladze E, Jojua N. The efficacy of topical drugs in treatment of noninflammatory acne vulgaris. *Georgian Medical News.* Sep 2010(186):46–50.
43. Eichenfield LF, Fowler JF, Jr., Fried RG, Friedlander SF, Levy ML, Webster GF. Perspectives on therapeutic options for acne: An update. *Seminars in Cutaneous Medicine and Surgery.* Jun 2010;29(2 Suppl 1):13–16.
44. Lott R, Taylor SL, O'Neill JL, Krowchuk DP, Feldman SR. Medication adherence among acne patients: A review. *Journal of Cosmetic Dermatology.* Jun 2010;9(2):160–166.
45. Dutil M. Benzoyl peroxide: Enhancing antibiotic efficacy in acne management. *Skin Therapy Letter.* Nov-Dec 2010;15(10):5–7.
46. Patel VB, Misra A, Marfatia YS. Clinical assessment of the combination therapy with liposomal gels of tretinoin and benzoyl peroxide in acne. *AAPS PharmSciTech.* 2001;2(3):E-TN4.
47. Bettoli V, Sarno O, Zauli S et al. [What's new in acne? New therapeutic approaches]. *Annales de dermatologie et de venereologie.* Nov 2010;137 Suppl 2:S81–85.
48. Del Rosso J, Kircik L. Comparison of the tolerability of benzoyl peroxide microsphere wash versus a gentle cleanser, when used in combination with a clindamycin and tretinoin gel: A multicenter, investigator-blind, randomized study. *Journal of the American Academy of Dermatology.* Mar 2009;60(3):AB17–AB17.
49. Bikowski J, Del Rosso JQ. Benzoyl peroxide microsphere cream as monotherapy and combination treatment of acne. *Journal of Drugs in Dermatology.* Jun 2008;7(6):590–595.
50. Wester RC, Patel R, Nacht S, Leyden J, Melendres J, Maibach H. Controlled release of benzoyl peroxide from a porous microsphere polymeric system can reduce topical irritancy. *Journal of the American Academy of Dermatology.* May 1991;24(5):720–726.
51. Kinney MA, Yentzer BA, Fleischer AB, Jr., Feldman SR. Trends in the treatment of acne vulgaris: Are measures being taken to avoid antimicrobial resistance? *Journal of Drugs in Dermatology.* May 2010;9(5):519–524.
52. Ingram JR, Grindlay DJ, Williams HC. Management of acne vulgaris: An evidence-based update. *Clinical and Experimental Dermatology.* Jun 2010;35(4):351–354.
53. Shanmugam S, Song CK, Nagayya-Sriraman S et al. Physicochemical characterization and skin permeation of liposome formulations containing clindamycin phosphate. *Archives of Pharmacal Research.* Jul 2009;32(7):1067–1075.
54. Honzak L, Sentjure M. Development of liposome encapsulated clindamycin for treatment of acne vulgaris. *Pflugers Archiv: European Journal of Physiology.* 2000;440(5):R44–R45.

55. Skalko N, Cajkovac M, Jalsenjak I. Liposomes with clindamycin hydrochloride in the therapy of acne-vulgaris. *International Journal of Pharmaceutics.* Sep 1992;85(1–3):97–101.

56. Hagiwara Y, Arima H, Miyamoto Y, Hirayama F, Uekama K. Preparation and pharmaceutical evaluation of liposomes entrapping salicylic acid/gamma-cyclodextrin conjugate. *Chemical & Pharmaceutical Bulletin.* Jan 2006;54(1): 26–32.

57. Motwani MR, Rhein LD, Zatz JL. Deposition of salicylic acid into hamster sebaceous glands. *Journal of Cosmetic Science.* Nov-Dec 2004;55(6):519–531.

58. Yentzer BA, McClain RW, Feldman SR. Do topical retinoids cause acne to "flare"? *Journal of Drugs in Dermatology.* Sep 2009;8(9):799–801.

59. Gollnick H. Current concepts of the pathogenesis of acne—Implications for drug treatment. *Drugs.* 2003;63(15):1579–1596.

60. Castro GA, Coelho A, Oliveira CA, Mahecha GAB, Orefice RL, Ferreira LAM. Formation of ion pairing as an alternative to improve encapsulation and stability and to reduce skin irritation of retinoic acid loaded in solid lipid nanoparticles. *International Journal of Pharmaceutics.* Oct 2009;381(1):77–83.

61. Pardeike J, Hommoss A, Muller RH. Lipid nanoparticles (SLN, NLC) in cosmetic and pharmaceutical dermal products. *International Journal of Pharmaceutics.* Jan 2009;366(1–2):170–184.

62. Castro GA, Ferreira LAM, Orefice RL, Buono VTL. Characterization of a new solid lipid nanoparticle formulation containing retinoic acid for topical treatment of acne. *Powder Diffraction.* Jun 2008;23(2):S30–S35.

63. Carafa M, Marianecci C, Salvatorelli M et al. Formulations of retinyl palmitate included in solid lipid nanoparticles: Characterization and influence on light-induced vitamin degradation. *Journal of Drug Delivery Science and Technology.* Mar-Apr 2008;18(2):119–124.

64. Castro GA, Ferreira LAM. Novel vesicular and particulate drug delivery systems for topical treatment of acne. *Expert Opinion on Drug Delivery.* Jun 2008;5(6):665–679.

65. Castro GA, Orefice RL, Vilela JMC, Andrade MS, Ferreira LAM. Development of a new solid lipid nanoparticle formulation containing retinoic acid for topical treatment of acne. *Journal of Microencapsulation.* 2007;24(5):395–407.

66. Date AA, Naik B, Nagarsenker MS. Novel drug delivery systems: Potential in improving topical delivery of antiacne agents. *Skin Pharmacology and Physiology.* 2006;19(1):2–16.

67. Shah KA, Joshi MD, Patravale VB. Biocompatible microemulsions for fabrication of glyceryl monostearate solid lipid nanoparticles (SLN) of tretinoin. *Journal of Biomedical Nanotechnology.* Aug 2009;5(4):396–400.

68. Pariser D, Bucko A, Fried R et al. Tretinoin gel microsphere pump 0.04% plus 5% benzoyl peroxide wash for treatment of acne vulgaris: Morning/morning regimen is as effective and safe as morning/evening regimen. *Journal of Drugs in Dermatology.* Jul 2010;9(7):805–813.

69. Nighland M, Yusuf M, Wisniewski S, Huddleston K, Nyirady J. The effect of simulated solar UV irradiation on tretinoin in tretinoin gel microsphere 0.1% and tretinoin gel 0.025%. *Cutis.* May 2006;77(5):313–316.

70. Fleischer A, Leyden J, Lucky A, Nighland M. A double-blind randomized, vehicle-controlled, multicenter study to assess tretinoin gel microsphere 0.04% in the treatment of acne vulgaris in adults. *Journal of the American Academy of Dermatology.* Mar 2006;54(3):AB23–AB23.

71. Dosik JS, Homer K, Arsonnaud S. Cumulative irritation potential of adapalene 0.1% cream and gel compared with tretinoin microsphere 0.04% and 0.1%. *Cutis.* Apr 2005;75(4):238–243.

72. Nyirady J, Lucas C, Yusuf M, Mignone P, Wisniewski S. The stability of tretinoin in tretinoin gel microsphere 0.1%. *Cutis.* Nov 2002;70(5):295–298.

73. Torok HM, Pillai R. Safety and efficacy of micronized tretinoin gel (0.05%) in treating adolescent acne. *Journal of Drugs in Dermatology.* Jun 2011;10(6):647–652.

74. Lucky AW, Sugarman J. Comparison of micronized tretinoin gel 0.05% and tretinoin gel microsphere 0.1% in young adolescents with acne: A post hoc analysis of efficacy and tolerability data. *Cutis.* Jun 2011;87(6):305–310.

75. Ramos-e-Silva M, Carvalho J, Marques-Costa J, Goldsztajn K, Carneiro S. Tretinoin microsphere 0.1% gel for acne patients. *Journal of the American Academy of Dermatology.* Feb 2011;64(2):AB5–AB5.

76. Eichenfield LF, Matiz C, Funk A, Dill SW. Study of the efficacy and tolerability of 0.04% tretinoin microsphere gel for preadolescent acne. *Pediatrics.* Jun 2010;125(6):E1316–E1323.

77. Leyden JJ, Nighland M, Rossi AB, Ramaswamy R. Irritation potential of tretinoin gel microsphere pump versus adapalene plus benzoyl peroxide gel. *Journal of Drugs in Dermatology.* Aug 2010;9(8):998–1003.

78. Pannu J, Martin A, McCarthy A, Sutcliffe J, Ciotti S. NB-003 activity against *Propionibacterium acnes* in a pig skin model. *Journal of the American Academy of Dermatology.* Mar 2010;62(3):AB14–AB14.

79. Kang K, Polster AM, Nedorost, Susan T, Stevens SR, Cooper KD. Chapter 13–Atopic Dermatitis. In: Bolognia J, Jorizzo JL, Rapini RP, eds. *Dermatology.* London; New York: Mosby; 2003.

80. Laughter D, Istvan JA, Tofte SJ, Hanifin JM. The prevalence of atopic dermatitis in Oregon schoolchildren. *Journal of the American Academy of Dermatology.* 2000;43(4):649–655.

81. Luoma R, Koivikko A, Viander M. Development of asthma, allergic rhinitis and atopic dermatitis by the age of five years: A prospective study of 543 newborns. *Allergy.* 1983;38(5):339–346.

82. Kemp AS. Cost of illness of atopic dermatitis in children: A societal perspective. *PharmacoEconomics.* 2003;21(2):105–113.

83. Kelsay K. Management of sleep disturbance associated with atopic dermatitis. *Journal of Allergy and Clinical Immunology.* 2006;118(1):198–201.

84. Gonzalez S, Gonzalez E, White WM, Rajadhyaksha M, Anderson RR. Allergic contact dermatitis: Correlation of *in vivo* confocal imaging to routine histology. *Journal of the American Academy of Dermatology.* May 1999;40(5 Pt 1):708–713.

85. Richtig E, Ahlgrimm-Siess V, Arzberger E, Hofmann-Wellenhof R. Noninvasive differentiation between mamillary eczema and Paget disease by *in vivo* reflectance confocal microscopy on the basis of two case reports. *British Journal of Dermatology.* Aug 2011;165(2):440–441.

86. Zhang EZ, Povazay B, Laufer J et al. Multimodal photoacoustic and optical coherence tomography scanner using an all optical detection scheme for 3D morphological skin imaging. *Biomedical Optics Express.* Aug 1 2011;2(8): 2202–2215.

87. Braconi D, Bernardini G, Santucci A. Post-genomics and skin inflammation. *Mediators of Inflammation.* 2010;2010:364823.

88. Berardesca E, Barbareschi M, Veraldi S, Pimpinelli N. Evaluation of efficacy of a skin lipid mixture in patients with irritant contact dermatitis, allergic contact dermatitis or atopic dermatitis: A multicenter study. *Contact Dermatitis.* Nov 2001;45(5):280–285.
89. Wilsmann-Theis D, Hagemann T, Jordan J, Bieber T, Novak N. Facing psoriasis and atopic dermatitis: Are there more similarities or more differences? *European Journal of Dermatology.* Mar-Apr 2008;18(2):172–180.
90. Pople PV, Singh KK. Targeting tacrolimus to deeper layers of skin with improved safety for treatment of atopic dermatitis. *International Journal of Pharmaceutics.* Oct 15 2010;398(1–2):165–178.
91. Singh KK, Pople P. Safer than safe: Lipid nanoparticulate encapsulation of tacrolimus with enhanced targeting and improved safety for atopic dermatitis. *Journal of Biomedical Nanotechnology.* Feb 2011;7(1):40–41.
92. Vemula PK, Anderson RR, Karp JM. Animal models for nickel allergy. *Nature Nanotechnology.* 2011;6(9):533.
93. Vemula PK, Anderson RR, Karp JM. Nanoparticles reduce nickel allergy by capturing metal ions. *Nature Nanotechnology.* May 2011;6(5):291–295.
94. Aschberger K, Johnston HJ, Stone V et al. Review of fullerene toxicity and exposure—Appraisal of a human health risk assessment, based on open literature. *Regulatory Toxicology and Pharmacology: RTP.* Dec 2010;58(3):455–473.
95. Dellinger A, Zhou Z, Lenk R, MacFarland D, Kepley CL. Fullerene nanomaterials inhibit phorbol myristate acetate-induced inflammation. *Experimental Dermatology.* Dec 2009;18(12):1079–1081.
96. Gao J, Wang Y, Folta KM et al. Polyhydroxy fullerenes (fullerols or fullerenols): Beneficial effects on growth and lifespan in diverse biological models. *PLoS One.* 2011;6(5):e19976.
97. Henry TB, Petersen EJ, Compton RN. Aqueous fullerene aggregates (nC(60)) generate minimal reactive oxygen species and are of low toxicity in fish: A revision of previous reports. *Current Opinion in Biotechnology.* Aug 2011;22(4):533–537.
98. Kolosnjaj J, Szwarc H, Moussa F. Toxicity studies of fullerenes and derivatives. *Advances in Experimental Medicine and Biology.* 2007;620:168–180.
99. Uo M, Akasaka T, Watari F, Sato Y, Tohji K. Toxicity evaluations of various carbon nanomaterials. *Dental Materials Journal.* Jun 2 2011;30(3):245–263.
100. Kalariya M, Padhi BK, Chougule M, Misra A. Clobetasol propionate solid lipid nanoparticles cream for effective treatment of eczema: Formulation and clinical implications. *Indian Journal of Experimental Biology.* Mar 2005;43(3):233–240.
101. Berwick M. Melanoma epidemiology In: Bosserhoff A, ed. *Melanoma Development.* Vienna: Springer; 2011:pp. 35–55.
102. Whiteman DC, Pavan WJ, Bastian BC. The melanomas: A synthesis of epidemiological, clinical, histopathological, genetic, and biological aspects, supporting distinct subtypes, causal pathways, and cells of origin. *Pigment Cell & Melanoma Research.* October 2011;24(5):879–897.
103. SEER Cancer Statistics Review, 1975–2008, National Cancer Institute. http://seer.cancer.gov/csr/1975_2008/. Accessed posted to the SEER web site, 2011.
104. Geller AC, Miller DR, Annas GD, Demierre MF, Gilchrest BA, Koh HK. Melanoma incidence and mortality among US whites, 1969–1999. *JAMA-Journal of the American Medical Association.* Oct 9 2002;288(14):1719–1720.

105. Whiteman DC, Watt P, Purdie DM, Hughes MC, Hayward NK, Green AC. Melanocytic nevi, solar keratoses, and divergent pathways to cutaneous melanoma. *Journal of the National Cancer Institute.* Jun 4 2003;95(11):806–812.

106. Bastian BC, Olshen AB, LeBoit PE, Pinkel D. Classifying melanocytic tumors based on DNA copy number changes. *American Journal of Pathology.* Nov 2003;163(5):1765–1770.

107. Berry E, Handley JW, Fitzgerald AJ et al. Multispectral classification techniques for terahertz pulsed imaging: An example in histopathology. *Medical Engineering & Physics.* Jun 2004;26(5):423–430.

108. Hong H, Sun J, Cai W. Anatomical and molecular imaging of skin cancer. *Clinical, Cosmetic and Investigational Dermatology.* 2008;1:1–17.

109. Joseph CS, Yaroslavsky AN, Neel VA, Goyette TM, Giles RH. Continuous wave terahertz transmission imaging of nonmelanoma skin cancers. *Lasers in Surgery and Medicine.* Aug 2011;43(6):457–462.

110. Mitobe K, Manabe M, Yoshimura N, Kurabayashi T. Imaging of epithelial cancer in sub-terahertz electromagnetic wave. *Conference Proceedings: Annual International Conference of the IEEE Engineering in Medicine and Biology Society. IEEE Engineering in Medicine and Biology Society. Conference.* 2005;1:199–200.

111. Mogensen M, Jemec GB. Diagnosis of nonmelanoma skin cancer/keratinocyte carcinoma: A review of diagnostic accuracy of nonmelanoma skin cancer diagnostic tests and technologies. *Dermatologic Surgery.* Oct 2007;33(10):1158–1174.

112. Ney M, Abdulhalim I. Modeling of reflectometric and ellipsometric spectra from the skin in the terahertz and submillimeter waves region. *Journal of Biomedical Optics.* Jun 2011;16(6):067006.

113. Pickwell E, Cole BE, Fitzgerald AJ, Pepper M, Wallace VP. *In vivo* study of human skin using pulsed terahertz radiation. *Physics in Medicine and Bbiology.* May 7 2004;49(9):1595–1607.

114. Tewari P, Taylor ZD, Bennett D et al. Terahertz imaging of biological tissues. *Studies in Health Technology and Informatics.* 2011;163:653–657.

115. Wallace VP, Fitzgerald AJ, Pickwell E et al. Terahertz pulsed spectroscopy of human Basal cell carcinoma. *Applied Spectroscopy.* Oct 2006;60(10):1127–1133.

116. Wallace VP, Fitzgerald AJ, Shankar S et al. Terahertz pulsed imaging of basal cell carcinoma ex vivo and in vivo. *British Journal of Dermatology.* Aug 2004;151(2):424–432.

117. Woodward RM, Wallace VP, Pye RJ et al. Terahertz pulse imaging of ex vivo basal cell carcinoma. *Journal of Investigative Dermatology.* Jan 2003;120(1):72–78.

118. Forsea AM, Carstea EM, Ghervase L, Giurcaneanu C, Pavelescu G. Clinical application of optical coherence tomography for the imaging of non-melanocytic cutaneous tumors: A pilot multi-modal study. *Journal of Medicine and Life.* Oct-Dec 2010;3(4):381–389.

119. Gambichler T, Regeniter P, Bechara FG et al. Characterization of benign and malignant melanocytic skin lesions using optical coherence tomography in vivo. *Journal of the American Academy of Dermatology.* Oct 2007;57(4):629–637.

120. Hamdoon Z, Jerjes W, Upile T, Hopper C. Optical coherence tomography-guided photodynamic therapy for skin cancer: Case study. *Photodiagnosis and Photodynamic Therapy.* Mar 2011;8(1):49–52.

121. Jorgensen TM, Tycho A, Mogensen M, Bjerring P, Jemec GB. Machine-learning classification of non-melanoma skin cancers from image features

obtained by optical coherence tomography. *Skin Research and Technology.* Aug 2008;14(3):364–369.

122. Konig K, Speicher M, Buckle R et al. Clinical optical coherence tomography combined with multiphoton tomography of patients with skin diseases. *Journal of Biophotonics.* Jul 2009;2(6–7):389–397.

123. Mogensen M, Joergensen TM, Nurnberg BM et al. Assessment of optical coherence tomography imaging in the diagnosis of non-melanoma skin cancer and benign lesions versus normal skin: Observer-blinded evaluation by dermatologists and pathologists. *Dermatologic Surgery.* Jun 2009;35(6):965–972.

124. Mogensen M, Jorgensen TM, Thrane L, Nurnberg BM, Jemec GB. Improved quality of optical coherence tomography imaging of basal cell carcinomas using speckle reduction. *Experimental Dermatology.* Aug 2010;19(8):e293–295.

125. Mogensen M, Nurnberg BM, Forman JL, Thomsen JB, Thrane L, Jemec GB. *In vivo* thickness measurement of basal cell carcinoma and actinic keratosis with optical coherence tomography and 20-MHz ultrasound. *British Journal of Dermatology.* May 2009;160(5):1026–1033.

126. Mogensen M, Nurnberg BM, Thrane L, Jorgensen TM, Andersen PE, Jemec GB. How histological features of basal cell carcinomas influence image quality in optical coherence tomography. *Journal of Biophotonics.* Aug 2011;4(7–8): 544–551.

127. Mogensen M, Thrane L, Joergensen TM, Andersen PE, Jemec GB. Optical coherence tomography for imaging of skin and skin diseases. *Seminars in Cutaneous Medicine and Surgery.* Sep 2009;28(3):196–202.

128. Mogensen M, Thrane L, Jorgensen TM, Andersen PE, Jemec GB. OCT imaging of skin cancer and other dermatological diseases. *Journal of Biophotonics.* Jul 2009;2(6–7):442–451.

129. Morsy H, Kamp S, Thrane L et al. Optical coherence tomography imaging of psoriasis vulgaris: Correlation with histology and disease severity. *Archives of Dermatological Research.* Mar 2010;302(2):105–111.

130. Patel JK, Konda S, Perez OA, Amini S, Elgart G, Berman B. Newer technologies/techniques and tools in the diagnosis of melanoma. *European Journal of Dermatology.* Nov-Dec 2008;18(6):617–631.

131. Strasswimmer J, Pierce MC, Park BH, Neel V, de Boer JF. Polarization-sensitive optical coherence tomography of invasive basal cell carcinoma. *Journal of Biomedical Optics.* Mar-Apr 2004;9(2):292–298.

132. von Felbert V, Neis M, Megahed M, Spoler F. [Imaging of actinic porokeratosis by optical coherence tomography (OCT)]. *Hautarzt.* Nov 2008;59(11): 877–879.

133. Welzel J, Lankenau E, Birngruber R, Engelhardt R. Optical coherence tomography of the human skin. *Journal of the American Academy of Dermatology.* Dec 1997;37(6):958–963.

134. Piche E, Hafner HM, Hoffmann J, Junger M. [FOITS (fast optical *in vivo* topometry of human skin): New approaches to 3-D surface structures of human skin]. *Biomedizinische Technik. Biomedical Engineering.* Nov 2000;45(11):317–322.

135. Lang JM, Shennan M, Njauw JC et al. A flexible multiplex bead-based assay for detecting germline CDKN2A and CDK4 variants in melanoma-prone kindreds. *Journal of Investigative Dermatology.* Feb 2011;131(2):480–486.

136. Sharma S, Neale MH, Di Nicolantonio F et al. Outcome of ATP-based tumor chemosensitivity assay directed chemotherapy in heavily pre-treated recurrent ovarian carcinoma. *BMC Cancer.* Jul 3 2003;3:19.

137. Cree IA. Chemosensitivity testing as an aid to anti-cancer drug and regimen development. *Recent Results in Cancer Research. Fortschritte Der Krebsforschung. Progres Dans les recherches Sur le Cancer.* 2003;161:119–125.
138. Kurbacher CM, Cree IA. Chemosensitivity testing using microplate adenosine triphosphate-based luminescence measurements. *Methods in Molecular Medicine.* 2005;110:101–120.
139. Parker KA, Glaysher S, Polak M et al. The molecular basis of the chemosensitivity of metastatic cutaneous melanoma to chemotherapy. *Journal of Clinical Pathology.* Nov 2010;63(11):1012–1020.
140. Ugurel S, Tilgen W, Reinhold U. Chemosensitivity testing in malignant melanoma. *Recent Results in Cancer Research. Fortschritte Der Krebsforschung. Progres Dans Les Recherches sur le Cancer.* 2003;161:81–92.
141. Amiri H, Mahmoudi M, Lascialfari A. Superparamagnetic colloidal nanocrystal clusters coated with polyethylene glycol fumarate: A possible novel theranostic agent. *Nanoscale.* Mar 2011;3(3):1022–1030.
142. Caldorera-Moore ME, Liechty WB, Peppas NA. Responsive theranostic systems: Integration of diagnostic imaging agents and responsive controlled release drug delivery carriers. *Accounts of Chemical Research.* October 2011; 44(10):1061–1070.
143. Gittard SD, Miller PR, Boehm RD et al. Multiphoton microscopy of transdermal quantum dot delivery using two photon polymerization-fabricated polymer microneedles. *Faraday Discussions.* 2011;149:171–185; discussion 227–145.
144. Puri A, Blumenthal R. Polymeric lipid assemblies as novel theranostic tools. *Accounts of Chemical Research.* Sep 15 2011.
145. Yoo D, Lee JH, Shin TH, Cheon J. Theranostic magnetic nanoparticles. *Accounts of Chemical Research.* Aug 8 2011.
146. Lu W, Xiong C, Zhang G et al. Targeted photothermal ablation of murine melanomas with melanocyte-stimulating hormone analog-conjugated hollow gold nanospheres. *Clinical Cancer Research: An Official Journal of the American Association for Cancer Research.* Feb 1 2009;15(3):876–886.
147. Longo C, Gambara G, Espina V et al. A novel biomarker harvesting nanotechnology identifies Bak as a candidate melanoma biomarker in serum. *Experimental Dermatology.* Jan 2011;20(1):29–34.
148. Solassol J, Guillot B, Maudelonde T. [Circulating prognosis markers in melanoma: Proteomic profiling and clinical studies]. *Annales de Biologie Clinique.* Mar-Apr 2011;69(2):151–157.
149. Seki T, Fang J, Maeda H. Enhanced delivery of macromolecular antitumor drugs to tumors by nitroglycerin application. *Cancer Science.* Dec 2009;100(12): 2426–2430.
150. Bal SM, Kruithof AC, Zwier R et al. Influence of microneedle shape on the transport of a fluorescent dye into human skin in vivo. *Journal of Controled Release.* Oct 15 2010;147(2):218–224.
151. Donnelly RF, Morrow DI, Fay F et al. Microneedle-mediated intradermal nanoparticle delivery: Potential for enhanced local administration of hydrophobic pre-formed photosensitisers. *Photodiagnosis and Photodynamic Therapy.* Dec 2010;7(4):222–231.
152. Donnelly RF, Morrow DI, McCarron PA et al. Microneedle arrays permit enhanced intradermal delivery of a preformed photosensitizer. *Journal of Photochemistry and Photobiology.* Jan-Feb 2009;85(1):195–204.

153. Li X, Zhao R, Qin Z et al. Microneedle pretreatment improves efficacy of cutaneous topical anesthesia. *American Journal of Emergency Medicine.* Feb 2010;28(2):130–134.

154. Mikolajewska P, Donnelly RF, Garland MJ et al. Microneedle pre-treatment of human skin improves 5-aminolevulininc acid (ALA)- and 5-aminolevulinic acid methyl ester (MAL)-induced PpIX production for topical photodynamic therapy without increase in pain or erythema. *Pharmaceutical Research.* Oct 2010;27(10):2213–2220.

155. Song JM, Kim YC, Barlow PG et al. Improved protection against avian influenza H5N1 virus by a single vaccination with virus-like particles in skin using microneedles. *Antiviral Research.* Nov 2010;88(2):244–247.

156. Miller PR, Gittard SD, Edwards TL et al. Integrated carbon fiber electrodes within hollow polymer microneedles for transdermal electrochemical sensing. *Biomicrofluidics.* 2011;5(1):13415.

157. Kosoglu MA, Hood RL, Chen Y, Xu Y, Rylander MN, Rylander CG. Fiber optic microneedles for transdermal light delivery: Ex vivo porcine skin penetration experiments. *Journal of Biomechanical Engineering.* Sep 2010;132(9):091014.

158. Shapira O, Kuriki K, Orf ND et al. Surface-emitting fiber lasers. *Optics Express.* May 1 2006;14(9):3929–3935.

159. Chren M-M. Costs of therapy for dermatophyte infections. *Journal of the American Academy of Dermatology.* 1994;31(3, Part 2):S103–S106.

160. Arenas-Guzman R, Tosti A, Hay R, Haneke E. Pharmacoeconomics—an aid to better decision-making. *Journal of the European Academy of Dermatology and Venereology.* 2005;19:34–39.

161. Sobera JO, Elewski BE. Chapter 76–Fungal Diseases. In: Bolognia J, Jorizzo JL, Rapini RP, eds. *Dermatology.* London; New York: Mosby; 2003.

162. Adams BB. *Sports Dermatology.* New York, NY: Springer; 2006.

163. Mahendra R, Yadav A, Gade A. Silver nanoparticles as a new generation of anti-microbials. *Biotechnology Advances.* 2009;27:76–83.

164. Pal STY, Song JM. Does the antibacterial actiivty of silver nanoparticles depend on the shape of the nanoparticles? A study of the gram-negative bacterium *Escherechia coli. Applied and Environmental Microbiology.* 2007;27(6):1712–1720.

165. Sanpui P, Murugadoss A, Prasad PV, Ghosh SS, Chattopadhyay A. The antibac-terial properties of a novel chitosan-Ag-nanoparticle composite. *International Journal of Food Microbiology.* May 31 2008;124(2):142–146.

166. Ruparelia JP, Chatterjee AK, Duttagupta SP, Mukherji S. Strain specificity in antimicrobial activity of silver and copper nanoparticles. *Acta Biomaterialia.* May 2008;4(3):707–716.

167. Kim KJ, Sung WS, Suh BK et al. Antifungal activity and mode of action of silver nano-particles on Candida albicans. *Biometals.* Apr 2009;22(2):235–242.

168. Paulo CS, Vidal M, Ferreira LS. Antifungal nanoparticles and surfaces. *Biomacromolecules.* Oct 11 2010;11(10):2810–2817.

169. Panacek A, Kolar M, Vecerova R et al. Antifungal activity of silver nanoparticles against Candida spp. *Biomaterials.* Oct 2009;30(31):6333–6340.

170. Esteban-Tejeda L, Malpartida F, Esteban-Cubillo A, Pecharroman C, Moya JS. The antibacterial and antifungal activity of a soda-lime glass containing silver nanoparticles. *Nanotechnology.* Feb 2009;20(8).

171. Banergee M, Mallick S, Paul A, Chattopadhyay A, Ghosh S. Heightened reac-tive oxygen species generation in the antimicrobial activity of three component

iodinated chitosan-silver nanoparticle composite. *Langmuir.* 2010;26(8): 5901–5908.

172. Ma Y, Zhou T, Zhao C. Preparation of chitosan-nylon-6 blended membranes containing silver ions as antibacterial materials. *Carbohydrate Research.* Feb 4 2008;343(2):230–237.

173. Qi L, Xu Z, Jiang X, Hu C, Zou X. Preparation and antibacterial activity of chitosan nanoparticles. *Carbohydrate Research.* 2005;339:2693–2700.

174. Alburquenque C, Bucarey SA, Neira-Carrillo A, Urzua B, Hermosilla G, Tapia CV. Antifungal activity of low molecular weight chitosan against clinical isolates of Candida spp. *Medical Mycology.* Dec 2010;48(8):1018–1023.

175. Albasarah YY, Somavarapu S, Stapleton P, Taylor KMG. Chitosan-coated antifungal formulations for nebulisation. *Journal of Pharmacy and Pharmacology.* Jul 2010;62(7):821–828.

176. Li RC, Guo ZY, Jiang PA. Synthesis, characterization, and antifungal activity of novel quaternary chitosan derivatives. *Carbohydrate Research.* Sep 2010;345(13):1896–1900.

177. Kulikov SN, Tiurin Iu A, Fassakhov RS, Varlamov VP. [Antibacterial and antimycotic activity of chitosan: Mechanisms of action and role of the structure]. *Zhurnal mikrobiologii, epidemiologii, i immunobiologii.* Sep-Oct 2009(5):91–97.

178. Kwak S, H. KS. Hybrid Organic/Inorganic reverse osmosis (RO) membrane for bactericidal anti-fouling. 1. Preparation and characterization of TiO nanoparticle self-assembled aromatic polyamide thin-film-composite (TFC) membrane. *Environmental Science and Technology.* 2001;35(11):2388–2394.

179. Kim SH, Kwak S, Sohn B, Park TH. Design of TiO$_2$ nanoparticle self-assembled aromatic polyamide thin-film-composite (TFC) membrane as an approach to solve biofouling problem. *Journal of Membrane Science.* 2003;211:157–165.

180. Martinez-Gutierrez F, Olive PL, Banuelos A et al. Synthesis, characterization, and evaluation of antimicrobial and cytotoxic effect of silver and titanium nanoparticles. *Nanomedicine.* Oct 2010;6(5):681–688.

181. Karthikeyan R, Amaechi BT, Rawls HR, Lee VA. Antimicrobial activity of nanoemulsion on cariogenic Streptococcus mutans. *Archives of Oral Biology.* May 2011;56(5):437–445.

182. Ziani K, Chang YH, McLandsborough L, McClements DJ. Influence of surfactant charge on antimicrobial efficacy of surfactant-stabilized thyme oil nanoemulsions. *Journal of Agricultural and Food Chemistry.* Jun 2011;59(11):6247–6255.

183. Hemmila MR, Mattar A, Taddonio MA et al. Topical nanoemulsion therapy reduces bacterial wound infection and inflammation after burn injury. *Surgery.* Sep 2010;148(3):499–509.

184. Ciotti S, Eisma R, Ma L, Baker JR. In-vitro skin penetration of novel antimicrobial nanoemulsion formulations containing antifungal agents. *Journal of Investigative Dermatology.* Apr 2009;129:S78–S78.

185. Fothergill AW, McCarthy DI, Sutcliffe JA, Rinaldi MG. Antifungal activity of NB-002 a topical nanoemulsion, against rare fungal pathogens of onychomycosis. *Journal of the American Academy of Dermatology.* Mar 2009;60(3): AB117–AB117.

186. Jones T, Ijzerman M, Flack M. A randomized, double-blind, vehicle-controlled trial of a novel topical antifungal nanoemulsion (NB-002) in subjects with distal subungual onychomycosis. *Journal of the American Academy of Dermatology.* Mar 2009;60(3):AB102-AB102.

187. McCarthy A, Pannu J, Ciotti S, Hamouda T, Sutcliffe J, Baker JR. Antimicrobial activity of nanoemulsion against clinical isolates from cystic fibrosis patients. (Poster) 23th North American Cystic Fibrosis Conference, abstr. 364. Minneapolis, MN.

188. Pengon S, Limmatvapirat C, Limmatvapirat S. Preparation and evaluation of antimicrobial nanoemulsion containing herbal extracts. *Drug Metabolism Reviews.* Aug 2009;41:85–85.

189. Hamouda T, Flack M, Baker J. Development of a novel topically applied antifungal agent (NB-002) based on nanoemulsion technology. *Journal of the American Academy of Dermatology.* Feb 2008;58(2):AB90–AB90.

190. Teixeira PC, Leite GM, Domingues RJ, Silva J, Gibbs PA, Ferreira JP. Antimicrobial effects of a microemulsion and a nanoemulsion on enteric and other pathogens and biofilms. *International Journal of Food Microbiology.* Aug 2007;118(1):15–19.

191. Hamouda T, Myc A, Donovan B, Shih AY, Reuter JD, Baker JR. A novel surfactant nanoemulsion with a unique non-irritant topical antimicrobial activity against bacteria, enveloped viruses and fungi. *Microbiological Research.* 2001;156(1):1–7.

192. Hamouda T, Hayes MM, Cao ZY et al. A novel surfactant nanoemulsion with broad-spectrum sporicidal activity against Bacillus species. *Journal of Infectious Diseases.* Dec 1999;180(6):1939–1949.

193. Pannu J, McCarthy A, Martin A et al. NB-002, a Novel nanoemulsion with broad antifungal activity against dermatophytes, other filamentous fungi, and Candida albicans. *Antimicrobial Agents and Chemotherapy.* Aug 2009;53(8):3273–3279.

194. Pannu J, Sutcliffe J, Ma LF, Ciotti S. Antifungal activity and mechanism of action of NB-002, a novel topical antifungal, against the major pathogens of onychomycosis. *Journal of the American Academy of Dermatology.* Mar 2009;60(3):AB114–AB114.

195. Jones T, Flack M, Ijzerman M, Baker J. Safety, tolerance, and pharmacokinetics of topical nanoemulsion (NB-002) for the treatment of onychomycosis. *Journal of the American Academy of Dermatology.* Feb 2008;58(2):AB83–AB83.

196. Ijzerman M, Baker J, Flack M, Robinson P. Efficacy of topical nanoemulsion (NB-002) for the treatment of distal subungual onychomycosis: A randomized, double-blind, vehicle-controlled trial. *Journal of the American Academy of Dermatology.* Mar 2010;62(3):AB76–AB76.

197. Shim YH, Kim YC, Lee HJ et al. Amphotericin B aggregation inhibition with novel nanoparticles prepared with poly(epsilon-caprolactone)/poly(n,n-dimethylamino-2-ethyl methacrylate) diblock copolymer. *Journal of Microbiology and Biotechnology.* Jan 2011;21(1):28–36.

198. Sheikh S, Ali SM, Ahmad MU et al. Nanosomal Amphotericin B is an efficacious alternative to Ambisome for fungal therapy. *International Journal of Pharmaceutics.* Sep 15 2010;397(1–2):103–108.

199. Burgess BL, Cavigiolio G, Fannucchi MV, Illek B, Forte TM, Oda MN. A phospholipid-apolipoprotein A-I nanoparticle containing amphotericin B as a drug delivery platform with cell membrane protective properties. *International Journal of Pharmaceutics.* Oct 2010;399(1–2):148–155.

200. Shao K, Huang RQ, Li JF et al. Angiopep-2 modified PE-PEG based polymeric micelles for amphotericin B delivery targeted to the brain. *Journal of Controlled Release.* Oct 2010;147(1):118–126.

201. Jung SH, Lim DH, Lee JE, Jeong KS, Seong H, Shin BC. Amphotericin B-entrapping lipid nanoparticles and their *in vitro* and *in vivo* characteristics. *European Journal of Pharmaceutical Sciences*. Jun 28 2009;37(3–4):313–320.

202. Amaral AC, Bocca AL, Ribeiro AM et al. Amphotericin B in poly(lactic-co-glycolic acid) (PLGA) and dimercaptosuccinic acid (DMSA) nanoparticles against paracoccidioidomycosis. *Journal of Antimicrobial Chemotherapy*. Mar 2009;63(3): 526–533.

203. Fukui H, Koike T, Saheki A, Sonoke S, Tomii Y, Seki J. Evaluation of the efficacy and toxicity of amphotericin B incorporated in lipid nano-sphere (LNS (R)). *International Journal of Pharmaceutics*. Sep 2003;263(1–2):51–60.

204. Ritter J. Amphotericin B and its lipid formulations. *Mycoses*. 2002;45:34–38.

205. Bekersky I, Boswell GW, Hiles R, Fielding RM, Buell D, Walsh TJ. Safety, toxicokinetics and tissue distribution of long-term intravenous liposomal amphotericin B (AmBisome (R)): A 91-day study in rats. *Pharmaceutical Research*. Dec 2000;17(12):1494–1502.

206. Bekersky I, Boswell GW, Hiles R, Fielding RM, Buell D, Walsh TJ. Safety and toxicokinetics of intravenous liposomal amphotericin B (AmBisome (R)) in beagle dogs. *Pharmaceutical Research*. Nov 1999;16(11):1694–1701.

207. Johnson EM, Ojwang JO, Szekely A, Wallace TL, Warnock DW. Comparison of *in vitro* antifungal activities of free and liposome-encapsulated nystatin with those of four amphotericin B formulations. *Antimicrobial Agents and Chemotherapy*. Jun 1998;42(6):1412–1416.

208. Gulati M, Bajad S, Singh S, Ferdous AJ, Singh M. Development of liposomal amphotericin B formulation. *Journal of Microencapsulation*. Mar-Apr 1998;15(2):137–151.

209. Hiemenz JW, Walsh TJ. Lipid formulations of amphotericin B. *Journal of Liposome Research*. 1998;8(4):443–467.

210. Hillery AM. Supramolecular lipidic drug delivery systems: From laboratory to clinic—A review of the recently introduced commercial liposomal and lipid-based formulations of Amphotericin B. *Advanced Drug Delivery Reviews*. Mar 17 1997;24(2–3):345–363.

211. Anstey NM, Stewart LM, Packard M, Graney WF, Bartlett JA. Open-label titration study of the safety of RMP-7 in patients with the acquired immune deficiency syndrome. *International Journal of Antimicrobial Agents*. Apr 1996;6(4): 183–187.

212. Joly V, Farinotti R, Saintjulien L, Cheron M, Carbon C, Yeni P. In-vitro renal toxicity and in-vivo therapeutic efficacy in experimental murine cryptococcosis of amphotericin-b (fungizone) associated with intralipid. *Antimicrobial Agents and Chemotherapy*. Feb 1994;38(2):177–183.

213. Bekersky I, Fielding RM, Buell D, Lawrence I. Lipid-based amphotericin B formulations: From animals to man. *Pharmaceutical Science & Technology Today*. Jun 1999;2(6):230–236.

214. Gelfand JM, Weinstein R, Porter SB, Neimann AL, Berlin JA, Margolis DJ. Prevalence and Treatment of Psoriasis in the United Kingdom: A Population-Based Study. *Archives of Dermatology*. December 1, 2005;141(12):1537–1541.

215. Gelfand JM, Stern RS, Nijsten T et al. The prevalence of psoriasis in African Americans: Results from a population-based study. *Journal of the American Academy of Dermatology*. 2005;52(1):23–26.

216. Yip SY. The prevalence of psoriasis in the Mongoloid race. *Journal of the American Academy of Dermatology.* 1984;10(6):965–968.
217. Ferrándiz C, Pujol RM, García-Patos V, Bordas X, Smandía JA. Psoriasis of early and late onset: A clinical and epidemiologic study from Spain. *Journal of the American Academy of Dermatology.* 2002;46(6):867–873.
218. Duffy DL, Spelman LS, Martin NG. Psoriasis in Australian twins. *Journal of the American Academy of Dermatology.* 1993;29(3):428–434.
219. Griffiths CEM, Barker JNWN. Psoriasis. *Rook's Textbook of Dermatology:* Wiley-Blackwell; 2010:1–89.
220. Al Robaee AA. Molecular genetics of Psoriasis (Principles, technology, gene location, genetic polymorphism and gene expression). *International Journal of Health Sciences.* Nov 2010;4(2):103–127.
221. Aydin SZ, Ash Z, Del Galdo F et al. Optical coherence tomography: A new tool to assess nail disease in psoriasis? *Dermatology.* 2011;222(4):311–313.
222. D'Elios MM, Del Prete G, Amedei A. Targeting IL-23 in human diseases. *Expert Opinion on Therapeutic Targets.* Jul 2010;14(7):759–774.
223. Duffin KC, Krueger GG. Genetic variations in cytokines and cytokine receptors associated with psoriasis found by genome-wide association. *Journal of Investigative Dermatology.* Apr 2009;129(4):827–833.
224. Elder JT. Genome-wide association scan yields new insights into the immunopathogenesis of psoriasis. *Genes and Immunity.* Apr 2009;10(3):201–209.
225. Guttman-Yassky E, Lowes MA, Fuentes-Duculan J et al. Low expression of the IL-23/Th17 pathway in atopic dermatitis compared to psoriasis. *Journal of Immunology.* Nov 15 2008;181(10):7420–7427.
226. Kagami S, Rizzo HL, Lee JJ, Koguchi Y, Blauvelt A. Circulating Th17, Th22, and Th1 cells are increased in psoriasis. *Journal of Investigative Dermatology.* May 2010;130(5):1373–1383.
227. Tokura Y, Mori T, Hino R. Psoriasis and other Th17-mediated skin diseases. *Journal of UOEH.* Dec 1 2010;32(4):317–328.
228. Strange A, Capon F, Spencer CC et al. A genome-wide association study identifies new psoriasis susceptibility loci and an interaction between HLA-C and ERAP1. *Nature Genetics.* Nov 2010;42(11):985–990.
229. van Kuijk AW, DeGroot J, Koeman RC et al. Soluble biomarkers of cartilage and bone metabolism in early proof of concept trials in psoriatic arthritis: Effects of adalimumab versus placebo. *PLoS One.* 2010;5(9).
230. Baspinar Y, Keck CM, Borchert HH. Development of a positively charged prednicarbate nanoemulsion. *International Journal of Pharmaceutics.* Jan 4 2010;383(1–2):201–208.
231. Hofkens W, van den Hoven JM, Pesman GJ et al. Safety of glucocorticoids can be improved by lower yet still effective dosages of liposomal steroid formulations in murine antigen-induced arthritis: Comparison of prednisolone with budesonide. *International Journal of Pharmaceutics.* Sep 20 2011;416(2):493–498.
232. Zhang J, Smith E. Percutaneous permeation of betamethasone 17-valerate incorporated in lipid nanoparticles. *Journal of Pharmaceutical Sciences.* Mar 2011;100(3):896–903.
233. Kim ST, Jang DJ, Kim JH et al. Topical administration of cyclosporin A in a solid lipid nanoparticle formulation. *Pharmazie.* Aug 2009;64(8):510–514.

234. Barker JN. Methotrexate or fumarates: Which is the best oral treatment for psoriasis? *British Journal of Dermatology.* Apr 2011;164(4):695.
235. Concannon C, Hennelly DA, Noott S, Sarker DK. Nanoemulsion encapsulation and *in vitro* SLN models of delivery for cytotoxic methotrexate. *Current Drug Discovery Technologies.* Jun 1 2010;7(2):123–136.
236. Lin YK, Huang ZR, Zhuo RZ, Fang JY. Combination of calcipotriol and methotrexate in nanostructured lipid carriers for topical delivery. *International Journal of Nanomedicine.* 2010;5:117–128.
237. Majoros IJ, Williams CR, Becker A, Baker JR, Jr. Methotrexate delivery via folate targeted dendrimer-based nanotherapeutic platform. *Wiley Interdisciplinary Reviews. Nanomedicine and Nanobiotechnology.* Sep-Oct 2009;1(5):502–510.
238. Mukesh U, Kulkarni V, Tushar R, Murthy RS. Methotrexate loaded self stabilized calcium phosphate nanoparticles: A novel inorganic carrier for intracellular drug delivery. *Journal of Biomedical Nanotechnology.* Feb 2009;5(1):99–105.
239. Paliwal R, Rai S, Vyas SP. Lipid drug conjugate (LDC) nanoparticles as autolymphotrophs for oral delivery of methotrexate. *Journal of Biomedical Nanotechnology.* Feb 2011;7(1):130–131.
240. Singka GS, Samah NA, Zulfakar MH, Yurdasiper A, Heard CM. Enhanced topical delivery and anti-inflammatory activity of methotrexate from an activated nanogel. *European Journal of Pharmaceutics and Biopharmaceutics.* Oct 2010;76(2):275–281.
241. Luo J, Wu SJ, Lacy ER et al. Structural basis for the dual recognition of IL-12 and IL-23 by ustekinumab. *Journal of Molecular Biology.* Oct 8 2010;402(5):797–812.
242. Sobell JM, Kalb RE, Weinberg JM. Management of moderate to severe plaque psoriasis (part 2): Clinical update on T-cell modulators and investigational agents. *Journal of Drugs in Dermatology.* Mar 2009;8(3):230–238.
243. Benson JM, Sachs CW, Treacy G et al. Therapeutic targeting of the IL-12/23 pathways: Generation and characterization of ustekinumab. *Nature Biotechnology.* Jul 2011;29(7):615–624.
244. Ayroldi E, Bastianelli A, Cannarile L, Petrillo MG, Delfino DV, Fierabracci A. A Pathogenetic Approach to autoimmune skin disease therapy: Psoriasis and biological drugs, unresolved issues, and future directions. *Current Pharmaceutical Design.* Aug 25 2011.
245. Raval K, Lofland JH, Waters H, Piech CT. Disease and treatment burden of psoriasis: Examining the impact of biologics. *Journal of Drugs in Dermatology.* Feb 2011;10(2):189–196.
246. Reich AK, Burden AD, Eaton JN, Hawkins NS. Efficacy of biologics in the treatment of moderate to severe psoriasis: A network meta-analysis of randomised controlled trials. *British Journal of Dermatology.* 2012;166(1):179–188.
247. Bak RO, Mikkelsen JG. Regulation of cytokines by small RNAs during skin inflammation. *Journal of Biomedical Science.* 2010;17:53.
248. Leng RX, Pan HF, Tao JH, Ye DQ. IL-19, IL-20 and IL-24: Potential therapeutic targets for autoimmune diseases. *Expert Opinion on Therapeutic Targets.* Feb 2011;15(2):119–126.
249. Sun BK, Tsao H. Small RNAs in development and disease. *Journal of the American Academy of Dermatology.* Nov 2008;59(5):725–737; quiz 738–740.
250. Watt SA, Pourreyron C, Purdie K et al. Integrative mRNA profiling comparing cultured primary cells with clinical samples reveals PLK1 and C20orf20 as therapeutic targets in cutaneous squamous cell carcinoma. *Oncogene.* 2011;30(46):4666–4677.

251. Xu N, Brodin P, Wei T et al. MiR-125b, a microRNA downregulated in psoriasis, modulates keratinocyte proliferation by targeting FGFR2. *The Journal of Investigative Dermatology.* Jul 2011;131(7):1521–1529.

252. Alam MR, Ming X, Fisher M et al. Multivalent cyclic RGD conjugates for targeted delivery of small interfering RNA. *Bioconjugate Chemistry.* Aug 17 2011;22(8):1673–1681.

253. Davis ME, Zuckerman JE, Choi CH et al. Evidence of RNAi in humans from systemically administered siRNA via targeted nanoparticles. *Nature.* Apr 15 2010;464(7291):1067–1070.

254. Al-Hoqail IA. Personalized medicine in psoriasis: Concept and applications. *Current Vascular Pharmacology.* May 1 2010;8(3):432–436.

255. Woolf RT, Smith CH. How genetic variation affects patient response and outcome to therapy for psoriasis. *Expert Review of Clinical Immunology.* Nov 2010;6(6):957–966.

256. Galasso M, Elena Sana M, Volinia S. Non-coding RNAs: A key to future personalized molecular therapy? *Genome Medicine.* 2010;2(2):12.

257. Warren RB, Smith RL, Campalani E et al. Genetic variation in efflux transporters influences outcome to methotrexate therapy in patients with psoriasis. *The Journal of Investigative Dermatology.* Aug 2008;128(8):1925–1929.

258. Nasir A, Friedman A. Nanotechnology and the Nanodermatology Society. *Journal of Drugs in Dermatology.* Jul 2010;9(7):879–882.

259. Zippin JH, Friedman A. Nanotechnology in Cosmetics and Sunscreens: An Update. *Journal of Drugs in Dermatology.* Oct 2009;8(10):955–958.

260. Burnett ME, Wang SQ. Current sunscreen controversies: A critical review. *Photodermatology Photoimmunology & Photomedicine.* Apr 2011;27(2):58–67.

261. Berwick M. The Good, the Bad, and the Ugly of Sunscreens. *Clinical Pharmacology & Therapeutics.* Jan 2011;89(1):31–33.

262. EWG. Skin Deep Cosmetic Safety Database: Nanotechnology—Summary. 2010. http://www.cosmeticsdatabase.com/special/sunscreens/nanotech.php.

263. Faunce T, Murray, K., Nasu, H., Bowman, D. Sunscreen Safety: The precautionary principle, the Australian therapeutic goods administration and nanoparticles in sunscreens. *Nanoethics.* 2008;2:231–241.

264. TGA. A review of the scientific literature on the safety of nanoparticulate titanium dioxide or zinc oxide in sunscreens. *Australian Therapeutic Goods Administration.* http://www.tga.gov.au/pdf/sunscreens-nanoparticles-2009.pdf.

6

Nanoparticles for Drug Delivery of Small Molecules

Ana Sofia Macedo and Eliana B. Souto

CONTENTS

6.1 Introduction 131
6.2 Gene Delivery 133
6.3 Vaccine Delivery and Adjuvant 136
6.4 Conclusion 139
Acknowledgment 140
References... 140

6.1 Introduction

Nanotechnology has been applied in the field of medicine—the so-called nanomedicine, bringing along increased expectations for the improvement of healthcare. Nanomedicine aims to treat, prevent, and diagnose several diseases (e.g., cancer) and traumatic injuries. The basic principle behind this technology is the application of nanoscale particles that vary from a few nanometers to hundreds of nanometers in size to deliver drugs to specific target sites. Their small size allows them to cross biological barriers, such as tissues, cells, and organelles, as nanoparticles are engineered to have similar size and structure to biological molecules (Husseini and Pitt, 2008). It is thought that the particle size is determinant for particle uptake. Thus, those particles smaller than 200 nm suffer uptake by unspecialized cells, whereas particles smaller than 35 nm may enter the nucleus, and particles smaller than 30 nm are able to reach the central nervous system (CNS) via olfactory neuronal transport (Salvati et al., 2011). Small molecules reach the organs and cellular compartments, according to equilibrium principles. Therefore, small molecules that are used routinely (e.g., chemotherapeutic agents for cancer therapy) have limited clinical use due to low water solubility, nonspecific biodistribution, and targeting, which results in low therapeutic indices. In addition, the risk of drug resistance shortly after the treatment, not only decreases the efficacy of the conventional drug but also decreases the therapeutic efficacy of a newer targeted drug (Zhuo, 2010). However, nanoparticles are processed by cellular machinery and are trafficked by active processes, similar to drug biomolecules (Salvati et al., 2011). Nanoparticles for drug delivery should be physicochemically stable, have a high loading capacity, be able to incorporate both hydrophilic and hydrophobic drug molecules, and be feasible for several administration routes (e.g., oral, parenteral, nasal, and topical). Moreover, the advantages of nanoparticles go well beyond targeted delivery, since they also allow sustained drug release from the matrix, which results in the improvement of bioavailability, lower dosing frequency, and less side effects, ultimately resulting in better patient compliance (Fadeel and Garcia-Bennett, 2010).

In spite of the advantages of using nanoparticles as drug delivery systems, there are still safety issues that must be taken into account. The ultimate fate of nanoparticles after degradation and excretion is still not well understood, and neither is the potential release of degradation products that might cause toxicity (Fadeel and Garcia-Bennett, 2010).

Efforts have been focused on the targeting of specific disease sites to deliver the drugs. The target can be an organ, tissue, cell, or intracellular. In intracellular targeting, the drugs exert their pharmacological action on cellular organelles, and cellular uptake must take place to generate a therapeutic effect. The complexity of cellular compartments, uptake, and trafficking pathways compromise the success of pharmacological effect and may cause undesired exposure of the additional organelles (Choi et al., 2012, Sneh-Edri and Stepensky, 2011).

Cellular uptake begins with endocytosis. The endocytosis may occur by phagocytosis (i.e., when large particles are internalized) and by pinocytosis (i.e., when there is an uptake of fluids and solutes). Phagocytosis is very common in mammalian cells such as macrophages, which have a specialized endocytic receptor in the cell surface. The process begins with binding of macromolecules to the cell receptor in the plasma membrane, the clathrin-coated pits. These molecules are transformed into mildly acidic (pH 5.0–6.5) vesicles called endosomes that later fuse with more mature endosomes or lysosomes. Once in the lysosomes, they face lower pH and enzymatic degradation. One can take advantage of drug uptake and accumulation in lysosomes to address lysosomal disorders, such as lysosomal metabolic disorders and infections (Breunig et al., 2008, Hild et al., 2008).

However, the administration of macromolecules such as peptides, proteins, DNAzymes, and small interfering RNA (siRNA) suffers some limitations, since these molecules are only active after being released into the cytosol. Knowing that endocytosis is the first step of cellular uptake, most of these molecules accumulate in the endosomal and lysosomal compartments, and consequently lose their pharmacological effect (Breunig et al., 2008, Hild et al., 2008).

Several drug delivery systems have been proposed to overcome endosomal degradation, such as pH-responsive polymeric nanoparticles, fusogenic peptides, cell-penetrating peptides, and pH-responsive liposomes and micelles (Breunig et al., 2008).

Some polymers, for example, polyethylenimine (PEI) have the ability to escape endolysosomal activity by destroying the endolysosomal complex. PEI's endosomolytic effect is due to its ability to buffer the endolysosomal vesicle environment, causing osmotic swelling of the vesicle and consequent rupture (Breunig et al., 2008). A DNA/PEI complex, for instance, can be released into the cytoplasm without suffering endolysosomal degradation. Yang et al. (2006) used poly(2-hydroxyethyl aspartamide) (PHEA) as the polymer to which they attached histidine (His) by an esteric linkage to load with doxorubicin (DOX). Histidine acts as an endosomolytic agent. The authors reported by confocal microscopy that after 8 h of incubation, PHEA-g-C18-His was more uniformly distributed in HeLa cells than PHEA-g-C18, which was endorsed to the endolysomolytic activity of histidine. The DOX released from PHEA-g-C18-His was faster at pH 5, possibly enabling the access of DOX to HeLa cellular nucleus.

Gillies and Fréchet (2005) have also attempted to deliver DOX using polyethylene (PEG) dendrimer-based micelles, which are pH-sensitive. To develop pH-sensitive micelles, they attached hydrophobic groups to the dendrimer periphery by acetal linkage. When the acetal linkage hydrolysis occurs, the core-forming block becomes hydrophilic, thereby causing destabilization of the micelle and drug release (Gillies et al., 2004, Gillies and Fréchet, 2005).

In some studies, nanoparticles based on hydrophobically modified glycol chitosan (hydrophobic chitosan glycol [HCG]) have been reported to address the poor efficacy of passive-targeting systems in the treatment of tumors. A chitosan-based system conjugated with interleukin 4 receptor (I4R) was linked to an interleukin-4 (IL-4) receptor-binding peptide. The study showed that HCG-I4R nanoparticles yielded higher cellular uptake in tumors when compared to HCG nanoparticles, thus increasing the pharmacological effect (Kim et al., 2012).

Recently, PEG liposomes were produced as a drug delivery system for solid tumors, which were able to target the tumor cells by attaching transferrin to their surface (Kazuo, 2011). Transferrin–PEG liposomes remained in the blood circulation and maintained anticancer drugs in interstitial space for a long period of time, releasing the drug into the cytoplasm of tumor cells by transferrin receptor-mediated endocytosis (Kazuo, 2011).

6.2 Gene Delivery

Gene therapy is still underexploited, in spite of its great potential. In gene therapy, a gene is delivered to a specific targeted patient's tissue or cell. Once there, the encoded gene in the form of oligonucleotides or plasmid will induce the expression of proteins, or the encoded gene in the form of antisense oligonulceotides or siRNA will silence the expression of the target genes (Jayakumar et al., 2010, Liu et al., 2010, Xu et al., 2011).

Many attempts have been made to develop a gene delivery product to treat many diseases, such as cancer, acquired immunodeficiency syndrome (AIDS), cardiovascular diseases, inflammation, diabetes, cystic fibrosis, deaminase deficiency, and Parkinson's disease. However, until now there are no approved products by the regulatory authorities. The only exception is Gendicine®, a sole virus-based system only available in China. The lack of successful gene delivery systems in the market is due to the inability to produce safe and efficient delivery systems and absence of sustained gene expression after administration (Giger et al., 2011, Jayakumar et al., 2010). The major difficulty in the outcome from the cells is the ineffective crossing of the plasma membrane by nucleic acids, due to their hydrophilic polyanionic nature and high molecular weight. Within the cell, the nucleic acids must avoid destruction and elimination processes in the endosome and be transported to the nucleus. Degradation by serum nucleases is an obstacle to be overcome for a successful delivery system (Jayakumar et al., 2010, Liu et al., 2010). Consequently, a perfect carrier for gene delivery should protect the deoxyribonucleic acid (DNA) until it reaches the target site and carries the DNA without causing toxicity reactions and immune response. The transport of exogenous genes can be reached using viral and nonviral systems and naked DNA. Naked DNA (Figure 6.1) is unsuitable for systemic administration, since it is rapidly eliminated by serum nucleases. Furthermore, genetic expression is very low when naked DNA is used (del Pozo-Rodríguez et al., 2010). Viral systems (Figure 6.1) provide high transfection rate; however, they lack in target specificity and in their ability to incorporate foreign DNA sequences into their genome. Beyond that, they have high toxicological risk and may cause inflammatory reactions, inducing immune responses and potential oncogenic effects. Viral vectors mainly used nowadays are retroviruses, herpes simplex virus, lentivirus, adenovirus, and adeno-associated

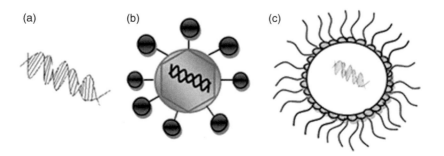

FIGURE 6.1
Representation of viral and nonviral vectors for DNA transfection: naked DNA (a), herpes simplex virus (b), and PEGylated nanoparticle (c).

virus (Jayakumar et al., 2010). Nonviral gene (Figure 6.1) delivery systems have raised growing interest since they can overcome some of the drawbacks pointed out for viral vectors, because they are safer, of low cost, and not constricted to DNA size. Despite their safety profile improvement, the transfection efficiency of nonviral systems is significantly lower when compared to viral systems, especially *in vivo*. In addition, gene delivery carriers are very toxic owing to their polycationic carrier nature, which limits their clinical application (Liu et al., 2010, Xu et al., 2011).

An ideal nonviral gene delivery system must have extensive uptake by the targeting spot, without affecting the surrounding tissues. The level of gene expression should be high enough to achieve noticeable phenotypic expression without causing toxicity. Furthermore, the phenotypic expression should persist during a lifetime in the treatment of chronic diseases and not suffer degeneration, as well as being feasible to administer through a noninvasive route. Ultimately, the ideal nonviral vector must not cause significant immune response, be well tolerated, and not cause any other adverse physiological side effects (Conley and Naash, 2010).

Most of nonviral systems are composed of cationic peptides, cationic polymers, or cationic lipids; however, blending a few of them is also feasible (Table 6.1). Lately, there has been a rising interest in cationic lipids to carry genes, which are regarded as immunologically inert and potential safety *in vivo* when compared to viral vectors (del Pozo-Rodríguez et al., 2010, Wasungu and Hoekstra, 2006). Cationic lipids are amphiphilic molecules, with a hydrophilic head group and a hydrophobic region. Geometry is an important property of cationic lipids that must be taken into account when the goal is to develop a gene delivery system. Like any amphiphilic molecule, cationic lipids can adopt several structural phases when they are suspended in an aqueous media, which might be micellar, lamellar, cubic, and inverted hexagonal phases (Wasungu and Hoekstra, 2006). Owing to the positive charge of cationic lipids, these molecules interact with cell surfaces and are internalized via endocytosis. Furthermore, cationic lipids self-assemble with DNA and form particles that are suitable for cellular uptake (Mark, 2002). In Table 6.2 are summarized the most important aspects of gene delivery nanosystems.

TABLE 6.1

Examples of Some Carriers Used to Deliver Genes

Nanoparticle Matrix		Drug/Gene	References
Polysaccharide	Chitosan	DNA	Gan et al. (2005)
Polymer	PGLA/PGA	DNA	Zou et al. (2009)
	PVA	DNA	Kimura et al. (2004)
Lipid	Steric acid and	DNA	Vighi et al. (2010)
	stearylamine	p53 tumor	Choi et al. (2012)
	DOPE and DC–Chol	suppressing gene	
Layered double hydroxides		DNA	Ladewig et al. (2010)

TABLE 6.2

Summary of Most Important Aspects of Gene Delivery

- Genes must be specifically delivered into a tissue or cell, without affecting the vicinity
- Genes will express or silence the expression of proteins
- Main drawbacks associated with genetic therapy are inefficient transfection and absence of expression
- Nonviral systems yield most of advantages such as improved safety and low toxicity, and they are not constricted by drug size
- Nonviral systems should have large uptake by the tissue of interest, not cause immune response and be preferentially administered by a noninvasive route
- Most systems used to produce/formulate nanoparticles are composed of cationic peptides, cationic polymers, or cationic lipids

---

Giger et al. (2011) successfully synthesized calcium phosphate–DNA nanoparticles coated with biphosphonate derivatives for DNA transfection. Their study showed that the nanoparticles were stable over time, providing efficient transfection and low toxicity. Solid lipid nanoparticles (SLN) are nanoparticles whose matrixes are made of solid lipid at both body and room temperatures, they are biodegradable, biocompatible, and present a low risk of toxicity reactions. Its many advantages have been extensively described elsewhere (Müller et al., 2000).

Del Pozo-Rodríguez et al. (2010) developed a solid lipid SLN–DNA system to deliver CMS plasmid labeled with a fluorescent marker termed EGFP. After successful transfection, results showed that the foreign protein was expressed in both the liver and spleen in mice, and was maintained for at least 7 days.

6.3 Vaccine Delivery and Adjuvant

Vaccines have been used for several years for the treatment and control of several infections and it is essential to develop innovative vaccine formulations to address deadly diseases, such as malaria, AIDS, cancer, and many others (Ho et al., 2011).

The first vaccines developed enclosed live attenuated or inactivated pathogens, which hold the disadvantage of severe side effects like inflammation, and in some cases, the pathogen reversed to its virulent form; for these reasons, second-generation vaccines rapidly emerged (Ho et al., 2011, Lambert and Laurent, 2008).

The second generation of developed vaccines enclosed pathogen subunits, such as protein antigens or recombinant protein components. The main advantages of these particles are their safety, reproducibility, and purity. Even so, these vaccines still require immune-stimulating agents to attain an effective immune response by the stimulation of presenting antigen cells.

To achieve a successful immunogenicity, an antigen must be released in a sustained manner, so that the interaction between the antigen and immune cells is extended for a period of time. Furthermore, the sustained release of antigen may in fact enable the immunization, as well as eliminate the need for booster immunizations. Furthermore, soluble antigens or antigen fragments often have weak immunogenicity and provide little protection. For these reasons, nanoparticles have been sought out as feasible vehicles for the delivery of antigens (Jain et al., 2009, Gordon et al., 2010).

Small-sized nanoparticles (20–200 nm) are feasible to high intracellular uptake, whereas antigens can be attached onto the nanoparticle surface. The intracellular uptake occurs by endocytosis. By attaching antigens onto the nanoparticle surface, CD4 and CD8 T-cells and antibody production are elicited (Ho et al., 2011).

This particle range is preferentially taken up by the modulators and initiators of immune response, the dendritic cells. These cells assist in the activation of major histocompatibility complex I and II pathways to process antigens. Interestingly, smaller particles (40–50 nm) in diameter induce exacerbated responses by CD8 T-cell and Th-1 cells, while Th-2 responses are stimulated by submicron particle size. On the other hand, larger particles of 0.5–5 µm are internalized via phagocytosis by macrophages (Ho et al., 2011).

Nanosystems have been sought out as feasible vehicles to deliver vaccines, especially through oral and mucosal routes. Oral administration is the route of choice for the administration of many drugs because of its easy access and noninvasive nature. In addition, there is no discomfort or pain associated with the administration and has very decreased risk of contamination when compared to the parenteral route (des Rieux et al., 2006). Nevertheless, to be effective, bioactive drugs must overcome the hostile environment of the gastrointestinal tract and remain in the intestinal lumen to adhere to cells and be transcytosed by intestinal cells. In this scenario, proteins and peptides administered orally have low bioavailability because of their low mucosal permeability and stability in the gastrointestinal tract, which results in the elimination of the compounds. To obtain effective immunization, the vaccine must be encapsulated in a carrier to allow absorption without losing its activity (des Rieux et al., 2006).

The intestinal epithelium is composed of different types of cells and structures. The first barrier to overcome is the villus. Villi epithelium is composed of enterocytes and goblet cells. Enterocytes are involved in the absorption of nutrients and prevent the passage of macromolecules and pathogens (Buda et al., 2005). Goblet cells secrete mucins, highly glycosylated proteins that form a viscous fluid. Lymphoid nodules called O-MALT (organized mucosa associated lymphoid tissue) are dispersed through the intestinal mucosa, both individually or combined with Peyer's patches. In the Peyer's patches are located macro-fold cells (M-cells). M-cells are responsible for the delivery of foreign molecules from the lumen to the underlying organized mucosa lymphoid tissues to induce an immune response. The uptake of particles by the M-cells occurs through endocytosis and phagocytosis (Clark et al., 2000, des Rieux et al., 2006).

The nasal mucosa is highly vascularized and provides large contact surface with low proteolytic activity. For these reasons, nasal mucosa is very attractive for the delivery of vaccines. The epithelial cells in the nasal cavity are tightly linked and form an impermeable barrier and also cover the nasal-associated lymphoid tissue (NALT) and the M-cells. The immune response, both locally and systemic, begins with the targeting of the NALT at the Walderyer's ring, at the base of the nasal cavity. Then, the M-cells uptake the antigen and deliver it to the submucosal lymphoid tissues (Illum et al., 2001). However, this administration route has several features that must be taken into account such as short residence time in the nasal cavity because of the mucociliary clearance. Thus, antigen-loaded nanoparticle formulations must overcome these difficulties with efficient absorption and uptake of the nanoparticles from the epithelium. Therefore, mucoadhesive delivery systems are desired to improve residence rate and absorption of the drugs without causing unrequired immunogenicity (Amidi et al., 2011). Table 6.3 describes the characteristics of oral and nasal routes of administration.

Polymeric nanoparticles, for instance, have emerged as possible vehicles since they are biodegradable without producing any toxic products; they release the drug in a sustained manner, and possess adjuvant properties in the stimulation of an immune response. Several studies have been made to attempt to develop a nanoparticulate polymeric vaccine (Almeida and Souto, 2007). Alongside polymeric vaccines, adjuvants too have emerged as potential helpful tools in the stimulation of an immune response. Compounds such as latex, polystyrene, gold, and silica have been sought out as possible inductors of immune response; nevertheless, they are not biodegradable. So, in recent years, there has been a rising interest in the use of biodegradable compounds as immune system stimulators, such as liposomes, biodegradable polymers, immunostimulating complexes (ISCOMs), particulates, and

TABLE 6.3

Characteristics of Oral and Nasal Routes

Oral Route	Nasal Route
• Noninvasive	• Noninvasive
• Particles must overcome extreme pH conditions, digestion by biliary salts and enzymes to be absorbed in the gut	• Highly vascularized
	• Low proteolytic activity
• Bioactives must overcome villi epithelium and mucins secreted by goblet cells for further uptake by M-cells in the Peyer's patches	• Short residence time by particles due to the mucociliary clearance
	• Epithelial cells tightly linked to the NALT and M-cells
	• Particles must be designed to target the NALT to suffer uptake by M-cells

TABLE 6.4

Summary of Most Important Aspects of Vaccine and Vaccine Adjuvant

---

- Nanoparticulate vaccines enclose protein antigens or recombinant protein components
- Efficient immunization can be achieved with sustained antigen release
- The immune response depends on the particle size: smaller particles induce exacerbated immune response, while larger particles are processed by endocytosis and phagocytosis
- Biodegradable polymers have been recognized as valuable materials for vaccine delivery, since they release the drug in a sustained manner, they stimulate immune response and have low toxicity

---

virus-like particles, among others. It was found that the immune response was more efficient when the antigen was covalently coupled to the carrier, instead of being simply adsorbed to the carrier surface (Ho et al., 2011). Singh et al. (2006) evaluated the possibility of using several polymers such as poly(caprolactone) (PCL), a poly(lactide-*co*-glycolide) (PLGA)–PCL blend and copolymer nanoparticles to encapsulate toxoid diphtheria. According to their results, the most hydrophobic nanoparticles had the higher uptake by intranasal administration, as well as the strongest specific toxoid diphtheria immunoglobulin G (IgG) antibody response. However, the cytokine type that was induced depended on the route of administration.

Chitosan is nowadays most valued due to its mucoadhesive nature and ability to enhance permeability. Moreover, chitosan is a natural polymer, which is biodegradable and has low toxicity. Illum et al. (2001) have explored chitosan-based vehicles to deliver very diverse drugs, such as insulin, parathyroid hormone, calcitonin, low-molecular-weight polar drugs, and drugs for the treatment of migraine and cancer pain. Moreover, the authors have evaluated the use of this polysaccharide for the delivery of influenza vaccine through mucosal route. Other research include successfully encapsulating bovine serum albumin (BSA) or vaccine tetanus toxoid (TT) in the chitosan nanoparticles. Table 6.4 sums up the most important aspects of vaccine delivery systems and adjuvant.

6.4 Conclusion

Applications of nanotechnology in healthcare have been rising in the recent years. The use of nanoparticles promises to be a good approach in addressing several diseases that lack specific targeting strategies. Nanoparticles are internalized by tissues or cells due to their small size, which enables target drugs into cellular compartments. Therapeutic schemes (e.g., gene delivery, vaccine delivery, and/or intracellular targeting) could benefit from nanotechnology. Gene delivery is still underexploited, but has great potential for the treatment of genetic diseases. Gene-based nanoparticles are still lacking in the market, mainly due to low transfection and expression rates. Nanoparticle-based formulations to deliver vaccines are more advantageous when compared to conventional formulations, because of low toxicity and safety profiles. Furthermore, the treatment of some diseases based on cellular trafficking targeting could benefit from nanoparticle systems, which can specifically target a cellular compartment and release the drug in a sustained manner without causing toxicity to the other compartments. The main advantages of these systems are high specificity to the target, whether it is a tissue, cell, or organelle, sustained release, low toxicity, and less adverse side effects. However, there is still not much information about nanoparticle hazards after their metabolization and excretion, and whether toxic substances are produced. The use of nanoparticles as drug carriers to address several diseases is well established. The goal is to deliver small drug molecules into a specific target, without compromising the surrounding tissues. Nanoparticles can be designed to have affinity to specific targets, which make them an interesting strategy to address genetic diseases, to deliver vaccines, and to treat cancer, among others. Still, many questions remain about the ultimate fate of nanoparticles following drug release and excretion. For that reason, studies must be conducted to fully understand nanoparticle effects.

Acknowledgment

The authors wish to acknowledge Fundação para a Ciência e Tecnologia do Ministério da Ciência e Tecnologia, under the reference ERA—Eula/002/2009.

References

Almeida, A. J. and Souto, E. 2007. Solid lipid nanoparticles as a drug delivery system for peptides and proteins. *Advanced Drug Delivery Reviews*, 59, 478–490.

Amidi, M., De Raad, M., Crommelin, D. J., Hennink, W. E., and Mastrobattista, E. 2011. Antigen-expressing immunostimulatory liposomes as a genetically programmable synthetic vaccine. *Systems and Synthetic Biology*, 5, 21–31.

Breunig, M., Bauer, S., and Goepferich, A. 2008. Polymers and nanoparticles: Intelligent tools for intracellular targeting? *European Journal of Pharmaceutics and Biopharmaceutics*, 68, 112–128.

Buda, A., Sands, C., and Jepson, M. A. 2005. Use of fluorescence imaging to investigate the structure and function of intestinal M cells. *Advanced Drug Delivery Reviews*, 57, 123–134.

Choi, S. H., Jin, S.-E., Lee, M.-K., Lim, S.-J., Park, J.-S., Kim, B.-G., AHN, W. S., and Kim, C.-K. 2008. Novel cationic solid lipid nanoparticles enhanced p53 gene transfer to lung cancer cells. *European Journal of Pharmaceutics and Biopharmaceutics*, 68, 545–554.

Choi, K. Y., Saravanakumar, G., Park, J. H., and Park, K. 2012. Hyaluronic acid-based nanocarriers for intracellular targeting: Interfacial interactions with proteins in cancer. *Colloids and Surfaces B: Biointerfaces*, 99, 82–94.

Clark, M. A., Hirst, B. H., and Jepson, M. A. 2000. Lectin-mediated mucosal delivery of drugs and microparticles. *Advanced Drug Delivery Reviews*, 43, 207–223.

Conley, S. M. and Naash, M. I. 2010. Nanoparticles for retinal gene therapy. *Progress in Retinal and Eye Research*, 29, 376–397.

Del Pozo-Rodríguez, A., Delgado, D., Solinís, M. Á., Pedraz, J. L., Echevarría, E., Rodríguez, J. M., and Gascón, A. R. 2010. Solid lipid nanoparticles as potential tools for gene therapy: *In vivo* protein expression after intravenous administration. *International Journal of Pharmaceutics*, 385, 157–162.

des Rieux, A., Fievez, V., Garinot, M., Schneider, Y.-J., and Préat, V. 2006. Nanoparticles as potential oral delivery systems of proteins and vaccines: A mechanistic approach. *Journal of Controlled Release*, 116, 1–27.

Fadeel, B. and Garcia-Bennett, A. E. 2010. Better safe than sorry: Understanding the toxicological properties of inorganic nanoparticles manufactured for biomedical applications. *Advanced Drug Delivery Reviews*, 62, 362–374.

Gan, Q., Wang, T., Cochrane, C., and Mccaron, P. 2005. Modulation of surface charge, particle size and morphological properties of chitosan–TPP nanoparticles intended for gene delivery. *Colloids and Surfaces B: Biointerfaces*, 44, 65–73.

Giger, E. V., Puigmartí-Luis, J., Schlatter, R., Castagner, B., Dittrich, P. S., and Leroux, J.-C. 2011. Gene delivery with bisphosphonate-stabilized calcium phosphate nanoparticles. *Journal of Controlled Release*, 150, 87–93.

Gillies, E. R. and Fréchet, J. 2005. pH-Responsive copolymer assemblies for controlled release of doxorubicin. *Bioconjugate Chemistry*, 16, 361–368.

Gillies, E., Goodwin, A., and Fréchet, J. 2004. Acetals as pH-sensitive linkages for drug delivery. *Bioconjugate Chemistry*, 15, 1254–1263.

Gordon, S., Teichmann, E., Young, K., Finnie, K., Rades, T., and Hook, S. 2010. *In vitro* and *in vivo* investigation of thermosensitive chitosan hydrogels containing silica nanoparticles for vaccine delivery. *European Journal of Pharmaceutical Sciences*, 41, 360–368.

Hild, W. A., Breunig, M., and Goepferich, A. 2008. Quantum dots—Nano-sized probes for the exploration of cellular and intracellular targeting. *European Journal of Pharmaceutics and Biopharmaceutics*, 68, 153–168.

HO, J., AL-Deen, F. M. N., AL-Abboodi, A., Selomulya, C., Xiang, S. D., Plebanski, M., and Forde, G. M. 2011. N,N′-Carbonyldiimidazole-mediated functionalization of superparamagnetic nanoparticles as vaccine carrier. *Colloids and Surfaces B: Biointerfaces*, 83, 83–90.

Husseini, G. A. and Pitt, W. G. 2008. Micelles and nanoparticles for ultrasonic drug and gene delivery. *Advanced Drug Delivery Reviews*, 60, 1137–1152.

Illum, L., Jabbal-Gill, I., Hinchcliffe, M., Fisher, A. N., and Davis, S. S. 2001. Chitosan as a novel nasal delivery system for vaccines. *Advanced Drug Delivery Reviews*, 51, 81–96.

Jain, A. K., Goyal, A. K., Gupta, P. N., Khatri, K., Mishra, N., Mehta, A., Mangal, S., and Vyas, S. P. 2009. Synthesis, characterization and evaluation of novel triblock copolymer based nanoparticles for vaccine delivery against hepatitis B. *Journal of Controlled Release*, 136, 161–169.

Jayakumar, R., Chennazhi, K. P., Muzzarelli, R. A. A., Tamura, H., Nair, S. V., and Selvamurugan, N. 2010. Chitosan conjugated DNA nanoparticles in gene therapy. *Carbohydrate Polymers*, 79, 1–8.

Kazuo, M. 2011. Intracellular targeting delivery of liposomal drugs to solid tumors based on Epr effects. *Advanced Drug Delivery Reviews*, 63, 161–169.

Kim, J.-H., Bae, S. M., NA, M.-H., Shin, H., Yang, Y. J., Min, K. H., Choi, K. Y. et al. 2012. Facilitated intracellular delivery of peptide-guided nanoparticles in tumor tissues. *Journal of Controlled Release*, 157, 493–499.

Kimura, T., Okuno, A., Miyazaki, K., Furuzono, T., Ohya, Y., Ouchi, T., Mutsuo, S. et al. 2004. Novel PVA–DNA nanoparticles prepared by ultra high pressure technology for gene delivery. *Materials Science and Engineering: C*, 24, 797–801.

Ladewig, K., Niebert, M., Xu, Z. P., Gray, P. P., and Lu, G. Q. 2010. Controlled preparation of layered double hydroxide nanoparticles and their application as gene delivery vehicles. *Applied Clay Science*, 48, 280–289.

Lambert, P. H. and Laurent, P. E. 2008. Intradermal vaccine delivery: Will new delivery systems transform vaccine administration? *Vaccine*, 26, 3197–3208.

Liu, G., Swierczewska, M., Lee, S., and Chen, X. 2010. Functional nanoparticles for molecular imaging guided gene delivery. *Nano Today*, 5, 524–539.

Mark E. D. 2002. Non-viral gene delivery systems. *Current Opinion in Biotechnology*, 13, 128–131.

Müller, R. H., Mäder, K., and Gohla, S. 2000. Solid lipid nanoparticles (Sln) for controlled drug delivery—a review of the state of the art. *European Journal of Pharmaceutics and Biopharmaceutics*, 50, 161–177.

Salvati, A., Åberg, C., Dos Santos, T., Varela, J., Pinto, P., Lynch, I., and Dawson, K. A. 2011. Experimental and theoretical comparison of intracellular import of polymeric nanoparticles and small molecules: Toward models of uptake kinetics. *Nanomedicine: Nanotechnology, Biology and Medicine*, 7, 818–826.

Singh, J., Pandit, S., Bramwell, V. W., and Alpar, H. O. 2006. Diphtheria toxoid loaded poly-(ε-caprolactone) nanoparticles as mucosal vaccine delivery systems. *Methods*, 38, 96–105.

Sneh-Edri, H. and Stepensky, D. 2011. 'IntraCell' plugin for assessment of intracellular localization of nano-delivery systems and their targeting to the individual organelles. *Biochemical and Biophysical Research Communications*, 405, 228–233.

Vighi, E., Ruozi, B., Montanari, M., Battini, R., and Leo, E. 2010. pDNA condensation capacity and *in vitro* gene delivery properties of cationic solid lipid nanoparticles. *International Journal of Pharmaceutics*, 389, 254–261.

Wasungu, L. and Hoekstra, D. 2006. Cationic lipids, lipoplexes and intracellular delivery of genes. *Journal of Controlled Release*, 116, 255–264.

Xu, J., Ganesh, S., and Amiji, M. 2011. Non-condensing polymeric nanoparticles for targeted gene and siRNA delivery. *International Journal of Pharmaceutics*, 427, 21–34.

Yang, S. R., Lee, H. J., and Kim, J.-D. 2006. Histidine-conjugated poly(amino acid) derivatives for the novel endosomolytic delivery carrier of doxorubicin. *Journal of Controlled Release*, 114, 60–68.

Zhuo, C. 2010. Small-molecule delivery by nanoparticles for anticancer therapy. *Trends in Molecular Medicine*, 16, 594–602.

Zou, W., Liu, C., Chen, Z., and Zheng, N. 2009. Studies on bioadhesive PLGA nanoparticles: A promising gene delivery system for efficient gene therapy to lung cancer. *International Journal of Pharmaceutics*, 370, 187–195.

7

Nanoparticle Therapies for Wounds and Ulcer Healing

Chiara Gardin, Letizia Ferroni, Luca Lancerotto, Vincenzo Vindigni, Chiara Rigo, Marco Roman, Warren R. L. Cairns, and Barbara Zavan

CONTENTS

7.1 Overview of the Wound Healing Process 144
7.2 Inflammatory Phase 145
    7.2.1 Detailed Description of the Inflammatory Phase 145
    7.2.2 Applications of Nanotechnologies in Modulating and
        Modifying the Inflammatory Phase 147
        7.2.2.1 Direct Interaction between Nano-Structured
            Drugs and Inflammatory Cells 148
        7.2.2.2 Direct Interaction between Nanotechnology-
            Based Drugs and Inflammatory Enzymes 150
        7.2.2.3 Modification of the Wound Environment: Use of
            Nanoparticles to Avoid Bacterial Colonization 150
7.3 Proliferative Phase 164
    7.3.1 Detailed Description of the Proliferative Phase 164
    7.3.2 Applications of Nanotechnologies in Modulating and
        Modifying the Proliferative Phase 165
        7.3.2.1 Nanostructured Biomaterials 165
        7.3.2.2 Surfaces Modification of Nanostructured
            Biomaterials 169
        7.3.2.3 Drug-Delivering Nanostructured Biomaterials 171
7.4 Remodeling Phase 174
    7.4.1 Detailed Description of the Remodeling Phase 174
    7.4.2 Applications of Nanotechnologies in Modulating and
        Modifying the Remodeling Phase 175
7.5 Conclusions 176
References 176

Nanotechnology is the branch of technology that manipulates matter on an atomic or molecular scale. Materials, devices, or structures are defined as "nano" when they have at least one dimension that ranges from 1 to 100 nm. Nanomaterials often have different physical (mechanical, electrical, optical, etc.) properties compared to the same material at macrodimensions. Nanostructured biomaterials have the advantage of small size, high porosity, and most importantly a high surface-area-to-volume ratio (Ngiam et al. 2011). The increased surface-area-to-volume ratio alters the mechanical, thermal, and catalytic properties of materials. These new properties allow unique and innovative applications of nanomaterials in many fields.

Nanomedicine is the medical application of nanotechnologies (Freitas 2005); examples of nanomedical applications are the use of nanomaterials in developing new and more efficient drug delivery systems, the application of nanoelectronic biosensors, and *in vivo* imaging.

7.1 Overview of the Wound Healing Process

One of the key applications of nanomedicine is in the field of healing skin wounds and ulcers.

The skin is the largest organ of the human body, representing about 10% of its total weight. It plays a crucial role in many functions, such as protection against the external environment, fluid homeostasis, sensory detection, and self-healing (Zhong et al. 2010). Anatomically, skin is composed of two different tissues, the epidermis and the dermis, separated by the basement membrane. The outer tissue, the epidermis, is a multilayered flattened epithelium composed of keratinocytes, rising from the basal layer and migrating to the surface of the skin. The function of the epidermis is to maintain the anatomical integrity of the skin and act as a barrier against the noxae of the outside world. The dermis is relatively acellular and composed mainly of an extracellular matrix (ECM) made of collagen fibrils, elastin, and glycosaminoglycans (GAGs). Fibroblasts, the major cellular component of the dermis, produce and maintain most of the ECM. The role of the dermis is to provide resistance as well as elasticity to the skin and support the extensive vasculature, lymphatic system, and nerve bundles (Pomahac et al. 1998).

By definition, a wound is an injury to living tissue, causing a break or a discontinuity in the epithelium. Injuries can occur in soft tissues like skin or intestine, as well as in hard tissues like bones or cartilage and can be provoked by exogenous (trauma, compression, burns) or endogenous causes (metabolic diseases). The wound healing process is a cascade of orderly events, leading to the repair of damaged tissue and its eventual replacement. The final aim of the wound healing process is not only the reconstruction of the damaged tissue but also the recovery of its complete functionality, with a minimum of scarring. Alterations in wound healing processes and deviations from the normal pathways result in excessive or insufficient wound repair.

Independently from the tissue involved, the healing process always occurs through a series of molecular, biochemical, and cellular events that can be grouped in three overlapping phases: inflammation, proliferation, and remodeling (Singer and Clark 1999).

Inflammation spontaneously begins immediately after injury and lasts for 1–4 days. It is characterized by clotting in the wound, the release of signal molecules to recruit immune cells, and the release of specific enzymes (matrix metalloproteinases, MMPs) that clean the wound. The proliferative phase takes place between 4 and 21 days after wounding. In this phase, fibroblasts are stimulated to invade the wound site and to produce ECM components. Highly vascularized granulation tissue is formed and the gap is closed. The last phase is remodeling, which can take up to 1 year. The immature scar is transformed into a stable, less vascularized tissue, exhibiting good mechanical properties (Martin 1997).

Local and systemic factors can affect these three phases, resulting in bad healing. For example, infection of the wound can lead to an excessive or prolonged inflammation, and this obstructs the progression to the proliferative phase. If the cell metabolism is limited due to systemic conditions, the proliferative phase can also be negatively affected, resulting in a chronicization of wound. Chronic wounds often lead to loss of functional ability, increased pain, and reduced quality of life for the patients, as well as being a burden for health system resources. Hypertrophic or keloidal scars can occur in cases of excessive proliferation or during impairment in the remodeling process (Lindblad 2008).

Since the 1980s, in order to modulate and improve the whole wound healing process, and eventually correct the irregular and dysfunctional cellular pathways present in chronic wounds, researchers have focused their work on developing new nanotechnology-based therapies, such as drug release systems, biological and active dressings, and skin substitutes. Most effort has been concentrated in the modulation of the inflammatory phase, probably because it is the first step in the events cascade of the healing pathway. A positive ending of the whole healing process strictly depends on a favorable conclusion of this phase.

7.2 Inflammatory Phase

7.2.1 Detailed Description of the Inflammatory Phase

Immediately after injury, the first event that takes place in the inflammatory phase is the formation of a fibrin clot in the wound. This is a hemostatic early barrier to protect the exposed tissues, and comprises of coagulated platelets and blood protein webbed in a fibrin network, that is used as a scaffold in the cellular events to follow. The fibrin clot also acts as a matrix in guiding the homing of the cells involved in the repair process (platelets, monocytes, granulocytes, fibroblasts, endothelial cells, keratinocytes) and is a local reservoir of cytokines (tumor necrosis factor-α, TNF-α; interleukin-1β, IL-1β; interleukin-6, IL-6) and growth factors that are released from the platelets (platelet-derived growth factor, PDGF; insulin-like growth factor, IGF; epidermal growth factor, EGF; fibroblast growth factor, FGF; transforming growth factor-α, TGF-α; transforming growth factor-β, TGF-β) (Assoian and Sporn 1986; Lynch et al. 1989; Pierce et al. 1991; Schultz et al. 1991; Gartner et al. 1992; Shaw and Martin 2009).

A key element in the formation of the fibrin clot is thrombin; it is a hematic enzyme responsible for the conversion of fibrinogen into fibrin, and is essential for aggregation of blood platelets in forming the "platelet plug," as well as for activation of other hemostatic factors. Moreover, thrombin plays a pivotal role in all the events leading to increased vascular permeability and promotes immune cell migration into damaged tissue. In light of this, local administration of thrombin could appear useful and opportune. Unfortunately, thrombin is strictly controlled by protease inhibitors and several components of the vessel wall, so the half-life of this important molecule is less than 15 s in plasma (Kimball 1995). With the aim of developing long-lasting thrombin-based drugs that provide sufficient protection of the molecule from its natural inhibitors and degradation processes, it has been suggested that this enzyme could be conjugated to nanoparticles (NPs). In the laboratory of Ziv-Polat et al., thrombin was conjugated to iron oxide nanoparticles (Ziv-Polat et al. 2010); the product was tested during the treatment of incisional wounds in an *in vivo* rat skin model (Figure 7.1). The results demonstrated that conjugated thrombin maintained a good clotting activity, exhibited a high inhibitor resistance, and can persist in the wound for up to 14 days. Tensile strength and mechanical properties of the wounds were tested 28 days after treatment, and showed that thrombin-conjugated nanoparticles accelerated the healing of incisional wounds significantly compared to free thrombin or untreated wounds, with the benefit that minimal residual iron could be detected in the scars. These positive results highlighted a possible use of this conjugated product in medical applications to reduce possible surgical complications.

During the inflammatory phase, immune cells are recruited and migrate to the wound site. The process involves the migration first of neutrophils, followed immediately by macrophages, and later by lymphocytes. All these cells take part in the complex and fundamental process of wound cleansing. In the site of wound, the continuity of the physiological skin barrier is interrupted. The gap must be closed as soon as possible to reduce bacterial entrance and microorganisms already present must be eliminated, to avoid infection. The damaged or broken ECM must be removed and rapidly

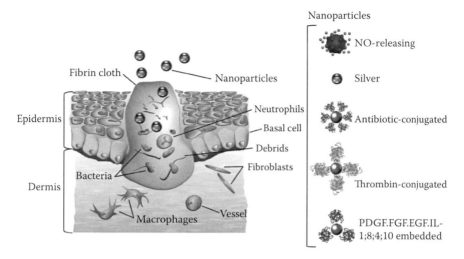

FIGURE 7.1
Applications of nanoparticles in the wound healing process.

substituted with a new one. All these activities are performed through phagocytosis, production of reactive oxygen species (ROS), and the release of lytic enzymes such as polymorphonuclear (PMN) elastase and MMPs. This early phase must be strictly time limited, as prolonged inflammation leads to the enlargement of the wound size and damage of surrounding healthy tissues due to an excessive activity of these proteolytic enzymes. The excessive action of elastase leads to considerably reduced amounts of growth factors and protease inhibitors, leaving unchecked MMPs to cleave collagens, elastin, and fibronectin, leading to the destruction of the ECM, chronicization of wounds, or a delayed onset of the proliferative phase (Barrick et al. 1999; Trengove et al. 1999).

7.2.2 Applications of Nanotechnologies in Modulating and Modifying the Inflammatory Phase

To limit excessive or prolonged inflammation, a possible strategy is the systemic or local administration of corticosteroids or nonsteroidal anti-inflammatory drugs (NSAIDs).

Unfortunately, steroidal drugs have strong systemic metabolic effects, their use is contraindicated in diabetic patients, and finally they have a negative effect on fibroblasts and keratinocytes. NSAIDs instead are not indicated for local administration in patients with open wounds due to the inhibitory activity of these pharmaceuticals on cyclooxygenase enzymes, leading to the prolongation of coagulation times.

Recently, interesting new alternatives have emerged from research in nanomedicine. The inflammatory phase can be modulated through direct interactions between drugs and inflammatory cells, between drugs and inflammatory signal molecules or enzymes, and finally through modification of the wound environment, by eliminating bacteria or other inflammatory stimuli.

7.2.2.1 Direct Interaction between Nano-Structured Drugs and Inflammatory Cells

Direct interactions between inflammatory cells and a nanoparticle-based drugs was investigated in 2011 by Norling and coworkers (Norling et al. 2011). These researchers first studied the temporal generation and properties of endogenous microparticles (MPs) produced during an *in vivo* induced inflammatory process and then investigated the possibility of constructing a novel biomimetic system using humanized nanoparticles to resolve inflammation.

MPs are vesicles physiologically released from PMNs. Originally, these vesicles were thought to be empty and inert, but recently, their multiple roles and functional significance during inflammation are beginning to be appreciated. In particular, potent specialized chemical mediators derived from fatty acids have been identified in these vesicles that have been demonstrated to actively promote inflammation resolution via novel proresolving and anti-inflammatory cascades. Norling and colleagues initiated peritonitis in male mice, and peritoneal lavages were collected to obtain exudate MPs. The vesicles collected were purified, characterized, and profiled to assess and confirm their phospholipid content. In particular, the authors discovered that endogenous MPs formed in inflammatory exudates contain esterified biosynthetic precursors of specialized proresolving lipid mediators (LM) and that these vesicles can act as intercellular communicators able to deliver the precursors to inflammatory loci.

Using human neutrophil-derived MPs, the authors synthesized innovative nanoparticles containing two potent LMs, aspirin-triggered resolvin D1 (AT-RvD1) and a lipoxin A_4 (LXA_4) analog. These humanized nanoparticles (alone or carried with LMs) were administered intravenously or intraperitoneally, prior to the induction of peritonitis in mice. At regular time intervals, peritoneal leukocytes were collected and assessed. The humanized NPs were found to be inherently anti-inflammatory; they were able to counterregulate PMN infiltration in acute peritonitis and to reduce PMN numbers and recruitment in a dose-dependent manner. The positive effect was greater when using AT-RvD1- and LXA_4-enriched NPs. Moreover, they found an inhibitory action on PMN recruitment when NPs were administered directly into the peritoneum, suggesting a direct action on resident macrophages that dampened their inflammatory response.

The authors also demonstrated the capacity of AT-RvD1- and LXA_4-enriched NPs to enhance wound closure rates when evaluated in a keratinocyte wound-healing assay and their role in preventing excessive neutrophilic infiltration during inflammation of an temporomandibular joint (TMJ), induced in a mouse model using complete Freund's adjuvant (CFA). CFA is a solution of antigen emulsified in mineral oil and used as an immunopotentiator. The complete form, Freund's complete adjuvant (CFA or FCA) is composed of inactivated and dried mycobacteria.

In the same time period, a novel site-directed drug delivery system based on liposomes was employed to target specifically inflamed cells (Kang et al. 2011). Liposomes are artificial microscopic vesicles consisting of an aqueous core enclosed in one or more phospholipid layers. Liposomes have been recently used to convey bioactive substances such as vaccines, drugs, and enzymes to target cells or organs (Vanniasinghe et al. 2009; Tan et al. 2010). In this research work, the authors delivered celasterol, a potent anti-inflammatory, antioxidative, and antiproliferative drug, to inflamed cells by loading this molecule into home-made liposomes and exploited a physiological molecular interaction between an inducible intracellular adhesion molecule-1 (ICAM-1) and a lymphocyte function-associated antigen-1 (LFA-1) integrin to target in a specific manner only the cells expressing high levels of ICAM-1. LFA-1 integrin is a physiological receptor for ICAM-1 and upregulated localized expression of ICAM-1 is known to be associated with most of the cellular players in acute and chronic inflammation and can be induced upon inflammatory stimuli in both immune and nonimmune cells.

In this work, the authors identified a specific domain of LFA-1 (Id-HA) and demonstrated that this domain among all those investigated possessed the highest affinity for ICAM-1. Id-HA was recombinantly produced, purified, and then attached via noncovalent binding to home-assembled liposomes. To verify the presence of Id-HA on the surface of the liposomes, the diameter of these molecules was measured before and after coupling. After protein conjugation, the liposome diameter was verified to increase from 107 to 115 nm, corresponding to a single layer of Id-HA.

With the aim of inducing inflammation and to monitor the upregulation of ICAM-1 expression, the researchers treated human dermal microvascular endothelial cells (HMEC-1) and human monocytic leukemia (THP-1) cells with lipopolysaccharides (LPS). The authors chose to challenge with LPS HMEC-1 and THP-1 cells because these cellular lines represent the main non-immune and immune cells present in an inflammatory milieu. In this work, the researchers first demonstrated that free colesterol could exert an inhibitory effect on LPS-induced gene expression of various proinflammatory mediators such as various cytokines and chemokines. It was found that cell surface molecules like ICAM-1 were greatly upregulated after HMEC-1 and THP-1 cells had been challenged with LPS but a pretreatment with free celasterol reduced considerably the expression of these proinflammatory markers. At the same time, the researchers assessed the ability of Id-HA/liposomes to target specifically and comprehensively LPS-treated HMEC-1 and THP-1 cells, and subsequently, Kang and colleagues identified the optimal Id-HA/lipids ratio to assemble liposomes able to target inflamed cells but not resting cells. Finally, the concentration of celasterol to be loaded into the liposomes was optimized to obtain an anti-inflammatory effect with a minimum cytotoxicity. Once the optimal mass ratio of Id-HA to phospholipid and dosage of celasterol were determined, the researchers investigated the inhibitory effect of colesterol-Id-HA/liposomes by targeted delivery on the expression of proinflammatory markers in HMEC-1 and THP-1 cells. In both cell lines, targeted delivery of colesterol-Id-HA/liposomes was demonstrated to be as effective or superior to the same dosage of free calesterol in down-regulating the expression of proinflammatory markers, including cell surface expression of ICAM-1. The lower amount of ICAM-1 on the cell surface was also proved to reduce effectively THP-1 cell adhesion to endothelial HMEC-1 cells and inhibited the continuing accumulation of immune cells in inflamed vasculature. This is an important feature that anti-inflammatory therapies should possess to be effective. The results achieved by this research group are very important and promising because they have cleared the way to ensure specific delivery of drug carriers to inflamed cells but not to normal cells, while maintaining potent therapeutic effects without causing cytotoxicity.

7.2.2.2 Direct Interaction between Nanotechnology-Based Drugs and Inflammatory Enzymes

The direct interaction between drugs and inflammatory enzymes was employed by Schmutz and coworkers (Schmutz et al. 2008) to treat locally venous leg ulcers. The researchers applied nano-oligosaccharide factor (NOSF), a synthesized component recently produced by the Urgo Laboratories Research Unit (France). NOSF is a healing accelerator with a chemical structure derived from the oligosaccharide family of compounds; it is shown to inhibit MMPs (MMP-1 in particular) in experimental cell culture models and increases the local residential time of various growth factors. NOSF can be incorporated within a lipido-colloid matrix (NOSF matrix) and is locally released into the wound site. The authors compared the performance of the NOSF matrix with a collagen oxidized regenerated cellulose (collagen-oxidized regenerated cellulose (ORC)) matrix; this is another dressing composed of bovine collagen (55%) and of ORC (45%) that is already known to be able to efficiently adsorb and inhibit various MMPs. The authors demonstrated that this NOSF matrix was superior to collagen-ORC for both the primary efficacy criterion (percentage relative wound reduction) and secondary endpoints (wound absolute reduction, healing rate, and percentage of wounds with 40% or more reduction compared with mean wound area at baseline).

7.2.2.3 Modification of the Wound Environment: Use of Nanoparticles to Avoid Bacterial Colonization

An alternative way to modulate and control the inflammatory phase is modifying the wound environment by reducing or eliminating inflammatory stimuli. Bacterial colonization is one of the most important problems to avoid in wound treatment, and until a few years ago, the use of antibiotics alone was enough to prevent or settle the occurrence of this negative complication. Although antibiotics are still of great importance, their widespread overuse and misuse has contributed to the rise of resistant bacteria. Multidrug-resistant nosocomial pathogens (*Pseudomonas aeruginosa*, *Acinetobacter baumannii*, methicillin-resistant staphylococci, and vancomycin-resistant enterococci) can induce systemic infections in hospitalized people, representing one of the major causes of the high mortality and morbidity of burn-wound patients. In last few years, many researchers have focused on developing new strategies to combat multidrug-resistant microorganisms. Nanoparticle-bearing antibiotics were successfully employed in multiple studies. For example, microparticles containing vancomycin have been developed (Hachicha et al. 2006) for intraocular continuous-release injection. This novel product was able to maintain the antibiotic concentration sufficiently high for 24 h, preventing microbial growth. Chakraborty et al. (2010) prepared folic acid-tagged chitosan nanoparticles to be used as Trojan horses to deliver vancomycin into bacterial cells. These vancomycin-loaded nanoparticles were physicochemically characterized and possessed a strong bactericidal effect on vancomycin-resistant *Staphylococcus aureus*. Turos and coauthors (Turos et al. 2007; Greenhalgh and Turos 2009; Garay-Jimenez et al. 2009) have focused their research work on identifying an effective drug delivery system that would enhance the water solubility of N-methylthiolated β-lactams, a new group of antibacterial agents able to kill *Staphylococcus* bacteria, including methicillin-resistant *S. aureus* (MRSA); however, they are virtually insoluble in water. First, the authors converted the antibiotic drug into an acrylated derivative, and then dissolved it to homogeneity in a liquid acrylate monomer. The mixture was preemulsified and treated with a water-soluble radical initiator to induce polymerization. The resulting emulsion contained uniformly sized polyacrylate nanoparticles in which the antibiotic drug was covalently incorporated. The drug-loaded nanoparticles proved to have a potent antibacterial activity against MRSA, were nontoxic to human dermal fibroblasts, and were stable for more than 24 h at moderately high temperatures (up to 60°C) and in blood serum.

Recently, many elements have been discovered to possess antibacterial properties as nanoparticles, including silver (Ag), titanium (Ti), copper (Cu), zinc (Zn), and manganese (Mg).

Among these elements, silver is probably the most investigated and employed. Silver in ionic form has been used as an antibacterial agent since medieval times, and recently a renewed interest in its properties has increased due to the rise of antibiotic-resistant bacteria. In 1965, Moyer obtained silver sulfadiazine (SSD) by combining silver nitrate ($AgNO_3$) and sulfadiazine, a sulfa drug that had been recently discovered. Silver complexes with the antibiotic were introduced as creams to combine the antibacterial action of the two components, and in the last few decades it has been the most widely used Ag-based product for the first treatment of burns. In recent years, a wide variety of silver-containing dressings have entered into commerce, innovating the care of burns, skin ulcers, and other cutaneous wounds. The dressings are generally composed of a polymeric scaffold coated or impregnated with silver salts or silver metal in nanoparticulate form. The chemical form of silver has antibacterial effects by acting on different cellular components: it has been demonstrated that silver nanoparticles and silver ions are able to bind to microbial DNA, altering the structure; they can bind to the cell wall and block respiratory enzyme pathways, causing the collapse of the proton motive force (Castellano et al. 2007); they can interact with ribosome, inhibiting RNA translation and protein production (Yamanaka et al. 2005); and they can cause the generation of ROS (Le Pape et al. 2004). It has been recently demonstrated that silver nanoparticles are able to reduce the growth of biofilms, by binding to and inhibiting the enzymatic activity of tryptophanase, a bacterial enzyme with no counterpart in eukaryotic cells, that is involved in bacteria multiplication and biofilm formation (Scherzer et al. 2009; Wigginton et al. 2010). A biofilm is an aggregate of microorganisms in which the cells adhere to each other on a surface. These adherent cells are frequently embedded within a self-produced matrix of extracellular polymeric substances and are generally more resistant to conventional drug therapies, disinfectants, and the immune response of the host than their planktonic counterparts (Kalishwaralal et al. 2010; Jefferson 2004).

Multiple research works have been performed to demonstrate the effectiveness of silver dressings as antimicrobial agents. The studies were conducted mainly *in vitro* (Wright et al. 1998; Parsons et al. 2005; Ip et al. 2006; Castellano et al. 2007; Cavanagh et al. 2010; Aramwit et al. 2010) but some *in vivo* studies have also been carried out (Luo et al. 2008; Uygur et al. 2009; Acar et al. 2011). In all cases, silver dressings were proven to be effective in reducing the microbial load.

Actually, numerous silver-containing dressings have been commercialized and are widely employed in wound and burn care. In most cases, when evaluating the effectiveness of silver dressings, researchers generally compare the healing results obtained using commercially available or home-developed silver dressings with the well-known and globally available SSD creams.

For example, in 2007, Tian and coworkers (Tian et al. 2007) compared the healing properties of a silver-nanoparticle-coated dressing with that of an adsorbent gauze impregnated with SSD in a thermal injury *in vivo* model. The authors demonstrated that silver nanoparticles can modulate local and systemic inflammatory responses after a burn injury by cytokine modulation.

This was done by scalding 20-week-old male mice, causing a deep partial thickness thermal injury to 10% of the total body surface of genetically diabetic and nondiabetic mice. They were then treated with commercially available silver nanoparticle-coated dressing or with a 1% SSD cream applied to a piece of a sterile nonadherent adsorbent dressing. The quantity of cream applied contained the equivalent amount of silver to a piece of silver nanoparticle-coated dressing. At regular time intervals, the mice were sacrificed and skin and blood samples were collected to monitor healing rate, bacterial colonization, and perform histological and proteomic analysis, as well as RNA extraction for cytokine evaluation. The authors observed that wound healing was accelerated by silver nanoparticles (also in genetically diabetic mice), and that the worst cosmetic appearance was obtained with SSD treatment. Histological sections from the SSD-treated group showed thickened epidermis and no evidence of hair growth, while wounds treated with silver nanoparticles showed the most resemblance to normal skin. Treatment with silver nanoparticles prevented microbial growth for up to 7 days, whereas bacteria were found in SSD-treated wounds 3 days after injury, confirming that silver nanoparticles are effective long-term antibacterial agents. The authors also investigated if silver could modulate the expression patterns of some cytokines, signal molecules that play an important role in the inflammatory phase and wound healing process. Using quantitative real-time reverse transcription-polymerase chain reaction (RT PCR), they found that silver nanoparticles and SSD can modify the expression patterns of IL-6, TGF-β1, IL-10, vascular endothelial growth factor (VEGF), and interferon γ (IFN-γ) in a dose-dependent manner. In the wound areas treated with silver nanoparticles, levels of IL-6 mRNA were maintained at statistically significantly lower levels throughout the healing process, while at the beginning of the healing process, mRNA levels of TGF-β1 were significantly higher and then decreased and maintained a lower level during the latter phases. For IL-10, VEGF and IFN-γ mRNA, at all time points during the experiment, these signal molecules stayed higher in the silver nanoparticle-treated group relative to those of the SSD-treated group. Observing histological sections of the burn wounds, after an initial influx of neutrophils into the wounds, the authors found significantly fewer neutrophils in the silver nanoparticle-treated group. This result suggests a diminished inflammatory response at the wound site. Proteomic analyses were conducted to monitor serum markers of injury. Serum expression of acute-phase proteins was dramatically stimulated by burn injury: for the first few days after injury, sera from both the silver nanoparticle-treated group and SSD-treated group showed augmented expression of hemopexin, haptoglobin, and serum amyloid protein component P. After 10 days, the levels of these proteins in the silver nanoparticle-treated group returned to nearly normal levels, whereas the levels in the SSD group were still elevated. It appears from these findings that silver nanoparticle treatment not only acts as a dampener on the inflammation processes but it also promotes scarless wound healing.

The construction of a novel wound dressing composed of silver nanoparticles and chitosan (SNC) has been reported (Lu et al. 2008), the authors evaluated its effectiveness in treating deep partial thickness wounds compared to SSD. Chitosan is a linear polysaccharide composed of randomly distributed β-(1-4)-linked D-glucosamine (deacetylated unit) and N-acetyl-D-glucosamine (acetylated unit), which remains positively charged in acidic and neutral solutions. Chitosan is produced commercially by deacetylation of chitin, which is the structural element in the exoskeleton of crustaceans (such as crabs and shrimp) and cell walls of fungi. Chitosan has many applications in the cosmetic, food, and medical industries. It is already well known that this compound can act as a painkiller, inhibit microbial growth, and facilitate tissue regeneration by promoting hemostasis and epidermal cell growth. In this work, Lu and colleagues fabricated an SNC wound dressing by immersing a homemade sterile chitosan film in a silver nanoparticle (60 nm in diameter) solution. The silver content in the SNC was determined by flame atomic absorption spectroscopy, and the surface morphology was determined using atomic force microscopy and scanning electron microscopy. The authors also assessed the SNC's biosafety: the novel dressing was verified as sterile and pyrogen negative. The SNC efficacy was evaluated in an *in vivo* model: 56 rats were anesthetized and in each one, a deep partial-thickness wound involving 10–13% of the total body surface area was produced using a dermatome. The 56 rats were randomly divided into four equal groups, and each group was treated with SNC, SSD, chitosan film, or nothing (negative control group). The wound dressings were applied and covered with sterilized gauze with stainless-steel wire gauze on top. On the 6th postoperative day, skin samples were taken and stained with hematoxylin and eosin for histological examination. The wound healing rate was assessed on postoperative days 10 and 13. To determine silver concentrations, venous blood samples were collected at regular time intervals after surgery and at 45 days postoperation, silver concentrations were measured in blood samples collected from the liver, brain, and kidney. Compared to the chitosan and negative control group, SNC significantly increased the rate of wound healing without causing argyria, and SNC-treated rats exhibited blood and tissue silver concentrations lower than SSD-treated rats. According to the evidence, the authors concluded that SNC dressings can promote wound healing and reduce the risk of infection and silver absorption when compared with SSD dressings.

In recent years, SSD and silver-containing dressings have been widely employed in the case of limb ulcers. In 2010, Carter and colleagues (Carter et al. 2010) published a systematic review and a meta-analysis of silver treatments and silver-impregnated dressings used in the healing of leg wounds and ulcers. The authors searched multiple databases using the term "silver" in combination with "wound" or "ulcer" (and in plural version), over a time span ranging from June 1950 to December 2008. Randomized controlled trial (RCT) studies were eligible for inclusion if the participants had any kind of leg ulcer or wound, if the experimental group had been treated topically with silver-based agents (SSD, or silver-impregnated dressings) while the control group received a placebo or a silver-free conservative wound care or treatment. Studies focusing on burns or other body parts were excluded. Studies were eligible for inclusion only if they reported at least one wound healing parameter as an outcome measure (complete wound healing, reduction of wound size or depth, healing rate, or time to heal) as the authors analyzed only these parameters. The quality of each RCT was then assessed, using Downs and Black's method (Downs and Black 1998) with some modifications (Carter et al. 2009) employing a score sheet comprising of five sections. Meta-analysis was then carried out only on those studies that used silver-impregnated dressings and whose outcomes were complete wound healing, wound size reduction, and healing rate. The search found approximately 1600 citations, of which only 10 studies were selected for inclusion in the analysis: three studies involved SSD and seven used silver-impregnated dressings. According to the authors, none of the three selected SSD-based RCTs showed any consistently significant wound healing differences between the experimental and the control groups, whereas the meta-analysis on seven selected silver dressing-based RCTs provided strong evidence for wound healing based on wound size reduction but no evidence based on complete wound healing or healing rates. It is necessary to highlight that the authors suggested that probably these results were due to the short period of time in which these selected RCTs were conducted (usually 4 weeks). Complete healing of wounds and ulcers generally takes several weeks or months, and to accumulate sufficient data for analysis, the RCTs should be conducted for several months. Unfortunately, in most cases, silver treatments and silver-impregnated dressings are typically used only for few weeks, and conducting RCTs for months is unfeasible due to the difficulties and the high costs of these studies. The authors speculate that if longer follow-up times were employed, the results could be reversed, demonstrating the efficacy of silver-based medical devices in complete wound healing. Similar results and conclusions were reported in 2009 by Toy and colleagues (Toy and Macera 2011).

Worldwide, many research projects have focused on the synthesis of silver nanoparticles and novel polymeric organic scaffolds to develop and commercialize novel silver dressings and medical devices. In 2009, Jain and colleagues (Jain et al. 2009) synthesized silver nanoparticles (Ag-NPs) using a proprietary process that involved photoassisted reduction of ionic silver to metallic nanoparticles followed by their stabilization (Paknikar 2012). The authors tested a gel formulation containing Ag-NPs (ranging in size from 7 to 20 nm) to identify the minimum inhibitory concentration and the minimum bactericidal concentration against standard reference cultures, and against multidrug-resistant organisms. As reported by other authors (Amato et al. 2011), Gram-negative bacteria were eliminated by Ag-NPs more efficiently than Gram-positive. Moreover Ag-NPs were proved to have good antifungal activity, exhibit synergism with commonly used antibiotics (ceftazidime), possess additive effects when associated with streptomycin, kanamicin, ampiclox, polymyxin B, and possess antagonistic effects with chloramphenicol.

Similarly, in 2011 Nguyen and colleagues (Nguyen et al. 2011) focused their research work on developing a novel polymeric organic scaffold to carry and deliver Ag-NPs. The authors synthesized a poly(vinyl alcohol) (PVA) mat and then loaded it with Ag-NPs. The novel PVA Ag-NP mat was proved experimentally to possess high tensile stress, excellent antimicrobial activity against both Gram-positive and Gram-negative bacteria, and very satisfactory Ag-NP surface distribution. PVA is a nontoxic, degradable material, known for its high mechanical stability and excellent thermostability and chemical resistance. The authors obtained the Ag-NP-loaded PVA mat by adding a $AgNO_3$ solution to a PVA solution and then irradiating the mix for a few seconds in a microwave oven. The irradiated solution was loaded into a plastic syringe equipped with a metal needle and then electrospun using a specific high-voltage power supply. Electrospinning is the simplest process available to fabricate a continuous small-diameter (typically on the micro- or nanoscale) fiber from a liquid. The generated nanofibers are characterized by a high surface area, small pore size, and good mechanical properties. During electrospinning, nanofibers are created from a polymeric solution by means of an electrostatic force. The solvent system used plays two crucial roles. First of all, it allows solvation of the polymer molecules, so that the polymer solution can form an electrified jet. The second role of the solvent is to carry the solvated polymer molecules toward the collector, enabling rapid vaporization of the solvent molecules and their departure from the polymer fibers (Hsu et al. 2010). The electrospinning process is versatile, cost-effective, and there are a wide range of materials that can be spun. Materials typically used in electrospinning are natural, synthetic biopolymers, or a combination of the two, and various substances (such as proteins and growth factors) can be incorporated into the spun materials (Wei and Ma 2008).

In this work, irradiation in a kitchen microwave oven and electrospinning were employed to evenly disperse the Ag-NPs inside the PVA fibers. The electrospun nanofiber mats were collected and then heated with the aim of increasing the number of Ag-NPs on the surface of the PVA fibers. The structure of the Ag-NP-loaded PVA fibers was observed using both scanning electron microscopy (SEM) and transmission electron microscopy (TEM), and the average diameter of the nanofibers was determined by analyzing the SEM images with an image analysis program. The electrospun PVA fibers appeared homogeneous and their diameters were verified to range between 100 and 200 nm. The presence of Ag-NPs was confirmed in solution after microwave treatment by x-ray diffraction and UV-Vis absorption spectroscopy; absorption spectra was measured in a wavelength ranging from 300 to 800 nm, and a maximum absorption peak located at 416 nm, which is a characteristic for Ag-NPs, was observed. High-resolution TEM images of the heated nanofibers demonstrated that Ag-NPs were spherically dispersed on the entire surface of the fibers and were present as single nanoparticles (diameters ranging between 5 and 15 nm) or as aggregates (diameter of 100 nm).

The authors investigated by differential scanning calorimetry and Fourier transform–infrared spectroscopy (FT-IR) the interactions between PVA and Ag. The authors experimentally verified the existence of interactions between Ag-NPs and the –OH groups of the PVA chain. Finally, the authors assessed the tensile strength of the fibers and demonstrated it to be very satisfactory. The antibacterial properties of the PVA/Ag-NP mat were tested against *S. aureus* and *Escherichia coli* using the disk diffusion method. The PVA/Ag-NP mat displayed a high antibacterial activity against both Gram-positive and Gram-negative bacteria, and *S. aureus* was found to be more sensitive than Gram-negative *E. coli*. In light of these results, Nguyen and colleagues developed a PVA/Ag-NP mat characterized by very promising properties by combining three simple methods (electrospinning, microwave treatment, and low-temperature aging) and optimizing the process parameters (time and the temperature of heating and of microwave irradiation).

Despite the great commercial success of silver-coated/impregnated dressings and their worldwide use, some concerns have arisen about their safety, their possible local toxic effects on human skin cells, or even systemic toxic effects due to silver absorption. Another worry is the possible existence and spread of silver-resistant bacteria.

In the last decade, silver-resistant bacteria have been isolated and genetically characterized by different researchers (Silver 2003; Lok et al. 2008; Woods et al. 2009; Glasser et al. 2010) but the clinical relevance of these strains is debated.

Many research works and clinical studies have focused on the possible toxic effects of the absorption of huge amounts of silver by treated patients. Until the advent of silver dressings, only SSD cream and diluted $AgNO_3$ solutions were used to treat burn patients. In burns units, SSD is commonly applied twice a day and $AgNO_3$ up to 12 times a day, with all of the mechanical trauma and discomfort that this can be caused to a patient (Dunn and Edwards-Jones 2004). Frequent dressing changes are necessary because silver ions are rapidly inactivated by organic matter and chloride present in wound fluids. The silver-impregnated or silver-coated dressings were developed to overcome these limitations and particularly the rapid inactivation of silver. These dressings need to be changed less frequently because they are designed to release additional silver as it is consumed by interaction with cells, proteins, or anions resulting theoretically in a sustained, steady supply of active silver. Considering the amount of time the silver-containing dressings are left in place and the amount of silver continuously released into the wound environment (Vlachou et al. 2007), this aspect is now being investigated in more detail.

The systemic absorption of silver and its effects in 30 patients treated with a commercially available nanocrystalline silver dressing have been investigated in a clinical study (Vlachou et al. 2007). The patients were eligible for the study if they had a deep partial-thickness or a full-thickness burn of at least 2% of their total body surface area, requiring autografting. The skin grafts, the superficial nongrafted burns, and the donor sites were covered with nanocrystalline silver dressings. Every 3 days, the dressings were changed and the wounds and patients were assessed, until complete healing of the wounds (graft site, donor site, and nongrafted burned area) up to 28 days after grafting. Silver dressings were no longer applied once wounds had healed. Photographs of the wounds and blood samples were taken at day 3 and 6, at the assessment when the donor or graft sites first healed and once treatment was discontinued, 28 days after grafting or when the silver treatment was stopped. After completion of treatment during the follow-up, blood samples and photographs were taken after 3 and 6 months. Blood biochemistry and hematological assays were performed to identify any indications of adverse effects arising from absorption of silver, and subsequent elevated serum silver concentrations. It should be noted that it is recommended that silver biological monitoring is carried out on whole blood as there is "an ill defined association between the metal and red blood cells" (Armitage et al. 1996) meaning that systemic analytical biases may be found when analyzing serum or plasma levels. The authors carried out the measurements by inductively coupled plasma mass spectroscopy (ICP-MS) and demonstrated that the use of nanocrystalline silver dressings caused an increase in serum silver levels that was dependent on the wound area exposed and the number of dressings employed during treatment. They found that the median maximum serum silver level during treatment was 57.8 µg/L and the median time to maximum silver level was 9 days. In the majority of participants, serum silver levels returned to near baseline by the 3-month follow-up. Six months after treatment the serum silver concentrations returned to very low levels similar to those measurable in unexposed patients (0.4 µg/L). Despite the increase in serum silver levels, no biochemical or hematological indicators of toxicity were found to be associated with silver absorption. In light of this research work, the use of nanocrystalline silver dressings seems safe and secure for patients.

In 2006, a case of silver toxicity was reported for the first time (Trop et al. 2006) in a patient who was treated with nanocrystalline silver dressings. The patient was a young, previously healthy 17-year-old boy with 30% mixed depth burns; he exhibited symptoms of silver toxicity after 1 week of treatment with these dressings. The patient showed signs of hepatotoxicity and a grayish discoloration of the face (argyria), as well as a change in lip color to pale blue. The serum silver and urine levels were elevated and an alteration in the pattern of hepatic enzymes was evident, suggesting that a liver insult had occurred as a consequence of the treatment. After cessation of nanocrystalline silver dressing use, the liver enzymes rapidly returned to normal values, the discoloration of the face faded with time, but the serum silver levels remained elevated for several weeks. Probably in this specific case, the adverse reaction was due to *sensitivity to* silver.

More recently, silver deposits were observed in a porcine deep dermal partial thickness burn model. The researchers (Wang et al. 2009) scalded eight pigs (four burns per pig, and two on each side in the thoracic rib region) and then covered the wound (debrided or not) with a nanocrystalline silver dressing until completion of wound reepithelialization. The dressings were changed twice a week for the first 3 weeks, and then once a week for the 3 weeks afterwards. Six weeks after injury, the researchers collected scar and normal uncovered tissues to measure silver levels by ICP-MS, or conduct histological analysis to observe changes in skin color or the presence of silver deposition by light microscopy. Wang and coworkers verified that after reepithelialization, numerous wounds had a gray appearance and brown-black pigments were detectable mostly in the middle and deep dermis within the scars. According to the authors, the skin discoloration caused by silver can be reasonably considered permanent, and because no effective therapies are available to reverse this adverse effect, caution should be taken when applying silver dressings, particularly in sensitive areas and for prolonged periods of time.

There is clearly a need for further studies in the light of these results and others obtained in recent research works. When testing the safety and the cytotoxicity of various silver-containing wound dressings, ointments and creams commonly employed in burn units, several authors have independently demonstrated by *in vitro* and *in vivo* models that silver can exert antiproliferative effects on human keratinocytes and fibroblasts, delaying wound healing or wound reepithelialization (Burd et al. 2007; Kempf et al. 2011; Zanette et al. 2011).

Other elements in nanoparticulate form possess bactericidal activity similar to silver, for instance, titanium dioxide nanoparticles (TiO_2-NPs) have been employed commonly as a photobactericide, deodorant, and antiviral agent (Budde 2010).

TiO_2-NPs have been homogeneously dispersed in a chitosan with collagen to form a nanotitanium dioxide collagen artificial skin (NTCAS) (Peng et al. 2008). The researchers produced and characterized their NTCAS by SEM, and determined the oxygen permeability of the skin substitute, the apparent density, the water absorptivity, the percent biodegradability, and the biodegradation rate. A bactericidal test verified the antimicrobial properties of NTCAS, which was further confirmed by an *in vivo* open wound model. The healing properties of NTCAS were assessed using three groups of wounded animals: the first group was treated with NTCAS, a second group with a commercialized market product known to promote healing, and a third group was left untreated to assess the course of wound healing without any treatment. On days 0, 7, and 14 postwounding, the inflammatory outcomes were assessed; the authors tracked the time course of wound healing daily and measured serum levels of TNF-α and IL-6 using an enzyme-linked immunosorbent assay (ELISA) kit to investigate if NTCAS or the positive control skin substitute were able to modulate serum concentrations of cytokines. Peng and coworkers demonstrated that NTCAS had promising and interesting characteristics as well as moderate water absorptivity, fine thickness, low density, and moderate as well as favorable time-dependent biodegradability. NTCAS has been showed to exhibit potent bactericidal properties against *S. aureus*, which was positively correlated with the amount of incorporated TiO_2-NPs. According to the authors, the extremely effective bactericidal activity can be attributed to the prominent photocatalytic activity of TiO_2-NPs. Immediately after injury, serum levels of TNF-α and IL-6 increases. In the first 7 days of the healing process, both NTCAS and a positive control skin-substitute-treated group exhibited significantly different IL-6 serum levels, compared to the untreated group. In this research work, NTCAS was proved to have a better effect than the market product in modulating the acute inflammatory response. Finally, it was verified that 12 days after wounding, both NTCAS-treated group and commercial-product-treated group showed a good wound healing and the group showing the best recovery was the NTCAS-treated group.

Copper is well known to be a broad-spectrum biocide, able to inhibit the growth of bacteria, fungi, and algae (Borkow and Gabbay 2004, 2005; Washington State Department of Ecology 2008). The Roman Empire used copper nails to stop fouling of its ships (Redfield et al. 1952; Hellio and Yebra 2009) and the Royal Navy clad their ships in copper (Bingeman et al. 2000) in the eighteenth century to prevent marine invertebrate parasites boring through the wood. Copper at lower concentrations is an essential element occurring naturally in all organisms (Festa and Thiele 2011) and plays a number of important roles in human health, including cellular energy production (Wikström 2004), balance of essential elements (e.g., zinc) (Castilloduran et al. 1990), and maintenance of signal molecules [estrogen (Fishman and Fishman 1987) and neurotransmitters (Prasad et al. 2011)]. Copper also supports key catalytic and structural roles in proteins (superoxide dismutase) and biomolecules (Messerschmidt 2010) and with respect to unessential elements, it shows a lower toxicity to humans due to the presence of mechanisms for protection against copper toxicity at the cellular, tissue, and organ levels (Turnlund 1998; Kim et al. 2008). Recently, copper nanoparticles (Cu-NPs) have been combined with a wide variety of materials to obtain novel products exhibiting antimicrobial properties. Two recent studies (Hamilton et al. 2010; Mikolay et al. 2010) demonstrated that in hospital settings, the incorporation of metallic copper-containing alloys into touch surfaces and the use of copper-containing detergents to clean working environments were shown to reduce hospital-acquired infections and the number of colony-forming units growing on the treated surfaces. The use of copper-containing surfaces and detergents resulted in a definite decrease in bacterial contamination of hospital surfaces. In 2011, Cady and colleagues (Cady et al. 2011) reported the construction of a copper-based nanostructured coating on natural cellulose and tested its effectiveness in killing *A. baumannii*, a multidrug-resistant wound-associated bacterium. The authors verified the safety and biocompatibility of the novel product by an *in vitro* test on embryonic fibroblast stem cells. First, the original fibers were converted into carboxymethyl cotton fiber using chloroacetic acid, and then this carboxymethylated cotton was used to chelate cationic copper (Cu^{2+}). In the following step, the authors reduced the

Cu^{2+} carboxymethyl cellulose complex with sodium borohydride to produce copper nanoparticles (Cu-NPs) that coated the cotton composite. An identical reaction sequence was employed to produce a Ag-NP-coated cotton dressing to compare the antimicrobial properties. The presence of nanoparticles on the surface of the dressings was verified by SEM analysis while copper and silver quantification in the dressings was performed by ICP-MS, the total copper content was found to range between 0.303% and 0.507% w/w, and the total silver content ranged between 0.115% and 0.248% w/w.

Zone inhibition tests were carried out for both Ag-NP- and Cu-NP-coated dressings and the results showed a strong difference in the diffusion properties of the two metal NP-coated dressings. When observing the inhibition zone sizes, Ag-NP-coated dressings exhibited a moderate diffusion of the antibacterial agent, while the Cu-NP-coated cellulose showed an apparent absence of diffusion and antimicrobial activity.

A liquid-based dynamic contact assay on bacteria in a liquid culture medium of trypticase soy broth showed that the Cu-NP-coated cotton was unexpectedly able to significantly reduce *A. baumannii* growth after 10 min of contact. A comparative silver-based material showed a marked lower bactericidal effect both after a contact period of 10 min and after 24 h. The Cu-NP-coated sample was also more effective at killing *A. baumannii* than one of the most commonly employed commercially available nanocrystal silver dressings. To try and explain this apparent activity difference, the authors carried out a liquid diffusion test by immersing the dressings in phosphate-buffered solution (PBS) for 3 h and the supernatants were assayed to see if they were able to inhibit the growth of *A. baumannii*. The results verified the zone inhibition test results; as the PBS exposed to Ag was able to reduce the number of viable bacteria by 60–90% (depending on the dressing), the supernatant exposed to Cu had no growth inhibitory effect. ICP-MS analysis of the supernatant solutions demonstrated the presence of Ag in solution at significant concentrations while copper was only present at trace ($\mu g/L$) levels. Analysis of the copper-based dressing after the leaching test showed that the copper levels were reduced from 0.57 to 0.42 weight%, and copper was also detected inside the bacterial cells. The authors suggest that the bacteria are able to uptake Cu-NPs at nonlethal levels.

The authors compared the antibacterial ability of Cu^{2+} ions with that of their Cu-cotton composite to gain insight into possible mechanisms of activity. They found that concentrations >600 mg/L of Cu^{2+} caused a 7 log reduction in growth, while an 8 log reduction was achieved with a concentration of 30 mg/L of Cu-NPs. The authors concluded that the interaction is not simply "due to copper release" but that there is a contact killing mechanism.

Cytotoxicity tests on mouse fibroblast cells showed that after a 24 h incubation period with exposure to either Ag-NP- or Cu-NP-coated dressings, there was no effect on cell viability. But at longer exposure times, Ag-NP-coated cotton proved to be fatal to mammalian cells, while at the same time, the Cu-NP-coated sample did not alter cell viability. Finally, in this work, the authors confirmed the absence of toxicity of Cu-NP-coated cotton by a cell adhesion test: mouse fibroblasts were supplemented with fetal bovine serum to facilitate cell adhesion and were allowed to adhere to the plate prior to exposure to metal NP samples. After an incubation time of 48 h, healthy mammalian fibroblasts were observed on the Cu-NP-coated fibers while few living cells were detectable on Ag-NP-coated cellulose, confirming the marked difference in the toxicity of the novel copper-based dressing for bacterial or mammalian cells.

Interestingly, zinc compounds in particulate form have been shown to possess antibacterial properties as well. Recently, Shalumon and collaborators (Shalumon et al. 2011) produced and incorporated zinc oxide nanoparticles (ZnO-NPs) in a sodium alginate (SA)/PVA fibrous mat. Alginate is an anionic polysaccharide distributed widely in the cell walls of brown algae. It is a linear copolymer with homopolymeric blocks of (1–4)-linked β-D-mannuronate (M) and (1-4)-linked α-L-guluronate (G) residues, covalently linked together in different sequences or blocks (Yang et al. 2011). SA is the sodium salt of alginate and possesses the following useful properties: it is of biological origin, nontoxic, biocompatible, biodegradable, and low-cost (d'Ayala et al. 2008). Owing to these characteristics, it has been widely used in many biomedical fields, including tissue engineering, regeneration of multiple tissues such as skin (Hashimoto et al. 2004), cartilage (Dausse et al. 2003; Thorvaldsson et al. 2008), bone (Alsberg et al. 2001), and liver (Wang et al. 2003) as well as the treatment of exuding wounds to enhance the healing process (Qin 2008). Recently, an SA has been developed as a controlled drug delivery system. This interest is hampered because SA occurs mainly in a nonflexible fragile gelatinous form that makes it difficult to process into nonspherical forms such as films and filaments. To overcome this problem, one possible solution is to blend SA with a compatible flexible vinyl polymer, such as PVA. The researchers prepared a 2% w/v SA solution and a 16% w/v PVA solution and found the optimum SA-to-PVA solution ratio to be 1:1 v/v. Subsequently, they added ZnO-NPs to the polymer combination at concentrations of 0.5%, 1.0%, 2.0%, and 5% w/w and the modified polymer was electrospun to obtain a mat. The solutions and fibers were characterized and their antimicrobial ability was verified. The antibacterial activity of the electrospun nanocomposite fibrous mats were studied against *E. coli* and *S. aureus* using the disk diffusion method and the zone of inhibition was analyzed. Cell adhesion studies, chromatin coloring (4′,6-diamidino-2-phenylindole (DAPI) staining) and cytotoxicity studies were also carried out using mouse fibroblasts cells to evaluate possible toxic effects of SA/PVA/ZnO-NPs mat on skin cells. After 24 h of incubation, an inhibition zone around SA/PVA/ZnO-NPs mat was clearly detectable and the size of the inhibition zone positively correlated with the amount of ZnO-NPs present in the mats. Compared with *S. aureus*, *E. coli* showed a slightly smaller inhibition zone, indicating that ZnO-NPs were more effective against Gram-positive rather than Gram-negative bacteria. In cell attachment studies, ZnO-NPs were verified to be slightly toxic at higher concentrations. As the nanoparticles concentration in the mats increased beyond 2%, cells showed a slightly rounded morphology that may be attributed to the toxic effect of ZnO-NPs. This result was supported by the results from the DAPI nuclear staining and cytotoxicity tests.

Interestingly, recent studies have demonstrated that dissolved Zn^{2+} plays a major role in the toxic effect of ZnO particles (Miao et al. 2010; Song et al. 2010), differently from what has been proved for Ag-NPs (Powers et al. 2011; Beer et al. 2012) and Cu-NPs (Cady et al. 2011). Ag-NP and Cu-NP effects are distinct from those of their respective ions, indicating that NP effects are not simply due to the release of ions into the surrounding environment.

Another element displaying antibacterial properties is magnesium. Magnesium oxide has been widely employed in many areas. Recently, it has been demonstrated that magnesium oxide possesses a good bactericidal performance in aqueous environments, and that magnesium oxide in nanoparticulate form exhibits high activity against bacteria, spores, and viruses (Shi et al. 2010) and this property increases after the adsorption of halogen gases (Stoimenov et al. 2002; Koper et al. 2002; Stoimenov et al. 2003). Compared with TiO_2-NPs, Ag-NPs, and Cu-NPs, magnesium oxide nanoparticles (MgO-NPs) have the advantages of being synthesized from readily available and low-cost precursors as well as being safe and nontoxic for humans.

In 2005, Huang and collaborators (Huang et al. 2005) synthesized MgO-NPs of seven different sizes by four methods and verified the bactericidal properties of the nanoparticles. The antibacterial tests were carried out using germs or spores of *S. aureus* and *Bacillus subtilis*. MgO-NPs exhibited an excellent bactericidal efficacy against *S. aureus*, which is relatively easy to destroy. The bactericidal effectiveness against *B. subtilis* was demonstrated to be good and in general it was observed to increase with decreasing nanoparticle size, but MgO-NPs smaller than 26 nm in diameter formed aggregates that showed a minimal bactericidal efficacy. The authors investigated the bactericidal mechanisms of MgO-NPs: in solution, magnesium oxide is very readily hydrated, forming a layer of $Mg(OH)_2$ on the surface. Superoxide anions (O_2^-) can be generated by single-electron reduction of oxygen dissolved in solution, and are stable in a basic environment. Superoxide ions exist on the surface of MgO-NPs at high concentrations due to this hydrolyzed surface. Quantitative FT-IR analysis revealed that O_2^- damages the secondary amide links in the proteins constituting the cell walls of bacteria and spores, leading to their gradual destruction.

The interest in using nitric oxide (NO)-releasing particles as local antibacterial agents has risen recently. These studies have deepened the antimicrobial properties of NO, a reactive free radical produced by neutrophils and macrophages during the inflammatory phase in the presence of bacterial infection (Weller 2009; Gusarov et al. 2009). NO has been proved to be able to efficiently kill both Gram-positive and Gram-negative bacteria, and can effectively destroy biofilms. For example, Hetrik and coworkers (Hetrick et al. 2009) published a research work investigating the antibacterial properties of chemically modified silica NPs able to release NO. A NO donor, diazeniumdiolate, was synthesized on aminoalkoxysilane precursors prior to NP construction and was then incorporated into the NP scaffold (Shin and Schoenfisch 2007; Shin et al. 2007), enabling the formation of particles with a superior NO release ability. Compared to small-molecule NO donors, NO-releasing silica nanoparticles showed enhanced bacterial efficacy against planktonic *P. aeruginosa* cells and were effective in destroying biofilms of *P. aeruginosa, E. coli, S. aureus, Staphylococcus epiderimidis,* and *Candida albicans.* According to the authors, the rapid diffusion characteristics of NO means that this highly reactive molecule can penetrate into a biofilm, meaning that it has a high effectivity against biofilm-embedded bacteria. In this research work, the authors verified that the NO released causes less cytotoxic effects on fibroblasts compared to commonly used antiseptics.

7.3 Proliferative Phase

7.3.1 Detailed Description of the Proliferative Phase

The first event in the proliferative phase is represented by the reepithelialization process, which begins about 24 h after wound formation. During this stage, the keratinocytes from the wound edges are stimulated by the release of several growth factors (EGF, FGF, TGF-α) to produce specific MMPs able to degrade the existing ECM components (Saarialhokere et al. 1994). In addition, keratinocytes produce a series of factors used to create a passage between the dermis and the fibrin clot. These factors are urokinase plasminogen activator (uPA) and tissue plasminogen activator (tPA), enzymes responsible for the conversion of plasminogen into plasmin, one of the most efficient substances for fibrin degradation (Jensen and Lavker 1996). As a result, keratinocytes begin to migrate and proliferate, forming an advancing epithelium above the dermis. Once the epidermal barrier is completely reestablished, keratinocyte migration stops and the epithelial cells pass into the proliferative phase. Approximately 4 days after injury, macrophages, fibroblasts, and endothelial cells move into the wound bed and form the so-called granulation tissue. FGF, TGF-β, and PDGF derived from macrophages cause fibroblast infiltration (Singer and Clark 1999). Activated fibroblasts invade the wound site and produce new ECM components, such as elastin, GAGs, and type III collagen. These components form an amorphous, gel-like connective tissue matrix necessary for cell migration. Fibroblasts also secrete FGF and, along with VEGF that is secreted by platelets and neutrophils during the inflammatory phase, they promote endothelial cell migration and proliferation (Nissen et al. 1998). This induces vascularization at the healing site, which is necessary for the supply of oxygen and nutrients, which is required for the synthesis, deposition, and organization of a new ECM. Later, some of the fibroblasts are phenotypically converted into myofibroblasts. These contractile cells, expressing α-smooth muscle actin and vimentin, facilitate the wound closure (Gabbiani 2003; Kondo and Ishida 2010).

7.3.2 Applications of Nanotechnologies in Modulating and Modifying the Proliferative Phase

The migration and proliferation of multiple cell types are key events during the proliferative phase of the wound healing process. These events are critically dependent on communications between cells and their environment, which are in turn influenced by cell–ECM interactions and cell stimulation by growth factors or cytokines. In recent years, the advent of nanotechnologies has allowed enormous progress in the field of biomaterial science and in the development of efficient drug delivery systems, aimed at improving cell migration and proliferation (Wei and Ma 2008).

7.3.2.1 Nanostructured Biomaterials

Important advances have been made in the production of materials made of nanofibers, especially biodegradable polymer nanofibers. This class of biomaterials should be an ideal scaffold for wound dressing. Compared to micrometer-scale fibers, nanofibers have a greater water retention capacity because of their very high surface-area-to-volume ratio and are very soft so that the dressing will not chafe the wound. In addition, nanofiber materials mimic the characteristics of the native ECM, thereby improving cell adhesion, proliferation, and differentiation as well as ECM deposition. There are three common methods for the fabrication of polymeric nanofibers: self-assembly, phase separation, and electrospinning (Ngiam et al. 2011). Self-assembly consists of the spontaneous aggregation of molecules, mainly peptides and phospholipids, under thermodynamic equilibrium conditions into well-organized and stable structures maintained by multiple noncovalent interactions (Zhang 2002). Among these techniques, self-assembly is the most complex technique, but has the advantage of creating nanofibers with very small diameters, ranging from a few to 100 nm. Phase separation is much simpler than self-assembly and generates polymers with diameters of 50–500 nm. In this technique, the temperature of a homogeneous multi-component system (made of a polymer, a solvent, and water) is gradually decreased. As a consequence, a phase separation is induced, which results in the formation of a polymer-rich phase and a polymer-lean phase. When the solvent is removed, the polymer-rich phase solidifies and a porous structure is obtained (Ma and Zhang 1999). Both self-assembly and phase separation have the disadvantage of creating only short strands of nanofibers. Electrospinning, on the contrary, represents the most reliable method to simply fabricate long continuous strands of nanofibers with diameters ranging from nanometers to micrometer (50–1000 nm). In addition, electrospun nanofibers possess the advantages of a very high surface-area-to-volume ratio and pore sizes ranging from several to tens of micrometers. The high surface-area-to-volume ratio and porosity of electrospun scaffolds facilitate oxygen permeability and allow fluid accumulation, which are highly desirable in the wound healing process (Zhong et al. 2010). Natural materials from which nanofibers have been created include collagen, chitin, fibrinogen, silk, gelatin, and dextran. The advantage of using natural biopolymers is that they are nonimmunogenic, nontoxic, and tend to have a greater cell binding capability (Hromadka et al. 2008).

Type I collagen is the main ECM component of the skin dermis; it is a fibrillar protein with a long and stiff triple-helix structure. The nanoscaled structure of collagen fibrils, with a diameter ranging from 50 to 500 nm, has been found to enhance cell–matrix interactions. Indeed, fibrils interact with cells via several receptor families, thus participating in the regulation of their proliferation, migration, and differentiation. In particular, it is now well recognized that type I collagen, as well as many other ECM proteins (laminin, fibronectin, and vitronectin), contain arginine–glycine–aspartic acid (RGD) sequences. These are responsible for the interactions with integrin receptors, which are expressed in a variety of cell types (Balasundaram and Webster 2007). Collagen has been widely used in a variety of clinical applications, such as wound dressing and scaffold for tissue engineering because of these properties. In the study of Rho and colleagues (Rho et al. 2006), a nanofibrous matrix of type I collagen was produced by electrospinning. This collagen nanofibrous matrix was then cross-linked using glutaraldehyde (GA) vapor for 12 h. Cross-linking of collagen is necessary to maintain the structural integrity of the scaffold during the desired implantation time, before cells repopulate and new tissue regenerates (Pieper et al. 2000). The cross-linked collagen nanofibrous scaffold was then used alone or after treatment with a coating of ECM proteins (type I collagen, laminin, fibronectin) to evaluate human keratinocyte adhesion and spreading. As explained later, surface modifications are often key for improving the natural properties of nanostructured biomaterials. Collagen nanofibers without ECM coating showed a low level of cell attachments, probably as a consequence of denaturing of the collagen conformation induced by electrospinning or cross-linking. Conversely, the coating of electrospun collagen nanofibers with ECM proteins was found to improve keratinocyte adhesion and spreading. This may be explained by the restoration of natural biological and structural properties of ECM proteins. In the same work, the effect of collagen nanofibers was examined on open wound healing in a rat model. Two full-thickness square wounds of 1×1 cm were made on the back of 12 rats, in parallel with the vertebral column. One of the wounds was covered with electrospun collagen nanofibers without ECM protein coating; the other one was treated with cotton gauze and used as a control. Seven days after injuries, the wound surface of the control group was covered by fibrinous tissue debris, and below that layer, infiltration of inflammatory cells was seen. In the collagen nanofiber group, the surface tissue debris had disappeared, and there was significant proliferation of young capillaries and fibroblasts. The authors concluded that collagen nanofibrous matrices were very effective as wound-healing accelerators, in particular, in the early stages of wound healing.

Glycosaminoglycans represent the other major class of ECM components. GAGs are glycoproteins with a protein core and polysaccharide branches composed of repeating disaccharide units containing carboxylic and/or sulfate ester groups. Endogenous GAGs are heparin, heparan sulfate, keratin sulfate, dermatan sulfate, chondroitin sulfate, and hyaluronic acid (Saliba 2001). It has been demonstrated that the combination of GAGs with collagen greatly enhances wound healing; in particular, GAGs have been reported to positively affect cellular response, morphology, and stiffness of the resultant matrix (Osborne et al. 1999). Zhong and coworkers (Zhong et al. 2005) have produced electrospun collagen–GAGs scaffolds based on collagen and 4% chondroitin sulfate. These scaffolds exhibited a uniform nanofibrous and porous structure with a mean diameter of 260 nm, similar to that found in native ECM (50–500 nm). The resultant nanofibrous collagen–GAG matrices were then cross-linked by GA vapor. The cross-linked collagen–GAG scaffolds showed greater biostability compared with the non-cross-linked counterparts, as resulting from a collagen digestion test. The biocompatibility of collagen–GAG scaffolds was evaluated in *in vitro* cultures of rabbit conjunctiva fibroblasts. Cross-linked collagen matrices with incorporated GAG exhibited higher fibroblasts proliferation with respect to the non-cross-linked scaffolds. This can be attributed to the fact that cross-linking not only increases the biostability of the scaffolds but also provides a better physical support for cell proliferation.

Among GAGs, hyaluronic acid (HA) is a fundamental carbohydrate component of the ECM. HA is a biological macromolecule with a highly conserved structure between mammalian species, and it has unique physiochemical properties. HA is one of the most hygroscopic molecules in nature, it is highly viscoelastic and shows excellent biocompatibility and biodegradability (Chen and Abatangelo 1999). These single characteristics probably explain the role of HA in many biological processes, including wound healing. It is well documented that HA participates in the regulation of the tissue repair process, from the early inflammatory response through to granulation tissue formation and to the reepithelialization process. For example, the presence of HA in the granulation tissue facilitates water recruitment and thus dilates the matrix, creating spaces among the fibers through which cells can migrate.

HA can be manufactured in a number of forms, such as gels, sheets of solid material, or lightly woven meshes. Recently, Uppal and colleagues (Uppal et al. 2011) produced HA nanofibers through electrospinning, and compared the efficacy of these fibers with that of an adhesive bandage, a sterilized solid HA, an antibiotic dressing, and gauze with Vaseline, using a pig wound model. The HA nanofiber scaffolds resulted as the best type of dressing out of the five types compared. The HA nanofiber dressing showed much greater air permeability than the sterilized solid HA; in addition, this dressing could act as a scaffold, thus improving cell migration, proliferation, angiogenesis, and consequently accelerated the wound healing process.

A nanofiber matrix composed of a combination of collagen and HA through electrospinning has been prepared, using a mixture of 1,1,1,3,3,3-hexafluoro-2-propanol and formic acid (70/30 vol.%) as solvent (Hsu et al. 2010). The fiber diameter was approximately 200 nm, a dimension that is similar to that of native fibrous proteins within the ECM. Foreskin fibroblasts were then seeded onto collagen–HA matrices, and adhesion, proliferation, and expression of the ECM-related gene were evaluated. Proliferation tests revealed that HA concentrations above 1.5% strongly inhibited adhesion and growth of fibroblasts. This result is in agreement with a previous work, which describes how only low concentrations of HA are able to stimulate fibroblast proliferation when added to cell cultures (Greco et al. 1998). Proteinases (especially MMPs) and tissue inhibitors of metalloproteinases (TIMPs) are implicated in epidermal repair during wound healing. MMP1, in particular, is primarily produced by dermal fibroblasts, and it has a high specificity for type I collagen. Its proteolytic function is specifically inhibited by TIMPs. Hsu and colleagues evaluated the expression of these enzymes in foreskin cells cultured on collagen–HA nanofiber matrices, and measured a lower ratio of TIMP to MMP1 compared with those grown on the collagen nanofibrous matrix alone. This decreased ratio is known to be a characteristic of scarless wounds (Dang et al. 2003), thus suggesting a possible role of such composite nanofibrous dressings for scarless skin regeneration.

Synthetic polymers have also been widely used to manufacture nanofibers. The main advantages of these synthetic polymers are their favorable mechanical properties, with degradation rates matched to the healing rate in damaged tissues. Scherer and colleagues (Scherer et al. 2009) developed a bioactive scaffold-like membrane based on new biodegradable nanofibers. These nanofibers were obtained through gamma radiation of native diatom-derived poly-N-acetyl-glucosamine fibers (sNAG). The authors tested these membranes in *in vitro* cultures of endothelial cells and fibroblasts, and *in vivo* in a diabetic mouse wound healing model. The sNAG nanofibers interacted with fibroblasts and endothelial cells *in vitro*, stimulating their migration and metabolic activity. *In vivo*, sNAG membranes significantly enhanced diabetic wound healing, through enhancement of angiogenesis, cell proliferation, and reepithelialization. Genes related to angiogenesis (VEGF), cell migration (uPA-receptor), tissue remodeling (MMP3, MMP9), and inflammatory response (IL-1β) were upregulated by sNAG membranes in wounds. The membrane was completely integrated into wounds, and in long-term follow-ups (3 and 6 months), sNAG fibers were no longer identifiable in the wounds.

Polyurethane (PU) nanofibrous membranes have been prepared by electrospinning (Khil et al. 2003) and their efficacy as wound dressings was evaluated. For this purpose, full-thickness wounds 1 × 1 cm were created on the back of 30 adult guinea pigs. The nanofibrous PU scaffolds were then laid down on the wounds of 15 adult guinea pigs; 15 other guinea pigs were used as controls and their wounds treated with a commercial product for wound healing. Wound reepithelialization occurred in 15 days after injury in both groups. Nevertheless, the dermis of the wound covered with the commercial product was still somewhat inflammatory, whereas the dermis in the group treated with PU nanofibrous membranes appeared well organized. In addition, the porous structure of electrospun membranes ensured a better oxygen permeability, a more controlled evaporative water loss, and inhibited exogenous microorganism invasion.

7.3.2.2 Surfaces Modification of Nanostructured Biomaterials

Surface modification of nanostructured biomaterials is an efficient way to improve cellular interactions with the nanofiber scaffolds (Wei and Ma 2008). Indeed, contact surfaces can influence cell fate through changing the shape and mechanical status of the cells.

Parkinson and coworkers (Parkinson et al. 2009) investigated the effect of nanotopography on cell response and the ability to elicit control over cells using surface details. Anodic aluminum oxide (AAO) is a potential scaffold that is formed through the oxidation of aluminum in acidic electrolytes and possesses a highly regular porous structure. It is inert, stable, nonreactive, and biocompatible. By changing its macroscopic parameters, such as the anodization time and voltage, the anodizing electrolyte, and the time of postchemical etching, it is possible to achieve different pore geometries. The authors developed highly regular nanoporous AAO films with a range of pore sizes between 40 and 500 nm, and tested the influence of different pore sizes on keratinocyte proliferation and migration, important aspects of cell behavior during wound healing. Significantly, 3 days after culturing, fewer cells were identified on 125 nm pore size membranes compared to other AAO membranes, suggesting that this particular pore size inhibits cell proliferation or adhesion. Also, migratory capacity was affected by pore size; in particular, cells migrated faster across the membrane with 500 nm pores than the 65 and 200 nm membranes. Overall, these results suggested the possibility of controlling cell behavior through nanotopography, which may optimize a membrane for rapid growth and enhancement of repair, or on the contrary, inhibit cell migration and proliferation and help modulate scarring.

Another example of surface modification of nanostructured biomaterials is reported in the paper of Liu and colleagues (Liu et al. 2010). In this work, various synthetic polymers (PVA, poly(e-caprolatone) (PCL), poly(acrylonitrile) (PAN), poly(vinylidene fluoride-co-hexafluoropropene) (PVdF-HFP), and PAN-poly(urethane) (PEU)) were used for the fabrication of nanofiber membranes through electrospinning. The diameter of all the nanofibers was in the range between 200 and 800 nm, and the porosity of the electrospun membranes was at least 60%. The nanofiber membranes were treated with a wool protein by means of dip-coating or coelectrospinning, to explore the effect of protein-based nutrients on wound healing efficiency. Untreated membranes were used as controls. All the dressings were tested on a rat wound model (5 animals per 11 treatment groups). The membranes containing wool protein had higher wound healing rates compared with the pure dressings. The authors hypothesized that wool protein may have supported the healing of wounds, both providing proteinaceous material to the wound and improving surface wettability. Among all the polymers, PVA nanofiber membranes performed better than PCL and PVdF-HFP. It should be noticed that PVA is a hydrophilic polymer, whereas PCL and PVdF-HFP are hydrophobic. A hydrophilic membrane surface enables proper contact to the wound, which enhances the protection functions of the wound dressing on the wound. On the contrary, significant fluid accumulation occurred under the hydrophobic dressings, thus increasing the chance of infections. Other important aspects affecting the healing process are the membranes porosity and permeability to air. In general, higher porosity and permeability of membranes to air led to better wound healing performance. Also, in this case, the healing rate was higher for the hydrophilic polymers compared with the hydrophobic ones.

Furthermore, the authors tested the efficacy of Ag coating on all nanofiber membranes. The PVA-Ag dressing had the strongest antibacterial ability; nevertheless, it did not show the best performance in the wound healing model. The authors speculated that there is no direct relationship between the antibacterial ability and the wound healing performance. Rather, as the interconnected nanofibers create pores in nanofiber membranes that are typically smaller than bacteria, the nanofiber membrane itself could prevent bacterial invasion, therefore effectively avoiding exogenous infections.

As reported elsewhere in the text, growth factors play a fundamental role in modulating the wound healing process at different levels. During the proliferative phase, the release of growth factors in the wound area significantly stimulates numerous cellular activities. Growth factors promote cell migrations at the wound site; stimulate keratinocytes and fibroblasts proliferation, as well as the formation of new blood vessels and new ECM. Several reports describe the promising potential of growth factors for effective wound healing (Tredget et al. 2005; Faler et al. 2006; Barrientos et al. 2008). The employment of growth factors has become possible by the rapid advance in recombinant technology and the availability on a large scale of purified recombinant polypeptides and proteins (Wei and Ma 2008). In the work of Choi and colleagues (Choi et al. 2008), recombinant human EGF (rhEGF) was chemically conjugated to electrospun nanofibers, obtained from a mixture of PCL and PCL-PEG (poly(ethyleneglycol)). EGF is a small protein that binds with a high affinity to EGF receptors (EGFR). This causes EGFR dimerization and phosphorylation, which in turn triggers the signal transduction pathways leading to increased cell proliferation and migration (Hardwicke et al.

2008). To evaluate the effects of rhEGF conjugated to nanofibers (rhEGF nanofibers) on cell proliferation and differentiation, human keratinocytes were seeded onto these scaffolds. Electrospun nanofibers with rhEGF in solution and pure nanofibers were used as controls. The expression levels of keratinocyte-specific genes, such as keratin1 and loricrin, in the keratinocytes cultivated on the rhEGF-nanofibers were much higher than those on nanofibers with rhEGF in solution or controls. It has been postulated that keratinocytes seeded on the rhEGF-nanofibers were continuously stimulated by rhEGF because the growth factor was chemically attached to the nanofibers and not in solution. The rate of wound closure after 7 and 14 days from injury was evaluated when rhEGF-nanofibers were applied to wounds in a diabetic mouse model. In this case, rhEGF-nanofibers performed better when compared with other treatments. The authors concluded that conjugation of EGF to nanofibers protected from degradation by proteolytic enzymes, allowing a continuous stimulation of keratinocyte proliferation and differentiation.

7.3.2.3 Drug-Delivering Nanostructured Biomaterials

As already discussed, growth factors play a pivotal role in stimulating cellular activity and regulating tissue regeneration; nevertheless, their clinical application is limited by a short half-life in the circulatory system and rapid digestion by numerous proteolytic enzymes (Wei and Ma 2008). Chemical conjugation to nanostructured biomaterials represents a useful way to maintain the functionality of growth factors, but the opportunity to control their release is often minimal. Conversely, a drug delivery system would be a more promising strategy to achieve the high therapeutic efficacy of such molecules. In this sense, nanotechnology has revolutionized drug delivery. By incorporating growth factors or other biological factors into appropriate devices, protein structure and biological activity can be stabilized, with the consequences of prolonging the time period over which these molecules are released at the delivery site (Kang and Schwendeman 2007; Wischke and Schwendeman 2008).

Polymeric nanoparticles, such as nanospheres and nanocapsules, have been demonstrated to be useful delivery matrices. In addition, nanoparticles have received more attention than liposomes because of their therapeutic potential and greater stability in biological fluids as well as during storage. Nanoparticles have in general dimensions ranging from 10 to 1000 nm, and can be produced from the following natural and synthetic polymers: gelatin, chitosan, sodium alginate, poly(D,L-glycolide) (PLG), poly(L-lactic acid) (PLLA), poly(lactide-co-glycolide) (PLGA), and poly(cyanoacrylate) (PCA). Nanoparticles can be prepared by different methods involving either a polymerization of dispersed monomers or a dispersion of polymers. The biological factor can be incorporated during the nanoparticle formation, so it is entrapped or dissolved within it, or absorbed at the surface after nanoparticle formation. The release of factors from nanoparticles is controlled first of all by diffusion and secondarily by degradation of the polymer matrix (Soppimath et al. 2001).

Zavan and coworkers (Zavan et al. 2009) have recently demonstrated the incorporation of PDGF in hyaluronan-based nanoparticles, by designing a growth factor–nanocarrier complex in which both the components are well-known active players in wound healing. HA, indeed, is a major constituent of ECM, whose deposition during wound healing is strongly regulated by PDGF; this growth factor also acts as a promoter of reepithelialization and granulation tissue formation. In this work, a benzyl ester of HA (Fidia Advanced Biopolymer, Italy), was used to prepare micro- and nanoparticles through a high-pressure gas antisolvent (GAS) precipitation process. Different to other more conventional techniques, such as double emulsion-solvent evaporation, the GAS system is environmentally safe and preserves the properties of thermally labile compounds. In the GAS precipitation process, a polymeric organic solution is pressurized with a dense gas or supercritical antisolvent (typically CO_2), resulting in fast precipitation of the polymer from organic solution, resulting in micro- and nanoparticles. By varying different parameters, such as temperature and pressure, different particle morphologies can be produced (Elvassore et al. 2001). Zavan and colleagues produced particles with sizes in the micro (900–1000 nm) and nano (300–400 nm) ranges. PDGF was absorbed into these particles after their production, by exploiting the properties of water as a vehicle for drug transport inside the polymeric matrix. Coprecipitation of the growth factor and benzyl ester of HA resulted in a poor loading and inactivation of PDGF, probably due to its denaturation during the GAS process. The growth factor release was mainly driven by the polymeric matrix erosion process in the presence of an alkaline environment, obtained by the addition of 5% Na_2CO_3. Indeed, under physiological conditions, the high affinity of the growth factor for the polymer did not allow its release into solution. PDGF micro- and nanoparticles were then used for treating skin ulcers. For this purpose, three full-thickness wounds (1 cm in diameter) were created on the back of 18 rats. One injury was treated with PDGF-embedded microparticles; the other two were treated with carrier inert gel only and inert gel plus untreated microparticles. At day 7, wounds treated with PDGF-embedded microparticles showed an increased reepithelialization with respect to other treatments. In addition, increase in breaking strength and collagen content was observed in PDGF-treated injuries, indicating a positive effect of this growth factor in the modulation of the healing process.

Shortly afterward, Chu and colleagues (Chu et al. 2010) used PLGA as the carrier for the production of rhEGF nanoparticles by means of a modified double-emulsion solvent evaporation method. This process implies that the polymer is dissolved in an organic solvent, like dichloromethane, chloroform, or ethyl acetate. The growth factor is then dispersed into this preformed polymeric solution, which is in turn emulsified into an aqueous solution, making the primary emulsion. A second emulsion is added to the first and sonicated, to obtain the double emulsion. Afterwards, the organic solvent is evaporated by increasing the temperature under pressure or by continuous stirring, and nanoparticles are recovered by centrifugation (Zambaux et al. 1998). The drawbacks associated with this technique are excessive use of organic solvent, which leads to pollution of the product and waste disposal problems, toxicity due to incomplete solvent removal, and thermal/chemical degradation of bioactive molecules. Morphological analyses of the nanoparticles produced with this method by Chu and coworkers revealed that they were spherical, uniform, and well dispersed, with a mean diameter of 193.5 nm. The release time of rhEGF in PBS was calculated to be 24 h, indicating that the nanoparticles can induce a controlled release of the growth factor. The rhEGF nanoparticles were used to determine their effect on fibroblasts proliferation in comparison with three other treatments: rhEGF stock solution, empty nanoparticles, and PBS. The rhEGF nanoparticle group showed the highest levels of cell proliferation. In addition, Chu and coworkers examined the effect of nanoparticles on wound healing in animal experiments. For this purpose, full-thickness wounds (1.8 cm in diameter) were created on the backbone of 130 diabetic rats, and the same four treatments listed before were applied onto these wounds (32 animals per four treatment groups). Within each group, four different time points were considered: 3, 7, 14, and 21 days. The healing effects of rhEGF nanoparticles were not any better than other groups on the third day of treatment. However, treatments of 7, 14, and 21 days accelerated the healing rate in the rhEGF nanoparticle group with respect to all of the other groups. These results suggested that rhEGF has no effects at the acute inflammatory stage of the wound healing because the cells are mainly composed of inflammatory cells. Rather, the effect of rhEGF is superior at intermediate and advanced stages of wound healing, when the granulation tissue forms and the fibroblasts become predominant. The authors also considered that the controlled release of the nanoparticles allows a continuous contact between rhEGF and the wound area, which maintains an effective concentration that promotes wound healing.

Wei and colleagues (Wei et al. 2006) have developed an interesting approach for drug delivery, which integrates scaffolds and growth factors. They combined the efficacy of nanostructured biomaterials in stimulating cell adhesion and proliferation with the potential of micro- and nano-carriers to modulate the release of growth factors. For this purpose, they incorporated microspheres containing growth factor into a nanofiber scaffold. First, PDGF encapsulated into PLGA microspheres (with a diameter of <1 µm) were fabricated through the double-emulsion technique. Then, PLLA macroporous nanofiber (pore diameters of 250–425 µm, fiber diameters of 50–500 nm) scaffolds were obtained by the combination of phase separation and sugar-leaching techniques. Finally, PLGA microspheres with rhPDGF were incorporated into the PLLA scaffolds using a postseeding method. The authors studied the release kinetics of the growth factor from scaffolds *in vitro*. The amounts of released rhPDGF from the scaffolds could be modulated either by the amount of the growth factor encapsulated in the microspheres or the amount of microspheres incorporated into the scaffolds. However, the main factor controlling the release of rhPDGF from the scaffolds was the degradation of the incorporated microspheres. In general, high-molecular-weight (HMW) PLGA microspheres containing PDGF took a longer time to degrade and consequently, released PDGF more slowly than their low-molecular-weight (LMW) counterparts. In addition, no loss of bioactivity was found for rhPDGF during encapsulation into PLGA microspheres, as was demonstrated by human gingival fibroblast DNA synthesis *in vitro*. These results overall demonstrated that the encapsulation of proteins into microspheres, which are then incorporated into the scaffolds, emerges as a promising strategy to achieve controlled release of growth factors from scaffolds while maintaining their biological activity.

In a following work by the same research group (Jin et al. 2008), these PDGF-delivering scaffolds were implanted subcutaneously in midsagittal incisions of a total of 27 rats. The animals were subjected to nine different treatments that can be grouped into three subgroups: (high dose or low dose) PDGF encapsulated in (HMW or LMW) PLGA microspheres incorporated into PLLA nanofibers, (HMW or LMW) PLGA microspheres incorporated into PLLA nanofibers, and (high dose or low dose) PDGF-coated coating PLLA nanofibers. Empty PLLA nanofibers were used as controls. At different time points, the scaffold implants were harvested to evaluate cell penetration, vasculogenesis, and tissue neogenesis. At 7 days, PDGF encapsulated in PLGA microspheres showed both significantly more tissue penetration and blood vessel formation when compared to scaffolds with a simple coating of PDGF or the controls. In particular, the nanofiber scaffolds containing HMW microspheres exhibited more blood vessels formation with respect to the LMW group, at both low and high doses of PDGF. Gene expression experiments were also performed to identify the potential genes related to PDGF function *in vivo*. The enhanced tissue neogenesis and neovascularization by continuous PDGF release were found to be associated with changes in PDGF-induced gene expression profiles of chemokine family members, actin and interleukins.

7.4 Remodeling Phase

7.4.1 Detailed Description of the Remodeling Phase

The last phase of the wound healing process is remodeling; this consists of a gradual conversion of granulation tissue to scar tissue. This step, which usually begins while tissue proliferation is still occurring, can continue for up to 1 year, and is associated with the apoptosis of myofibroblasts, endothelial cells, and macrophages that leave a relatively acellular scar tissue (Cross and Mustoe 2003). As a scar matures, it becomes less red, reflecting a change in the density of capillaries within the wound (Baum and Arpey 2005). At the same time, ECM components are modified by the balanced mechanism of proteolysis and new matrix secretion. In particular, immature type III collagen is gradually replaced by mature type I collagen (Rodero and Khosrotehrani 2010). The degradation of collagen in the wound is controlled by several MMPs, and the activity of these enzymes is balanced by the presence of inhibitors called TIMPs. The new collagen fibers are rearranged in a more organized structure that progressively continues to increase tensile strength in the wound area. Nevertheless, long-term strength at the injury site arrives at approximately 80% of the strength of the normal dermis 6 months after wounding and it never reaches the basal level (Baum and Arpey 2005). Another characteristics associated with mature scars is the absence of appendages, including hair follicles, sebaceous glands, and sweat glands (Werner and Grose 2003).

7.4.2 Applications of Nanotechnologies in Modulating and Modifying the Remodeling Phase

Numerous efforts aiming at the development of therapeutic strategies for effective skin repair have been made in recent years. From what has emerged so far, nanotechnologies have massively contributed to the modulation of the initial stages of the healing process, that is, the inflammatory and proliferative phases. In contrast, very little has been reported on the regulation of the last step of wound healing, the remodeling phase. A useful approach for improving the results of the remodeling phase would rely on the regulation of enzymatic activity of MMPs and TIMPs to control scar tissue formation. In this case, nanotechnologies could take advantage of the ability of nanoparticles to quantitatively and temporally modulate the delivery of biological active molecules to the wound site. Chellat and coworkers (Chellat et al. 2005) performed a preliminary study for evaluating the effect of chitosan–DNA nanoparticles on the behavior of THP-1 human macrophages (Figure 7.2). Chitosan is known for its biodegradability and biocompatibility. Its role in modulating the inflammatory response in conjunction with silver dressings has been reported earlier in this text. Macrophages are the first cells that intercept foreign bodies, which can even be introduced nanoparticles, with the effect of releasing inflammatory cytokines and MMPs. In this work, THP-1 human macrophages were incubated with chitosan–DNA nanoparticles, and the release of different cytokines and MMPs was assessed by ELISA. Surprisingly, internalization of chitosan–DNA nanoparticles by macrophages was related to the absence of TNF-α, IL-1β, IL-6, and anti-inflammatory interleukin-10 (IL-10) in cell supernatants, and with an increased secretion of MMP-9 after 24 and 48 h of incubation. Chellat and coauthors concluded that chitosan–DNA nanoparticles could be a promising drug delivery system since they do not induce an inflammatory response while promoting the release of MMP-9, which is a key regulator of tissue

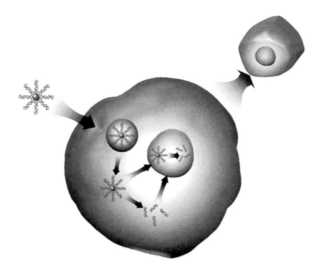

FIGURE 7.2
(**See color insert.**) Chitosan–DNA nanoparticles on the behavior of THP-1 human macrophages. Macrophages are the first cells that intercept foreign bodies, which can even be introduced nanoparticles, with the effect of releasing inflammatory cytokines and MMPs.

remodeling. However, more studies need to be done in the future to develop efficient therapeutic strategies that can influence the remodeling phase of wound healing.

7.5 Conclusions

Nanomedicine is still a new-born branch of science in its applications but appears to offer promising and innovative tools that may overcome some of the limits of traditional treatments in wound care. It may improve our capacity for direct intervention on the phases of wound healing, and more in general, may provide better solutions for wound dressings that induce favorable wound healing environments. However, as our knowledge of new nanodrugs is still limited, pharmacokinetic and toxicological studies are advisable to ensure the safety of the products that are available.

References

Acar, A., F. Uygur, H. Diktaş, R. Evinç, E. Ülkür, O. Öncül, and L. Görenek. 2011. Comparison of silver-coated dressing (Acticoat®), chlorhexidine acetate 0.5%

(Bactigrass®) and nystatin for topical antifungal effect in Candida albicans-contaminated, full-skin-thickness rat burn wounds. *Burns* 37 (5):882–885.

Alsberg, E., K. W. Anderson, A. Albeiruti, R. T. Franceschi, and D. J. Mooney. 2001. Cell-interactive alginate hydrogels for bone tissue engineering. *Journal of Dental Research* 80 (11):2025–2029.

Amato, E., Y. A. Diaz-Fernandez, A. Taglietti, P. Pallavicini, L. Pasotti, L. Cucca, C. Milanese et al. 2011. Synthesis, characterization and antibacterial activity against Gram positive and Gram negative bacteria of biomimetically coated silver nanoparticles. *Langmuir* 27 (15):9165–9173.

Aramwit, P., P. Muangman, N. Namviriyachote, and T. Srichana. 2010. *In vitro* evaluation of the antimicrobial effectiveness and moisture binding properties of wound dressings. *International Journal of Molecular Sciences* 11 (8):2864–2874.

Armitage, S. A., M. A. White, and H. K. Wilson. 1996. The determination of silver in whole blood and its application to biological monitoring of occupationally exposed groups. *Annals of Occupational Hygiene* 40 (3):331–338.

Assoian, R. K. and M. B. Sporn. 1986. Type β transforming growth factor in human platelets: Release during platelet degranulation and action on vascular smooth-muscle cells. *Journal of Cell Biology* 102 (4):1217–1223.

Balasundaram, G. and T. J. Webster. 2007. An overview of nano-polymers for orthopedic applications. *Macromolecular Bioscience* 7 (5):635–642.

Barrick, B., E. J. Campbell, and C. A. Owen. 1999. Leukocyte proteinases in wound healing: Roles in physiologic and pathologic processes. *Wound Repair Regeneration* 7 (6):410–422.

Barrientos, S., O. Stojadinovic, M. S. Golinko, H. Brem, and M. Tomic-Canic. 2008. Growth factors and cytokines in wound healing. *Wound Repair and Regeneration* 16 (5):585–601.

Baum, C. L. and C. J. Arpey. 2005. Normal cutaneous wound healing: Clinical correlation with cellular and molecular events. *Dermatologic Surgery* 31 (6):674–686.

Beer, C., R. Foldbjerg, Y. Hayashi, D. S. Sutherland, and H. Autrup. 2012. Toxicity of silver nanoparticles—Nanoparticle or silver ion? *Toxicology Letters* 208 (3):286–292.

Bingeman, J. M., J. P. Bethell, P. Goodwin, and A. T. Mack. 2000. Copper and other sheathing in the Royal Navy. *The International Journal of Nautical Archaeology* 29 (2):218–229.

Borkow, G. and J. Gabbay. 2004. Putting copper into action: Copper-impregnated products with potent biocidal activities. *FASEB Journal* 18 (14):1728–1730.

Borkow, G. and J. Gabbay. 2005. Copper as a biocidal tool. *Current Medicinal Chemistry* 12 (18):2163–2175.

Budde, F. E. 2010. Self-cleaning, odor reducing, and water shedding properties of titanium dioxide (TiO$_2$) photocatalytic oxidizing coatings. *Metal Finishing* 108 (1):34–36.

Burd, A., C. H. Kwok, S. C. Hung, H. S. Chan, H. Gu, W. K. Lam, and L. Huang. 2007. A comparative study of the cytotoxicity of silver-based dressings in monolayer cell, tissue explant, and animal models. *Wound Repair and Regeneration* 15 (1):94–104.

Cady, N. C., J. L. Behnke, and A. D. Strickland. 2011. Copper-based nanostructured coatings on natural cellulose: Nanocomposites exhibiting rapid and efficient inhibition of a multi-drug resistant wound pathogen, *A. baumannii*, and mammalian cell biocompatibility in vitro. *Advanced Functional Materials* 21 (13):2506–2514.

Carter, M. J., C. E. Fife, D. Walker, and B. Thomson. 2009. Estimating the applicability of wound care randomized controlled trials to general wound-care populations by estimating the percentage of individuals excluded from a typical wound-care population in such trials. *Advances in Skin & Wound Care* 22 (7):316–324.

Carter, M. J., K. Tingley-Kelley, and R. A. Warriner III. 2010. Silver treatments and silver-impregnated dressings for the healing of leg wounds and ulcers: A systematic review and meta-analysis. *Journal of the American Academy of Dermatology* 63 (4):668–679.

Castellano, J. J., S. M. Shafii, F. Ko, G. Donate, T. E. Wright, R. J. Mannari, W. G. Payne, D. J. Smith, and M. C. Robson. 2007. Comparative evaluation of silver-containing antimicrobial dressings and drugs. *International Wound Journal* 4 (2):114–122.

Castilloduran, C., P. Vial, and R. Uauy. 1990. Oral copper supplementation-effect on copper and zinc balance during acute gastroenteritis in infants. *American Journal of Clinical Nutrition* 51 (6):1088–1092.

Cavanagh, M. H., R. E. Burrell, and P. L. Nadworny. 2010. Evaluating antimicrobial efficacy of new commercially available silver dressings. *International Wound Journal* 7 (5):394–405.

Chakraborty, S. P., S. K. Sahu, S. K. Mahapatra, S. Santra, M. Bal, S. Roy, and P. Pramanik. 2010. Nanoconjugated vancomycin: New opportunities for the development of anti-VRSA agents. *Nanotechnology* 21 (10):105103.

Chellat, F., A. Grandjean-Laquerriere, R. Le Naour, J. Fernandes, L. Yahia, M. Guenounou, and D. Laurent-Maquin. 2005. Metalloproteinase and cytokine production by THP-1 macrophages following exposure to chitosan-DNA nanoparticles. *Biomaterials* 26 (9):961–970.

Chen, W. Y. J. and G. Abatangelo. 1999. Functions of hyaluronan in wound repair. *Wound Repair and Regeneration* 7 (2):79–89.

Choi, J. S., K. W. Leong, and H. S. Yoo. 2008. *In vivo* wound healing of diabetic ulcers using electrospun nanofibers immobilized with human epidermal growth factor (EGF). *Biomaterials* 29 (5):587–596.

Chu, Y. J., D. M. Yu, P. H. Wang, J. Xu, D. Q. Li, and M. Ding. 2010. Nanotechnology promotes the full-thickness diabetic wound healing effect of recombinant human epidermal growth factor in diabetic rats. *Wound Repair and Regeneration* 18 (5):499–505.

Cross, K. J. and T. A. Mustoe. 2003. Growth factors in wound healing. *Surgical Clinics of North America* 83 (3):531–545.

d'Ayala, G. G., M. Malinconico, and P. Laurienzo. 2008. Marine derived polysaccharides for biomedical applications: Chemical modification approaches. *Molecules* 13 (9):2069–2106.

Dang, C. M., S. R. Beanes, H. Lee, X. L. Zhang, C. Soo, and K. Ting. 2003. Scarless fetal wounds are associated with an increased matrix metalloproteinase-to-tissue-derived inhibitor of metalloproteinase ratio. *Plastic and Reconstructive Surgery* 111 (7):2273–2285.

Dausse, Y., L. Grossin, G. Miralles, S. Pelletier, D. Mainard, P. Hubert, D. Baptiste et al. 2003. Cartilage repair using new polysaccharidic biomaterials: Macroscopic, histological and biochemical approaches in a rat model of cartilage defect. *Osteoarthritis and Cartilage* 11 (1):16–28.

Downs, S. H. and N. Black. 1998. The feasibility of creating a checklist for the assessment of the methodological quality both of randomised and non-randomised studies of health care interventions. *Journal of Epidemiology and Community Health* 52 (6):377–384.

Dunn, K. and V. Edwards-Jones. 2004. The role of Acticoat (TM) with nanocrystalline silver in the management of burns. *Burns* 30:S1–S9.

Elvassore, N., A. Bertucco, and P. Caliceti. 2001. Production of insulin-loaded poly(ethylene glycol)/poly(l-lactide) (PEG/PLA) nanoparticles by gas antisolvent techniques. *Journal of Pharmaceutical Sciences* 90 (10):1628–1636.

Faler, B. J., R. A. Macsata, D. Plummer, L. Mishra, and A. N. Sidawy. 2006. Transforming growth factor-beta and wound healing. *Perspectives in Vascular Surgery and Endovascular Therapy* 18 (1):55–62.

Festa, R. A. and D. J. Thiele. 2011. Copper: An essential metal in biology. *Current Biology* 21 (21):R877–R883.

Fishman, J. H. and J. Fishman. 1987. Copper and the estradiol receptor. *Biochemical and Biophysical Research Communications* 144 (1):505–511.

Freitas, R. A. 2005. What is nanomedicine? *Nanomedicine-Nanotechnology Biology and Medicine* 1 (1):2–9.

Gabbiani, G. 2003. The myofibroblast in wound healing and fibrocontractive diseases. *Journal of Pathology* 200 (4):500–503.

Garay-Jimenez, J. C., D. Gergeres, A. Young, D. V. Lim, and E. Turos. 2009. Physical properties and biological activity of poly(butyl acrylate-styrene) nanoparticle emulsions prepared with conventional and polymerizable surfactants. *Nanomedicine-Nanotechnology Biology and Medicine* 5 (4):443–451.

Gartner, M. H., J. D. Benson, and M. D. Caldwell. 1992. Insulin-like growth factors I and II expression in the healing wound. *Journal of Surgical Research* 52 (4):389–394.

Glasser, J. S., C. H. Guymon, K. Mende, S. E. Wolf, D. R. Hospenthal, and C. K. Murray. 2010. Activity of topical antimicrobial agents against multidrug-resistant bacteria recovered from burn patients. *Burns* 36 (8):1172–1184.

Greco, R. M., J. A. Iocono, and H. P. Ehrlich. 1998. Hyaluronic acid stimulates human fibroblast proliferation within a collagen matrix. *Journal of Cellular Physiology* 177 (3):465–473.

Greenhalgh, K. and E. Turos. 2009. *In vivo* studies of polyacrylate nanoparticle emulsions for topical and systemic applications. *Nanomedicine-Nanotechnology Biology and Medicine* 5 (1):46–54.

Gusarov, I., K. Shatalin, M. Starodubtseva, and E. Nudler. 2009. Endogenous nitric oxide protects bacteria against a wide spectrum of antibiotics. *Science* 325 (5946):1380–1384.

Hachicha, W., L. Kodjikian, and H. Fessi. 2006. Preparation of vancomycin microparticles: Importance of preparation parameters. *International Journal of Pharmaceutics* 324 (2):176–184.

Hamilton, D., A. Foster, L. Ballantyne, P. Kingsmore, D. Bedwell, T. J. Hall, S. S. Hickok, A. Jeanes, P. G. Coen, and V. A. Gant. 2010. Performance of ultramicrofibre cleaning technology with or without addition of a novel copper-based biocide. *Journal of Hospital Infection* 74 (1):62–71.

Hardwicke, J., E. L. Ferguson, R. Moseley, P. Stephens, D. W. Thomas, and R. Duncan. 2008. Dextrin-rhEGF conjugates as bioresponsive nanomedicines for wound repair. *Journal of Controlled Release* 130 (3):275–283.

Hashimoto, T., Y. Suzuki, M. Tanihara, Y. Kakimaru, and K. Suzuki. 2004. Development of alginate wound dressings linked with hybrid peptides derived from laminin and elastin. *Biomaterials* 25 (7–8):1407–1414.

Hellio, C. and D. Yebra. 2009. *Advances in Marine Antifouling Coatings and Technologies.* Cambridge: Woodhead Publishing.

Hetrick, E. M., J. H. Shin, H. S. Paul, and M. H. Schoenfisch. 2009. Anti-biofilm efficacy of nitric oxide-releasing silica nanoparticles. *Biomaterials* 30 (14):2782–2789.

Hromadka, M., J. B. Collins, C. Reed, L. Han, K. K. Kolappa, B. A. Cairns, T. Andrady, and J. A. van Aalst. 2008. Nanofiber applications for burn care. *Journal of Burn Care & Research* 29 (5):695–703.

Hsu, F. Y., Y. S. Hung, H. M. Liou, and C. H. Shen. 2010. Electrospun hyaluronate-collagen nanofibrous matrix and the effects of varying the concentration of hyaluronate on the characteristics of foreskin fibroblast cells. *Acta Biomaterialia* 6 (6):2140–2147.

Huang, L., D. Q. Li, Y. J. Lin, M. Wei, D. G. Evans, and X. Duan. 2005. Controllable preparation of Nano-MgO and investigation of its bactericidal properties. *Journal of Inorganic Biochemistry* 99 (5):986–993.

Ip, M., S. L. Lui, V. K. M. Poon, I. Lung, and A. Burd. 2006. Antimicrobial activities of silver dressings: An *in vitro* comparison. *Journal of Medical Microbiology* 55 (1):59–63.

Jain, J., S. Arora, J. M. Rajwade, P. Omray, S. Khandelwal, and K. M. Paknikar. 2009. Silver nanoparticles in therapeutics: Development of an antimicrobial gel formulation for topical use. *Molecular Pharmacology* 6 (5):1388–1401.

Jefferson, K. K. 2004. What drives bacteria to produce a biofilm? *FEMS Microbiology Letters* 236 (2):163–173.

Jensen, P. J. and R. M. Lavker. 1996. Modulation of the plasminogen activator cascade during enhanced epidermal proliferation *in vivo. Cell Growth & Differentiation* 7 (12):1793–1804.

Jin, Q. M., G. B. Wei, Z. Lin, J. V. Sugai, S. E. Lynch, P. X. Ma, and W. V. Giannobile. 2008. Nanofibrous Scaffolds incorporating PDGF-BB microspheres induce chemokine expression and tissue neogenesis *in vivo. Plos One* 3 (3):e1729.

Kalishwaralal, K., S. BarathManiKanth, S. R. K. Pandian, V. Deepak, and S. Gurunathan. 2010. Silver nanoparticles impede the biofilm formation by *Pseudomonas aeruginosa* and *Staphylococcus epidermidis. Colloids and Surfaces B-Biointerfaces* 79 (2):340–344.

Kang, J. C. and S. P. Schwendeman. 2007. Pore closing and opening in biodegradable polymers and their effect on the controlled release of proteins. *Molecular Pharmaceutics* 4 (1):104–118.

Kang, S., T. Park, X. Y. Chen, G. Dickens, B. Lee, K. Lu, N. Rakhilin, S. Daniel, and M. M. Jin. 2011. Tunable physiologic interactions of adhesion molecules for inflamed cell-selective drug delivery. *Biomaterials* 32 (13):3487–3498.

Kempf, M., R. M. Kimble, and L. Cuttle. 2011. Cytotoxicity testing of burn wound dressings, ointments and creams: A method using polycarbonate cell culture inserts on a cell culture system. *Burns* 37 (6):994–1000.

Khil, M. S., D. I. Cha, H. Y. Kim, I. S. Kim, and N. Bhattarai. 2003. Electrospun nanofibrous polyurethane membrane as wound dressing. *Journal of Biomedical Materials Research Part B-Applied Biomaterials* 67B (2):675–679.

Kim, B. E., T. Nevitt, and D. J. Thiele. 2008. Mechanisms for copper acquisition, distribution and regulation. *Nature Chemical Biology* 4 (3):176–185.

Kimball, S. D. 1995. Thrombin active site inhibitors. *Current Pharmaceutical Design* 1 (4):441–468.

Kondo, T. and Y. Ishida. 2010. Molecular pathology of wound healing. *Forensic Science International* 203 (1–3):93–98.

Koper, O. B., J. S. Klabunde, G. L. Marchin, K. J. Klabunde, P. Stoimenov, and L. Bohra. 2002. Nanoscale powders and formulations with biocidal activity toward spores and vegetative cells of Bacillus species, viruses, and toxins. *Current Microbiology* 44 (1):49–55.

Le Pape, H., F. Solano-Serena, P. Contini, C. Devillers, A. Maftah, and P. Leprat. 2004. Involvement of reactive oxygen species in the bactericidal activity of activated carbon fibre supporting silver bactericidal activity of ACF(Ag) mediated by ROS. *Journal of Inorganic Biochemistry* 98 (6):1054–1060.

Lindblad, W. J. 2008. 41—Essential elements of wound healing. In *Principles of Regenerative Medicine*. San Diego: Academic Press.

Liu, X., T. Lin, J. A. Fang, G. Yao, H. Q. Zhao, M. Dodson, and X. G. Wang. 2010. *In vivo* wound healing and antibacterial performances of electrospun nanofibre membranes. *Journal of Biomedical Materials Research Part A* 94A (2):499–508.

Lok, C. N., C. M. Ho, R. Chen, P. K. H. Tam, J. F. Chiu, and C. M. Che. 2008. Proteomic identification of the Cus system as a major determinant of constitutive *Escherichia coli* silver resistance of chromosomal origin. *Journal of Proteome Research* 7 (6):2351–2356.

Lu, S., W. Gao, and H. Y. Gu. 2008. Construction, application and biosafety of silver nanocrystalline chitosan wound dressing. *Burns* 34 (5):623–628.

Luo, G., J. Tang, W. He, J. Wu, B. Ma, X. Wang, X. Chen et al. 2008. Antibacterial effect of dressings containing multivalent silver ion carried by zirconium phosphate on experimental rat burn wounds. *Wound Repair and Regeneration* 16 (6):800–804.

Lynch, S. E., R. B. Colvin, and H. N. Antoniades. 1989. Growth factors in wound healing. Single and synergistic effects on partial thickness porcine skin wounds. *The Journal of Clinical Investigation* 84 (2):640–646.

Ma, P. X. and R. Y. Zhang. 1999. Synthetic nano-scale fibrous extracellular matrix. *Journal of Biomedical Materials Research* 46 (1):60–72.

Martin, P. 1997. Wound healing—Aiming for perfect skin regeneration. *Science* 276 (5309):75–81.

Messerschmidt, A. 2010. 8.14—Copper metalloenzymes. In *Comprehensive Natural Products II*, eds. M. Editors-in-Chief: Lew and L. Hung-Wen. Oxford: Elsevier.

Miao, A. J., X. Y. Zhang, Z. Luo, C. S. Chen, W. C. Chin, P. H. Santschi, and A. Quigg. 2010. Zinc oxide-engineered nanoparticles: Dissolution and toxicity to marine phytoplankton. *Environmental Toxicology and Chemistry* 29 (12):2814–2822.

Mikolay, A., S. Huggett, L. Tikana, G. Grass, J. Braun, and D. H. Nies. 2010. Survival of bacteria on metallic copper surfaces in a hospital trial. *Applied Microbiology and Biotechnology* 87 (5):1875–1879.

Ngiam, M., L. T. H. Nguyen, S. Liao, C. K. Chan, and S. Ramakrishna. 2011. Biomimetic nanostructured materials—Potential regulators for osteogenesis? *Annals Academy of Medicine Singapore* 40 (5):213–222.

Nguyen, T. H., Y. H. Kim, H. Y. Song, and B. T. Lee. 2011. Nano Ag loaded PVA nanofibrous mats for skin applications. *Journal of Biomedical Materials Research Part B: Applied Biomaterials* 96 (2):225–233.

Nissen, N. N., P. J. Polverini, A. E. Koch, M. V. Volin, R. L. Gamelli, and L. A. DiPietro. 1998. Vascular endothelial growth factor mediates angiogenic activity during the proliferative phase of wound healing. *American Journal of Pathology* 152 (6):1445–1452.

Norling, L. V., M. Spite, R. Yang, R. J. Flower, M. Perretti, and C. N. Serhan. 2011. Cutting edge: Humanized nano-proresolving medicines mimic inflammation-resolution and enhance wound healing. *The Journal of Immunology* 186 (10):5543–5547.

Osborne, C. S., W. H. Reid, and M. H. Grant. 1999. Investigation into the biological stability of collagen/chondroitin-6-sulphate gels and their contraction by fibroblasts and keratinocytes: The effect of crosslinking agents and diamines. *Biomaterials* 20 (3):283–290.

Paknikar, K. M. 2012. United States Patent: 7514600 Stabilizing solutions for submicronic particles, methods for making the same and methods of stabilizing submicronic particles. http://patft.uspto.gov/netacgi/nph-Parser?Sect1=PT O1&Sect2=HITOFF&d=PALL&p=1&u =%2Fnetahtml%2FPTO%2Fsrchnum. htm&r=1&f=G&l=50&s1=7514600.PN.&OS=PN/7514600&RS=PN/7514600.

Parkinson, L. G., N. L. Giles, K. F. Adcroft, M. W. Fear, F. M. Wood, and G. E. Poinern. 2009. The potential of nanoporous anodic aluminium oxide membranes to influence skin wound repair. *Tissue Engineering Part A* 15 (12):3753–3763.

Parsons, D., P. G. Bowler, V. Myles, and S. Jones. 2005. Silver antimicrobial dressings in wound management: A comparison of antibacterial, physical, and chemical characteristics. *Wounds* 17 (8):222–232.

Peng, C. C., M. H. Yang, W. T. Chiu, C. H. Chiu, C. S. Yang, Y. W. Chen, K. C. Chen, and R. Y. Peng. 2008. Composite nano-titanium oxide-chitosan artificial skin exhibits strong wound-healing effect-an approach with anti-inflammatory and bactericidal kinetics. *Macromolecular Bioscience* 8 (4):316–327.

Pieper, J. S., T. Hafmans, J. H. Veerkamp, and T. H. van Kuppevelt. 2000. Development of tailor-made collagen-glycosaminoglycan matrices: EDC/NHS crosslinking, and ultrastructural aspects. *Biomaterials* 21 (6):581–593.

Pierce, G. F., T. A. Mustoe, B. W. Altrock, T. F. Deuel, and A. Thomason. 1991. role of platelet-derived growth-factor in wound-healing. *Journal of Cellular Biochemistry* 45 (4):319–326.

Pomahac, B., T. Svensjo, F. Yao, H. Brown, and E. Eriksson. 1998. Tissue engineering of skin. *Critical Reviews in Oral Biology & Medicine* 9 (3):333–344.

Powers, C. M., A. R. Badireddy, I. T. Ryde, F. J. Seidler, and T. A. Slotkin. 2011. Silver nanoparticles compromise neurodevelopment in PC12 cells: Critical contributions of silver ion, particle size, coating, and composition. *Environmental Health Perspectives* 119 (1):37–44.

Prasad, A. N., S. Levin, C. A. Rupar, and C. Prasad. 2011. Menkes disease and infantile epilepsy. *Brain & Development* 33 (10):866–876.

Qin, Y. M. 2008. Alginate fibres: An overview of the production processes and applications in wound management. *Polymer International* 57 (2):171–180.

Redfield, A. C., L. W. Hutchins, E. S. Deevy, J. C. Ayers, H. J. Turner, F. B. Laidlaw, J. D. Ferry, and D. Todd. 1952. Marine fouling and its prevention. *Contribution 580 from the Woodshole Oceanographic Institution.* United States Naval Institute. Annapolis, Maryland.

Rho, K. S., L. Jeong, G. Lee, B. M. Seo, Y. J. Park, S. D. Hong, S. Roh, J. J. Cho, W. H. Park, and B. M. Min. 2006. Electrospinning of collagen nanofibers: Effects on the behavior of normal human keratinocytes and early-stage wound healing. *Biomaterials* 27 (8):1452–1461.

Rodero, M. P. and K. Khosrotehrani. 2010. Skin wound healing modulation by macrophages. *International Journal of Clinical and Experimental Pathology* 3 (7):643–653.

Saarialhokere, U. K., A. P. Pentland, H. Birkedalhansen, W. C. Parks, and H. G. Welgus. 1994. Distinct populations of basal keratinocytes express stromelysin-1 and stromelysin-2 in chronic wounds. *Journal of Clinical Investigation* 94 (1):79–88.

Saliba, M. J. 2001. Heparin in the treatment of burns: A review. *Burns* 27 (4):349–358.

Scherer, S. S., G. Pietramaggiori, J. Matthews, S. Perry, A. Assmann, A. Carothers, M. Demcheva et al. 2009. Poly-*N*-acetyl glucosamine nanofibers a new bioactive material to enhance diabetic wound healing by cell migration and angiogenesis. *Annals of Surgery* 250 (2):322–330.

Scherzer, R., G. Y. Gdalevsky, Y. Goldgur, R. Cohen-Luria, S. Bittner, and A. H. Parola. 2009. New tryptophanase inhibitors: Towards prevention of bacterial biofilm formation. *Journal of Enzyme Inhibition and Medicinal Chemistry* 24 (2):350–355.

Schmutz, J. L., S. Meaume, S. Fays, Z. Ourabah, B. Guillot, V. Thirion, M. Collier et al. 2008. Evaluation of the nano-oligosaccharide factor lipido-colloid matrix in the local management of venous leg ulcers: Results of a randomised, controlled trial. *International Wound Journal* 5 (2):172–182.

Schultz, G., D. S. Rotatori, and W. Clark. 1991. EGF and TGF-alpha in wound-healing and repair. *Journal of Cellular Biochemistry* 45 (4):346–352.

Shalumon, K. T., K. H. Anulekha, S. V. Nair, K. P. Chennazhi, and R. Jayakumar. 2011. Sodium alginate/poly(vinyl alcohol)/nano ZnO composite nanofibers for antibacterial wound dressings. *International Journal of Biological Macromolecules* 49 (3):247–254.

Shaw, T. J. and P. Martin. 2009. Wound repair at a glance. *Journal of Cell Science* 122 (18):3209–3213.

Shi, L. E., L. Xing, B. Hou, H. Ge, X. Guo, and Z. Tang. 2010. Inorganic nano mental oxides used as anti-microorganism agents for pathogen control. *Current Research Education Technology Topics in Applied Microbiology, Microbial Biotechnology.* 1:361–368. Badajoz: Formatex Research Center.

Shin, J. H., S. K. Metzger, and M. H. Schoenfisch. 2007. Synthesis of nitric oxide-releasing silica nanoparticles. *Journal of the American Chemical Society* 129 (15):4612–4619.

Shin, J. H. and M. H. Schoenfisch. 2007. Inorganic/organic hybrid silica nanoparticles as a nitric oxide delivery scaffold. *Chemistry of Materials* 20 (1):239–249.

Silver, S. 2003. Bacterial silver resistance: Molecular biology and uses and misuses of silver compounds. *FEMS Microbiology Reviews* 27 (2–3):341–353.

Singer, A. J. and R. A. Clark. 1999. Cutaneous wound healing. *The New English Journal of Medicine* 341 (10):738–746.

Song, W., J. Zhang, J. Guo, J. Zhang, F. Ding, L. Li, and Z. Sun. 2010. Role of the dissolved zinc ion and reactive oxygen species in cytotoxity of ZnO nanoparticles. *Toxicology Letters* 199 (3):389–397.

Soppimath, K. S., T. M. Aminabhavi, A. R. Kulkarni, and W. E. Rudzinski. 2001. Biodegradable polymeric nanoparticles as drug delivery devices. *Journal of Controlled Release* 70 (1–2):1–20.

Stoimenov, P. K., R. L. Klinger, G. L. Marchin, and K. J. Klabunde. 2002. Metal oxide nanoparticles as bactericidal agents. *Langmuir* 18 (17):6679–6686.

Stoimenov, P. K., V. Zaikovski, and K. J. Klabunde. 2003. Novel halogen and interhalogen adducts of nanoscale magnesium oxide. *Journal of the American Chemical Society* 125 (42):12907–12913.

Tan, M. L., P. F. M. Choong, and C. R. Dass. 2010. Recent developments in liposomes, microparticles and nanoparticles for protein and peptide drug delivery. *Peptides* 31 (1):184–193.

Thorvaldsson, A., H. Stenhamre, P. Gatenholm, and P. Walkenström. 2008. Electrospinning of highly porous scaffolds for cartilage regeneration. *Biomacromolecules* 9 (3):1044–1049.

Tian, J., K. K. Wong, C. M. Ho, C. N. Lok, W. Y. Yu, C. M. Che, J. F. Chiu, and P. K. Tam. 2007. Topical delivery of silver nanoparticles promotes wound healing. *ChemMedChem* 2 (1):129–136.

Toy, L. W. and L. Macera. 2011. Evidence-based review of silver dressing use on chronic wounds. *Journal of the American Academy of Nurse Practitioners* 23 (4):183–192.

Tredget, E. B., J. Demare, G. Chandran, E. E. Tredget, L. J. Yang, and A. Ghahary. 2005. Transforming growth factor-beta and its effect on reepithelialization of partial-thickness ear wounds in transgenic mice. *Wound Repair and Regeneration* 13 (1):61–67.

Trengove, N. J., M. C. Stacey, S. MacAuley, N. Bennett, J. Gibson, F. Burslem, G. Murphy, and G. Schultz. 1999. Analysis of the acute and chronic wound environments: The role of proteases and their inhibitors. *Wound Repair and Regeneration* 7 (6):442–452.

Trop, M., M. Novak, S. Rodl, B. Hellbom, W. Kroell, and W. Goessler. 2006. Silver coated dressing Acticoat caused raised liver enzymes and argyria-like symptoms in burn patient. *Journal of Trauma-Injury Infection and Critical Care* 60 (3):648–652.

Turnlund, J. R. 1998. Human whole-body copper metabolism. *American Journal of Clinical Nutrition* 67 (5):960S–964S.

Turos, E., J. Y. Shim, Y. Wang, K. Greenhalgh, G. S. K. Reddy, S. Dickey, and D. V. Lim. 2007. Antibiotic-conjugated polyacrylate nanoparticles: New opportunities for development of anti-MRSA agents. *Bioorganic & Medicinal Chemistry Letters* 17 (1):53–56.

Uppal, R., G. N. Ramaswamy, C. Arnold, R. Goodband, and Y. Wang. 2011. Hyaluronic acid nanofiber wound dressing-production, characterization, and *in vivo* behavior. *Journal of Biomedical Materials Research Part B-Applied Biomaterials* 97B (1):20–29.

Uygur, F., O. Öncül, R. Evinç, H. Diktas, A. Acar, and E. Ülkür. 2009. Effects of three different topical antibacterial dressings on Acinetobacter baumannii-contaminated full-thickness burns in rats. *Burns* 35 (2):270–273.

Vanniasinghe, A. S., V. Bender, and N. Manolios. 2009. The potential of liposomal drug delivery for the treatment of inflammatory arthritis. *Seminars in Arthritis and Rheumatism* 39 (3):182–196.

Vlachou, E., E. Chipp, E. Shale, Y. T. Wilson, R. Papini, and N. S. Moiemen. 2007. The safety of nanocrystalline silver dressings on burns: A study of systemic silver absorption. *Burns* 33 (8):979–985.

Wang, X. Q., H. E. Chang, R. Francis, H. Olszowy, P. Y. Liu, M. Kempf, L. Cuttle, O. Kravchuk, G. E. Phillips, and R. M. Kimble. 2009. Silver deposits in cutaneous burn scar tissue is a common phenomenon following application of a silver dressing. *Journal of Cutaneous Pathology* 36 (7):788–792.

Wang, W. J., X. H. Wang, Q. L. Feng, and F. Z. Cui. 2003. Sodium alginate as a scaffold material for hepatic tissue engineering. *Journal of Bioactive and Compatible Polymers* 18 (4):249–257.

Washington State Department of Ecology. 2008. Supplemental Environment Impact Statement Assessments of Aquatic Herbicides: Risk Assessment for Copper. Study No. 00713. http://www.ecy.wa.gov/programs/wq/pesticides/seis/risk_assess.html#seis

Wei, G. B., Q. M. Jin, W. V. Giannobile, and P. X. Ma. 2006. Nano-fibrous scaffold for controlled delivery of recombinant human PDGF-BB. *Journal of Controlled Release* 112 (1):103–110.

Wei, G. B. and P. X. Ma. 2008. Nanostructured biomaterials for regeneration. *Advanced Functional Materials* 18 (22):3568–3582.

Weller, R. B. 2009. Nitric oxide-containing nanoparticles as an antimicrobial agent and enhancer of wound healing. *Journal of Investigative Dermatology* 129 (10): 2335–2337.

Werner, S. and R. Grose. 2003. Regulation of wound healing by growth factors and cytokines. *Physiological Reviews* 83 (3):835–870.

Wigginton, N. S., A. De Titta, F. Piccapietra, J. Dobias, V. J. Nesatty, M. J. F. Suter, and R. Bernier-Latmani. 2010. Binding of silver nanoparticles to bacterial proteins depends on surface modifications and inhibits enzymatic activity. *Environmental Science & Technology* 44 (6):2163–2168.

Wikström, M. 2004. Cytochrome c oxidase: 25 years of the elusive proton pump. *Biochimica et Biophysica Acta (BBA)—Bioenergetics* 1655:241–247.

Wischke, C. and S. P. Schwendeman. 2008. Principles of encapsulating hydrophobic drugs in PLA/PLGA microparticles. *International Journal of Pharmaceutics* 364 (2):298–327.

Woods, E. J., C. A. Cochrane, and S. L. Percival. 2009. Prevalence of silver resistance genes in bacteria isolated from human and horse wounds. *Veterinary Microbiology* 138 (3–4):325–329.

Wright, J. B., D. L. Hansen, and R. E. Burrell. 1998. The comparative efficacy of two antimicrobial barrier dressings: In-vitro examination of two controlled release of silver dressings. *Wounds* 10 (6):179–188.

Yamanaka, M., K. Hara, and J. Kudo. 2005. Bactericidal actions of a silver ion solution on *Escherichia coli*, studied by energy-filtering transmission electron microscopy and proteomic analysis. *Applied and Environmental Microbiology* 71 (11):7589–7593.

Yang, J. S., Y. J. Xie, and W. He. 2011. Research progress on chemical modification of alginate: A review. *Carbohydrate Polymers* 84 (1):33–39.

Zambaux, M. F., F. Bonneaux, R. Gref, P. Maincent, E. Dellacherie, M. J. Alonso, P. Labrude, and C. Vigneron. 1998. Influence of experimental parameters on the characteristics of poly(lactic acid) nanoparticles prepared by a double emulsion method. *Journal of Controlled Release* 50 (1–3):31–40.

Zanette, C., M. Pelin, M. Crosera, G. Adami, M. Bovenzi, F. Filon Larese, and C. Florio. 2011. Silver nanoparticles exert a long-lasting antiproliferative effect on human keratinocyte HaCaT cell line. *Toxicology In Vitro* 25 (5):1053–1060.

Zavan, B., V. Vindigni, K. Vezzu, G. Zorzato, C. Luni, G. Abatangelo, N. Elvassore, and R. Cortivo. 2009. Hyaluronan based porous nano-particles enriched with growth factors for the treatment of ulcers: A placebo-controlled study. *Journal of Materials Science-Materials in Medicine* 20 (1):235–247.

Zhang, S. G. 2002. Emerging biological materials through molecular self-assembly. *Biotechnology Advances* 20 (5–6):321–339.

Zhong, S. P., W. E. Teo, X. Zhu, R. Beuerman, S. Ramakrishna, and L. Y. L. Yung. 2005. Formation of collagen-glycosaminoglycan blended nanofibrous scaffolds and their biological properties. *Biomacromolecules* 6 (6):2998–3004.

Zhong, S. P., Y. Z. Zhang, and C. T. Lim. 2010. Tissue scaffolds for skin wound healing and dermal reconstruction. *Wiley Interdisciplinary Reviews-Nanomedicine and Nanobiotechnology* 2 (5):510–525.

Ziv-Polat, O., M. Topaz, T. Brosh, and S. Margel. 2010. Enhancement of incisional wound healing by thrombin conjugated iron oxide nanoparticles. *Biomaterials* 31 (4):741–747.

8

Nanoparticles in Bioimaging

Javier L. Pou Ucha

CONTENTS

8.1 Introduction...187
8.2 Nanotechnology-Oriented Medical Imaging 189
8.3 Nanoparticles and Nuclear Medicine..191
8.4 Radioisotopes for the Distribution of Nanoparticles and Drug
     Transport Visualization 193
8.5 Nanoparticles and Magnetic Resonance..196
8.6 Nanoparticles and Computed Tomography 199
8.7 Nanoparticles and Ultrasonography 200
8.8 Nanoparticles and Molecular Imaging 202
8.9 Nanoparticles and Optical Imaging 205
8.10 Nanoparticles and International Regulatory Agencies.......................205
References..206

8.1 Introduction

Currently on the market are different types of diagnostic imaging techniques that are widely used such as basic ultrasound (US), echocardiography, Doppler, angiography, multidetector computed tomography (MDCT), dynamic magnetic resonance imaging (Dynamic MRI), diffusion-weighted imaging (DWI), perfusion magnetic resonance imaging (Perfusion MRI), scintigraphy, single photon emission computed tomography (SPECT), positron emission tomography (PET). Although these techniques provide excellent anatomical and morphological characterization of the disease, they are obtained in advanced stages, presenting a poor therapeutic response and poor prognosis.

To optimize the diagnostic accuracy, different types of contrast agents for each imaging technique have been developed, most of them of intravenous administration. These contrast agents, widely used in clinical practice, are iodinated agents in CT scans, magnetic substances such as gadolinium for MRI, and multiple radiopharmaceuticals for PET and SPECT studies.

Despite the major contribution to the improvement in diagnostic performance, these substances have drawbacks such as adverse reactions, mostly seen in CT and MRI agents (anaphylactic reaction, nephrotoxicity, etc.), low intravascular free time, and little specificity toward the target tissue.

Good medical images require adequate signal enhancement at the site of interest to obtain good contrast with the surrounding normal tissue and must be able to make routine use of these agents for the early detection and localization of several pathologies in different tissues.

It is important to look for ways to provide a solution to improve the diagnostic sensitivity, the specific uptake of the contrast agent by the pathologic site, and the design of different types of energy to yield the diagnosis (light, sound, electron beam, etc.).

During the last decade, we have seen a boom in the number of nanotechnology-based agents, which have focused on biological and medical applications.

A promising direction was in the development of molecular images. These molecular imaging agents consist of nanometer-sized particles called "nanoparticles."

Nanoparticles have revolutionized medicine in the study of individual variability that patients experience with a predisposition to a disease, or in their responses to certain drug therapies, either in their efficacy or in their side effects. This is called personalized medicine.

They are currently designing an extensive list of nanoparticles of different sizes, shapes, and materials, and with multiple properties and chemical properties.[1] The most commonly used nanoparticles in the pharmaceutical industry with greater therapeutic utilities are

- Carbon nanotubes
- Buckyballs
- Liquid nanocrystals
- Nanoshells
- Quantum dots
- Superparamagnetic nanoparticles
- Microbubbles
- Dendrimers
- Liposomes

Nanoparticles have emerged as agents for diagnosis and treatment with the distinction of being manipulated in their surface structure, thereby allowing a longer intravascular circulation period, physical and chemical manipulation of energy, and being directed specifically to the target, achieving a target cell-specific uptake, allowing increased detection sensitivity through pathological signal amplification.

8.2 Nanotechnology-Oriented Medical Imaging

To achieve optimized medical imaging using targeted nanoparticles directly or indirectly to the target, a number of requirements have to be met:

- Easy preparation, easy handling, and stable storage
- No toxicity or immunogenicity
- Biocompatible and biodegradable
- Provide adequate intravascular circulation time to be studied properly by imaging techniques
- Have the ability to accumulate immediately on the site of interest, with minimal accumulation in nontarget tissue

These nanoparticles can be manipulated in their surface to reach the target. There are two ways of being targeted:

Passive Targeting: This depends on the pathophysiological features of tumor blood vessels. The incomplete tumor vasculature results in leaky vessels with enlarged gap junctions of 100 nm to 2 μm; hence, macromolecules easily access the tumor interstitium. Tumor lacks a well-defined lymphatic system, so the compounds will have a retention time higher than in the normal tissue. Those defects are called "enhanced permeability and retention (EPR) effect" and that effect is an important mechanism for the passive targeting and selective accumulation of nanoparticles in the tumor interstitium. The disadvantages of passive targeting are that the EPR is different in each tumor type, the cancer cells can reduce a number of specific interactions, the PEGylated surfaces can reduce nanoparticle–surface cell interaction, and the lack of control generates a multidrug resistance.

Active Targeting: This occurs by attaching targeting moieties to the nanoparticle surface that can bind through ligand–receptor interactions, which induce receptor-mediated endocytosis. The receptor must be expressed exclusively on target cancer cells (10^4–10^5 copies per cell) relative to normal cells and expression should be homogenous across all targeted cells. The advantages of the active targeting are the high targeting specificity and delivery efficiency avoiding nonspecific binding and the multidrug resistance reflux mechanism. Some examples are transferrin receptor-targeted cytotoxic platinum-based oxaliplatin in a liposome (MBP-426); transferring receptor-targeted cyclodextrin-containing nanoparticles with siRNA payload (CALAH-01); and prostate-specific membrane antigen (PSMA)-targeted polymeric nanoparticles containing docetaxel (BIND-014).

The nanoparticle surface can be conjugated with different targeting moieties: genes, antibodies, peptides, small molecules, aptamers, drugs, and fluorescence dyes.

Special mention goes to liposomatic nanoparticles (Figure 8.1).[2] First described in 1965, they are one of the first structures built in nanometer scale for medical application.[3] Liposomatic nanoparticles have become very important since the 1980s. They have a spherical lipid shape containing a liquid space inside. Depending on its design and composition, the size can range from tens of nanometer to micrometer.[4]

The characteristics that are given great importance at present are

- Excellent biocompatibility
- Manipulation of ligands on the surface to modify its pharmacokinetic characteristics

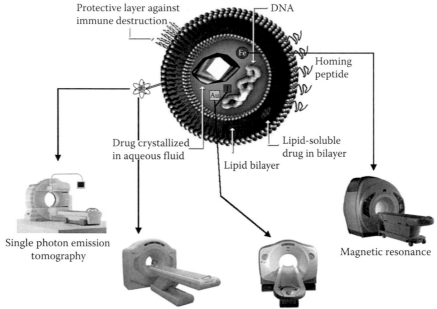

FIGURE 8.1
Image of a liposome visualized by multiple radiological and nuclear medicine imaging techniques (SPECT, PET, CT, MRI). On the liposomatic surface, a radioisotope is attached to be viewed by the gamma camera detector; polyethylene glycol is also observed as being able to avoid liposomatic destruction by immune cells and to remain for a longer time period in intravascular circulation; peptides design an active target. The lipid shell is observed embedding lipophilic therapeutic drugs. Inside the liposome, therapeutic particles are transported in aqueous solution (drug, DNA, iron, iodine, and gold). (Image modified from http://en.wikipedia.org/wiki/File:Liposome.jpg.)

- Transport of diagnostic and therapeutic agents on the surface, within their lipid bilayer, or into intraliposomatic space
- Protection of agents against inactivating plasmatic components

8.3 Nanoparticles and Nuclear Medicine

Nuclear medicine is a medical specialty that uses radiopharmaceuticals for diagnosis and treatment purpose. Drugs have a special biodistribution and are marked with different types of radioisotopes to obtain physiological images and to identify pathophysiologic and metabolic changes.

These scintigraphic images offer multiple advantages over morphological images of high definition (CT, MRI):

- Whole-body visualization for the detection of all sites of increased uptake
- Noninvasive quantification of radioisotope concentration in the pathologic site with respect to the total injected
- Ability to perform a dynamic study to monitor the kinetics and physical behavior of the radioisotope over time
- Administration of a low concentration of radioisotope (in nanograms), which does not interfere with the physiological process, and thus reduces the risk of an adverse reaction induced by the same agent
- Diagnostic functional images precede the diagnosis of tumor or infectious disease by the anatomical images (US, Rx, MRI, CT) (Figure 8.2)

Nuclear medicine also includes morphological studies such as ventilation–perfusion scintigraphy in patients with suspected pulmonary embolism (PE), performing a double study with intravenous administration of radiolabeled particles, albumin macroaggregates (size of 10–40 μm) labeled with Tc-99m, which will impact the pulmonary vascular network to give an overall picture of the two silhouettes lung and identifying nonperfused and thrombosed sites (Figure 8.3).

In the area of nuclear medicine, liposomes play an important role. They can be functionalized with target agents such as antibodies and protective polymers such as polyethylene-glycol (PEG) to prevent opsonization by the immune system and increase circulation time and diagnostic markers such as radioisotopes,[4] which would allow viewing and monitoring pathologies by SPECT and PET cameras.

They are currently used experimentally in the fields of nuclear oncology, atherosclerosis, and neurodegenerative disease.

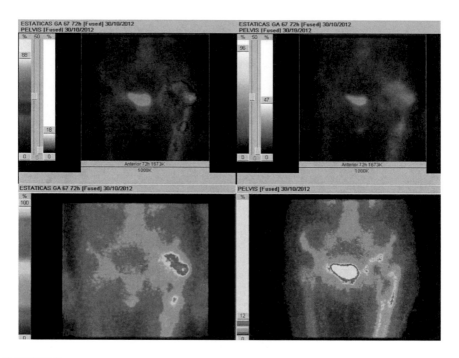

FIGURE 8.2
(See color insert.) Fusion image of two scintigraphic studies with double tracer, Tc-99m-DPD + Ga-67-citrate. It shows increased uptake in periprosthetic bone of Tc-99m-DPD radio-tracer (gray scale) at the left hip and left femoral diaphysis with an accumulation of Ga-67-citrate (color scale, left panel; red scale, right panel) in the same site related to periprosthetic infectious-inflammatory process.

The current strength of nanoparticles within the field of nuclear medicine focuses on the *highly specific identification of different physiological processes*, from changes in the metabolism of glucose, fatty acids, and proteins, to the demonstration of gene expression and signal changes due to an increased or decreased concentration of receptors on cell surface or intracellular space (Figure 8.4).

Another area of great importance in nuclear medicine is the detection of the sentinel node by peritumoral or intratumoral injection of radiolabeled nanocolloid (80 nm in diameter), which shows a very good visualization of lymphatic drainage to the first node responsible for the disease site and thus we can improve the pathological staging process (Figure 8.5).

Nowadays, nuclear medicine centers are performing the novel techniques radioguided occult lesion localization (ROLL) and radioguided sentinel node and occult lesion localization (SNOLL) not only to locate the sentinel node but also to allow optimum extraction of the primary tumor lesion with less nontumor tissue invasion by the addition of macroaggregated albumin with Tc-99m labeled (MAA) and their location with an intraoperative gamma probe.

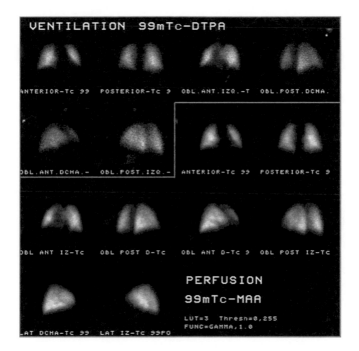

FIGURE 8.3
Ventilation–perfusion scintigraphy normal study. Above: the ventilation images (anterior, posterior, and anterior and posterior oblique projections); below: the perfusion images (anterior, posterior, oblique, and lateral projections). (Image courtesy of Dr. Luis Campos and Andrew Serena.)

8.4 Radioisotopes for the Distribution of Nanoparticles and Drug Transport Visualization

The gamma photon emission images, both PET and SPECT,[5] are the predominant methods for further *in vivo* biodistribution of particles. In the case of PET, two annihilation photons of 511 keV (products of the collision between a positron and an electron) and emitted in opposite poles are detected and used to locate the particles.[6] In contrast, the SPECT uses single photon emission with a combined collimation system to predict the photon path and thus the particle to be located within the body.

The selection of the radioisotope depends on a number of features, including the platform type of nanoparticle, simplicity of preparation, and stability of the radioisotope–nanoparticle conjugation, as well as their availability and the decay characteristic of the radioisotope[7]:

- *Technetium-99m* is available in almost all centers and comprises 80% of nuclear medicine studies[8] and it is frequently used for nanoparticle labeling. It has a half-life of 6.05 h.

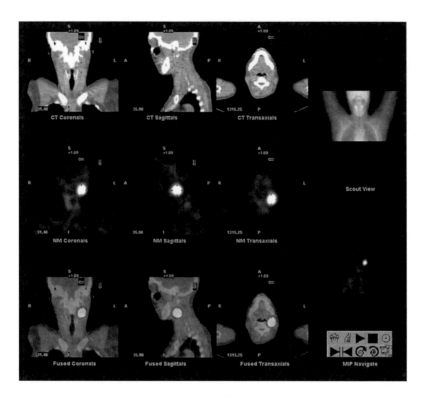

FIGURE 8.4
SPECT/CT study with somatostatin analog labeled with In-111 (In-111 Octreoscan). CT image at the top line, SPECT image in the middle line, and merged SPECT/CT images at the bottom line, projected on three axes (left to right: coronal, sagittal, and axial). CT scout image at the top right, SPECT MIP image at the bottom right. Scintigraphic visualization of high somatostatin receptor expression at the level of the lesion in left cervical region in correspondence to carotid paraganglioma.

- *Carbon-14* was one of the first elements used to track the nanoparticles by measuring urinary excretion of the radioisotope.[9] It has a half-life greater than 5000 years.
- *Tritium* has a long history of use in tracing particles.[10,11] It has a half-life of 12.5 years.

Since 1990, SPECT and PET studies have been the most useful techniques for intracorporeal tracking of the biodistribution and uptake quantification of the radiotracer:

- *Copper-64* is a frequently used agent for PET imaging. It can be incorporated into a variety of nanoparticles for *in vivo* monitoring.[12–17] This presents a simple conjugation process.

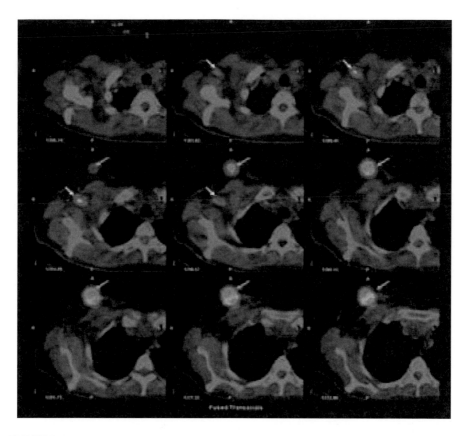

FIGURE 8.5
(**See color insert.**) Sentinel node scintigraphy. Multimodal image, SPECT/CT (nine axial slices focused on right chest), showing a focal uptake in right axillary region, posterior to the pectoral muscles, in correspondence with sentinel node (yellow arrow). The injection site is observed in the right mammary tissue (green arrow).

- *Indio-111 and technetium–99m*: Both have a long history of use for the development of drugs such as SPECT imaging agents (Figures 8.3 through 8.5).[7,18–23]

- *Iodine-123, 124, 125, and 131* have been used for whole-body planar (Figure 8.6) and SPECT images (Figure 8.7).[24–30]

- *Gallium-68*: This is the PET agent currently in use.[7,31] It is widely used in the clinic for diagnosis, staging, and posttreatment control of neuroendocrine tumors as well as other high somatostatin receptor expression tumors, when it is labeled with somatostatin hormone analog (DOTA-NOC) (Figure 8.8).

Lazarova et al.[32] performed work that consisted in designing a dual-modality nanoparticle about the microbubble labeled with Tc-99m radioisotope and in viewing their biodistribution *in vivo* by ultrasound and SPECT/CT techniques.

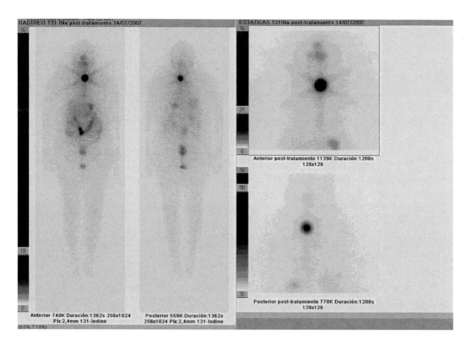

FIGURE 8.6
Whole-body scintigraphy with I-131 (103 mCi) for differentiated thyroid cancer (DTC) follow-up. Viewing only high uptake lesion in the thoracic anterior slightly lateralized to the left with respect to the mid-line. Study showing viable tumor cells related to thoracic metastasis in post-treatment control.

New studies show the utility of multimodal images with SPECT/MRI agents for the localization of the sentinel node. Madru et al.[33] designed nanoparticles with an iron oxide core coated with polyethylene glycol and labeled with Tc-99m achieving an efficiency of 97% at 24 h after labeling in both water and serum plasma and observed an accumulation of contrast agent in the sentinel node of 100% and in liver and spleen of 2%.

8.5 Nanoparticles and Magnetic Resonance

Within the field of magnetic resonance, nanoparticles are composed of iron oxide that acts as a negative contrast agent. There are two types currently approved for clinical use, superparamagnetic particles of iron oxide (SPIO) and ultrasmall superparamagnetic iron oxide (USPIO) particles.

SPIO agents (Feridex IV®, Endorem®) are captured by cells of the reticulo-endothelial system (RES) of the normal liver parenchyma; hence, increasing

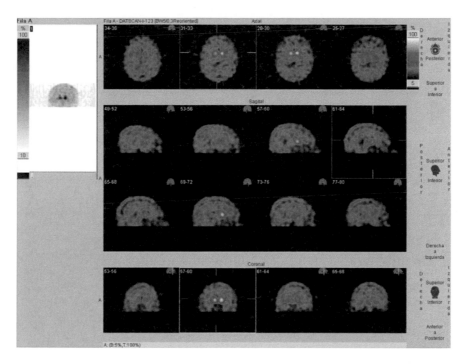

FIGURE 8.7
(**See color insert.**) SPECT study with 123I-ioflupane. Images displaying axial, sagittal, and coronal (top to bottom) projections. Specific uptake was observed at presynaptic dopamine subcortical level in the caudate nuclei (color scale). Severe decrease in uptake in both putamens in relation to Parkinson's disease.

the contrast between it and the pathological liver tissue is very useful for the diagnosis of hepatocellular carcinoma and intrahepatic metastatic lesions.[34,35] Currently under experimental study, the SPIO agent is used as a cell therapy agent, which represents a major challenge for noninvasive monitoring due to the limited incorporation of stem cells that occurs in the presence of massive cell death.[36] The stem cells should be labeled with SPIO, which will give good contrast in MRI images. The standard technique for labeling is based on the molecular biology transfection method.[37]

USPIO agents (Sinerem®, Combidex®, Clariscan®) are captured by macrophages; thus, this agent is useful to differentiate between inflammatory and metastatic nodes. There is an emerging role of USPIO agents in MRI images in atherosclerotic disease, where these nanoparticles are captured by macrophages in atherosclerotic plaques being displayed as areas of signal loss in MRI images. New superparamagnetic particles are being developed for the visualization of other cells responsible for the atherosclerotic plaque formation.[38]

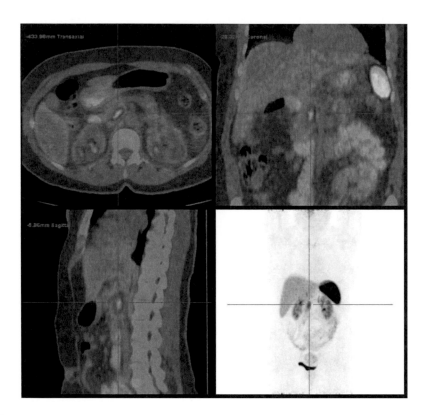

FIGURE 8.8
PET study with Ga-68-DOTA-NOC focused on abdominal region. It shows increased focal uptake at the pancreatic uncus level in correspondence with focal physiological increased somatostatin receptors expression. Rest of the body uptake corresponds to the physiological biodistribution of the radiopharmaceutical. (Image courtesy of Dr. Stefano Fanti and Dr. Paolo Castellucci from University of Bologna, Italy.)

There is also a third type of iron particles of larger diameter with respect to the two mentioned earlier; these are called micrometer-sized iron oxide (MPIO) particles used for experimental studies and early identification of the intracoronary activation of platelets while it is also useful for cell labeling.[39]

Although SPIO nanoparticles are still the most common contrast agents used for MRI images, there is a need to develop new types of nanoparticles to increase relaxation in MRI and to increase the contrast enhancement in MRI applied to various medical conditions, including cancer[40]. Taylor et al.[41] have described the synthesis of superparamagnetic iron and platinum particles (SIPPs) and then superficially PEGylated them to create immunomicelles (DSPE-SIPPs), which can be specifically targeted to the tumor cell lines of human prostate and detected using MRI and immunofluorescence images.

8.6 Nanoparticles and Computed Tomography

In radiological practice, iodinated contrast agents have been used for over 20 years for the optimization of radiological images. But these agents impose serious limitations in current medical imaging: short viewing time period, the need for catheterization in several cases, occasional renal toxicity, and poor contrast images in patients with elevated body surface that still require a high dose of iodine contrast agent.

Many experiments with other radiological contrast agents show promise as a blood pool agent, including standard iodinated agents encapsulated in liposomes,[42,43] polymers of dysprosium–DTPA–dextran,[44] PEGylated polymeric micelles containing iodine,[45] perfluoroctyl bromide,[46] linked to polylysine-derivatized iodine,[47] and iodine bound to a polycarboxylate core.[48]

Liposomes loaded with iodine can be used for optimized detection of tumors, inflammations, and infections. These have the advantage of a membranous structure and can be manipulated to add molecules such as polyethylene glycol (PEG) to the surface liposome area to increase their plasma circulation time and labeling antibodies (immunoliposomes) to find specific target tissue achieving an increase of the contrast medium in the lesion site. This preparation of immunoliposomes showed formidable challenges, including the avoidance of the reticuloendothelial system, an extended period of free movement of the contrast agent, avoidance of steric hydration, access of extravascular target, selective binding to the target, and an appropriate contrast lesion/normal tissue.

Since several years, much work has been carried out with gold nanoparticles.[49–51] With a higher atomic number (Au, 79 vs. I, 53) and a higher absorption coefficient (at 100 keV: gold: 5.16 cm^2/g; iodine: 1.94 cm^2/g; soft tissue: 0.169 cm^2/g; and bone: 0.186 cm^2/g), gold provides approximately 2.7 times greater contrast per unit weight than iodine. Gold has less bone and tissue interference and therefore achieves better contrast with lower doses of x-rays. It has a lower retention by the liver and spleen. Both kidney and tumor tissue were visualized with unusual clarity and with high spatial resolution. The renal clearance of nanoparticles is slower compared to iodinated agents allowing more viewing time. Blood vessels less than 100 μm diameter could be delineated, allowing a vascular casting *in vivo*. Regions with increased vascularization and angiogenesis could be distinguished.

There are several works with gold nanoparticles. To visualize *in vivo* the biodistribution of gold nanoparticles for the effective transport of therapeutic agent, Sanchez et al. are designing gold-loaded gelatin nanoparticles (Figure 8.9). Fayad et al., in an experimental study with rats, developed gold nanoparticles bound to high density lipoprotein (HDL) to identify the atherosclerotic plaque composition, visualizing them *in vivo* by CT scans, which provided useful information.[51] Kim et al.[52] designed multifunctional theranostics gold nanoparticles adding RNA aptamers on

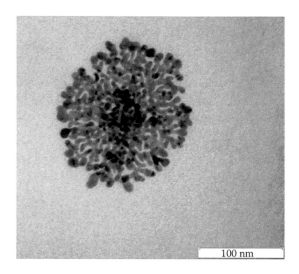

FIGURE 8.9
Gold-loaded gelatin nanoparticle. (From Professor Begoña Seijo and Alejandro Sanchez Laboratory at University of Santiago de Compostela, Spain.)

its surface that bind to prostate-specific membrane antigen (PSMA) and loaded with doxorubicin obtaining a tomographic signal with a strength greater than four times that of the standard.

8.7 Nanoparticles and Ultrasonography

Ultrasound is a field with many advantages, especially for its low cost, convenience, and real-time capability of ultrasound images, features that can provide significant improvements in diagnosis and posttreatment control. Many years ago, with the advent of Doppler US technique,[53] it has strengthened the field of flow and perfusion evaluation, especially useful in areas like cardiovascular disease.

Later, the concept of targeted contrast ultrasound imaging has been proposed. Several materials have been designed for ultrasound viewing as targeted microbubbles, with a spherical design and multiple applications.[54] One of the advantages of these microbubbles over other conventional contrast agents in other imaging techniques (CT, MRI) is that they have a longer intravascular circulation allowing a prolonged intravascular contrast time period for visualization. Another significant advantage is the opportunity to evaluate the parameters of real-time contrast enhancement without having to predefine scan times or bolus-tracking, and furthermore, the possibility of repeating tests because of it being tolerated well by the patient.[55]

Transpulmonary contrast agents currently marketed in Europe are

- Levovist®: its indications include heart, abdomen, including vesico-ureteral reflux, and transcranial
- Optison®: cardiac indication
- SonoVue®: cardiac, macrovascular, liver, and breast indications

Levovist agent contains air while SonoVue (sulfur hexafluoride) and Optison (perflutren) contain gases of low solubility, enhancing the stability of the microbubbles.

Generally, microbubbles are extremely safe and have very low incidence of adverse effects. Those are not nephrotoxic or cardiotoxic and the incidence of hypersensitivity or allergy appear in smaller numbers than CT and MRI contrast agents. No need for renal studies to be conducted prior to the administration of microbubbles. There is a theoretical possibility that the interaction between ultrasound and ultrasound contrast agent could produce biological effects. Animal studies have shown that microvascular ruptures can exist when agents are insonated. This could be of great importance in cases of ultrasound in tissues with high clinical impact as ocular ultrasonography and neonatal brain.[54]

It is useful for screening tests, interpretation and evaluation of focal liver lesions,[56] as well as local ablative liver posttreatment control.[57]

Multiple studies have been conducted with the agent SonoVue®. In a multicenter study, a total of 23,188 investigations were reported by Piscaglia et al. and their safety as ultrasound contrast agent in indications for abdominal pathology was proved.[58] Kalantarinia et al. also demonstrated that not only the myocardial perfusion can be measured but the microbubbles are also useful for monitoring the renal plasma volume, flow, and speed without showing severe adverse effects.[59] The contrast-enhanced ultrasound is easily performed in clinical practice and allows improved characterization of some renal tumors compared to other cross-sectional imaging techniques (Figure 8.10).

To increase the specificity of lesional detection, antibodies, peptides, and carbohydrates can be added as special target ligands to the microbubble's layer. Willmann et al.[60] developed an ultrasound contrast agent with dual signaling, adding to the surface of the microbubbles the antiendothelial growth factor antibodies (anti-VEGF Ab) and anti-$\alpha v\beta 3$ integrin Ab, which are useful to enhance the ultrasound imaging visualization of tumor angiogenesis.

The active targeted US contrast agents are intravenously administered into the body and they accumulate in the pathological lesion. The acoustically active contrast agents are also being widely used for clinical applications such as improved definition of the cardiac chambers[61] (Figure 8.11) and assessment of myocardial perfusion.[62]

There are also studies that have demonstrated the utility of the microbubbles to detect inflammation between lipid components and the immune coat located on the surface of the inflamed endothelium. The ultrasound contrast

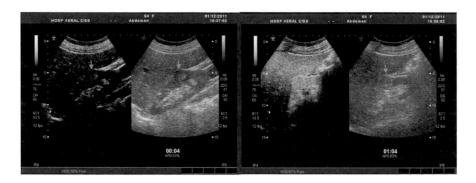

FIGURE 8.10
(**See color insert.**) Right renal ultrasound images (longitudinal axis) enhanced with SonoVue®
(microbubbles contrast agent) of the cortical renal hypervascularized tumor (green arrow). The
figure is divided in two panels composed with two images per panel. The enhanced US images
with SonoVue®, displayed at the right in both panels, were taken at 4 seconds and 1 minute
postinjection time respectively and compared with those respective non-enhanced US images (left
images in both panels) visualizing the hypervascularization of the renal tumor. (Image courtesy of
Dra. María Milagros Otero from Hospital Xeral-Cies, Spain.)

agents that incorporate sophisticated peptides or high-affinity antibodies in
their lipid layer can display markers of inflammation, thrombosis, and neovascularization in the arterial wall of atherosclerotic animal models.

Current studies also show the usefulness of the microbubbles in the detection and assessment of cerebrovascular diseases. Meairs et al.[63] have described
multiple uses of microbubbles in the assessment of stroke patients. These agents
have signed up new ultrasound perspectives in the diagnosis and monitoring
of both ischemic and hemorrhagic strokes. Additionally, it allows the assessment of atherosclerotic plaques in the carotid arteries and their probability of
rupture. There is also a particular interest in the use of ultrasound as a therapeutic application, particularly in the field of sonothrombolysis. The treatment
of ischemic stroke can be optimized with the use of ultrasound and microbubbles loaded with thrombolytic drugs.[63,64] New therapeutic ways include
opening of the blood brain barrier (BBB) with microbubbles and ultrasound to
facilitate the release of the drugs into the brain. Microbubbles are also assum-
ing a central role in molecular imaging with multiple targets of interest for the
evaluation of pathophysiological processes associated with cerebrovascular
disease, including angiogenesis, inflammation, and thrombus formation.[63]

8.8 Nanoparticles and Molecular Imaging

Nanoparticles have received considerable attention over the past decade
because of their potential use in molecular imaging.

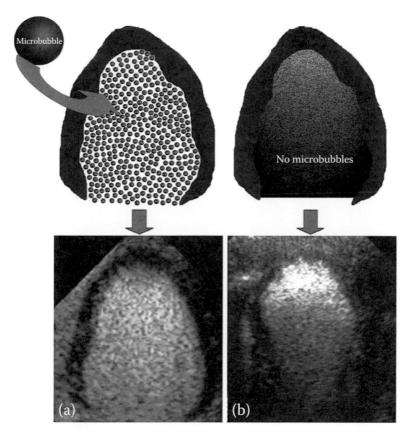

FIGURE 8.11
Four cardiac chamber ultrasound images centered in the left ventricle. (a) displays an increased acoustic contrast between the ventricular wall and intraventricular space due to the high concentration of microbubbles in the LV chamber. In (b), there is a normal noncontrast echocardiography with nonenhanced LV chamber and less LV wall/chamber contrast. (Image courtesy of Dra. Barbara Suarez from University of Vigo, Spain.)

With the optimization of the active targeting specificity, detection methods should improve simultaneously, leading to early detection of pathologies such as neoplastic disease and cardiovascular disease.

While liposomatic radiolabeled nanoparticles have been studied for a long time, only recently have researchers developed imaging agents for their potential use in humans. Active works done in this area are consistent with PET imaging, SPECT, MRI, and Quantum Dots.

Molecular imaging has evolved considerably in recent decades, and one of the most intriguing aspects of molecular imaging with nanoparticles is the potential for the particle combination design to be used as a multifaceted imaging agent.

Carriers are designed in different forms; they are of a single, double, and even triple mode.

- *Single-Mode Carriers*: There are good reasons to functionalize the nanoparticles with nuclear imaging agents for PET and SPECT visualization. While glucose analogs as FDG show the tumor uptake by Warburg effect,[5,65] its specificity could be increased by means of enhanced permeability and retention (EPR) effect.[66] Additionally, nanocarriers could be functionalized with specific ligands to improve the specificity of the target.[1] Despite its widespread use in clinical care, it is difficult to functionalize the F-18 with nanoparticles. Elements such as copper-64 are easier to be functionalized with nanoparticles because of its long half-life (12.7 h). Chakrabarti et al.[67] designed a peptide nucleic acid probe radiolabeled with copper-64 mutant KRAS mRNA for signaling. KRAS is mutated at high levels in pancreatic cancer. To achieve the cellular uptake of nanoparticles, they were combined with peptide analogs of IGF-1 peptides to allow for internalization by endocytosis through IGF-1 receptors (these IGF-1 receptors are highly increased in pancreatic carcinomas). Experimentally, Petersen et al.[68] designed liposomatic nanoparticles radiolabeled with copper-64 for PET imaging in mouse models. Authors have labeled nanoparticles to visualize tumor neovasculature by PET and SPECT cameras. Hu et al. designed perfluorocarbon nanoparticles labeled with In-111 targeted toward $\alpha v \beta 3$ integrin characteristically overexpressed in tumor neovasculature. Ruggiero et al. visualized tumor vasculature using carbon nanotubes marked with zirconium-89 for displaying the monomeric epitope of vascular endothelial cadherin, which is frequently overexpressed in tumor vasculature.[69]

- *Dual-Mode Carriers*: Several investigators have described multifaceted nanoparticles for imaging with both PET or SPECT cameras in combination with quantum dots. Cai et al. designed cadmium quantum dots functionalized with RGD peptide, $\alpha v \beta 3$ antagonist, and radiolabeled with Cu-64. This allowed dual-mode images with simultaneous display of near-infrared fluorescence (NIRF) and PET. The probe was tested in a mouse model of glioblastoma and showed an excellent correlation between *in vivo* PET imaging and *ex vivo* NIRF. On histological examination, the nanoparticles exhibited specificity for tumor neovasculature. This study allowed an accurate determination of the biodistribution of the probe. The biggest advantage of this probe may be the gain in sensitivity with PET. This allows the use of low levels of cadmium quantum dots to achieve a precise image. Works about SPECT agents in combination with quantum dots have also been described.[70] But a better combination to assess the *in vivo* biodistribution is the combination of SPECT-MRI[71–74] and PET-MRI.[75] Researchers are also designing nanoparticles of iron oxide radiolabeled with Cu-64.[76–78]

- *Triple-Modality Carriers*: Multiple investigators have described tri-modal nanoparticle images used for PET, MRI, and fluorescence imaging.[79–82] Xing et al. are also designing nanoparticles for cancer cell visualization by fluorescence, MRI, and CT cameras.[83] Arifin et al. designed microcapsules loaded with gadolinium and gold nanoparticles and pancreatic cells for DM type I treatment and their corporeal biodistribution obtaining encouraging results.[84]

8.9 Nanoparticles and Optical Imaging

In recent years, the area that is gaining great interest has been the field of optical imaging.

The field of fluorescence has gained great importance for the impact it could have at the surgical level. Tumor-specific intraoperative fluorescence imaging may improve staging and debulking efforts in cytoreductive surgery and thereby improve prognosis. Van Dam et al. proved that intraoperative tumor-specific fluorescence imaging with an FR-α-targeted fluorescent agent showcased the potential applications in patients with ovarian cancer for improved intraoperative staging and more radical cytoreductive surgery.[85] There are some tumors whose growth depend on the transforming growth factor beta1 (TGF-beta1) molecule. A special work by Li et al.[86] suggested that inhibition of TGF-beta1 signaling pathway by siRNA could be beneficial in the treatment of patients with metastatic bladder cancer (Figure 8.12).

Newly introduced nanoparticles are called quantum dots (QDs). QDs are conductive colloid particles at nanoscale levels. They have unique electronic and optical properties such as light-dependent emission color depending on their size, brightness signal optimized, fotobleaching resistance, and simultaneous fluorescent colors excitation. These properties make QDs an ideal type of nanoparticles to characterize different types of pathologic processes, with great promise in oncology.

However, the QDs have many disadvantages such as *ex vivo* visualization of the biodistribution, limited tissue penetration, lack of spatial resolution in the depth of tumor, location, and fear of potential toxicity. For clinical applications, the biggest obstacle is the potential toxicity of QD probes, which have become a topic of discussion and debate.

For these reasons, the optical images remain in the field of research.

8.10 Nanoparticles and International Regulatory Agencies

Finally, we must mention the importance of international regulatory agencies in the stability concerns of nanoparticles. The release of volatile toxic

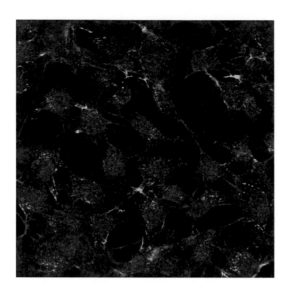

FIGURE 8.12
FITC-labeled gelatin nanoparticles associated with siRNA. Fibroblastic cell W3T3 (core DAPI, membrane Bodipy. Nps FITC). (From Professor Begoña Seijo and Alejandro Sanchez Laboratory at University of Santiago de Compostela, Spain.)

metals in certain physiological conditions, with changes in pH, temperature, and osmolarity, is a topic of great interest. Furthermore, the particles have to be biodegraded and must present an appropriate route of elimination. It is likely that those inert particles are not adequately removed from the organ and thus they will not be temporarily approved by the regulatory agencies. Quantum dots are the current example of nanoparticles that are not approved for the current clinical practice.

References

1. Wang AZ, Gu F, Zhang L, Chan JM, Radovic-Moreno A, Shaikh MR, Farokhzad OC. Biofunctionalized targeted nanoparticles for therapeutic applications. *Expert Opin Biol Ther.* 2008 Aug;8(8):1063–70.
2. Liposome. http://en.wikipedia.org/wiki/Liposome.
3. Bangham AD. Liposomes: The Babraham connection. *Chem Phys Lipids.* 1993 Sep;64(1–3):275–85.
4. Torchilin VP. Recent advances with liposomes as pharmaceutical carriers. *Nat Rev Drug Discov.* 2005 Feb;4(2):145–60.
5. Racker E, Spector M. Warburg effect revisited: Merger of biochemistry and molecular biology. *Science.* 1981 Jul 17;213(4505):303–7.
6. Chen K, Conti PS. Target-specific delivery of peptide-based probes for PET imaging. *Adv Drug Deliv Rev.* 2010 Aug 30;62(11):1005–22.

7. Phillips WT, Goins BA, Bao A. Radioactive liposomes. *Wiley Interdiscip Rev Nanomed Nanobiotechnol.* 2009 Jan–Feb;1(1):69–83.

8. IAEA 2011 Report. Production and Supplies of Mo-99: Lesons Learnt and New Options within Research Reactors and Neutron Sources Community. http://www.iaea.org/OurWork/ST/NE/NEFW/Technical_Areas/RRS/documents/mo99/NR_Mo99_Lessons_2011.pdf.

9. Bazile DV, Ropert C, Huve P, Verrecchia T, Marlard M, Frydman A, Veillard M, Spenlehauer G. Body distribution of fully biodegradable [14C]-poly(lactic acid) nanoparticles coated with albumin after parenteral administration to rats. *Biomaterials.* 1992;13(15):1093–102.

10. Kukowska-Latallo JF, Candido KA, Cao Z, Nigavekar SS, Majoros IJ, Thomas TP, Balogh LP, Khan MK, Baker JR Jr. Nanoparticle targeting of anticancer drug improves therapeutic response in animal model of human epithelial cancer. *Cancer Res.* 2005 Jun 15;65(12):5317–24.

11. Takahama H, Minamino T, Asanuma H, Fujita M, Asai T, Wakeno M, Sasaki H, et al. Prolonged targeting of ischemic/reperfused myocardium by liposomal adenosine augments cardioprotection in rats. *J Am Coll Cardiol.* 2009 Feb 24;53(8):709–17.

12. Fukukawa K, Rossin R, Hagooly A, Pressly ED, Hunt JN, Messmore BW, Wooley KL, Welch MJ, Hawker CJ. Synthesis and characterization of core-shell star copolymers for *in vivo* PET imaging applications. *Biomacromolecules.* 2008 Apr;9(4):1329–39.

13. Pressly ED, Rossin R, Hagooly A, Fukukawa K, Messmore BW, Welch MJ, Wooley KL, Lamm MS, Hule RA, Pochan DJ, Hawker CJ. Structural effects on the biodistribution and positron emission tomography (PET) imaging of well-defined (64)Cu-labeled nanoparticles comprised of amphiphilic block graft copolymers. *Biomacromolecules.* 2007 Oct;8(10):3126–34.

14. Rossin R, Pan D, Qi K, Turner JL, Sun X, Wooley KL, Welch MJ. 64Cu-labeled folate-conjugated shell cross-linked nanoparticles for tumor imaging and radiotherapy: Synthesis, radiolabeling, and biologic evaluation. *J Nucl Med.* 2005 Jul;46(7):1210–8.

15. Schipper ML, Cheng Z, Lee SW, Bentolila LA, Iyer G, Rao J, Chen X, Wu AM, Weiss S, Gambhir SS. MicroPET-based biodistribution of quantum dots in living mice. *J Nucl Med.* 2007 Sep;48(9):1511–8.

16. Xie H, Wang ZJ, Bao A, Goins B, Phillips WT. *In vivo* PET imaging and biodistribution of radiolabeled gold nanoshells in rats with tumor xenografts. *Int J Pharm.* 2010 Aug 16;395(1–2):324–30.

17. Xie J, Chen K, Huang J, Lee S, Wang J, Gao J, Li X, Chen X. PET/NIRF/MRI triple functional iron oxide nanoparticles. *Biomaterials.* 2010 Apr;31(11):3016–22.

18. DeNardo SJ, DeNardo GL, Natarajan A, Miers LA, Foreman AR, Gruettner C, Adamson GN, Ivkov R. Thermal dosimetry predictive of efficacy of 111In-ChL6 nanoparticle AMF-induced thermoablative therapy for human breast cancer in mice. *J Nucl Med.* 2007 Mar;48(3):437–44.

19. Elbayoumi TA, Pabba S, Roby A, Torchilin VP. Antinucleosome antibody-modified liposomes and lipid-core micelles for tumor-targeted delivery of therapeutic and diagnostic agents. *J Liposome Res.* 2007;17(1):1–14.

20. Masuda H, Takakura Y, Hashida M. Pharmacokinetics and disposition characteristics of recombinant decorin after intravenous injection into mice. *Biochim Biophys Acta.* 1999 Feb 2;1426(3):420–8.

21. Lin YY, Li JJ, Chang CH, Lu YC, Hwang JJ, Tseng YL, Lin WJ, Ting G, Wang HE. Evaluation of pharmacokinetics of 111In-labeled VNB-PEGylated liposomes after intraperitoneal and intravenous administration in a tumor/ascites mouse model. *Cancer Biother Radiopharm*. 2009 Aug;24(4):453–60.

22. Natarajan A, Gruettner C, Ivkov R, DeNardo GL, Mirick G, Yuan A, Foreman A, DeNardo SJ. NanoFerrite particle based radioimmunonanoparticles: Binding affinity and *in vivo* pharmacokinetics. *Bioconjug Chem*. 2008 Jun;19(6):1211–8.

23. Natarajan A, Xiong CY, Gruettner C, DeNardo GL, DeNardo SJ. Development of multivalent radioimmunonanoparticles for cancer imaging and therapy. *Cancer Biother Radiopharm*. 2008 Feb;23(1):82–91.

24. Chrastina A, Schnitzer JE. Iodine-125 radiolabeling of silver nanoparticles for *in vivo* SPECT imaging. *Int J Nanomedicine*. 2010 Sep 7;5:653–9.

25. Gèze A, Chau LT, Choisnard L, Mathieu JP, Marti-Batlle D, Riou L, Putaux JL, Wouessidjewe D. Biodistribution of intravenously administered amphiphilic beta-cyclodextrin nanospheres. *Int J Pharm*. 2007 Nov 1;344(1–2):135–42.

26. Gratton SE, Pohlhaus PD, Lee J, Guo J, Cho MJ, Desimone JM. Nanofabricated particles for engineered drug therapies: A preliminary biodistribution study of PRINT nanoparticles. *J Control Release*. 2007 Aug 16;121(1–2):10–8.

27. Kennel SJ, Woodward JD, Rondinone AJ, Wall J, Huang Y, Mirzadeh S. The fate of MAb-targeted Cd(125 m)Te/ZnS nanoparticles *in vivo*. *Nucl Med Biol*. 2008 May;35(4):501–14.

28. Kumar R, Roy I, Ohulchanskky TY, Vathy LA, Bergey EJ, Sajjad M, Prasad PN. *In vivo* biodistribution and clearance studies using multimodal organically modified silica nanoparticles. *ACS Nano*. 2010 Feb 23;4(2):699–708.

29. Malik N, Wiwattanapatapee R, Klopsch R, Lorenz K, Frey H, Weener JW, Meijer EW, Paulus W, Duncan R. Dendrimers: Relationship between structure and biocompatibility *in vitro*, and preliminary studies on the biodistribution of 125I-labelled polyamidoamine dendrimers *in vivo*. *J Control Release*. 2000 Mar 1;65(1–2):133–48.

30. Medina OP, Pillarsetty N, Glekas A, Punzalan B, Longo V, Gönen M, Zanzonico P, Smith-Jones P, Larson SM. Optimizing tumor targeting of the lipophilic EGFR-binding radiotracer SKI 243 using a liposomal nanoparticle delivery system. *J Control Release*. 2011 Feb 10;149(3):292–8.

31. Helbok A, Decristoforo C, Dobrozemsky G, Rangger C, Diederen E, Stark B, Prassl R, von Guggenberg E. Radiolabeling of lipid-based nanoparticles for diagnostics and therapeutic applications: A comparison using different radiometals. *J Liposome Res*. 2010 Sep;20(3):219–27.

32. Lazarova N, Causey PW, Lemon JA, Czorny SK, Forbes JR, Zlitni A, Genady A, Foster FS, Valliant JF. The synthesis, magnetic purification and evaluation of 99mTc-labeled microbubbles. *Nucl Med Biol*. 2011 Nov;38(8):1111–8.

33. Madru R, Kjellman P, Olsson F, Wingårdh K, Ingvar C, Ståhlberg F, Olsrud J, Lätt J, Fredriksson S, Knutsson L, Strand SE. 99mTc-Labeled Superparamagnetic iron oxide nanoparticles for multimodality SPECT/MRI of sentinel lymph nodes. *J Nucl Med*. 2012 Mar;53(3):459–63.

34. Reimer P, Tombach B. Hepatic MRI with SPIO: Detection and characterization of focal liver lesions. *Eur Radiol*. 1998;8(7):1198–204.

35. Tanimoto A, Kuribayashi S. Application of superparamagnetic iron oxide to imaging of hepatocellular carcinoma. *Eur J Radiol*. 2006 May;58(2):200–16.

36. Bulte JW, Kraitchman DL. Monitoring cell therapy using iron oxide MR contrast agents. *Curr Pharm Biotechnol*. 2004 Dec;5(6):567–84.

37. Lakshmipathy U, Pelacho B, Sudo K, Linehan JL, Coucouvanis E, Kaufman DS, Verfaillie CM. Efficient transfection of embryonic and adult stem cells. *Stem Cells*. 2004;22(4):531–43.

38. Corot C, Petry KG, Trivedi R, Saleh A, Jonkmanns C, Le Bas JF, Blezer E, Rausch M, Brochet B, Foster-Gareau P, Balériaux D, Gaillard S, Dousset V. Macrophage imaging in central nervous system and in carotid atherosclerotic plaque using ultrasmall superparamagnetic iron oxide in magnetic resonance imaging. *Invest Radiol*. 2004 Oct;39(10):619–25.

39. Duerschmied D, Meisner M, Peter K, Neudorfer I, Roming F, Zirlik A, Bode C, von Elverfeldt D, von Zur Muhlen C. Molecular magnetic resonance imaging allows the detection of activated platelets in a new mouse model of coronary artery thrombosis. *Invest Radiol*. 2011 Oct;46(10):618–23.

40. Koike N, Cho A, Nasu K, Seto K, Nagaya S, Ohshima Y, Ohkohchi N. Role of diffusion-weighted magnetic resonance imaging in the differential diagnosis of focal hepatic lesions. *World J Gastroenterol*. 2009 Dec 14;15(46):5805–12.

41. Taylor RM, Huber DL, Monson TC, Ali AM, Bisoffi M, Sillerud LO. Multifunctional iron platinum stealth immunomicelles: Targeted detection of human prostate cancer cells using both fluorescence and magnetic resonance imaging. *J Nanopart Res*. 2011 Oct 1;13(10):4717–29.

42. Kao CY, Hoffman EA, Beck KC, Bellamkonda RV, Annapragada AV. Long-residence-time nano-scale liposomal iohexol for x-ray-based blood pool imaging. *Acad Radiol*. 2003;10:475–83.

43. Schmiedl UP, Krause W, Leike J, Sachse A. CT blood pool enhancement in primates with lopromide-carrying liposomes containing soy phosphatidyl glycerol. *Acad Radiol*. 1999;6:164–9.

44. Vera DR, Mattrey RF. A molecular CT blood pool contrast agent. *Acad Radiol* 2002;9:784–92.

45. Torchilin VP. 45. PEG-based micelles as carriers of contrast agents for different imaging modalities. *Adv Drug Deliv Rev*. 2002;54:235–52.

46. Fruman SA, Harned RK 2nd, Marcus D, Kaufman S, Swenson RB, Bernardino ME. Perfluoroctyl bromide as a blood pool contrast agent for computed tomographic angiography. *Acad Radiol*. 1994;1:151–3.

47. Torchilin VP, Frank-Kamenetsky MD, Wolf GL. CT visualization of blood pool in rats by using long-circulating, iodine-containing micelles. *Acad Radiol*. 1999;6:61–5.

48. Idée JM, Port M, Robert P, Raynal I, Prigent P, Dencausse A, Le Greneur S, et al. Preclinical profile of the monodisperse iodinated macromolecular blood pool agent P743. *Invest Radiol*. 2001;36:41–9.

49. Hainfeld JF, Slatkin DN, Focella TM, Smilowitz HM. Gold nanoparticles: A new x-ray contrast agent. *Br J Radiol*. 2006 Mar;79(939):248–53.

50. Popovtzer R, Agrawal A, Kotov NA, Popovtzer A, Balter J, Carey TE, Kopelman R. Targeted gold nanoparticles enable molecular CT imaging of cancer. *Nano Lett*. 2008 Dec;8(12):4593–6.

51. Cormode DP, Roessl E, Thran A, Skajaa T, Gordon RE, Schlomka JP, Fuster V, Fisher EA, Mulder WJ, Proksa R, Fayad ZA. Atherosclerotic plaque composition: Analysis with multicolor CT and targeted gold nanoparticles. *Radiology*. 2010 Sep;256(3):774–82.

52. Kim D, Jeong YY, Jon S. A drug-loaded aptamer-gold nanoparticle bioconjugate for combined CT imaging and therapy of prostate cancer. *ACS Nano*. 2010 Jul 27;4(7):3689–96.

53. Kremkau FW. Doppler color imaging. Principles and instrumentation. *Clin Diagn Ultrasound.* 1992;27:7–60.
54. Xu HX. Contrast-enhanced ultrasound: The evolving applications. *World J Radiol.* 2009 Dec 31;1(1):15–24.
55. Albrecht T, Blomley M, Bolondi L, Claudon M, Correas JM, Cosgrove D, Greiner L, et al. Guidelines for the use of contrast agents in ultrasound. January 2004. *Ultraschall Med.* 2004 Aug;25(4):249–56.
56. Salvatore V, Borghi A, Piscaglia F. Contrast-enhanced ultrasound for liver imaging: Recent advances. *Curr Pharm Des.* 2012;18(15):2236–2252.
57. Meloni MF, Livraghi T, Filice C, Lazzaroni S, Calliada F, Perretti L. Radiofrequency ablation of liver tumors: The role of microbubble ultrasound contrast agents. *Ultrasound Q.* 2006 Mar;22(1):41–7.
58. Piscaglia F, Bolondi L. Italian society for ultrasound in medicine and biology (SIUMB) study group on ultrasound contrast agents. The safety of Sonovue in abdominal applications: Retrospective analysis of 23188 investigations. *Ultrasound Med Biol.* 2006;32(9):1369–75.
59. Kalantarinia K, Belcik JT, Patrie JT, Wei K. Real-time measurement of renal blood flow in healthy subjects using contrast-enhanced ultrasound. *Am J Physiol Renal Physiol.* 2009 Oct;297(4):F1129–34.
60. Willmann JK, Lutz AM, Paulmurugan R, Patel MR, Chu P, Rosenberg J, Gambhir SS. Dual-targeted contrast agent for US assessment of tumor angiogenesis *in vivo. Radiology.* 2008 Sep;248(3):936–44.
61. Nucifora G, Faletra FF. Current applications of contrast echocardiography. *Minerva Cardioangiol.* 2011 Oct;59(5):519–32.
62. Porter TR, Xie F. Myocardial perfusion imaging with contrast ultrasound. *JACC Cardiovasc Imaging.* 2010 Feb;3(2):176–87.
63. Meairs S, Culp W. Microbubbles for thrombolysis of acute ischemic stroke. *Cerebrovasc Dis.* 2009;27 Suppl 2:55–65.
64. Soltani A, Singhal R, Obtera M, Roy RA, Clark WM, Hansmann DR. Potentiating intra-arterial sonothrombolysis for acute ischemic stroke by the addition of the ultrasound contrast agents (Optison™ & SonoVue(®)). *J Thromb Thrombolysis.* 2011 Jan;31(1):71–84.
65. Gatenby RA, Gillies RJ. Why do cancers have high aerobic glycolysis? *Nat Rev Cancer.* 2004 Nov;4(11):891–9.
66. Noguchi Y, Wu J, Duncan R, Strohalm J, Ulbrich K, Akaike T, Maeda H. Early phase tumor accumulation of macromolecules: A great difference in clearance rate between tumor and normal tissues. *Jpn J Cancer Res.* 1998 Mar;89(3):307–14.
67. Chakrabarti A, Zhang K, Aruva MR, Cardi CA, Opitz AW, Wagner NJ, Thakur ML, Wickstrom E. Radiohybridization PET imaging of KRAS G12D mRNA expression in human pancreas cancer xenografts with [(64)Cu]DO3A-peptide nucleic acid-peptide nanoparticles. *Cancer Biol Ther.* 2007; 6(6):948–56.
68. Petersen AL, Binderup T, Rasmussen P, Henriksen JR, Elema DR, Kjær A, Andresen TL. 64Cu loaded liposomes as positron emission tomography imaging agents. *Biomaterials.* 2011 Mar;32(9):2334–41.
69. Ruggiero A, Villa CH, Holland JP, Sprinkle SR, May C, Lewis JS, Scheinberg DA, McDevitt MR. Imaging and treating tumor vasculature with targeted radiolabeled carbon nanotubes. *Int J Nanomedicine.* 2010 Oct 5;5:783–802.

70. Lijowski M, Caruthers S, Hu G, Zhang H, Scott MJ, Williams T, Erpelding T, et al. High sensitivity: High-resolution SPECT-CT/MR molecular imaging of angiogenesis in the Vx2 model. *Invest Radiol.* 2009 Jan;44(1):15–22.

71. Liang S, Wang Y, Yu J, Zhang C, Xia J, Yin D. Surface modified superparamagnetic iron oxide nanoparticles: As a new carrier for bio-magnetically targeted therapy. *J Mater Sci Mater Med.* 2007 Dec;18(12):2297–302.

72. Park SI, Kwon BJ, Park JH, Jung H, Yu KH. Synthesis and characterization of 3-[131I]iodo-L-tyrosine grafted Fe$_3$O$_4$@SiO$_2$ nanocomposite for single photon emission computed tomography (SPECT) and magnetic resonance imaging (MRI). *J Nanosci Nanotechnol.* 2011 Feb;11(2):1818–21.

73. Torres Martin de Rosales R, Tavaré R, Glaria A, Varma G, Protti A, Blower PJ. (^{99}m)Tc-bisphosphonate-iron oxide nanoparticle conjugates for dual-modality biomedical imaging. *Bioconjug Chem.* 2011 Mar;16;22(3):455–65.

74. Zielhuis SW, Seppenwoolde JH, Mateus VA, Bakker CJ, Krijger GC, Storm G, Zonnenberg BA, van het Schip AD, Koning GA, Nijsen JF. Lanthanide-loaded liposomes for multimodality imaging and therapy. *Cancer Biother Radiopharm.* 2006 Oct;21(5):520–7.

75. Cheon J, Lee JH. Synergistically integrated nanoparticles as multimodal probes for nanobiotechnology. *Acc Chem Res.* 2008 Dec;41(12):1630–40.

76. Glaus C, Rossin R, Welch MJ, Bao G. *In vivo* evaluation of (64)Cu-labeled magnetic nanoparticles as a dual-modality PET/MR imaging agent. *Bioconjug Chem.* 2010 Apr 21;21(4):715–22.

77. Jarrett BR, Gustafsson B, Kukis DL, Louie AY. Synthesis of 64Cu-labeled magnetic nanoparticles for multimodal imaging. *Bioconjug Chem.* 2008 Jul;19(7):1496–504.

78. Patel D, Kell A, Simard B, Xiang B, Lin HY, Tian G. The cell labeling efficacy, cytotoxicity and relaxivity of copper-activated MRI/PET imaging contrast agents. *Biomaterials.* 2011 Feb;32(4):1167–76.

79. Devaraj NK, Keliher EJ, Thurber GM, Nahrendorf M, Weissleder R. 18F labeled nanoparticles for *in vivo* PET-CT imaging. *Bioconjug Chem.* 2009 Feb;20(2):397–401.

80. Ko HY, Choi KJ, Lee CH, Kim S. A multimodal nanoparticle-based cancer imaging probe simultaneously targeting nucleolin, integrin αvβ3 and tenascin-C proteins. *Biomaterials.* 2011 Feb;32(4):1130–8.

81. Nahrendorf M, Zhang H, Hembrador S, Panizzi P, Sosnovik DE, Aikawa E, Libby P, Swirski FK, Weissleder R. Nanoparticle PET-CT imaging of macrophages in inflammatory atherosclerosis. *Circulation.* 2008 Jan 22;117(3):379–87.

82. Zhou J, Yu M, Sun Y, Zhang X, Zhu X, Wu Z, Wu D, Li F. Fluorine-18-labeled Gd3+/Yb3+/Er3+ co-doped NaYF4 nanophosphors for multimodality PET/MR/UCL imaging. *Biomaterials.* 2011 Feb;32(4):1148–56.

83. Xing H, Bu W, Zhang S, Zheng X, Li M, Chen F, He Q, Zhou L, Peng W, Hua Y, Shi J. Multifunctional nanoprobes for upconversion fluorescence, MR and CT trimodal imaging. *Biomaterials.* 2012 Feb;33(4):1079–89.

84. Arifin DR, Long CM, Gilad AA, Alric C, Roux S, Tillement O, Link TW, Arepally A, Bulte JW. Trimodal gadolinium-gold microcapsules containing pancreatic islet cells restore normoglycemia in diabetic mice and can be tracked by using US, CT, and positive-contrast MR imaging. *Radiology.* 2011 Sep;260(3):790–8.

85. van Dam GM, Themelis G, Crane LM, Harlaar NJ, Pleijhuis RG, Kelder W, Sarantopoulos A, et al. Intraoperative tumor-specific fluorescence imaging in ovarian cancer by folate receptor-α targeting: First in-human results. *Nat Med.* 2011 Sep 18;17(10):1315–9.

86. Li Y, Yang K, Mao Q, Zheng X, Kong D, Xie L. Inhibition of TGF-beta receptor I by siRNA suppresses the motility and invasiveness of T24 bladder cancer cells via modulation of integrins and matrix metalloproteinase. *Int Urol Nephrol.* 2010 Jun;42(2):315–23.

9

Nanoparticles in Anticancer Drug Delivery

Frederic Lagarce

CONTENTS

9.1 Introduction 213
9.2 Bioavailability Enhancement 214
  9.2.1 Oral Route 215
  9.2.2 Blood–Brain Barrier Crossing 217
  9.2.3 Delivery of Fragile Biomolecules 218
9.3 Targeting 219
  9.3.1 Passive Targeting in Cancer Therapy 219
  9.3.2 Active Targeting 221
9.4 Overcoming Drug Resistance 223
  9.4.1 Drug Diffusion in the Tumor Microenvironment 223
  9.4.2 Efflux Pump Inhibition 225
  9.4.3 Overcoming Deregulation of Apoptosis 226
9.5 Diagnostics and Cancer Therapy: Rise of Theranostics 228
9.6 Conclusion 231
References 231

9.1 Introduction

Despite many therapeutic breakthroughs, cancer remains one of the worst killer. In 2008, more than 12.6 m new cases of cancer were recorded and the number of cancer deaths in the same year was 7.5 m (Ferlay et al., 2010).

In view of this health problem, one of the proposed solutions is to enhance the efficiency of the existing anticancer drugs. Nanotechnology is one of the most promising strategies to change the fate of the drug in the body. In 2004, the National Cancer Institute launched the alliance for nanotechnology in cancer, and a new interdisciplinary field called nanomedicine emerged (Kim et al., 2010b). Encapsulated in the heart of a nanosized drug delivery system (NDDS) or attached to its surface, the anticancer molecule displays new pharmacological properties. For example, its residence time in the body can be enhanced, it can be guided actively or passively to the tumor site, and the NDDS can sometimes help the drug to avoid resistance of the tumor cell. In fact, nanoparticles

TABLE 9.1

Approved Nanoparticles for Anticancer Therapy in Europe or United States

Type of NDDS	Trade Name	Drug	Tumor Target	Company
Protein nanoparticle	Abraxane	Paclitaxel	Breast	Abraxis Bioscience
Pegylated liposome	Doxyl/Caelix	Doxorubicin	Breast, ovary, multiple myeloma	OrthoBiotech/ Janssen Cilag
Liposome	Myocet	Doxorubicin	Breast	Zeneus Pharma/ Cephalon
Liposome	Daunoxome	Daunorubicin	Kaposi's sarcoma	Gilead Sciences
Multivesicular lipid particles	Depocyte	Cytarabine	Lymphomatous meningitis	Skye Pharma/ Pacira Limited

have a long story since the first idea of "magic bullets," that is, drug targeting using nanocarriers, raised by Paul Erlich in the 1950s (Kreuter, 2007).

Today, a few NDDSs are already available to treat cancer (Table 9.1) and many are under clinical trial (Heidel and Davis, 2011). In November 2011, 399 trials with both keywords "liposomes" and "cancer" and 80 trials with "nanoparticles" and "cancer" were found in the web database clinicaltrials.gov.

NDDS is a big and diverse family. Under the term nanoparticle, one finds many different entities in the nanosize range (mainly 10–200 nm). Liposomes are aqueous vesicles surrounded by one or several phospholipid bilayers; nanoparticles can be made of inorganic atoms such as gold or silver, or from lipids that are solid at room temperature—these are called solid lipid nanoparticles; one also found nanocapsules often composed of lipid or aqueous core surrounded by a crown often containing surfactants. Other very small nano-objects such as quantum dots, dendrimers, polymersomes, or carbon nanotubes are described. Because of their different physicochemical properties, NDDSs display a wide range of advantages and are adapted to a broad variety of drugs from the small molecules to the large biological molecules such as proteins. In this chapter, the advantages and limits of the NDDSs will be listed in function of their awaited pharmacological properties: bioavailability enhancement, targeting, drug resistance suppression, and imaging. Because of their unique properties, nanoparticles are a great hope to improve cancer therapy, we will try to determine how promising this new drug device can be.

9.2 Bioavailability Enhancement

Encapsulation of a molecule in a nanocarrier or association to its surface can change the fate of this active drug in the body. For example, the two main parameters (solubility and permeability) raised by Amidon and coworkers as the main determinant of bioavailability after oral administration (Amidon et al., 1995) can be dramatically changed by drug association with NDDSs. The stability of the drug can also be enhanced as long as it stays protected in the core of the nanoparticle. Thus, nanotechnology can be a way to enhance bioavailability or to obtain a formulation compatible with the desired route of administration. To illustrate this point, we will take examples from oral delivery and central nervous system delivery. Pulmonary, transdermal and ocular delivery will be described respectively in Chapters 3, 5 and 11 of this book. Encapsulation in NDDSs is also a way to deliver fragile molecules such as biomolecules into cancer cells.

9.2.1 Oral Route

Oral route is not the main route for chemotherapies because these molecules are often not well absorbed, belonging to the class II and IV of the biophar-maceutical classification system (Amidon et al., 1995). It is, for example, the case of paclitaxel, which has a very low solubility (LogP = 3.5) and perme-ability across enterocytes because it is subjected to efflux mediated by P glycoproteins (PgP) (Sparreboom et al., 1997) and can undergo metabolism by cytochrome P-450 3A4 (Malingre et al., 2001). The absolute bioavailabil-ity of paclitaxel after oral administration was reported to be less than 7% (Sparreboom et al., 1997). Because paclitaxel is one of the main drugs used against breast cancer or non-small-cell lung cancer, oral formulations, which are more convenient for patients, were sought (Singh and Dash, 2009). Lipid nanocapsules (Peltier et al., 2006), poly(anhydride) nanoparticles containing cyclodextrins (Figure 9.1) (Agueros et al., 2010), hydrotropic polymer micelles (Kim et al., 2008), chitosan nanoparticles containing paclitaxel nanocrystals (Lv et al., 2011), solid lipid nanoparticles (Jain et al., 2011a) among many other formulations have shown very promising results to enhance bioavailability and efficacy of paclitaxel administered orally. Thus, oral bioavailability of PTX was raised to more than 80% (Agueros et al., 2010) after its encapsula-tion into nanoparticles. Poly(amido amine) (PAMAM) dendrimers have been used to enhance the bioavailability of doxorubicin by a 200-fold factor in rats (Ke et al., 2008). In fact, it was also demonstrated *in vitro* that doxorubicin–PAMAM complexes display a higher ability to cross a caco-2 cell monolayer, a well-known *in vitro* model of intestinal barrier. Similar results were found after permeability studies performed on freshly excised small intestinal mucosa of rats.

NDDSs were also used to enhance the bioavailability of anticancer drugs such as Sn38 (Roger et al., 2011), tamoxifen (Jain et al., 2011a), and many other chemotherapies (Roger et al., 2010a). Using NDDS to allow a better oral drug delivery is, however, not a very simple task. The involved phenomena are very complex, and so the fate of the nanoparticles after oral delivery depends on many parameters (Roger et al., 2010a): the stability of the NDDS in gastric

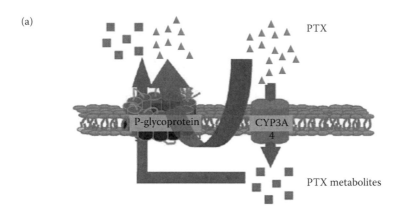

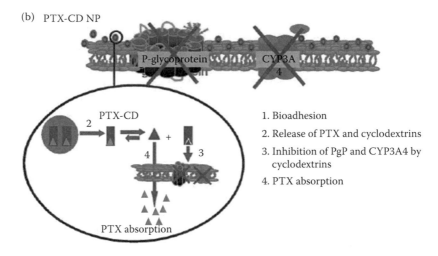

FIGURE 9.1
(a) Mechanisms of paclitaxel (PTX) degradation by cyp 3A4 and efflux mediated by PgP raised to explain its poor oral bioavailability. (b) Scheme showing how nanoparticles containing PTX included in cyclodextrins can suppress these mechanisms of PTX degradation and efflux. (Reprinted from *J Control Release*, 145, Agueros, M. et al., Increased oral bioavailability of paclitaxel by its encapsulation through complex formation with cyclodextrins in poly(anhydride) nanoparticles, 2–8, Copyright 2010, with permission from Elsevier.)

or intestinal fluids (Roger et al., 2009a), its diffusion possibilities across the mucus layer (Crater and Carrier, 2010), its permeability across enterocytes (Roger et al., 2009b), and its interaction with PgP (Roger et al., 2010b) are examples of what has to be studied to optimize and understand the behavior of nanoparticulate systems in the gastrointestinal tract. Many *in vitro* models can be used besides animal studies; in the case of nanoparticulate system evaluation, it is important to validate the models for this task as they were not always designed initially for it. The best example is with caco-2 cells, widely used for nanoparticle uptake studies but having some pitfalls for this task (Lagarce and Roger, 2011).

Not many papers describe the mechanisms of nanoparticle uptake in the enterocytes. There are in fact different possibilities:

- The drug can be released from the NDDS and then be absorbed passively or actively via transcellular route.
- The NDDS can diffuse passively across the enterocyte lipid bilayer and then in the cytosol of the cell.
- The NDDS can be internalized in the enterocytes by active transport in a vacuole (cytosis).
- The NDDS can release some materials that open the tight junctions between the enterocytes and allow the drug to pass through paracellular pathway.

The size and surface properties of the nanoparticle are of primary importance to determine its uptake mechanisms. See Roger et al. (2010a) for a review.

It is important to note that nanotechnology is only one of the possibilities to enhance drug bioavailability after oral delivery. In fact, many other strategies such as emulsions, prodrugs, solid dispersions, lipid suspensions, and absorption enhancers can be proposed (Fasinu et al., 2011).

9.2.2 Blood–Brain Barrier Crossing

Another important feature that NDDSs can provide to chemotherapies is the ability to cross the blood–brain barrier (BBB) (Garcia-Garcia et al., 2005). This barrier protects the central nervous system from toxic molecules. Only a few drugs such as irinotecan or temozolomide can cross the BBB and thus can be easily used to treat brain tumors or brain metastases from other tumor sites such as the lung (Juillerat-Jeanneret, 2008). Encapsulation in nanoparticles can help to actively target the central nervous system and also to overcome the BBB (Beduneau et al., 2007). Polysorbate 80 was initially used by Kreuter and his team to obtain a significant passage in mice brain of peptides encapsulated in nanoparticles (Kreuter et al., 1995). More than 15 years later, many NDDSs able to cross the BBB have been proposed. For example, lipid nanocapsules conjugated with the OX26 monoclonal antibody directed against the transferrin receptor expressed on the cerebral endothelium have shown interesting properties of brain targeting: concentrations of these immunonanocapsules were twofold more important in the brain than that of regular nanocapsules (Beduneau et al., 2008). After encapsulation in nanoparticles, the drug can reach therapeutic concentration and can be used to treat brain tumors such as gliomas (Caruso et al., 2011). This has been, for example, demonstrated in rats with doxorubicin, a drug that normally does not diffuse in the brain parenchyma. Doxorubicin poly(lactic-*co*-glycolic acid) (PLGA) nanoparticles coated with poloxamer 188 have shown efficacy on glioma-bearing rats after intravenous injection (Wohlfart et al., 2011).

9.2.3 Delivery of Fragile Biomolecules

DNA or small interfering RNA (SiRNA) is often viewed as promising future treatments for cancer therapy because of their specific pharmacological targets. However, these molecules are very difficult to deliver to cell with a good efficiency because of their instability and their inability to reach intracellular targets.

SiRNA can be used to silence oncogene expression involved in deregulated functions of the cancer cell (proliferation, survival, invasion, inhibition of apoptosis, etc.) (Aagaard and Rossi, 2007). Small double-stranded RNAs are recognized by Dicer, an endonuclease, and cleaved into two SiRNAs. The antisense strand becomes associated with the RNA-induced silencing complex (RISC), which targets mRNA. Then, mRNA is cleaved by Ago2 leading to a shutdown of protein expression. Tumors display a relatively low Dicer level, in this condition, the interaction is favorable only with small 21–23-nucleotide-long RNAs. Delivering such RNAs to cell for oncogene-silencing purpose needs to be done with a nanocarrier to help the RNAs to enter the cell and to avoid degradation by nucleases and rapid renal clearance after systemic administration (Ozpolat et al., 2010). SiRNAs are negatively charged as cell membranes explaining the low uptake of these molecules. Cationic nanocarriers have been used to transport SiRNAs at their surface and let them enter the cell where they could meet the Dicer endonuclease. The delivery of negatively charged DNA suffers the same limitations (negatively charged, poor uptake, poor stability, etc.); in this case, the target is the nucleus of the cell. Thus, the proposed solutions for the delivery of SiRNA or DNA will often be similar.

Cationic lipids such as 1,2-dioleyl-3-trimethylammonium-propane (DOTAP) form lipoplexes with SiRNA or DNA. Lipoplexes can then be encapsulated into liposomes (Landen et al., 2005, Zimmermann et al., 2006), nanoparticles (Li and Szoka, 2007), or nanocapsules (Morille et al., 2010). The use of cationic liposomes has been limited by dose-dependent toxicity and pulmonary inflammation (Dokka et al., 2000); lipid nanocapsules display a better toxicity profile and good transfection properties (Morille et al., 2011).

Only a few SiRNA-based therapeutics are currently under clinical trials for various diseases, including cancer (Tiemann and Rossi, 2009). The more promising strategy to date is proposed by Calando Pharmaceuticals, Inc., with the targeting of the M2 subunit of a ribonucleotide reductase using SiRNA encapsulated in a complex nanocarrier. This delivery system, called RONDEL®, used three components: cyclodextrin-containing polycation, pegylated adamantine, and pegylated adamantane conjugated to a human transferrin targeting ligand. It has been effectively delivered to mice and showed specific gene knockdown (Hu-Lieskovan et al., 2005) and has been safely administered in monkeys (Heidel et al., 2007), and is now proposed to patients in clinical trials (Davis et al., 2010). The first results show that this NDDS accumulated in melanoma cancer cells in a dose-dependent manner after systemic administration (Davis et al., 2010). It is important to note that in the proof of concept of RNA interference utilization for therapeutic purposes, it is mandatory to avoid siRNA off-target effects. Thus, off-target effects due to a lack of siRNA specificity can lead to toxicity and can complicate the interpretation of phenotypic effects in gene-silencing experiments (Jackson and Linsley, 2010).

9.3 Targeting

Besides their ability to overcome biological barriers and to protect fragile molecules from degradation, nanoparticles are used to reach pharmacological targets. This property, called targeting, is very useful in cancer therapy: the tumor is often not easily reachable and it is particularly difficult for a drug to diffuse deeply in its microenvironment. In fact, a successful targeting allows most of the drug to reach the tumor cells and avoid healthy tissue, which limits the numerous side effects of the anticancer drugs. There are two possibilities: passive or active targeting. In passive targeting, the physical properties of the nanocarrier (mostly its size) are used to help the nanocarrier to reach its targets. In active targeting, the NDDS is able to interact actively with the tissues or cells to deliver its drug at the right place. This property is, for example, obtained by linking an antibody to the surface of the NDDS, which is able to recognize a tumor antigen. In both active and passive targeting, the diffusion of the drug in the body does not depend anymore on its physicochemical properties but depends on the physicochemical properties of the nanocarrier. Active and passive targeting have their own supporters; there is still a controversy of what strategy could be the most effective in cancer therapy (Huynh et al., 2010). We will address this point in the following sections.

9.3.1 Passive Targeting in Cancer Therapy

Passive targeting of solid tumors is based on the enhanced permeation and retention (EPR) effect. Discovered by Matsumara in 1986, originally for macromolecules (Matsumura and Maeda, 1986), the EPR effect is due to the leaky structure of blood vessels in tumors and the reduced clearance of macromolecules from tumor microenvironment due to a lack of lymphatic drainage (Fang et al., 2011). Very recently, the discovery of EPR effect was commented as "a crucial step" in cancer therapy by V. Torchilin in an editorial of *Advanced Drug Delivery Reviews* (Torchilin, 2011) because it facilitates the tumor delivery of macromolecules and nanoparticles by passive targeting. The EPR effect allows the drug to accumulate into the tumor. To permeate into the tumor using the permeabilized vasculature, nanoparticles should have a size below 500 nm, preferably below 200 nm. In fact, the size of the pore varies as per the function of the tumor; smaller in cranial tumors and larger in subcutaneous tumors (Hobbs et al., 1998). But also to have a chance to diffuse and reach the tumor site, the nanoparticles should avoid the recognition by mononuclear phagocytic system (MPS) after opsonization. Such stealth nanoparticles can be obtained by modifying the surface of the NDDS by grafting water-soluble polymers to avoid the adhesion of opsonins. This strategy was first applied with doxorubicin liposomes. Caelix® is a doxorubicin pegylated liposome formulation of a size below 100 nm (Figure 9.2). In comparison to free doxorubicin, the area under the curve after IV injection is multiplied by a 300-fold factor (Gabizon et al., 2003). This allows the drug to display a prolonged residence time in the body and to diffuse in the tumor by EPR effect. This accumulation in tumors was demonstrated after biopsies of Kaposi's sarcoma lesions treated by these stealth liposomes. In fact, 48–96 h after administration, the accumulation of doxorubicin was 10–15-fold higher in lesions than in normal adjacent skin (Northfelt et al., 1997). More interestingly, similar results (10-fold increase doxorubicin concentration in tumor) were found in bone metastasis from breast cancer (Symon et al., 1999); this

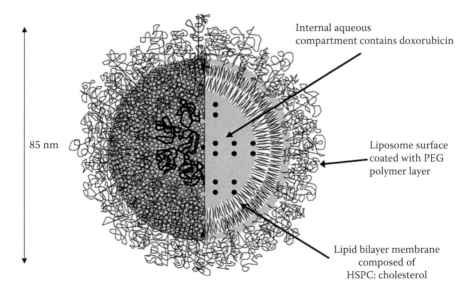

FIGURE 9.2
Structure of CAELIX®/DOXIL®. (From Gabizon, A., Shmeeda, H. and Barenholz, Y. 2003. Pharmacokinetics of pegylated liposomal doxorubicin: Review of animal and human studies. *Clin Pharmacokinet*, 42, 419–36. With permission.)

result was important because diffusion of anticancer drugs into bone is not often achieved. Radiolabeled pegylated liposomes have been shown to accumulate in solid tumors (lung, breast, gliomas) (Harrington et al., 2001).

Many pegylated nanoparticles such as liposomes or PLGA nanoparticles containing paclitaxel, docetaxel, or doxorubicin, cisplatin, or campotecin analogs have been used in preclinical studies in anticancer therapy (Huynh et al., 2010) for their passive targeting properties due to the polyethylene glycol polymers at their surface.

The passive targeting allowing drug accumulation in the tumor is very promising, but surprisingly not many drugs encapsulated in pegylated NDDS are approved worldwide. This may be due to the fact that passive targeting suffers from some limitations (Huynh et al., 2010):

- Certain tumors do not exhibit EPR effect due to a lack of blood irrigation or because the pore size of the vessels is too narrow.
- The diffusion of the drugs is modified and so its toxicity is different, for example, doxorubicin pegylated liposomes display a particular skin toxicity.
- The intracellular uptake can be limited in case of a too hydrophilic surface brought by PEG.

9.3.2 Active Targeting

Active targeting is a very promising strategy to accumulate the anticancer drug where it should display a therapeutic efficacy and to avoid healthy tissue. Different ligands can be used to recognize the tumor or to help the nanocarrier to enter the cancer cell. As in passive targeting, active nanocarriers should display stealth properties to avoid MPS and thus display a prolonged circulation half-life. Active nanocarriers are thus often pegylated and tumor recognition ligands can be attached at the end of the PEG molecules.

Monoclonal antibodies have been used to target cancer cells. Antibodies have been attached to liposomes (to obtain what are called immunoliposomes) or to nanoparticles such as PLGA nanoparticles. Many tumor antigens have been targeted, for example, EGF receptor-2 (HER2) overexpressed at the surface of breast cancer cells has been a target for immunoliposome-containing doxorubicin. No such active nanocarrier has reached the market yet. This could be due to different factors:

- The immunogenicity of nanoparticle-bearing antibodies at their surface has to be addressed because it could seriously impair the tolerance of the NDDS.
- In the same manner, circulating antibodies, released by the NDDS, could be the source of immunologic reactions.

- It is difficult to produce large batches of such complex nanodevices with industrial constraints.
- Evidence of the superiority of active targeting using monoclonal antibodies is not fully demonstrated.

Besides monoclonal antibodies, peptides have been used to help the nano-carrier to enter the cancer cell. The best-known example is the integrin receptor binding peptides, including arginine–glycine–aspartate (RGD) domains. First published in 1980 by Pierschbacher and Ruoslahti, these peptides have been widely used for tumor targeting (Ruoslahti, 2002). Some other peptides bind to fibrin–fibronectin complexes and home to tumors; this is due to the fact that tumor blood vessels contain products of blood clotting. Cell surface and tumor vessels targets also comprise endosialin, aminopeptidase N, fibro-nectin ED-B, interleukin-11 receptor α, αvβ3, and αvβ5 integrins (Ruoslahti et al., 2010). A tumor-penetrating peptide named iRGD was used as a per-meation tumor enhancer (Sugahara et al., 2010). This peptide binds to αv integrins specifically expressed in tumor vessels. Nab-paclitaxel (Abraxane®) was chemically bound to iRDG and injected intravenously to mouse. The drug accumulation in orthotopic BT474 human breast tumor was 12-fold higher than the drug given alone. In the same paper, the authors describe an enhanced tumor penetration after the administration of iRGD with doxo-rubicin liposomes (10-fold). Interestingly, iRGD was also combined with an approved monoclonal antibody (trastuzumab) and this enhanced its tumor activity significantly. Cell-penetrating peptides have also been attached to quantum dots to enhance their potential for intracellular delivery, thus allow-ing improved tumor tracking and cellular imaging (Liu et al., 2010).

The peptide GE11 (sequence: YHWYGYTPQNVIGGGGC) was success-fully bound to PLA-PEG and then inserted in poly(ε-caprolactone) nanopar-ticles. These modified nanoparticles thus acquired the ability to target the epithelial growth factor receptor (EGFR) overexpressed at the surface of multidrug-resistant (MDR) cells. Safety and efficacy of these nanoparticles loaded with paclitaxel or lonidamine (1-[(2,4-dichlorophenyl)methyl]-1*H*-in-dazole-3-carboxylicacid), an hexokinase-2 inhibitor that has been shown to induce apoptosis in MDR cells, were demonstrated on an orthotopic breast cancer model (Milane et al., 2011a). Moreover, the pharmacokinetic profile of these targeted nanoparticles was found superior to the profile observed with nonencapsulated drugs: the half-life of encapsulated paclitaxel or lonidam-ine was increased and the area under the curve of lonidamine was enhanced (Milane et al., 2011b).

Small molecules such as folic acid or sugar molecules have also been used. Folate receptors are overexpressed in many cancer cells for their proliferation. Folate receptor targeting has been used not only with nanoparticles for tumor imaging properties (Hou et al., 2011) but also for therapeutic properties. For example, methotrexate loaded folate conjugated albumin nanoparticles (Jain et al., 2011b), or paclitaxel folate targeted nanoparticles (Werner et al., 2011) have very recently shown interesting properties in cancer therapy. Mannose receptors have also been targeted to improve the efficacy of vaccine or chemotherapies. Mannose has been conjugated to nanoparticles, liposomes, and niosomes (Irache et al., 2008).

9.4 Overcoming Drug Resistance

Drug resistance to anticancer drugs can be from different origins. First of all, the tumor microenvironment is important to consider. In fact, one of the main reasons for drug resistance is the lack of diffusion of the therapeutic drug in the mass of solid tumors. The cancer cells also display general mechanisms of resistance called multidrug resistance (MDR). MDR is an ensemble of mechanisms that diminish the sensitivity of cancer cells to chemotherapy. In MDR, the mechanisms of resistance are not specific of the structure or mechanism of action of the drug. MDR is mainly mediated by proteins from the cell membrane, the cytoplasm, or the nucleus and is often not specific of an anticancer drug. The major mechanisms are

- Decrease drug influx
- Activation of efflux by membrane protein such as PgP
- Activation of the enzymes of the glutathione detoxification system
- Alteration of the proteins (or directly the genes) involved in the control of apoptosis, for example, p53 or Bcl-2

Besides MDR, there is also specific drug resistance found (e.g., activation of DNA repair) with molecules such as platin salts or taxanes.

Nanotechnology was claimed as a solution to overpass one or several of these drug resistance mechanisms.

9.4.1 Drug Diffusion in the Tumor Microenvironment

On different models such as spheroids, multilayered cell cultures (Kyle et al., 2004), or *in vivo* implanted tumors, it has been clearly shown that some major anticancer drugs display insufficient diffusion/penetration properties. It is, for example, the case for doxorubicin, mitoxantrone, methotrexate, vincristine, or gemcitabin (Minchinton and Tannock, 2006). It has also been demonstrated for gemcitabin that after causing an almost complete cessation of tumor proliferation at clinical doses *in vivo*, a resurgence of cell proliferation distant to blood vessels was observed (Huxham et al., 2004). It is important to note that the results of the diffusion studies are only valid for the model used. Some differences exist between the *in vitro* models due to, for example, different culture conditions.

The tumor microenvironment is thus very important to consider in evaluating anticancer strategies. Drug development strategies set up to improve intratumor drug permeability would help the development of effective anticancer therapies (Minchinton and Tannock, 2006). Besides the defective blood vessels and the lack of functional lymphatics put to good use to accumulate drug into tumors via the EPR effect, tumors display abnormal interstitial properties such as increased stiffness of tumor extracellular matrix and high interstitial fluid pressure, which are known to be a barrier to drug diffusion in the tumor mass (Holback and Yeo, 2011).

The drug moves into the cancer tissue by extracellular diffusion and also by cellular uptake and efflux, thus penetrating in the tumor mass by diffusing from one cell to the other (Baguley, 2010). This transcellular diffusion was the rationale to develop tumor-penetrating peptides that were previously discussed in this chapter. The entrapment of a drug in a nanocarrier may also help its diffusion into the tumor by extracellular pathway. The nanosized device allowing a good tumor penetration can be very complex. This is, for example, the case of multistage 100 nm gelatin nanoparticles releasing 10 nm nanoparticles after extravasation from vasculature in tumors via the EPR effect. The 10 nm nanoparticles having a size suitable for a good diffusion in tumor are produced by the proteases present in the tumor microenvironment, which degrade the gelatin cores of the particles (Wong et al., 2011). In fact, the size of the carrier is one of the key points for diffusion into the tumor mass. Different studies have shown that a nanocarrier size under 40 nm and preferably under 25 nm could be a condition for deep diffusion into solid tumors (Lee et al., 2010, Goodman et al., 2008). For size, the things are clear, and it seams that the lower the size, the better the diffusion. This is not the case for surface charge of nanoparticles. For a prolonged circulation time, the neutral particles are claimed to be better, but cationic nanoparticles interact more with cell membrane and thus could theoretically display more ability to diffuse. The effect of surface charge was studied with 6 nm gold nanoparticles on cylindroidal cell aggregates (Kim et al., 2010a). Cationic gold nanoparticles (+30 mV) stayed on the periphery of the cylindroids while anionic nanoparticles (−36 mV) were able to penetrate into the cell mass. This result was partly explained by *in vitro* diffusion studies performed in a tumor extracellular matrix material (Matrigel) in which cationic nanoparticles showed a reduced diffusion coefficient in comparison to anionic nanoparticles. Some diffusion studies show that anionic particles also display limited diffusion ability in comparison to pegylated particles that shield electrostatic surface charges from the interaction with biomolecules of the extracellular matrix (Lieleg et al., 2009). Neutral particles that interact less with the microenvironment should display better diffusion properties (Stylianopoulos et al., 2010). It is worth noting that ligands used for tumor targeting purposes, as seen previously, contribute to modify the diffusion of NDDS in the tumor mass. A good affinity for tumor cell membrane can be a good way to target the NDDS to the solid tumors but could hinder its diffusion into the tumor (Jang et al., 2003). On 3D diffusion models, it has been shown that the diffusion of paclitaxel, a drug that binds to protein and thus has a limited intratumor penetration, was dependent on the induced apoptosis (Jang et al., 2001a,b). This interesting result could be useful to improve the penetration of nanoparticles into tumor and improve the performance of NDDS.

9.4.2 Efflux Pump Inhibition

PgP is an efflux pump belonging to the human ATP-binding cassette (ABC) transporter superfamily. PgP is present at the surface of the cancer cell but also in healthy cells such as the enterocytes. Other efflux pumps in ABC family include multidrug resistance-associated proteins (MRP) and breast cancer resistance proteins (BCRP). PgP can be inhibited by small molecules such as verapamil or cyclosporine. Surfactants such as Pluronic® have demonstrated PgP inhibition properties.

There are three different strategies using NDDS to inhibit efflux pumps. First, it is possible to induce the silencing of the genes involved in the production of the protein-composing efflux pumps. The most studied transporter genes are *ABCB1* and *ABCC1* coding for PgP (MDR1) and *MRP1*. This strategy of gene silencing was discussed earlier in Section 9.2.3.

The second possibility is to target directly the drug efflux proteins; this was done with nanoemulsions, polymeric nanoparticles, copolymeric nanoparticles conjugated to quantum dots, liposomes, and surfactant–polymer nanoparticles (Shapira et al., 2011). For example, direct PgP inhibition has been observed with lipid nanocapsules (LNC). A formulation of LNC-containing solutol HS15, a pegylated hydroxystearate, has shown PgP inhibition properties that were used to enhance anticancer activity of paclitaxel against glioma cells (Garcion et al., 2006) and was also effective to improve the efficacy of etoposide on the same cells (Lamprecht and Benoit, 2006). Etoposide and paclitaxel are both known as substrates for the PgP and thus suffer from high efflux from the cancer cell impairing their cytotoxic effects. This mechanism of interaction of LNC with PgP is very complex. A reciprocal competition between PgP and LNC has recently been demonstrated on Caco-2 cells displaying different PgP activity levels, after experiments involving paclitaxel-loaded LNC, blank LNC, and known PgP inhibitors verapamil and vinblastin (Roger et al., 2010b).

The third possibility is to design NDDS that evade drug efflux pumps. Nanoparticles have the potential to bypass MDR mediated by PgP as they enter in the cell via endocytosis (Davis et al., 2008) and then in the cytosol, they shield the encapsulated anticancer drug from the efflux pump.

Nanoparticle endocytosis is not alone responsible for MDR inhibition by overpassing drug efflux mediated by PgP. In fact, degradation products of the nanoparticles can play a role in overcoming MDR. This property was demonstrated with poly(alkylcyanoacrylate) (PACA) nanoparticles containing doxorubicin on P388 leukemia cell culture (Vauthier et al., 2003): it was observed that PLGA or alginate nanoparticles were unable to reverse MDR on this cell model, whereas after PACA nanoparticle treatment, the sensitivity of the resistant cell lines reached the parent sensitive cell lines suggesting that PACA nanoparticles could reverse MDR entirely. The proposed mechanism to explain this surprising result is based on the adhesion of the nanoparticle to the resistant cancer cell surface, followed by the release of the drug and nanoparticle degradation products, which form an ion pair that is able to cross the cell membrane without being recognized by PgP (Colin de Verdiere et al., 1997).

9.4.3 Overcoming Deregulation of Apoptosis

One of the main pharmacological mechanisms of anticancer drugs is to drag the cancer cell into apoptotic death. In the mechanism of apoptosis, the point of no return is defined by mitochondrial outer membrane permeabilization, which is regulated by the bcl-2, a prosurvival family protein (Danial, 2007). In cancer cell, bcl-2 can be overexpressed preventing apoptosis. The balance of bcl-2 activity is modulated by proteins (p53, PTEN) and by the RAS/RAF pathway (Baguley, 2010). Silencing the expression of bcl-2 with SiRNA, NDDS has been a strategy used in the last few years. For example, mesoporous silica nanoparticles were used to deliver doxorubicin and SiRNA against bcl-2 proteins (Chen et al., 2009). The nanoparticles were modified with amine-terminated PAMAM dendrimers to allow the complexation with SiRNA. Then the nanoparticles were delivered into multidrug-resistant A2780/AD human ovarian cancer cells. This new NDDS allowed an increased efficacy of doxorubicin of 132 times in comparison to free doxorubicin.

Nuclear factor kappa B (NF-κB), a transcription factor involved in the cell response to various external stimuli such as cytokines or free radicals, has been shown to regulate the expression of bcl-2 and other cellular inhibitors of apoptosis. Cancer progression and chemoresistance have been related to NF-κB deregulation. Doxorubicin is known to induce NF-κB expression, which leads to resistance. Inhibitors of NF-κB, such as pyrrolidine dithiocarbamate, have recently been coencapsulated with doxorubicin in micellar nanoparticles self-assembled from copolymer folate–chitosan with success (Fan et al., 2010). These very interesting new NDDS have demonstrated Hegp-2 cell uptake via folate receptor endocytosis and codelivery of the anticancer drug with NF-κB inhibitor (Figure 9.3). However, this complex drug delivery system remains to be evaluated *in vivo*.

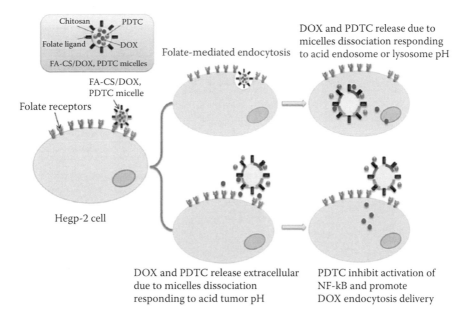

FIGURE 9.3
Scheme of pyrrolidine dithiocarbamate (PDTC) doxorubicin micellar nanoparticle behavior in the presence of Hegp-2 cells. (Reprinted from *Biomaterials*, 31, Fan, L. et al., Co-delivery of PDTC and doxorubicin by multifunctional micellar nanoparticles to achieve active targeted drug delivery and overcome multidrug resistance, 5634–42, Copyright 2010, with permission from Elsevier.)

Hypoxia is characteristic of tumor tissues. Under hypoxia, some specific genes are activated to help the cell to resist harsh conditions and promote cell survival and growth. Hypoxic tumor cell also acquires resistance to chemotherapy and to radiotherapy. Among these genes, one finds hypoxia-inducible factors (HIFs). Hypoxia-inducible factor alpha (HIF1α) gene encodes for a transcription factor involved in cellular response to hypoxia. The role of hypoxic tumor microenvironment has been shown to be responsible for resistance to antiangiogenic therapy. The inhibition of HIF1α by topotecan has led to an enhanced activity of bevacizumab, a monoclonal antibody directed against vascular endothelial growth factor A, in mice bearing U251-HRE xenografts (Rapisarda et al., 2009). The cytotoxicity of doxorubicin immunoliposomes targeted against RON receptor tyrosine kinase overexpressed in breast and colon cancers has been tested against hypoxic colon HCT116 and SW620 cancer cells (Guin et al., 2011). The resistance of these cells to doxorubicin was verified (high IC50) and a partial removal of this resistance was observed with immunoliposome (reduced IC50); a link was also observed between efficiency of treatment and RON expression in cells under hypoxic conditions.

9.5 Diagnostics and Cancer Therapy: Rise of Theranostics

As previously explained in Section 9.3, nanoparticles display very interesting properties to target cancer cells and to penetrate deeply into the tumor microenvironment if correctly labeled and functionalized. Nanoparticles can also be used for diagnostics as they can help tumor imaging because of their targeting properties associated with the capacity to transport imaging agents. The strategy of targeting in view of tumor imaging was recently reviewed extensively (Yu et al., 2012). For example, superparamagnetic iron oxide nanoparticles (SPIONs) have been successfully used to detect splenic metastasis more than 20 years ago by magnetic resonance with an enhanced signal intensity of tumor and a decreased intensity of spleen in 18 patients. The improved contrast-to-noise ratio allowed the detection of metastasis in 4 patients out of 18 versus 2 in the nonenhanced MR imaging group (Weissleder et al., 1988). These nanoparticles brought only an improved contrast due to a passive accumulation in the tumor; much better results can be obtained with an enhanced tumor targeting. Thus, functionalized lipid nanoparticles have shown interesting properties in fluorescence tumor imaging. The peptide cRGD that targets $\alpha v \beta 3$ integrin was used to help solid lipid nanoparticles made from Suppocire NCTM and containing a lipidic fluorescent dye, DID, to specifically target HEK293(ß3) cells implanted in nude mice (Goutayer et al., 2010). The tumor was implanted subcutaneously as a xenograft. After excitation by 660-nm light-emitting diodes, fluorescence images are acquired by a CCD camera. Images can also be obtained on the isolated organs after autopsy of the animals (Figure 9.4).

This example shows how targeting, if efficient, can allow tumor imaging. Many works with a great variety of ligands have described tumor-specific imaging. This is very interesting in diagnostics, particularly to highlight metastasis that can be very difficult to detect at an early stage. This is really important in cancer therapy as it was postulated that the earlier the metastasis or primary tumor is detected, the better the prognosis or remission. Because nanoparticles have been shown to be good vectors for imaging and on the other side, for cancer therapy, it was proposed to associate imaging and therapy in the same systems. This domain is called theranostics, a contraction word from therapeutics and diagnostics. Combining all of what was previously reviewed in this chapter, a new nanodelivery system consisted of SPIONs, allowing MRI monitoring, with a fluorescent dye (Cy 5.5) and SiRNA directed against the apoptotic gene BIRC5 was proposed in a recent study (Kumar et al., 2010). After intravenous injection of the nanoparticles in mice bearing BT-20 breast tumor, the tumors were detected by fluorescence, thanks to Cy 5.5, and within 2 weeks, a high level of necrosis and apoptosis was observed due to the action of the SiRNA (Figure 9.5). The change of tumor volume has been quantified over time by the monitoring

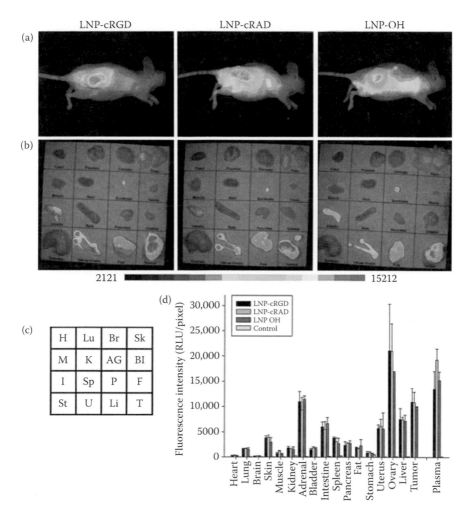

FIGURE 9.4
In vivo fluorescence imaging of tumors implanted subcutaneously using three different types of functionalized lipid nanoparticles in the living animal (a) and after autopsy (b) in different organs listed in (c). The fluorescence intensity is important in the tumor signing the efficiency of targeting (d). (Reprinted from *Eur J Pharm Biopharm*, 75, Goutayer, M. et al., Tumor targeting of functionalized lipid nanoparticles: Assessment by *in vivo* fluorescence imaging, 137–47, Copyright 2010, with permission from Elsevier.)

of fluorescence. The concomitant diagnosis and treatment have also been sought with pegylated gold nanoparticles containing phthalocyanine 4 (PC4), a drug used in photodynamic therapy, able to be detected by fluorescence. After IV injection in mice bearing a subcutaneous 9 L glioma xenograft, the gold nanoparticles have been shown to deeply accumulate

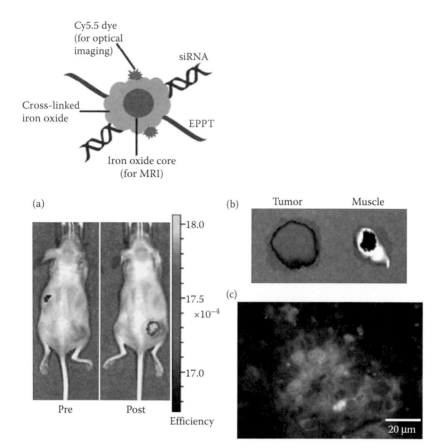

FIGURE 9.5
(**See color insert.**) Imaging of multifunctionalized nanoparticles targeted against cancer cells: in the mice (a), *ex vivo* in tumor and muscle (b), and in fluorescence microscopy (c). (From Kumar, M. et al. 2010. *Cancer Res*, 70, 7553–61. With permission from American Association for Cancer Research.)

in the tumor by flurorescence imaging by EPR effect, thus effectively and specifically delivering the PC4. The drug is then released from the nanoparticles because of its affinity to cell membranes (a raise in fluorescence is then observed). The best time to perform photodynamic therapy has been shown to be 6 h. The good clearance of the particles after 7 days has also been observed (Cheng et al., 2011).

These examples raise the huge potential of theranostics achieved by nanoparticles in cancer therapy; many examples of this new interesting strategy to highlight and destroy primary tumor or metastasis can be found in the literature (Yu et al., 2012).

9.6 Conclusion

As stated by Missoni and Foffani (2009), "the ultimate goal of developing and introducing new technologies should be to improve life conditions and health." So, it is legitimate to ask ourselves if nanotechnology will change the fate of cancer therapy because these technologies are still very expensive and have to provide a great benefit to a maximum of persons to worth the efforts made for their development. The aforementioned examples show that nanoparticles can target a drug to a tumor passively or actively with good efficiency. This allows in obtaining a higher concentration of the drug where it should act and not where it could harm. Moreover, nanoparticles have been shown to be very good tools for diagnostics, thus allowing a concomitant imaging of the tumor and its treatment. So, will nanomedicine win the fight against cancer? It is not sure for many reasons. First of all, the new effective nanodrugs have to be produced in adequate quantities with pharmaceutical quality constraints, which is very difficult to achieve in the case of complex formulations. Second, the efficiency of nanoparticles has often been studied but because the biodistribution of the drug is altered with nanoparticles, the toxicity could also be very important and difficult to assess. The field of nanotoxicology is new and rapidly growing, as shown in Chapter 12 of this book, but the road will be long to prove the lack of toxicity of nanomedicines. The case of immunotoxicity is particularly important to study for objects in the nanometer range. Nanoparticles should only contain generally-recognized-as-safe compounds, to avoid toxicity after their diffusion and/or destruction in the body (Hureaux et al., 2009). Finally, cancer cells are very adaptable and versatile; it is thus really possible that new mechanisms of resistance directed against nanoparticles will appear. Nevertheless, nanoparticles can thus be considered as a good new option to help drugs to better reach the tumor and to be more efficient; these new formulations are, however, not devoid of risk. This is why new effective drugs or therapeutic strategies are still needed to win the fight against cancer but nanotechnology remains a great hope for many patients. The road is still very long but the game is really worth the candle.

References

Aagaard, L. and Rossi, J. J. 2007. RNAi therapeutics: Principles, prospects and challenges. *Adv Drug Deliv Rev*, 59, 75–86.

Agueros, M., Zabaleta, V., Espuelas, S., Campanero, M. A., and Irache, J. M. 2010. Increased oral bioavailability of paclitaxel by its encapsulation through complex formation with cyclodextrins in poly(anhydride) nanoparticles. *J Control Release*, 145, 2–8.

Amidon, G. L., Lennernas, H., Shah, V. P., and Crison, J. R. 1995. A theoretical basis for a biopharmaceutic drug classification: The correlation of *in vitro* drug product dissolution and *in vivo* bioavailability. *Pharm Res*, 12, 413–20.

Baguley, B. C. 2010. Multiple drug resistance mechanisms in cancer. *Mol Biotechnol*, 46, 308–16.

Beduneau, A., Hindre, F., Clavreul, A., Leroux, J. C., Saulnier, P., and Benoit, J. P. 2008. Brain targeting using novel lipid nanovectors. *J Control Release*, 126, 44–9.

Beduneau, A., Saulnier, P., and Benoit, J. P. 2007. Active targeting of brain tumors using nanocarriers. *Biomaterials*, 28, 4947–67.

Caruso, G., Caffo, M., Alafaci, C., Raudino, G., Cafarella, D., Lucerna, S., Salpietro, F. M., and Tomasello, F. 2011. Could nanoparticle systems have a role in the treatment of cerebral gliomas? *Nanomedicine*, 7, 744–52.

Chen, A. M., Zhang, M., Wei, D., Stueber, D., Taratula, O., Minko, T., and He, H. 2009. Co-delivery of doxorubicin and Bcl-2 sirna by mesoporous silica nanoparticles enhances the efficacy of chemotherapy in multidrug-resistant cancer cells. *Small*, 5, 2673–7.

Cheng, Y., Meyers, J. D., Broome, A. M., Kenney, M. E., Basilion, J. P., and Burda, C. 2011. Deep penetration of a PDT drug into tumors by noncovalent drug-gold nanoparticle conjugates. *J Am Chem Soc*, 133, 2583–91.

Colin de Verdiere, A. C., Dubernet, C., Nemati, F., Soma, E., Appel, M., Ferte, J., Bernard, S., Puisieux, F., and Couvreur, P. 1997. Reversion of multidrug resistance with polyalkylcyanoacrylate nanoparticles: Towards a mechanism of action. *Br J Cancer*, 76, 198–205.

Crater, J. S. and Carrier, R. L. 2010. Barrier properties of gastrointestinal mucus to nanoparticle transport. *Macromol Biosci*, 10, 1473–83.

Danial, N. N. 2007. BCL-2 family proteins: Critical checkpoints of apoptotic cell death. *Clin Cancer Res*, 13, 7254–63.

Davis, M. E., Chen, Z. G., and Shin, D. M. 2008. Nanoparticle therapeutics: An emerging treatment modality for cancer. *Nat Rev Drug Discov*, 7, 771–82.

Davis, M. E., Zuckerman, J. E., Choi, C. H., Seligson, D., Tolcher, A., Alabi, C. A., Yen, Y., Heidel, J. D., and Ribas, A. 2010. Evidence of RNAi in humans from systemically administered siRNA via targeted nanoparticles. *Nature*, 464, 1067–70.

Dokka, S., Toledo, D., Shi, X., Castranova, V., and Rojanasakul, Y. 2000. Oxygen radical-mediated pulmonary toxicity induced by some cationic liposomes. *Pharm Res*, 17, 521–5.

Fan, L., Li, F., Zhang, H., Wang, Y., Cheng, C., Li, X., Gu, C. H., Yang, Q., Wu, H., and Zhang, S. 2010. Co-delivery of PDTC and doxorubicin by multifunctional micellar nanoparticles to achieve active targeted drug delivery and overcome multidrug resistance. *Biomaterials*, 31, 5634–42.

Fang, J., Nakamura, H., and Maeda, H. 2011. The EPR effect: Unique features of tumor blood vessels for drug delivery, factors involved, and limitations and augmentation of the effect. *Adv Drug Deliv Rev*, 63, 136–51.

Fasinu, P., Pillay, V., Ndesendo, V. M., Du Toit, L. C., and Choonara, Y. E. 2011. Diverse approaches for the enhancement of oral drug bioavailability. *Biopharm Drug Dispos*, 32, 185–209.

Ferlay, J, S. H., Bray, F., Forman, D., Mathers, C., and Parkin, D. M. 2010. GLOBOCAN 2008 v1.2, Cancer Incidence and Mortality Worldwide: IARC CancerBase No. 10 [Online]. Lyon: International Agency for Research on Cancer. Available: http://globocan.iarc.fr [Accessed September 2, 2011].

Gabizon, A., Shmeeda, H., and Barenholz, Y. 2003. Pharmacokinetics of pegylated liposomal doxorubicin: Review of animal and human studies. *Clin Pharmacokinet*, 42, 419–36.

Garcia-Garcia, E., Andrieux, K., Gil, S., and Couvreur, P. 2005. Colloidal carriers and blood-brain barrier (BBB) translocation: A way to deliver drugs to the brain? *Int J Pharm*, 298, 274–92.

Garcion, E., Lamprecht, A., Heurtault, B., Paillard, A., Aubert-Pouessel, A., Denizot, B., Menei, P., and Benoit, J. P. 2006. A new generation of anticancer, drug-loaded, colloidal vectors reverses multidrug resistance in glioma and reduces tumor progression in rats. *Mol Cancer Ther*, 5, 1710–22.

Goodman, T. T., Chen, J., Matveev, K., and Pun, S. H. 2008. Spatio-temporal modeling of nanoparticle delivery to multicellular tumor spheroids. *Biotechnol Bioeng*, 101, 388–99.

Goutayer, M., Dufort, S., Josserand, V., Royere, A., Heinrich, E., Vinet, F., Bibette, J., Coll, J. L., and Texier, I. 2010. Tumor targeting of functionalized lipid nanoparticles: Assessment by *in vivo* fluorescence imaging. *Eur J Pharm Biopharm*, 75, 137–47.

Guin, S., Ma, Q., Padhye, S., Zhou, Y. Q., Yao, H. P., and Wang, M. H. 2011. Targeting acute hypoxic cancer cells by doxorubicin-immunoliposomes directed by monoclonal antibodies specific to RON receptor tyrosine kinase. *Cancer Chemother Pharmacol*, 67, 1073–83.

Harrington, K. J., Mohammadtaghi, S., Uster, P. S., Glass, D., Peters, A. M., Vile, R. G., and Stewart, J. S. 2001. Effective targeting of solid tumors in patients with locally advanced cancers by radiolabeled pegylated liposomes. *Clin Cancer Res*, 7, 243–54.

Heidel, J. D. and Davis, M. E. 2011. Clinical developments in nanotechnology for cancer therapy. *Pharm Res*, 28, 187–99.

Heidel, J. D., Yu, Z., Liu, J. Y., Rele, S. M., Liang, Y., Zeidan, R. K., Kornbrust, D. J., and Davis, M. E. 2007. Administration in non-human primates of escalating intravenous doses of targeted nanoparticles containing ribonucleotide reductase subunit M2 siRNA. *Proc Natl Acad Sci USA*, 104, 5715–21.

Hobbs, S. K., Monsky, W. L., Yuan, F., Roberts, W. G., Griffith, L., Torchilin, V. P., and Jain, R. K. 1998. Regulation of transport pathways in tumor vessels: Role of tumor type and microenvironment. *Proc Natl Acad Sci USA*, 95, 4607–12.

Holback, H. and Yeo, Y. 2011. Intratumoral drug delivery with nanoparticulate carriers. *Pharm Res*, 28, 1819–30.

Hou, J., Zhang, Q., Li, X., Tang, Y., Cao, M. R., Bai, F., Shi, Q., Yang, C. H., Kong, D. L., and Bai, G. 2011. Synthesis of novel folate conjugated fluorescent nanoparticles for tumor imaging. *J Biomed Mater Res A*, 99, 684–9.

Hu-Lieskovan, S., Heidel, J. D., Bartlett, D. W., Davis, M. E., and Triche, T. J. 2005. Sequence-specific knockdown of EWS-FLI1 by targeted, nonviral delivery of small interfering RNA inhibits tumor growth in a murine model of metastatic Ewing's sarcoma. *Cancer Res*, 65, 8984–92.

Hureaux, J., Lagarce, F., Gagnadoux, F., Clavreul, A., Benoit, J. P., and Urban, T. 2009. The adaptation of lipid nanocapsule formulations for blood administration in animals. *Int J Pharm*, 379, 266–9.

Huxham, L. A., Kyle, A. H., Baker, J. H., Nykilchuk, L. K., and Minchinton, A. I. 2004. Microregional effects of gemcitabine in HCT-116 xenografts. *Cancer Res*, 64, 6537–41.

Huynh, N. T., Roger, E., Lautram, N., Benoit, J. P., and Passirani, C. 2010. The rise and rise of stealth nanocarriers for cancer therapy: Passive versus active targeting. *Nanomedicine (Lond)*, 5, 1415–33.

Irache, J. M., Salman, H. H., Gamazo, C., and Espuelas, S. 2008. Mannose-targeted systems for the delivery of therapeutics. *Expert Opin Drug Deliv*, 5, 703–24.

Jackson, A. L. and Linsley, P. S. 2010. Recognizing and avoiding siRNA off-target effects for target identification and therapeutic application. *Nat Rev Drug Discov*, 9, 57–67.

Jain, A. K., Swarnakar, N. K., Godugu, C., Singh, R. P., and Jain, S. 2011a. The effect of the oral administration of polymeric nanoparticles on the efficacy and toxicity of tamoxifen. *Biomaterials*, 32, 503–15.

Jain, S., Mathur, R., Das, M., Swarnakar, N. K., and Mishra, A. K. 2011b. Synthesis, pharmacoscintigraphic evaluation and antitumor efficacy of methotrexate-loaded, folate-conjugated, stealth albumin nanoparticles. *Nanomedicine (Lond)*, 6, 1733–54.

Jang, S. H., Wientjes, M. G., and Au, J. L. 2001a. Determinants of paclitaxel uptake, accumulation and retention in solid tumors. *Invest New Drugs*, 19, 113–23.

Jang, S. H., Wientjes, M. G., and Au, J. L. 2001b. Enhancement of paclitaxel delivery to solid tumors by apoptosis-inducing pretreatment: Effect of treatment schedule. *J Pharmacol Exp Ther*, 296, 1035–42.

Jang, S. H., Wientjes, M. G., Lu, D., and Au, J. L. 2003. Drug delivery and transport to solid tumors. *Pharm Res*, 20, 1337–50.

Juillerat-Jeanneret, L. 2008. The targeted delivery of cancer drugs across the blood-brain barrier: Chemical modifications of drugs or drug-nanoparticles? *Drug Discov Today*, 13, 1099–106.

Ke, W., Zhao, Y., Huang, R., Jiang, C., and Pei, Y. 2008. Enhanced oral bioavailability of doxorubicin in a dendrimer drug delivery system. *J Pharm Sci*, 97, 2208–16.

Kim, B., Han, G., Toley, B. J., Kim, C. K., Rotello, V. M., and Forbes, N. S. 2010a. Tuning payload delivery in tumour cylindroids using gold nanoparticles. *Nat Nanotechnol*, 5, 465–72.

Kim, S., Kim, J. Y., Huh, K. M., Acharya, G., and Park, K. 2008. Hydrotropic polymer micelles containing acrylic acid moieties for oral delivery of paclitaxel. *J Control Release*, 132, 222–9.

Kim, B. Y., Rutka, J. T., and Chan, W. C. 2010b. Nanomedicine. *N Engl J Med*, 363, 2434–43.

Kreuter, J. 2007. Nanoparticles—A historical perspective. *Int J Pharm*, 331, 1–10.

Kreuter, J., Alyautdin, R. N., Kharkevich, D. A., and Ivanov, A. A. 1995. Passage of peptides through the blood-brain barrier with colloidal polymer particles (nanoparticles). *Brain Res*, 674, 171–4.

Kumar, M., Yigit, M., Dai, G., Moore, A., and Medarova, Z. 2010. Image-guided breast tumor therapy using a small interfering RNA nanodrug. *Cancer Res*, 70, 7553–61.

Kyle, A. H., Huxham, L. A., Chiam, A. S., Sim, D. H., and Minchinton, A. I. 2004. Direct assessment of drug penetration into tissue using a novel application of three-dimensional cell culture. *Cancer Res*, 64, 6304–9.

Lagarce, F. and Roger, E. 2011. Nanocarrier absorption studies with Caco-2 cells. In: Shulz, M. A. (ed.) *Caco-2 Cells and Their Uses*. Nova Science Publishers, Inc., Hauppauge, New York.

Lamprecht, A. and Benoit, J. P. 2006. Etoposide nanocarriers suppress glioma cell growth by intracellular drug delivery and simultaneous P-glycoprotein inhibition. *J Control Release*, 112, 208–13.

Landen, C. N., Jr., Chavez-Reyes, A., Bucana, C., Schmandt, R., Deavers, M. T., Lopez-Berestein, G., and Sood, A. K. 2005. Therapeutic EphA2 gene targeting *in vivo* using neutral liposomal small interfering RNA delivery. *Cancer Res*, 65, 6910–8.

Lee, H., Fonge, H., Hoang, B., Reilly, R. M., and Allen, C. 2010. The effects of particle size and molecular targeting on the intratumoral and subcellular distribution of polymeric nanoparticles. *Mol Pharm*, 7, 1195–208.

Li, W. and Szoka, F. C., Jr. 2007. Lipid-based nanoparticles for nucleic acid delivery. *Pharm Res*, 24, 438–49.

Lieleg, O., Baumgartel, R. M., and Bausch, A. R. 2009. Selective filtering of particles by the extracellular matrix: An electrostatic bandpass. *Biophys J*, 97, 1569–77.

Liu, B. R., Huang, Y. W., Chiang, H. J., and Lee, H. J. 2010. Cell-penetrating peptide-functionalized quantum dots for intracellular delivery. *J Nanosci Nanotechnol*, 10, 7897–905.

Lv, P. P., Wei, W., Yue, H., Yang, T. Y., Wang, L. Y., and Ma, G. H. 2011. Porous quaternized chitosan nanoparticles containing paclitaxel nanocrystals improved therapeutic efficacy in non-small-cell lung cancer after oral administration. *Biomacromolecules*, 12, 4230–39.

Malingre, M. M., Beijnen, J. H., and Schellens, J. H. 2001. Oral delivery of taxanes. *Invest New Drugs*, 19, 155–62.

Matsumura, Y. and Maeda, H. 1986. A new concept for macromolecular therapeutics in cancer chemotherapy: Mechanism of tumoritropic accumulation of proteins and the antitumor agent smancs. *Cancer Res*, 46, 6387–92.

Milane, L., Duan, Z., and Amiji, M. 2011a. Therapeutic efficacy and safety of paclitaxel/lonidamine loaded EGFR-targeted nanoparticles for the treatment of multi-drug resistant cancer. *PLoS One*, 6, e24075.

Milane, L., Duan, Z. F., and Amiji, M. 2011b. Pharmacokinetics and biodistribution of lonidamine/paclitaxel loaded, EGFR-targeted nanoparticles in an orthotopic animal model of multi-drug resistant breast cancer. *Nanomedicine*, 7, 435–44.

Minchinton, A. I. and Tannock, I. F. 2006. Drug penetration in solid tumours. *Nat Rev Cancer*, 6, 583–92.

Missoni, E. and Foffani, G. 2009. Nanotechnologies and challenges for global health. *Studies Ethics Law Technol*, 3, 1–16.

Morille, M., Montier, T., Legras, P., Carmoy, N., Brodin, P., Pitard, B., Benoit, J. P., and Passirani, C. 2010. Long-circulating DNA lipid nanocapsules as new vector for passive tumor targeting. *Biomaterials*, 31, 321–9.

Morille, M., Passirani, C., Dufort, S., Bastiat, G., Pitard, B., Coll, J. L., and Benoit, J. P. 2011. Tumor transfection after systemic injection of DNA lipid nanocapsules. *Biomaterials*, 32, 2327–33.

Northfelt, D. W., Dezube, B. J., Thommes, J. A., Levine, R., Von Roenn, J. H., Dosik, G. M., Rios, A., Krown, S. E., Dumond, C., and Mamelok, R. D. 1997. Efficacy of pegylated-liposomal doxorubicin in the treatment of AIDS-related Kaposi's sarcoma after failure of standard chemotherapy. *J Clin Oncol*, 15, 653–9.

Ozpolat, B., Sood, A. K., and Lopez-Berestein, G. 2010. Nanomedicine based approaches for the delivery of siRNA in cancer. *J Int Med*, 267, 44–53.

Peltier, S., Oger, J. M., Lagarce, F., Couet, W., and Benoit, J. P. 2006. Enhanced oral paclitaxel bioavailability after administration of paclitaxel-loaded lipid nanocapsules. *Pharm Res*, 23, 1243–50.

Rapisarda, A., Hollingshead, M., Uranchimeg, B., Bonomi, C. A., Borgel, S. D., Carter, J. P., Gehrs, B. et al. 2009. Increased antitumor activity of bevacizumab in combination with hypoxia inducible factor-1 inhibition. *Mol Cancer Ther*, 8, 1867–77.

Roger, E., Lagarce, F., and Benoit, J. P. 2009a. The gastrointestinal stability of lipid nanocapsules. *Int J Pharm*, 379, 260–5.

Roger, E., Lagarce, F., and Benoit, J. P. 2011. Development and characterization of a novel lipid nanocapsule formulation of Sn38 for oral administration. *Eur J Pharm Biopharm*, 79, 181–98.

Roger, E., Lagarce, F., Garcion, E., and Benoit, J. P. 2009b. Lipid nanocarriers improve paclitaxel transport throughout human intestinal epithelial cells by using vesi-cle-mediated transcytosis. *J Control Release*, 140, 174–81.

Roger, E., Lagarce, F., Garcion, E., and Benoit, J. P. 2010a. Biopharmaceutical param-eters to consider in order to alter the fate of nanocarriers after oral delivery. *Nanomedicine (Lond)*, 5, 287–306.

Roger, E., Lagarce, F., Garcion, E., and Benoit, J. P. 2010b. Reciprocal competition between lipid nanocapsules and P-gp for paclitaxel transport across Caco-2 cells. *Eur J Pharm Sci*, 40, 422–9.

Ruoslahti, E. 2002. Specialization of tumour vasculature. *Nat Rev Cancer*, 2, 83–90.

Ruoslahti, E., Bhatia, S. N., and Sailor, M. J. 2010. Targeting of drugs and nanoparticles to tumors. *J Cell Biol*, 188, 759–68.

Shapira, A., Livney, Y. D., Broxterman, H. J., and Assaraf, Y. G. 2011. Nanomedicine for targeted cancer therapy: Towards the overcoming of drug resistance. *Drug Resist Updat*, 14, 150–63.

Singh, S. and Dash, A. K. 2009. Paclitaxel in cancer treatment: Perspectives and pros-pects of its delivery challenges. *Crit Rev Ther Drug Carrier Syst*, 26, 333–72.

Sparreboom, A., Van Asperen, J., Mayer, U., Schinkel, A. H., Smit, J. W., Meijer, D. K., Borst, P., Nooijen, W. J., Beijnen, J. H., and Van Tellingen, O. 1997. Limited oral bioavailability and active epithelial excretion of paclitaxel (Taxol) caused by P-glycoprotein in the intestine. *Proc Natl Acad Sci USA*, 94, 2031–5.

Stylianopoulos, T., Poh, M. Z., Insin, N., Bawendi, M. G., Fukumura, D., Munn, L. L., and Jain, R. K. 2010. Diffusion of particles in the extracellular matrix: The effect of repulsive electrostatic interactions. *Biophys J*, 99, 1342–9.

Sugahara, K. N., Teesalu, T., Karmali, P. P., Kotamraju, V. R., Agemy, L., Greenwald, D. R., and Ruoslahti, E. 2010. Coadministration of a tumor-penetrating peptide enhances the efficacy of cancer drugs. *Science*, 328, 1031–5.

Symon, Z., Peyser, A., Tzemach, D., Lyass, O., Sucher, E., Shezen, E., and Gabizon, A. 1999. Selective delivery of doxorubicin to patients with breast carcinoma metas-tases by stealth liposomes. *Cancer*, 86, 72–8.

Tiemann, K. and Rossi, J. J. 2009. RNAi-based therapeutics-current status, challenges and prospects. *EMBO Mol Med*, 1, 142–51.

Torchilin, V. 2011. Tumor delivery of macromolecular drugs based on the EPR effect. *Adv Drug Deliv Rev*, 63, 131–5.

Vauthier, C., Dubernet, C., Chauvierre, C., Brigger, I., and Couvreur, P. 2003. Drug delivery to resistant tumors: The potential of poly(alkyl cyanoacrylate) nanopar-ticles. *J Control Release*, 93, 151–60.

Weissleder, R., Hahn, P. F., Stark, D. D., Elizondo, G., Saini, S., Todd, L. E., Wittenberg, J., and Ferrucci, J. T. 1988. Superparamagnetic iron oxide: Enhanced detection of focal splenic tumors with MR imaging. *Radiology*, 169, 399–403.

Werner, M. E., Karve, S., Sukumar, R., Cummings, N. D., Copp, J. A., Chen, R. C., Zhang, T., and Wang, A. Z. 2011. Folate-targeted nanoparticle delivery of chemo- and radiotherapeutics for the treatment of ovarian cancer peritoneal metastasis. *Biomaterials*, 32, 8548–54.

Wohlfart, S., Khalansky, A. S., Gelperina, S., Maksimenko, O., Bernreuther, C., Glatzel, M., and Kreuter, J. 2011. Efficient chemotherapy of rat glioblastoma using doxorubicin-loaded PLGA nanoparticles with different stabilizers. *PLoS One*, 6, e19121.

Wong, C., Stylianopoulos, T., Cui, J., Martin, J., Chauhan, V. P., Jiang, W., Popovic, Z., Jain, R. K., Bawendi, M. G., and Fukumura, D. 2011. Multistage nanoparticle delivery system for deep penetration into tumor tissue. *Proc Natl Acad Sci USA*, 108, 2426–31.

Yu, M. K., Park, J., and Jon, S. 2012. Targeting strategies for multifunctional nanoparticles in cancer imaging and therapy. *Theranostics*, 2, 3–44.

Zimmermann, T. S., Lee, A. C., Akinc, A., Bramlage, B., Bumcrot, D., Fedoruk, M. N., Harborth, J. et al. 2006. RNAi-mediated gene silencing in non-human primates. *Nature*, 441, 111–4.

10

Formulations of Nanoparticles in Drug Delivery

Sushama Talegaonkar, Mohammad Tariq, and Zeenat Iqbal

CONTENTS

10.1 Introduction 240
    10.1.1 Advantages of Using Nanoparticles as a Drug Delivery
    System 241
        10.1.1.1 Disadvantages of Nanoparticles 241
10.2 Formulation Development 241
10.3 Formulation Techniques 246
    10.3.1 Dispersion of Preformed Polymers 247
        10.3.1.1 Single-Emulsion Solvent Evaporation Method 247
        10.3.1.2 Double-Emulsion (W/O/W) Solvent Evaporation
        Method 252
        10.3.1.3 Single-Emulsion Solvent Diffusion Method 255
        10.3.1.4 Spontaneous Emulsification or Modified Solvent
        Diffusion Method 259
        10.3.1.5 Salting Out 261
        10.3.1.6 Nanoprecipitation or Solvent Displacement
        Method 262
        10.3.1.7 Dialysis 264
        10.3.1.8 Supercritical Fluid Technology 267
        10.3.1.9 Ionic Gelation Method 270
    10.3.2 Polymerization Methods 270
        10.3.2.1 Emulsion Polymerization 271
        10.3.2.2 Miniemulsion Polymerization 273
        10.3.2.3 Microemulsion Polymerization 273
        10.3.2.4 Interfacial Polymerization 274
10.4 Conclusion 275
Abbreviations 275
References 276

10.1 Introduction

Nanotechnology is the science that deals with structures in the size range of nanometers. It has the potential to greatly impact our lives. The employment of nanotechnology has opened new vistas in the areas of personalized health care, drug delivery, gene therapy, diagnostics, imaging, and novel drug discovery techniques. Enormous research is going on in the field of nanotechnology to resolve various issues such as bioavailability, spatial and temporal delivery of drugs, and precise delivery of new molecules like genes and deoxyribonucleic acid (DNA). The delivery of therapeutic and diagnostic agents through the colloidal carriers is at the forefront of nanotechnology as it provides numerous opportunities for efficient exploitation of different formulations and routes of administration. In this perspective, first, solid-core nanoparticles (NPs) were reported as an alternative drug carrier. NPs are defined as particulate dispersions or solid particles with a size in the range of 10–200 nm, built from macromolecular and/or molecular assemblies, in which the active principle is dissolved, dispersed, encapsulated, or even adsorbed or attached to the external interface. NPs are divided into two main classes based on their structures: nanospheres and nanocapsules that can be obtained by varying the methods of preparation. Nanospheres are matrix systems in which the drug is physically and uniformly dispersed and have a homogeneous structure, whereas nanocapsules are the systems in which the drug is confined in a cavity surrounded by a unique polymer membrane exhibit a typical core–shell structure (Figure 10.1). Their higher kinetic stability and rigid morphology are the major advantages over other colloidal drug delivery systems (such as liposome, niosome, microemulsions, nanoemulsions, etc.). Pharmaceutical NPs are one of the colloidal vehicles that possess the ability to carry drugs, accumulate preferentially at the target site, or release drugs in a controlled way within the body, which leads to improved pharmacokinetics and biodistribution of therapeutic

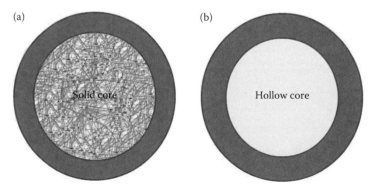

FIGURE 10.1
Illustration of polymeric nanoparticles: (a) nanosphere, the drug uniformly distributed into the solid matrix; (b) nanocapsule, the drug encapsulated within the hollow core.

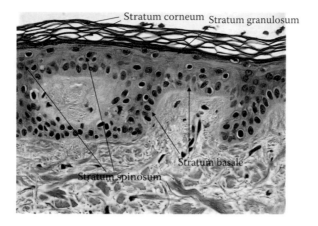

FIGURE 5.1
Histology of human skin.

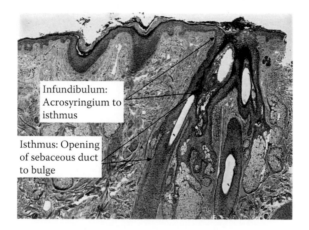

FIGURE 5.2
Histology of the pilosebaceous unit.

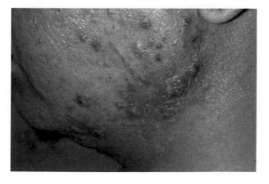

FIGURE 5.3
Nodulocystic acne vulgaris.

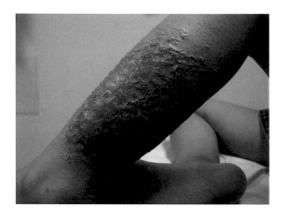

FIGURE 5.4
Atopic dermatitis.

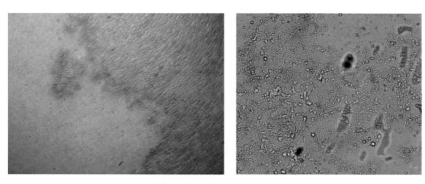

FIGURE 5.6
Dermatophytosis—annular, scaly erythematous plaques (left); potassium hydroxide wet prep demonstrating hyphae (right).

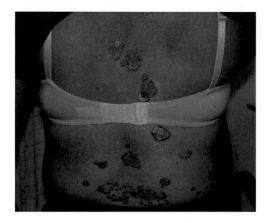

FIGURE 5.7
Psoriasis.

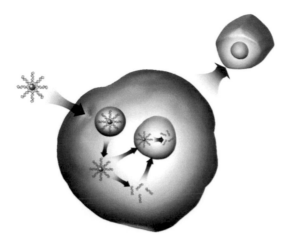

FIGURE 7.2
Chitosan–DNA nanoparticles on the behavior of THP-1 human macrophages. Macrophages are the first cells that intercept foreign bodies, which can even be introduced nanoparticles, with the effect of releasing inflammatory cytokines and MMPs.

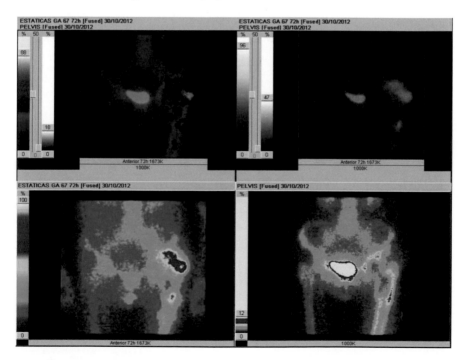

FIGURE 8.2
Fusion image of two scintigraphic studies with double tracer, Tc-99m-DPD + Ga-67-citrate. It shows increased uptake in periprosthetic bone of Tc-99m-DPD radiotracer (gray scale) at the left hip and left femoral diaphysis with an accumulation of Ga-67-citrate (color scale, left panel; red scale, right panel) in the same site related to periprosthetic infectious-inflammatory process.

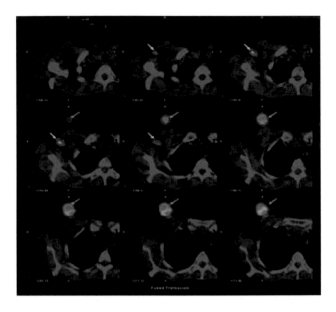

FIGURE 8.5

Sentinel node scintigraphy. Multimodal image, SPECT/CT (nine axial slices focused on right chest), showing a focal uptake in right axillary region, posterior to the pectoral muscles, in correspondence with sentinel node (yellow arrow). The injection site is observed in the right mammary tissue (green arrow).

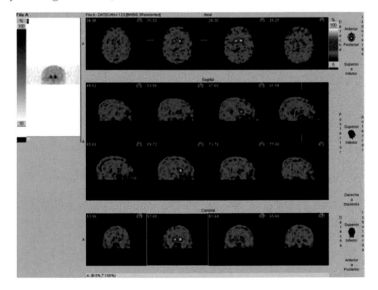

FIGURE 8.7

SPECT study with 123I-ioflupane. Images displaying axial, sagittal, and coronal (top to bottom) projections. Specific uptake was observed at presynaptic dopamine subcortical level in the caudate nuclei (color scale). Severe decrease in uptake in both putamens in relation to Parkinson's disease.

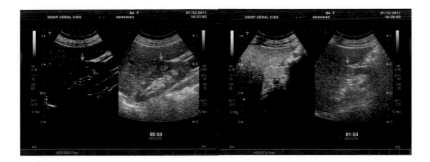

FIGURE 8.10
Right renal ultrasound images (longitudinal axis) enhanced with SonoVue® (microbubbles contrast agent) of the cortical renal hypervascularized tumor (green arrow). The figure is divided in two panels composed with two images per panel. The enhanced US images with SonoVue®, displayed at the right in both panels, were taken at 4 seconds and 1 minute postinjection time respectively and compared with those respective non-enhanced US images (left images in both panels) visualizing the hypervascularization of the renal tumor. (Image courtesy of Dra. María Milagros Otero from Hospital Xeral-Cies, Spain.)

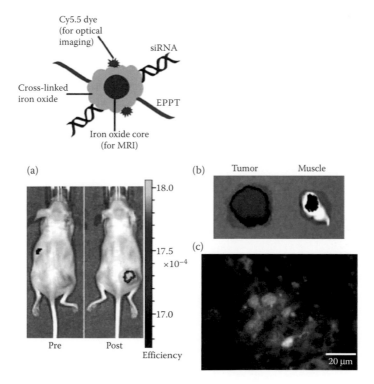

FIGURE 9.5
Imaging of multifunctionalized nanoparticles targeted against cancer cells: in the mice (a), *ex vivo* in tumor and muscle (b), and in fluorescence microscopy (c). (From Kumar, M. et al. 2010. *Cancer Res*, 70, 7553–61. With permission from American Association for Cancer Research.)

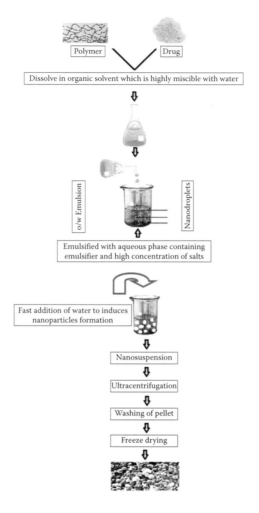

FIGURE 10.6
Schematic representation of the salting-out method.

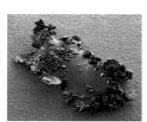

Different sizes of colloidal gold particles

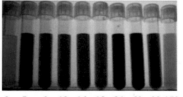

2   5   6   12   16   18   24   60   90 150 nm

FIGURE 12.1
Alteration in the optical properties of gold NPs as a function of size of the NPs. (From Erik C.D. et al. *Chem Soc Rev*, 2012, **41**(7), 274–79. http://www.ansci.wisc.edu/facstaff/Faculty/pages/albrecht/albrecht_web/Programs/microscopy/colloid.html.)

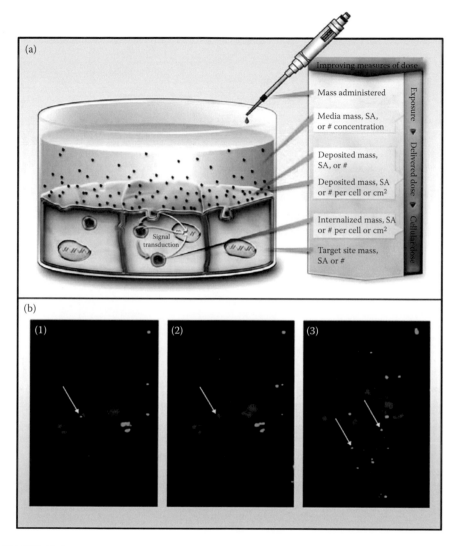

FIGURE 13.6

Dose for nanoparticles *in vitro* increases in specificity and relevancy as dose measures move from administered amount to amount delivered to cells or internalized by cells (a) SA, surface area; #, particle number. (b) Images of an alveolar epithelial cell (C10), grown in culture and exposed to fluorescence-tagged 500-nm amorphous silica particles, demonstrate the principles shown in (a). The cell membrane is marked (red) by a membrane-specific fluorescent marker (wheat germ agglutinin), which was also internalized over time as an integral part of endocytotic vesicles. (b.1) Illustrates delivered dose: a silica particle (green) on the apical surface of the cell. The particle is no longer visible as the focal plane moves into the interior of the cell (b.2). Silica particles taken up into the cell are observed as the focal plane moves farther into the interior of the cell (b.3). (Adapted with permission from Teeguarden, J. G. et al. 2007. Particokinetics *in vitro*: Dosimetry considerations for *in vitro* nanoparticle toxicity assessments. *Toxicol Sci*, 95, 300–12. Copyright 2006 Oxford University Press.)

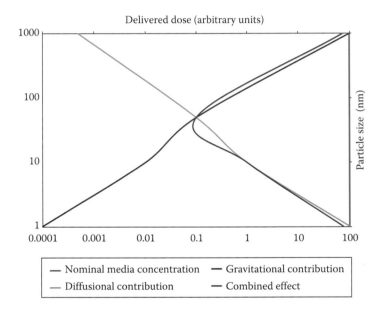

FIGURE 13.7
Generalized representation of the particokinetic contribution to delivered dose within an *in vitro* system. As particle size increases, the contribution of diffusion to delivered dose decreases while the contribution of gravitational settling increases. It is estimated that at about 50 nm, the effective contribution of diffusion and gravitational settling are near equilibrium.

agents with consequent reduction in systemic side effects and more efficient use of the therapeutic agents (Kreuter 1994; Alexis et al., 2008; Qi et al., 2012). They do not only allow the delivery of small drug molecules but are also expected to deliver peptides, proteins, and nucleic acids, hence opening the gate for gene therapy (Kim et al., 2005; Kommareddy et al., 2005; Jeon et al., 2012). NPs are usually administered through the parenteral route; however, because of their excellent barrier-crossing property, they are also being investigated for oral (Yin et al., 2007; Agueros et al., 2009; Kalaria et al., 2009; Jain et al., 2011), ocular (Motwani et al., 2008; Gupta et al., 2010; Basaran et al., 2011), nasal (Michael et al., 2009; Shahnaz et al., 2012), pulmonary (Ungaro et al., 2012), periodontal (Pinon-Segundo et al., 2005; Saboktakin et al., 2011), and transdermal (Elnaggar et al., 2011; Gupta and Vyas, 2012) routes. In spite of being a young technology, thousands of nanopharmaceuticals have been patented worldwide (Caruthers et al., 2007) and many have been approved by the Food and Drug Administration (FDA) for clinical purposes (Table 10.1).

10.1.1 Advantages of Using Nanoparticles as a Drug Delivery System

Particle size and surface characteristics of NPs can be easily manipulated; therefore, both passive and active drug targeting can be achieved.

NPs can be exploited for controlled and sustained release of drugs at the site of localization. They can also be employed for altering organ distribution of the drug and subsequent clearance to increase drug therapeutic efficacy and reduction in side effects. Controlled release and particle degradation characteristics can be readily modulated by altering the matrix constituents. Drug loading capacity is relatively higher than other colloidal drug delivery systems. Site-specific targeting can be achieved by surface modification with the help of targeting ligands or employing magnetic guidance.

10.1.1.1 Disadvantages of Nanoparticles

In spite of the various advantages, NPs have certain limitations. For example, their small size and large surface area can lead to particle–particle aggregation, making physical handling of NPs difficult in liquid and dry forms. In addition, small particle size and large surface area leads to limited drug loading and burst release. These practical problems have to be overcome before NPs can be used clinically or made commercially available.

10.2 Formulation Development

The development of nanoparticle formulations involves a basic understanding of various formulation components such as nature of the core material, polymers, stabilizers, and formulation techniques. These components affect

TABLE 10.1

FDA-Approved Nanopharmaceuticals for Clinical Purposes

Therapeutic/ Diagnostic Agents	Delivery System	Marketed Name	Route of Administration	Company	Indication	Year of Approval
Doxorubicin	Liposome	Myocet	IV	Zeneus Pharma, Sopherion Therapeutics	Late stage of metastatic breast cancer	July 2000
Propofol	Liposomes	Diprivan	IV	Zeneca Pharma	Anesthetic	October 1989
Doxorubicin	Pegylated liposomes	Doxil Caelyx	IV	OrthoBiotech Schering-Plough	Metastatic ovarian cancer and AIDS-related Kaposi's sarcoma	November 1995
Doxorubicin	Liposome	DaunoXome	IV	Gilead Sciences	Advanced HIV-related Kaposi's sarcoma	April 1996
Amphotericin B	Liposomes	Ambisome	IV	Gilead sciences	Fungal infections	August 1997
Cytarabine	Liposomes	Depocyt	IV	SkyePharma, Enzon	Lymphomatous meningitis	April 1999
Verteporfin	Liposomes	Visudyne	IV	Novartis AG	Photodynamic therapy for age-related macular degeneration	April 2000
Estradiol hemihydrates	Micelle	Estrasorb	Transdermal	Novavax	Reduction of vasomotor symptoms in menopausal women	October 2003
Docetaxel	Micelle	Taxotere	IV	Sanofi Aventis	Antineoplastic	May 1996
Paclitaxal	Nanoparticles	Abraxane	IV	Abraxis BioScience AstraZeneca	Metastatic breast cancer	January 2005

Drug	Formulation	Product	Route	Company	Indication	Date
Mexoryl SX	Nanoparticle (cream)	Anthelios 20	Topical	La Roche Posay	Sunscreen	October 2005
Ecamsule, avobenzone, octocryleneand, titanium dioxide	Nanoparticle	Helioblock SX	Topical	La Roche Posay	Sunscreen	March 2008
Sirolimus	Nanocrystal (tablets, solution)	Rapamune	Oral	Wyeth, Elan	Immunosuppressant for kidney transplant	September 1999
Aprepitant	Nanocrystal (capsule, injection)	Emend	Oral, IV	Merck, Elan	Chemotherapy-induced nausea and vomiting	March 2003
Fenofibrate	Nanocrystal	Tricor	Oral tablet	Abbot, Elan	Lipid disorders	November 2004
Fenofibrate	Nanocrystal	Triglide	Oral tablets	SkyePharma, First Horizon	Lipid disorders	May 2005
Megestrol acetate	Nanocrystal	Megace ES	Oral suspension	PAR Pharm, Strativa Pharmaceuticals	Anorexia, cachexia, or an unexplained significant weight loss in AIDS patients	July 2005
PEG–adenosine deaminase	Nanoconjugates	Adagen	IV	Enzon	Enzyme replacement therapy	March 1990
PEG–interferon α-2a	Nanoconjugates	PEGASYS	Subcutaneous	Nektar	Chronic hepatitis C virus infection	October 2002
PEG–hGH	Nanoconjugates	Somavert	Subcutaneous	Nektar, Pfizer	Acromegaly	March 2003
PEG–hG-CSF	Nanoconjugates	Neulasta	Subcutaneous	Amgen	Febrile neutropenia	January 2002
PEG–interferon α-2b	Nanoconjugates	PEGIntron	Subcutaneous	Enzon, Schering-Plough	Chronic hepatitis C virus infection	January 2001
PEG–asparginase	Nanoconjugates	Oncaspar	Subcutaneous	Enzon	Leukemia	February 1994
Amphotericin B	Nanoconjugates	Abelcet	IV	Enzon	Invasive fungal infections	November 1995

continued

TABLE 10.1 (continued)

FDA-Approved Nanopharmaceuticals for Clinical Purposes

Therapeutic/ Diagnostic Agents	Delivery System	Marketed Name	Route of Administration	Company	Indication	Year of Approval
Sevelamer hydrochloride	Cross-linked poly(allylamine) resin (tablet, capsule)	Renagel	Oral	Genzyme	Control of serum phosphorus in patients with chronic kidney disease on dialysis	October 1998
Amphotericin B	Lipid-based colloidal suspension	Amphotec	Subcutaneous	Sequus	Invasive fungal infection	November 1996
Estradiol	Nanoparticles-incorporated gel	Elestrin	Transdermal	BioSanté	Reduction of vasomotor symptoms in menopausal women	December 2006
Lanreotide	Nanotubes	Somatuline Deppot®	Subcutaneous	Beaufour Ipsen	Acromegaly	August 2007
Magnetite	Colloidal particles	Faraheme	IV	AMAG Pharmaceutical's	Iron deficiency	June 2009
Ferumoxides	Colloidal particles	Feridex	IV	AMAG Pharmaceutical's	MRI contrast agent	August 1996
Ferumoxsil	Colloidal suspension	Gastromark	Oral	AMAG Pharmaceutical's	Imaging of abdominal structure	December 1996

the characteristics, stability, and release profile of the developed systems, hence affecting their *in vitro* and *in vivo* performance. Before designing the blueprint of the system, consideration must be given to immunogenicity, clinical acceptance, and possible environmental hazards.

Polymers are the backbone in the successful formulation of nanoparticulate systems. They can be classified on the basis of their source, biodegradability, solubility, and mechanism/stimuli responsiveness (Table 10.2). The first reported NPs were based on nonbiodegradable polymers (such as polyacryl

TABLE 10.2

Classification of Polymer

I. Origin of Polymer	
Natural polymers	Gelatin, albumin, vicilin, lactin, legumin, dextran, pullulan, agarose, chitosan, alginate, and so on
Synthetic polymers	Poly-ε-caprolactone, polylactic acid, polylactide-*co*-glycolic acid, polyisobutylcyanoacrylates, polystyrene, polybutylcyanoacrylates, polyhexylcyanoacrylates, and polymethyl methacrylate
II. Degradation Profile	
Biodegradable polymers	Poly-ε-caprolactone, polylactic acid, polylactide-*co*-glycolic acid, polyisobutylcyanoacrylates, polybutylcyanoacrylates, polyhexylcyanoacrylates, and polymethyl methacrylate
Nonbiodegradable	Polystyrene, acrylic polymers (Eudragit®), cellulose esters, ethyl cellulose, cellulose acetate, cellulose acetate propionate, and cellulose acetate butyrate
III. Water Solubility	
Hydrophilic polymers	Gelatin, albumin, vicilin, lactin, legumin, dextran, pullulan, agarose, chitosan, and alginate
Hydrophobic polymers	Polystyrene, acrylic polymers (Eudragit), cellulose esters, ethyl cellulose, poly-ε-caprolactone, polylactic acid, polylactide-*co*-glycolic acid, polyisobutylcyanoacrylates, polybutylcyanoacrylates, polyhexylcyanoacrylates, and polymethyl methacrylate
IV. Mechanism/Stimuli/Response	
Mucoadhesive polymers	Alginate, chitosan, polyacrylic acid, and cyanoacrylates (commonly known as "super glues")
Photoresponsive polymers	Copolymer gels of N-isopropylacrylamide, cross-linked hyaluronic acid
pH-sensitive polymers	Mixture of acrylic acid and methacryl–amidopropyl–trimethyl ammonium chloride, poly(methacrylic acid–ethylene glycol) copolymer
Temperature-sensitive polymers	N-alkyl acrylamide homopolymers and their copolymers
Inflammation-responsive polymers	Cross-linked hyaluronic acid

amide, polystyrene, etc.) but due to the toxicity issues, their systemic administration was the matter of concern. Nowadays, various materials are being used for the preparation of NPs but the biodegradable polymers supersede the existing materials for human use as these materials afford good tissue compatibility and minimize the apprehension of hypersensitivity reactions. Biodegradable NPs have shown their advantages over other carriers due to their increased stability and controlled-release ability. Biodegradable NPs for pharmaceutical use are prepared from a variety of synthetic and natural polymers. Synthetic polymers such as polyacrylates, polycaprolactones, polylactides, and its copolymers with polyglycolides are widely used and discussed (Hans and Lowman, 2002).

Poly(lactic-*co*-glycolic acid) (PLGA) is one of the most widely used biodegradable polymers and has been approved by the FDA for certain human clinical uses. PLGA nanospheres have been suggested to be a good delivery carrier because of the safety and achieving sustained release (Prabha et al., 2002) and its degradation time can be altered from weeks to months by varying the molecular weight of the copolymer or the lactic acid to glycolic acid ratio in the copolymer (Kim et al., 2005).

Natural polymers including albumin (Langer et al., 2000), alginate (Zahoor et al., 2005), gelatin (Bajpai and Choubey, 2006), and probably the most studied natural polymer, chitosan (Agnihotri et al., 2004) are macromolecules have attracted wide interest as biomaterials due to their intrinsic biodegradability and biocompatibility. However, polymers of natural origin suffer from some disadvantages, including (a) batch-to-batch variation, (b) conditional biodegradability, and (c) antigenicity. Parenteral administration of polymeric NPs gets compromised mainly due to antigenicity. There is a need for extensive studies to generate the safety profile of carriers based on proteins and polysaccharides. Alginate-based delivery systems for oral and ophthalmic administrations have been approved (Al-Shamkhani et al., 1991) and it is also reported as homocompatible and convincingly acceptable system for parenteral administration of bioactives. In contrast, dextran, albumin, and gelatin, which are acceptable materials for parenteral administration, manifest immunogenicity due to the use of cross-linking agents, which are employed during their preparations. Chitosan, on the other hand, is a homo-noncompatible material and hence should be restricted to extracorporeal uses only (Pangburn et al., 1984). The selection of polymers for the NP development is done on the basis of the nature of drugs, desired size, and applications of interest.

10.3 Formulation Techniques

Methods available for the synthesis of NPs are based on two approaches: top-down and bottom-up (Alexis et al., 2008). The top-down process starts with a larger object and breaks it into nanostructures. However, the method is time consuming and often generates particles of broader size distribution (La-Van et al., 2003). Top-down techniques employ preformed polymers for the synthesis of NPs. In contrast, the bottom-up techniques, such as polymerizations, employ a monomer as a starting point and involved atom-by-atom or molecule-by-molecule arrangement in a controlled manner, which is regulated by thermodynamic means (Keck et al., 2008). Bottom-up techniques create heavily clustered masses of particles that do not break down on reconstitution (Shrivastava, 2008).

The method of preparation plays a vital role in determining the *in vitro* and *in vivo* fate of NPs. The selection of a suitable method is made on the basis of inherent properties of the drugs to be loaded (aqueous solubility and stability), matrix materials used, required size of NPs, surface characteristics such as charge and permeability, degree of biodegradability, biocompatibility, antigenicity, toxicity, desired release profile, and application of interest of the final product.

In this section, various methods of NP preparation are classified and discussed along with process variables, applications, and limitation.

10.3.1 Dispersion of Preformed Polymers

Dispersion of preformed polymers is a common technique used to prepare NPs of biodegradable material such as polylactic acid (PLA), polylactide-*co*-glycolic acid (PLGA), poly-ε-caprolactone (PCL), Eudragit® polybutylcyanoacrylate (PBCA), and so on. This technique can be used in various ways for the preparation of polymeric NPs and all the methods are described below.

10.3.1.1 Single-Emulsion Solvent Evaporation Method

Emulsion evaporation is the oldest and the most commonly used method for the preparation of polymeric NPs from preformed polymers. The method is based on the emulsification of an organic solution of the polymer in an aqueous phase followed by the evaporation of the organic solvent. The polymer and the drug are first dissolved in a water-immiscible volatile solvent, such as ethyl acetate, dichloromethane (DCM), or chloroform, which is then emulsified in an aqueous solution containing a stabilizer. The emulsification is brought about by subsequent exposure to a high-energy shearing source, such as an ultrasonic device or a homogenizer. The organic phase is evaporated under reduced pressure or vacuum, resulting in a fine aqueous dispersion of NPs. The NPs are collected by ultracentrifugation and washed with distilled water to remove stabilizer residues or any free drug, and then they are lyophilized for storage (Astete and Sabliov, 2006; Anton et al., 2008). The emulsion evaporation method is schematically represented in Figure 10.2. Normal emulsions, oil-in-water (o/w) or water-in-oil (w/o), and double emulsions such as water-in-oil-in-water (w/o/w) can be used to accommodate the

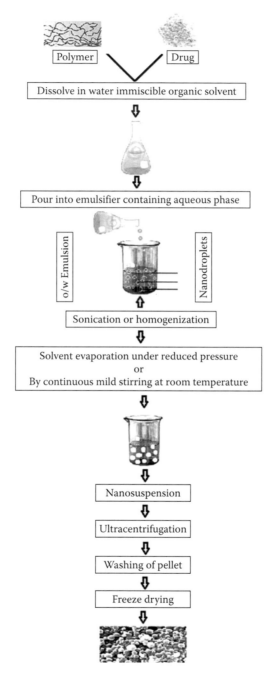

FIGURE 10.2
Schematic representation of the single-emulsion solvent evaporation method.

entrapment of active components with different physicochemical properties. The o/w emulsion is used for entrapment of hydrophobic compounds, whereas w/o/w double emulsion is used for the entrapment of hydrophilic compounds. The emulsion evaporation method can be used for the preparation of particles with sizes varying from a few nanometers to micrometers. Particle size was found to be influenced by the type and concentration of the stabilizer, homogenizer speed, and polymer concentration. It is the most suitable method for highly lipophilic drugs (Kwon et al., 2001; Mu and Feng, 2003; Feng, 2004; Chavanpatil et al., 2006). To produce small particle size, a high-speed homogenization or ultrasonication has to be employed, which is the main drawback of this method (Zambaux et al., 1998). The method is widely used for the preparation of microparticulate systems because it is easy to scale up and it does not require high shear stress for microencapsulation. NPs prepared by single-emulsion solvent evaporation have been reported in Table 10.3 along with their size and drug entrapment efficiency (EE)/drug loading.

The particle size, its distribution, and drug content are important characteristics that determine the release behavior of the drugs and these characteristics depend on the parameter employed for fabrication to make the particles (Seo et al., 2003). The general emulsification–solvent evaporation method employed to produce NPs involves a number of processing and material parameters: power and duration of energy applied, aqueous phase volume, pH of the aqueous phase, polymer and drug concentration in the organic phase, polymer molecular weight, polymer end groups, solvent volume, and surfactant concentration. Each of these processing and material parameters influences the size and/or the drug content of the NPs, which can be understood by applying appropriate scientific principles, as summarized here.

TABLE 10.3

Nanoparticles Prepared by Single-Emulsion Solvent Evaporation Method

Polymer	Drug	Mean Particle Size	EE/Drug Loading (%)	Reference
PLGA/ montmorillonite	Paclitaxel/ Coumarin-6	304.3–310.9 nm	46.5–52	Dong and Feng (2005)
PEG-PLGA-PEG	Mitoxantrone (DHAQ)	500 nm	90	Duan et al. (2012)
PLGA	Paclitaxel	80–150 nm	88.52	Jin et al. (2007)
PLGA	Paclitaxel	200–800 nm	85.5	Jin et al. (2008)
PLGA	Rapamycin	246.8 nm	77.53	Miao et al. (2008)
PLGA	Paclitaxel	318 ± 5.1 nm	88.52	Jin et al. (2009)
Eudagit RS 100	Naproxen	378 ± 48–644 ± 65 nm	0.120 ± 0.06– 0.238 ± 0.046	Adibkia et al. (2011)
PLGA	β-Aescin	<300 nm	14–22	Ven et al. (2012)

Budhian et al. (2007) prepared haloperidol-loaded PLGA NPs by three different methods: emulsification by homogenization–solvent evaporation (homogenization), emulsification by sonication–solvent evaporation (sonication), and nanoprecipitation. Homogenization and sonication involved the preparation of an organic phase consisting of polymer (such as PLGA or PLA, typical concentration) and drug (haloperidol) in DCM. This organic phase is added to an aqueous phase containing a surfactant, polyvinyl alcohol (PVA) to form an emulsion. This emulsion is broken down into nanodroplets by applying external energy (through a homogenizer or a sonicator) and which turn into NPs upon evaporation of the highly volatile organic solvent. The solvent is evaporated while magnetic stirring at 300 rpm under atmospheric conditions for 4 h, leaving behind a colloidal suspension of PLGA NPs in water. Nanoprecipitation is similar to homogenization and sonication, except that the organic solvent is acetone, a water-miscible solvent, and there is no application of external energy. Once the colloidal suspension of NPs is prepared using one of the above three methods, the free drug is removed to obtain the final nanoparticulate suspension containing the encapsulated drug. They studied the effect of various processing parameters on particle size and drug pay load. Gradual increment in NP size was observed upon increasing the polymer concentration from 5 to 66.6 mg/mL by keeping all other processing parameters at standard conditions. When external energy was applied in the form of sonication and homogenization, similar results were observed in terms of particle diameter while a unimodal size distribution turns into bimodal size distribution in case of homogenization. They also found that particle size increased on increasing the polymer concentration. Enhancement in the polymer concentration leads to an increase in the viscosity of the organic phase; hence, reduction in shear stress and resisting droplet breakdown consequently resulted in larger-size nanoparticle. Several researchers reported the similar effect of polymer concentration on the size of particles produced by the general emulsification process (Desgouilles et al., 2003; Zweers et al., 2003; Song et al., 2008). Drug content in NPs was also found to be increased with increasing polymer concentration in the organic phase; higher polymer concentration led to higher viscosity of the organic phase that increases the diffusional resistance to drug molecules from organic phase to the aqueous phase. Another probable reason was that increasing the polymer concentration resulted in larger particle size and consequently larger diffusional pathways into the aqueous phase, thereby reducing the loss of drug through diffusion (Budhian et al., 2007; Song et al., 2008).

Lemoine and Preat (1998) prepared NPs by utilizing DCM 1.0% (w/v) as the solvent and PVA and Span 40 as the stabilizing agents. They observed that increasing the PVA (stabilizer) concentration resulted in a marked decrease of the nanoparticle size, whereas the homogenizer speed, the evaporation rate and the freeze drying slightly influenced the nanoparticle size. Hence, a minimum number of surfactant molecules are required to achieve small particle size and narrow size distribution. At very low concentrations of PVA, the total amount of PVA, relative to PLGA, is insufficient to stabilize the emulsion droplets and causes larger particles. Zweers et al. (2003) have reported an increase in the size of PLGA NPs at high PVA concentrations (5–10%), while Allemann et al. (1992) have reported a continuous decrease in particle size. Initial reduction in particle size then reached a plateau upon increasing the surfactant concentration; after a certain point, further increment in the stabilizer concentration led to an increment in particle diameter (Budhian et al., 2007; Song et al., 2008). To resolve this contradiction, they propose that at higher stabilizer concentration, more stabilizer molecules can be oriented at the organic/aqueous phase interface that can reduce the interfacial tension more efficiently that resulted in smaller emulsion droplets formation, that is, smaller particle size. However, at higher PVA concentration, the viscosity of external aqueous internal phase increased, which resulted in increased size due to the reduction in the net shear stress. As the PVA concentration is increased, the drug content first decreases and then plateaus with a slight increase in particles size. The changes in drug content with PVA concentration are predominantly a result of changing the particle size. As discussed above, larger NPs have higher drug content because fewer drug molecules have sufficient time to diffuse into the aqueous phase.

Further, Budhian et al. (2007) investigated the effect of initial drug concentration and observed that as the initial haloperidol concentration is increased, the drug entrapment first increases, then plateaus, and then finally decreases. The drug entrapment in the NPs is affected by the drug–polymer interactions and the drug miscibility in the polymer. When the haloperidol concentration was increased above 2.5 mg/ml, the reduction in drug content was observed within the polymer matrix as more haloperidol molecules migrate to the aqueous phase and nucleate its crystals. The influence of drug miscibility for a hydrophobic drug–polymer system of dexamethasone or flutamide-loaded PLGA/PLA has also been discussed by Panyam et al. (2004). They reported that higher drug–polymer miscibility leads to higher drug incorporation. As the initial drug concentration or the drug input to the system increases, the drug incorporation process operates at its maximum efficiency and the drug content increases until it reaches its limiting value determined by the drug miscibility in the polymer at the given processing conditions and polymer characteristics, where it plateaus. Increasing the initial drug concentration beyond the limit of drug miscibility leads to constant drug content and a decrease in drug incorporation efficiency due to the fixed amount of drug going into the particles in spite of increasing the drug input. Mainardes and Evangelista used different organic solvents to prepare NPs of PLGA and studied their effect on the particle size; in this study, methylene chloride (water-immiscible solvent) and ethyl acetate (partially miscible with water) were employed and were observed that the NPs prepared with methylene chloride were larger than those prepared with ethyl acetate.

10.3.1.2 Double-Emulsion (W/O/W) Solvent Evaporation Method

The first step of the double-emulsion method is the formation of water-in-oil (w/o) emulsion where the aqueous solution contains the hydrophilic active component and the organic phase contains a polymer and a suitable surfactant (Span 80, Pluronic F 68, and others) with a low HLB. The primary emulsion is formed under strong shear stress (i.e., sonication, microfluidization, and high-speed homogenization). Next, the obtained primary w/o is emulsified in the aqueous phase containing surfactants of high HLB value. The formed w/o/w emulsion is sonicated or homogenized for droplet size reduction and should be controlled to minimize the hydrophilic active component diffusion to the external aqueous phase. Finally, the organic solvent is evaporated under vacuum to avoid the polymer and active component damage, and to promote final NP size reduction. A schematic representation of this method is shown in Figure 10.3.

The main drawback of the double-emulsion method is the large size of the NPs and low EE. The coalescence and Ostwald ripening are the two important mechanisms that destabilize the double-emulsion droplets, responsible for large particle size, and low EE because of high diffusion through the organic phase of the hydrophilic active component. Drug loading can be improved by employing a polymer of high molecular mass at high polymer concentration as well as increasing the viscosity of the inner water phase and the surfactant molecular mass (Domb et al., 1996). Few examples of polymeric NPs that have been prepared by the double-emulsion solvent evaporation method are listed in Table 10.4.

Jeong et al. (2008) prepared ciprofloxacin-loaded PLGA NPs by separately dissolving polylactide-*co*-glycolide in 7 mL of DCM and ciprofloxacin in 2 mL of deionized water. An aqueous solution of ciprofloxacin was poured drop by drop to DCM and was sonicated at 40 W for 1 min using an ultrasonicator. The prepared 1° emulsions were poured into 10 mL of 1% (w/v) aqueous PVA solution and the resultant solution was homogenized with a high-pressure homogenizer at 600 bars for 5 cycles/min and were sonicated once more at 40 W for 1 min to make the w/o/w emulsion. PLGA NPs showed spherical shapes with particle sizes around 100–300 nm. Loading efficiency was lower than 50% (w/w) because of the high water solubility of ciprofloxacin. Dillen et al. (2008) also developed Eudragit and PLGA by w/o/w emulsification solvent evaporation utilizing high-pressure homogenization as an external energy source and obtained a particle size in the range 150–250 nm. They also studied the effect of freeze drying and gamma sterilization on zeta potential.

Kalaria et al. (2009) prepared doxorubicin-loaded PLGA NPs for the oral delivery of doxorubicin and studied the effect of the types of stabilizer and their concentration on the particle size and EE. PVA, didodecyl dimethyl ammonium bromide (DMAB), and PF68 were used as stabilizers. PVA was found to be the choice among the stabilizers as it provided higher EE

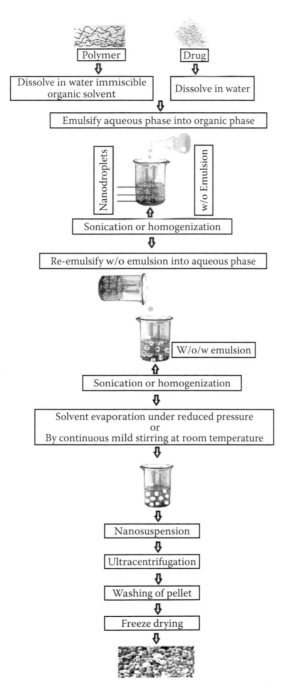

FIGURE 10.3
Schematic representation of the double-emulsion solvent evaporation method.

TABLE 10.4

Nanoparticles Prepared by Double-Emulsion Solvent Evaporation

Polymer	Drug	Mean Particle Size	EE/Drug Loading%	Reference
PLA–PEG	FITC	196 ± 20 nm	56.0 ± 2.07	Behrens et al. (2002)
Eudragit and PLGA	Ciprofloxacin	171.8 ± 2.3– 240 ± 3.0 nm	62–68	Dillen et al. (2008)
PLGA and PLA	Daunorubicin (DNR)	200–300 nm	>80	Liu et al. (2010)
PLGA	Doxorubicin	160.20 ± 0.99 nm	55.40 ± 2.30	Jain et al. (2011)
PEG–CH$_2$O CH$_2$–PEG	Insulin-2 and Insulin-5	>300 nm	70% and 30	Giovino et al. (2012)
PLGA	Minocycline	85–424 nm	4.7	Kashi et al. (2012)
PLGA	B-Aescin	<300 nm	22	Ven et al. (2012)

coupled with optimum particle size and polydispersity. On the contrary, smaller particle size and lower EE were obtained with DMAB. This may be attributed to the solubility enhancement of doxorubicin in the presence of DMAB that provides sink conditions due to which more number of drug molecules migrated to the aqueous phase rather than getting loaded in the hydrophobic polymeric matrix. PF-68 on the other hand gave particles with larger diameter, and polydispersity through encapsulation efficiency was appreciable. The effect of different concentrations of PVA on particle size and polydispersity index (PDI) was also investigated. An increase in PVA concentration in the external aqueous phase corresponded to a decrease in particle size and PDI. These results were corroborated with already available reported results (Niwa et al., 1993; Scholes et al., 1993). The initial drug concentration in the internal phase was varied to investigate its effect on NP characteristics, including size, PDI, and EE. The three concentrations tested were 2.5%, 5%, and 10% w/w and had minimum effect on particle size and polydispersity. A minor increase in particle size can be attributed to higher drug loading. Drug-loaded particles were very similar to blank particles. The EE of the drug in NPs was also found to be consistent. Hence, 10% w/w provided particles with optimum size, PDI, and entrapment.

Lemoine and Preat (1998) used single-emulsion and double-emulsion methods to prepare the NPs and studied the effect of experimental parameters on the particle size. They employed PVA and Span 40 as stabilizers in the double-emulsion method and observed that when PVA was used in the internal aqueous phase, the nanoparticle size was lower in comparison to that with Span 40. On the other hand, PVA concentration in the external aqueous phase, the homogenizer speed and the freeze drying slightly influenced the NP size. Similarly, PEG coated nanosphere with mean diameter of about 200 nm have also been prepared by double emulsion solvent evaporation method by using sodium cholate as a stabilizer in place of PVA

(Quellec eal al., 1999). Polymeric NPs of poly-L-lactic acid, PCL, and PLGA were prepared by employing sodium dodecyl sulfate as the surfactant and a smallest mean diameter of 76 nm obtained for PLGA, while the PCL particles were the largest (Musyanovych et al., 2008). Bilati et al. (2003) studied the influence of the sonication process on the characteristics of PLGA NPs. They investigated the duration and intensity of sonication with respect to size and size distribution. They found that the duration of the second mixing step is more crucial for the final mean particle size than the first step for the w/o emulsion; the mean particle size decreased to a certain level upon increasing the second emulsification time period. This study suggested that a threshold exists for the sonication intensity leading to a controlled particle size with a narrow distribution.

10.3.1.3 Single-Emulsion Solvent Diffusion Method

In this method (Figure 10.4), the polymer is dissolved in an organic phase that must be partially miscible in water (Moinard-Checot et al., 2006). The suitable solvents are benzyl alcohol, propylene carbonate, ethyl acetate, isopropyl acetate, methyl acetate, methyl ethyl ketone, benzyl alcohol, butyl lactate, and isovaleric acid. The organic phase is emulsified with an aqueous solution of suitable surfactants (i.e., anionic sodium dodecyl sulfate (SDS), nonionic polyvinyl alcohol (PVA), or cationic didodecyl dimethyl ammonium bromide (DMAB)) under stirring. Once the o/w emulsion is obtained, it is diluted with a large quantity of pure water. As a result of this dilution, the present within the diffuses out and the diffusion of the organic solvent and the counter diffusion of water into the emulsion droplets induce the precipitation of the polymer and lead to the formation of polymer NPs (Quintanar-Guerrero et al., 1998). This method has been used for the preparation of polymeric NPs of various drugs (Table 10.5). The method is similar to the solvent evaporation method except in the sense that the solvent must first diffuse out into the external aqueous dispersion medium before it can be removed from the system by evaporation (Vauthier and Bouchemal, 2009). The NPs are collected by ultracentrifugation and washed with distilled water to remove stabilizer residues or any free drug, and then lyophilized for storage.

There are many drawbacks of this method, as it requires large amounts of water for the formation of NPs, which makes the recovery of the formed particle difficult, requires large time of emulsion agitation, and the process does not use shear stress for size reduction (high-speed agitation or sonication); therefore, the size of NPs is highly sensitive to polymer concentration and low drug EE because hydrophilic components have a high migration tendency due to the diffusion of the polar solvent to the aqueous phase. The parameters that affect the nanoparticle's characteristics are: polymer concentration, solvent nature, surfactant, polymer molecular mass, viscosity, organic aqueous phase ratios, stirring rate, temperature, and the flow of water added.

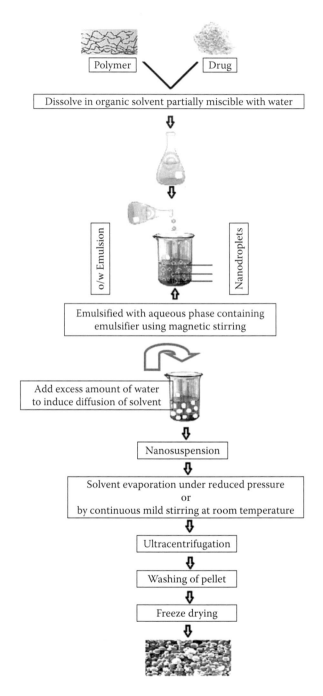

FIGURE 10.4
Schematic representation of the single-emulsion solvent diffusion method.

TABLE 10.5

Nanoparticles Prepared by Solvent Diffusion Method

Polymer	Drug	Mean Particle Size	EE/Drug Loading (%)	Reference
PMMA	Enalaprilat	297 ± 2–612 ± 45 nm	4.5 ± 2.3	Ahlin et al. (2002)
PLGA	Paclitaxel	72.0 ± 1.5–163.2 ± 3.6 nm	47 ± 6	Bhardwaj et al. (2009)
Pullulan acetate	Epirubicin	355.8 ± 2.9–537.5 ± 18.6 nm	38.9 ± 1.2–61.8 ± 0.3	Zhang et al. (2009)
PLGA	Temoxifen	168 ± 3.1–195.5 ± 9.2 nm	84.94 ± 1.55–86.20 ± 1.55	Jain et al. (2010)
PNIPAAm-PLA	Betamethasone disodium 21-phosphate	140 nm	NA	Ayano et al. (2011)
PLGA	Insulin–sodium deoxycholate complex	278 ± 13 nm	93.6 ± 2.81	Sun et al. (2011)
PLA	Oridonin	105.2 nm	28.24 ± 0.81	Xu et al. (2012)

Pinon-Segundo et al. (2005) prepared triclosan NPs for the treatment of periodontal diseases using the emulsification diffusion technique. The organic solvent (ethyl acetate or methyl ethyl ketone) and water were mutually saturated for at least 20 min before use, to ensure initial thermodynamic equilibrium of both liquids. Polymer and triclosan were dissolved in water-saturated organic solvent, and this organic solution was emulsified with a 5% (w/v) PVA solution saturated with organic solvent using a magnetic stirrer at 1700 rpm for 10 min. Distilled water was subsequently added to the emulsion to induce diffusion of organic solvent into the continuous phase, leading to the formation of NPs. The organic solvent was eliminated from the raw NP suspension by vacuum steam distillation at 35°C. NP suspension was centrifuged and obtained NPs were finally freeze dried. In this method, 20 mL of organic solvent, 40 mL of PVA solution, and 160 mL of distilled water were used per 400 mg of polymer. All NPs obtained were less than 500 nm in size. Process efficiency was higher than 99.0% and EE was found to be between 63.8% and 89.4%. They also studied the effect of the initial triclosan concentration on particle size and EE and found that the higher the initial quantity of triclosan, the higher the EE and the larger the mean particle size.

The solubility of drugs and polymers in solvents also affects the particle characteristics (Kristl et al., 1996). Ahlin et al. (2002) investigated many organic solvents such as acetone, chloroform, tetrahydrofuran (THF), and benzyl alcohol for the preparation of enalaprilat-loaded NPs, and benzyl alcohol was found to be the most suitable solvent.

Kwon et al. (2001) studied the effect of various stabilizers such as PEG 8000, Tween 80, gelatin, dextran (MW 6000), pluronic L-63, and PVA on the preparation of estrogen-loaded NPs by emulsion diffusion methods. They observed that particles were formed only when PVA and DMAB were used as stabilizers (Lourenco et al., 1996; Quintanar-Guerrero et al., 1996). The mean particle size was found to be decreased sharply when the concentration of DMAB and PVA were used in the range of 1–2% w/v and 2–4% w/v, respectively. However, no significant difference in particle size was observed when DMAB and PVA were used above 2% w/v and 4% w/v, respectively. The results were in agreement with those reported by Rafati et al. (1997) for the preparation of NPs by the w/o/w emulsion evaporation method using PVA as the stabilizer. The mean particle size of NPs prepared with DMAB was found to be smaller than that of PVA because DMAB has much lower CMC than PVA that indicated that DMAB forms aggregates at very low concentration and solubilizes the organic polymer solution more than PVA. They also studied the effect of polymer concentration on the development of NPs by varying it from 1.0 to 4.0% (w/v) keeping the PVA concentration at 2.5% w/v. Polymer concentration in the internal phase was found to be a crucial factor on the NP size; as the polymer concentration increases, the viscosity of the organic solution also increases, which imposes high viscous resistance to the shear forces that hinders droplets breakdown, resulting in larger particle size. The results were well corroborated with reported studies (Schlicher et al., 1997; Budhian et al., 2007; Song et al., 2008). Allemann et al. (1992) prepared PLGA NPs by varying the homogenization speed and keeping all the processing parameters constant, including homogenization time, and observed that increasing the homogenization speed led to the reduction in particle size; however, above 12,000 rpm, no significant difference was observed in particle size, which indicated that the final size of the NPs depends on the globule size throughout the emulsification process.

The rate of diffusion of the organic solvent from droplets is also an important factor that influences the particle size of the nanoparticle. The factors that affect the diffusion process can be explained by the Stokes–Einstein equation as follows:

$$D_{AB} = \frac{kT}{6pr\eta}$$

where D_{AB} is the mutual diffusion coefficient, k is the Boltzmann's coefficient, $T(K)$ is the Kelvin temperature, r is the hydrodynamic volume radius, and η is the viscosity of the continuous phase.

The diffusion coefficient is directly proportional to the Kelvin temperature of the system and inversely proportional to the viscosity of the continuous phase. The particle size decreases as the temperature of the added water is increased because high temperature promotes diffusion and rapid solvent exchange that precipitate the polymer more quickly.

10.3.1.4 *Spontaneous Emulsification or Modified Solvent Diffusion Method*

This is a modified version of the solvent diffusion method (Figure 10.5). In this method, the water-miscible solvents along with a small amount of the water-immiscible organic solvents are used as an oil phase. Owing to the spontaneous diffusion of solvents, an interfacial turbulence is created between the two phases, leading to the formation of small particles. Both solvent evaporation and solvent diffusion methods can be used for hydrophobic or hydrophilic drugs. Some examples of polymeric NPs prepared by the spontaneous emulsification method are summarized in Table 10.6.

Niwa et al. (1993) prepared PLGA NPs by the spontaneous emulsification solvent diffusion method. They employed the organic phase consisting of DCM and acetone, a water-immiscible and a freely water-miscible organic solvent, respectively. Song et al. (2008) also prepared vincristine sulfate and quercetine-loaded PLGA NPs by employing acetone and DCM in the ratio of 1:2 and obtained the particle size 139.5 ± 4.3 nm with EE $92.84 \pm 3.37\%$ and $32.66 \pm 2.92\%$ for vincristine sulfate and quercetine, respectively. In the above-discussed methods, NP formations took place via the following steps: when the polymeric solution is added into the aqueous phase, emulsion droplets are formed; acetone quickly diffuses out from each emulsion droplet that leads to the reduction of droplets into nanosize, followed by the removal of the remaining DCM; consequently, droplets solidified and turned into polymeric NPs. This method is associated with a drawback that due to a considerable amount of residual DCM, the particles are likely to aggregate during the solvent evaporation process. Therefore, when a larger amount of polymeric solution is used, the probability of collision among particles in the aqueous phase would increase and the aggregation cannot be prevented. With the intention to alleviate this drawback, one more water-miscible solvent such as ethanol or methanol can be incorporated along with acetone and DCM mixture to reduce the amount of DCM in the solvent system and to achieve smaller particles. This alteration prevents the aggregation of particles even at a high fed amount of polymeric solution, resulting in an improvement of yield that is acceptable for industrial purposes (Murakami et al., 1999; Esmaeili et al., 2008).

Esmaeili et al. (2008) prepared estradiol-loaded PLGA NPs and employed acetone, ethanol, and DCM as the organic solvent system and used factorial design to study the parameters affecting the formulation characteristics, including acetone and ethanol volume, PVA percentage, homogenization and mixing time, centrifugation time, and polymer/drug ratio. It was found that addition of a small volume of ethanol to the mixture of acetone/DCM leads to smaller estradiol NPs and this alteration can prevent the aggregation of particles effectively. The optimum ratio of the solvents used for the preparation of NPs (containing 200 mg PLGA/20 mg of estradiol valerate) was 10:5:25 (v/v) for DCM, ethanol, and acetone, respectively to ensure the production of particles 150–200 nm in size with a maximum standard

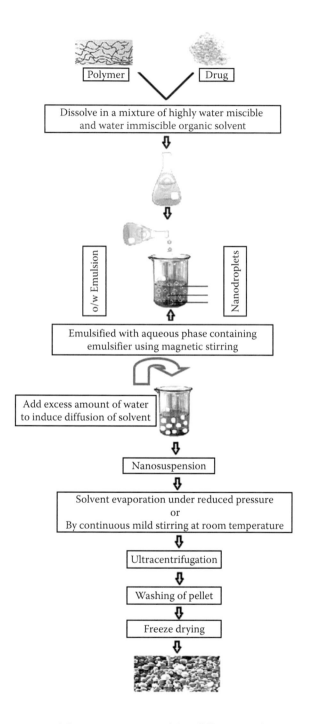

FIGURE 10.5
Schematic representation of the spontaneous-emulsion diffusion method.

TABLE 10.6

Nanoparticles Prepared by Spontaneous Solvent Emulsification and Modified Solvent Diffusion

Polymer	Drug	Mean Particle Size	EE/Drug Loading (%)	Reference
Poly(ε-caprolactone)	Rolipram	NA	<40	Lamprecht et al. (2001)
PLA	Triptolide	149.7 nm	74.27	Liu et al. (2004)
PLGA	Indocyanine green (ICG)	300–410 nm	74	Saxena et al. (2004)
PEG-PLGA	TNF-α-blocking peptide (TNF-BP)	79.7–126.1 nm	60.2	Yang et al. (2007)
PLGA	Rifampicin	209 ± 21–260 ± 23 nm	0.09 ± 0.001–5.08 ± 0.3	Esmaeili et al. (2007)

deviation of about 20 nm, indicating a quite narrow particle size distribution. Lowering the amount of acetone or ethanol resulted in larger particles and vice versa. However, a reduction in EE was noted upon employing a higher ratio of the acetone to DCM. This can be attributed to rapid diffusion of acetone into the aqueous phase, resulting in the migration of drug molecules in the dispersion media. Other process variables such as PVA and stabilizer concentration were also optimized with the intention to improve the EE of the drug. When the concentration of PVA was increased from 1% to 4%, EE of NPs dramatically decreased from 55% to 9% ($p < 0.05$), which is in agreement with the results of other studies (Jaiswal et al., 2004; Ricci et al., 2004). It might be due to higher surfactant concentration, which causes the migration of drug molecules to the continuous phase.

10.3.1.5 Salting Out

This method consists of dissolving the polymer in the organic phase that should be water miscible, such as acetone or THF. The organic phase is emulsified with an aqueous phase (under strong mechanical shear stress), and contains an emulsifier and a high concentration of salts that should be insoluble in the organic phase. The most commonly used electrolyte salts are magnesium chloride hexahydrate (Konan et al., 2002) or magnesium acetate tetrahydrate, sodium chloride, and nonelectrolyte such as sucrose, in a polymer-to-salt ratio of 1:3. In contrast to the emulsion diffusion method, there is no diffusion of the solvent due to the presence of salts. The fast addition of pure water to the o/w emulsion, under mild stirring, reduces the ionic strength and leads to the migration of the water-soluble organic solvent to the aqueous phase and induces nanosphere formation (Barrat et al., 2000). The final step is purification by cross-flow filtration or centrifugation to remove the salting-out agent. The main drawback of this method is the requirement of an extensive purification as it requires a high concentration of the salting-out agent. The salting-out method is schematically represented in Figure 10.6 and few examples of NPs prepared by this method are reported in Table 10.7.

Allemann et al. (1992) employed an aqueous solution containing electrolyte, nonelectrolyte, and PVA, the stabilizer as well as viscosity enhancer, added this solution into the solution of polymer in acetone under continuous stirring for the preparation of NPs. Electrolytes and nonelectrolytes present in aqueous solution prevented mixing of acetone with water by a salting-out process. After the preparation of an o/w emulsion, water was added in a sufficient amount to allow the complete diffusion of acetone into the aqueous phase, resulting in the formation of nanospheres. PLA NPs were also prepared with an average size of 295 nm by Leroux and coworkers by adding an aqueous gel containing magnesium acetate tetrahydrate and PVA to the solution of polymer in acetone (Leroux et al., 1996). Zhang et al. (2006) prepared NPs by both the single-emulsion method and the salting-out method and performed a comparative study on the effect of the stirring speed and polymer concentration on the nanoparticle size. They achieved particle size between 183 and 251 nm and found that stirring speed and polymer concentration significantly affect the nanoparticle size in the single-emulsion method than salting out and much smaller particles were obtained in the salting-out method under comparable conditions. These differences are probably due to the fact that the organic solvent (THF) used in the salting-out method is water miscible, whereas the single-emulsion method employed the water-immiscible solvent, DCM. The required energy for forming the droplet surface is therefore expected to be less in the salting-out method, which could be a probable reason for the production of NPs of smaller size than the single-emulsion method at comparable conditions.

10.3.1.6 Nanoprecipitation or Solvent Displacement Method

This method was developed by Fessi et al. for the preparation of polymeric NPs (Fessi et al., 1989). It is also known as the solvent displacement method (Figure 10.7). The technique is based on the interfacial deposition of a polymer after the displacement of a semipolar solvent from a lipophilic solution. In this method, solvents with high water miscibility such as acetone, acetonitrile, ethanol, or methanol are used. Rapid diffusion of these solvents into nonsolvent phase lowers the interfacial tension that in turn leads to an increase in surface area and formation of small droplets (Mishra et al., 2010). Acetone is one of the most commonly used solvent for the preparation of NPs by nanoprecipitation although some binary mixtures such as acetone with small amount of water or acetone and ethanol or methanol are also used. Typically, this method is used for hydrophobic drug entrapment, but it has been adapted for hydrophilic drugs as well. The polymer and the drug are dissolved in a polar, water-miscible solvent and poured in a controlled

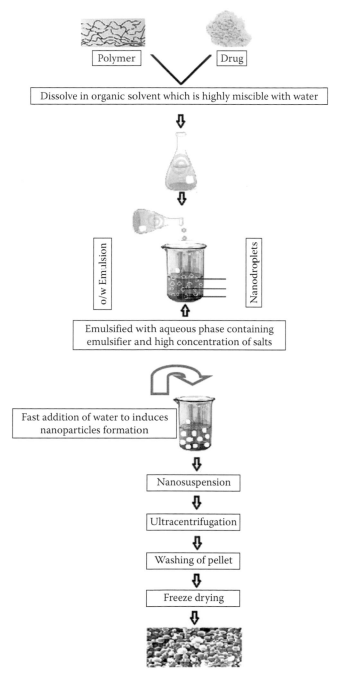

FIGURE 10.6
(See color insert.) Schematic representation of the salting-out method.

TABLE 10.7

Nanoparticles Prepared by Salting-Out Method

Polymer	Drug	Mean Particle Size	EE/Drug Loading%	Reference
PLA	Paclitaxel	171 ± 22 nm	78 ± 10	Cirstoiu-Hapca et al. (2009)
PLGA	5-Aminolevulinic acid/Nile red	150 nm	87 µg/mg	Donnelly et al. (2010)
PLGA	Meloxicam	170–231 nm	NA	Sengel-Türk et al. (2012)
PLGA	β-Aescin	<300 nm	14–22	Ven de Ven et al. (2012)

manner (i.e., drop-wise addition) into an aqueous solution containing the surfactant. NP formation takes place instantaneously due to rapid solvent diffusion. The prerequisite for this method is that the drug should be highly soluble in polar solvents (i.e., acetone, ethyl acetate) and should be slightly soluble in water to minimize the loss during solvent diffusion (De Jaeghere et al., 1999). Size is very much affected by the polymer concentration. NPs prepared by this method are given in Table 10.8.

Musumeci et al. (2006) prepared polymeric NPs of docetaxel, an anticancer agent by the solvent displacement method. They employed acetone as an organic solvent and a mixture of water and ethanol (1:1) containing 0.5% w/v of Tween 80 as the nonsolvent. Docetaxel (0.5% and 1% in weight, drug/polymers) and polymer (75 mg) were dissolved in 20 mL of acetone and poured into 40 mL of a nonsolvent phase under magnetic stirring that led to the formation of colloidal suspension. The organic solvent was then evaporated off under vacuum by a rotavapor. NPs were collected by employing centrifugation at $15,000 \times g$ for 1 h at 5°C. The obtained nanospheres were freeze dried and 5% HP-β cyclodextrin was used as a cryoprotectant. The obtained particles were in the size range from 100.7 ± 2.9 to 179.4 ± 1.7 nm and their entrapment efficiencies were in between 16.13 ± 1.3% and 23.09 ± 1.3%. Agüerosa also prepared polyanhydride particles by the solvent displacement method and the obtained particles were in the size range of 150–180 nm with a processing yield of 86.2–94.4%.

Nanoprecipitation is a simple, fast, and reproducible method and used for the preparation of both nanospheres and nanocapsules. It does not employ any external energy for size reduction; therefore, it is highly sensitive for processing and material parameters. The important parameters to be considered are polymer/surfactant ratio, polymer concentration, surfactant nature, viscosity, solvent nature, shear stress, evaporation, additives, and first-phase/second-phase ratios.

10.3.1.7 Dialysis

It offers a technique for the preparation of polymeric NPs of small size and with low polydispersity index. In this method, the polymer solution in an

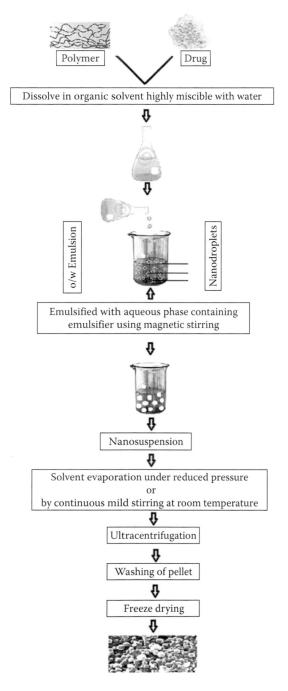

FIGURE 10.7
Schematic representation of the nanoprecipitation method.

TABLE 10.8

Nanoparticles Prepared by Nanoprecipitation Method

Polymer	Drug	Mean Particle Size	EE/Drug Loading%	Reference
Poly(o-caprolactone)	Tamoxifen	250–300 nm	64	Chawla and Amiji (2002)
PLGA	Flurbiprofen	185.1 ± 2.98–286.0 ± 6.1 nm	80.68 ± 0.69–7.53 ± 14	Vega et al. (2006)
PLGA	Flurbiprofen	380–910 nm	92.97–97.12	Sashmal et al. (2007)
Poly(anhydride)	Paclitaxel	≤300 nm	170 µg/mg	Agüeros et al. (2009)
PLA	Risperidone	78–184 nm	91–94	Muthu and Singh (2009)
PLGA	Minocycline	85–424 nm	0.8	Kashi et al. (2012)

organic solvent is placed inside a dialysis tube of proper molecular weight cutoff. Dialysis is conducted against a nonsolvent that would be miscible with organic solvent placed inside the dialysis tube. The displacement of the solvent inside the dialysis tube induces aggregation of the polymer due to the loss of solubility and results in the formation of homogeneous suspensions of NPs (Figure 10.8). The mechanism of polymeric NP formation by the dialysis method is still unclear but it looks like the nanoprecipitation method proposed

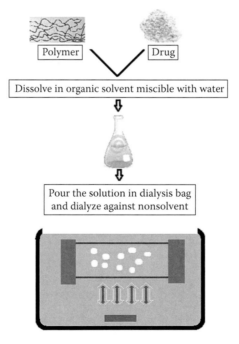

FIGURE 10.8
Schematic representation of the dialysis method.

TABLE 10.9

Nanoparticles Prepared by Dialysis Method

Polymer	Drug	Mean Particle Size	EE/Drug Loading (%)	Reference
Glycosal chitosan	Paclitaxel	200–416 nm	42 ± 8–94 ± 5	Kim et al. (2006)
PLA/PLGA	Paclitaxel	343 ± 19–437 ± 25 nm	51.8 ± 4.9–54.7 ± 6.8	Zhang and Feng (2006)
PLA and PLGA	Vlobetasol propionate	180–200 nm	100	Fontana et al. (2010)
Lactose-conjugated PLGA	Rifampicin	121–184 nm	38.4–42.2	Jain et al. (2010)
Dextran sulfate	Doxorubicin	250–500 nm	90	Yousefpour et al. (2011)
N-Trimethyl chitosan	Lactosyl-norcantharidin	120.6 ± 1.7 nm	69.29 ± 0.76	Guan et al. (2012)

by Fessi et al. (1989). The dialysis method has been employed for the preparation of NPs consisting of a variety of polymers and copolymers. Poly(γ-benzyl-L-glutamate)-b-poly(ethylene oxide) and poly(lactide)-b-poly(ethylene oxide) NPs were prepared using dimethylformamide (DMF) as a solvent (Oh et al., 1999; Lee et al., 2004). It was observed that the solvent used in the preparation of the polymer solution affects the NP size, and their distribution and morphology. Akagi et al. (2005) also studied the effect of different solvents such as dimethyl sulfoxide, dimethyl formamide, dimethyl acetamide, and N-methyl-2-pyrolidine on the polyglutamic acid NP formation. Spherical NPs with a size range of 100–200 nm and narrow size distribution were obtained with dimethyl sulfoxide whereas broader size distribution was obtained when N-methyl-2-pyrolidine was used as a solvent. Na et al. (2006) also developed poly(L-lactic acid)-b-poly(ethylene glycol) NPs with a size range of 90–330 nm by the dialysis method using dimethyl sulfoxide as a solvent. The results were in agreement with the results reported by Akagi et al. (2005). Dialysis methods have also been opted for the preparation of NPs of cellulose acetate and mixed cellulose acetate ester such as cellulose acetate propionate, cellulose acetate butyrate, and cellulose acetate phthalate (Hornig and Heinze, 2008). The polymeric solution in dimethyl acetamide was dialyzed against distilled water by employing a dialysis membrane with MMCO 3500 g/mol and the size of the obtained NPs was ranging from 166 to 399 nm. Few examples of NPs prepared by the dialysis method are shown in Table 10.9.

10.3.1.8 Supercritical Fluid Technology

It emerged as the most recent solvent-free technology for the preparation of polymeric microparticles and NPs (Figure 10.9). It is a safer method than all other methods previously discussed as it employs the ecofriendly solvent known as supercritical fluids and produces the solvent-free particle with high

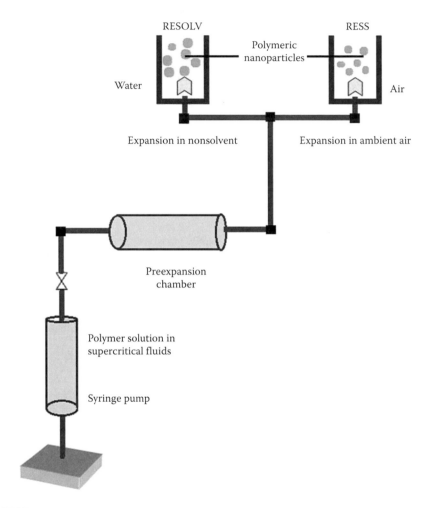

FIGURE 10.9
Schematic representation of supercritical fluid technology.

purity (Jung and Perrut, 2001). A supercritical fluid is a substance that shows the intermediate properties of gas and liquid at a temperature and pressure above its critical point, where distinct liquid and gas phases do not exist. It effuses like a gas and dissolves materials like a liquid. It has higher viscosity and density than the gases and lower than the liquids while its diffusivity is lower than the gases and higher than the liquids. SC fluids are ideal substitutes for organic solvents in a range of industrial and laboratory processes. Carbon dioxide and water are the most commonly used supercritical fluids. Supercritical CO_2 (SC CO_2) is widely used because of its mild critical conditions ($T_c = 31.1°C$, $P_c = 73.8$ bars), nontoxicity, nonflammability, and low price.

Technology has the potential to circumvent the shortcomings of traditional methods and the production of particles on a large scale. However, it is an expensive technology as it requires specially designed equipment. There are two basic methods, namely, rapid expansion of supercritical solution (RESS) and rapid expansion of supercritical solution into liquid solvent (RESOLV) used for the production of NPs.

10.3.1.8.1 Rapid Expansion of Supercritical Solution

RESS involves the dissolution of solutes in a supercritical fluid followed by rapid expansion of solution through a small nozzle into a region of lower pressure (Jung and Perrut, 2001). The reduction of solvent power of the supercritical fluid and high degree of supersaturation accompanied by the rapid reduction of pressure consequently results in homogeneous nucleation and formation of well-dispersed particles. The technique is also known as a clean technique as it produces solvent-free products (Sun et al., 2005).

The RESS experimental apparatus consists of three basic units: a high-pressure mixing cell, a syringe pump, and a preexpansion unit. A solution of polymer in the supercritical fluid such as CO_2 is prepared in a high-pressure mixing cell, then heated in the preexpansion unit at constant pressure to the preexpansion temperature, and finally allowed to expand through the nozzle using syringe pump at ambient pressure. The concentration and degree of saturation of the polymer have a considerable effect on the particle size and morphology.

Chernyak et al. (2001) employed this method and produced droplets from the rapid expansion of poly(perfluoropolyether diamide) CO_2 solutions. Lim et al. (2005) also studied the effect of polymer concentration on the size of particles and obtained the spherical particles in the size range of 50–500 nm by varying the concentration from 0.1 wt.% to 0.5 wt.% in CO_2 at preexpansion temperatures (40°C) and preexpansion pressures (27.6 Pa). Other factors such as material properties, processing conditions, molecular mass of the polymer, and so on also play a crucial role in determining the particle size.

10.3.1.8.2 Rapid Expansion of Supercritical Solution into Liquid Solvent

RESOLV is a modified form of RESS. It differs from RESS in employing the expansion of the supercritical solution into a liquid solvent instead of ambient air. This modified method was developed with the intention to achieve particles in nano range as it was expected that the liquid solvent suppresses the particle growth in the expansion chamber. Meziani et al. (2005) applied this technique for the preparation of NPs of an average size of 50 nm by dissolving poly(heptadecafluorodecylacrylate) in SC CO_2. At the initial period of rapid expansion, the aqueous NP suspension appeared clear and stable; however, as the rapid expansion progresses, clarity and stability of particles disappeared due to the aggregation of the already-formed small particles resulting in the formation of larger particles. To overcome this problem, water was replaced by an aqueous NaCl solution to increase the ionic strength of the suspension with a consequent improvement in stability.

Though green technologies, RESS, and RESOLV suffer from a limitation that most of the polymers and the drugs used for NP preparation are either poorly or even insoluble in supercritical fluids. To overcome this limitationThote and Gupta (2005) used a modified supercritical antisolvent (SAS) method for the formation of NPs containing the hydrophilic drug, dexamethasone phosphate. It employs a solvent, for example, methanol to dissolve the solute to be micronized as the solute is insoluble in the supercritical fluid. The liquid solvent used should be completely miscible with the supercritical fluid (SC CO_2) at the processing conditions. The extraction of the liquid solvent by supercritical fluid leads to the instantaneous precipitation of the solute, resulting in the formation of NPs (Reverchon and Adami, 2006). While working on the RESOLV processing of poly(methyl methyl acrylate) and poly-L-lactic acid in SC CO_2 cosolvent, Meziani's group observed that polymer concentration in the preexpansion supercritical solution plays a vital role in product morphology. Rapid expansion of the polymer solutions in SC CO_2 with low and high concentrations into an ambient aqueous sodium chloride solution produces exclusively NPs and nanofibers, respectively.

10.3.1.9 *Ionic Gelation Method*

This method is based on the interaction between two oppositely charged entities: one is polymer that can be either positively charged or negatively charged, and the other is an electrolyte. Electrostatic interaction between these two entities leads to the NP formation through material transition from liquid state to gel. The ionic gelation method is being used for the preparation of NPs of biodegradable hydrophilic polymers such as chitosan, gelatin, and sodium alginate. Some examples of NPs prepared by the ionic gelation method have been reported in Table 10.10. Calvo et al. (1997) developed an ionic gelation method for preparing NPs of the hydrophilic polymer, chitosan. Dustgania et al. (2008) also prepared dexamethasone sodium phosphate-loaded chitosan NPs using sodium tripolyphosphate as the electrolyte. The interaction between positively charged amino groups of chitosan with negatively charged tripolyphosphate led to the formation of particles in the size range of nanometers. Exploiting the same basic principle, Zahoor et al. (2005) prepared alginate NPs of antitubercular drugs by cation-induced controlled gelification of alginate.

10.3.2 Polymerization Methods

All the methods discussed in the previous section for the preparation of polymeric NPs are based on the precipitation of preformed polymers and do not involve the polymerization of monomers. In this method, monomers are polymerized to form NPs in an aqueous solution. The use of water as the dispersion medium serves two purposes, as it is ecofriendly and an excellent heat dissipater that is produced during the polymerization process. Drugs can be loaded either by dissolving in the polymerization medium

TABLE 10.10

Nanoparticles Prepared by Ionic Gelation Method

Polymer	Drug	Mean Particle Size	EE/Drug Loading (%)	Reference
Chitosan	FITC	290 ± 7 nm	92.3 ± 0.7	Behrens et al. (2002)
Chitosan	DNA	200 nm	≤100	Plapied et al. (2010)
Sodium alginate	Brimonidine tartrate	450 nm	4–18	Singh and Shinde (2010)
HTCC	PTHrP1-34	100–180 nm	78.4	Zhao et al. (2010)
Chitosan-thioglycolic acid	Trimethoprim	183–266 nm	37	Barthelmes et al. (2011)
Chitosan	Carvacrol	40–80 nm	14–31	Keawchaoon and Yoksan (2011)
Chitosan	Tea polyphenols	407 ± 50 nm	44–83	Liang et al. (2011)
Hyaluronan (HA)	Plasmid DNA (pDNA)	~400–600 nm	~75–85	Mahor et al. (2011)
Chitosan	Brimonidine tartrate	270–370 nm	36–49	Singh and Shinde (2011)
Trimethyl chitosan	Hyaluronic acid	250–350 nm	60	Verheul et al. (2011)

or by adsorption onto the formed NPs after completion of polymerization, which depends upon the thermal stability of active agents. Thermostable drugs may be added during polymerization but in the case of the thermolabile drug, the adsorptive method is employed. After the completion of polymerization, a nanosuspension is obtained that contains unused components such as monomers, stabilizers, and initiators that are generally removed by ultracentrifugation. The obtained particles are resuspended in an isotonic surfactant-free medium. The polymerization method has been exploited for preparing NPs of many polymers such as polybutylcyanoacrylate or poly(alkylcyanoacrylate) NPs (Boudad et al., 2001; Zhang et al., 2001). Polymerization methods that have been used for the production of polymeric NPs are briefly discussed in the following section.

10.3.2.1 Emulsion Polymerization

Emulsion polymerization is the most commonly used method and can be employed for a wide variety of materials for the production of NPs. On the basis of the use of surfactants, polymerization is categorized into conventional polymerization and surfactant-free emulsion polymerization (Asua, 2004; Thickett and Gilbert, 2007).

10.3.2.1.1 Conventional Emulsion Polymerization

Conventional emulsion polymerization is the most commonly used method for the production of polymeric NPs and the particles obtained are typically

100 nm in size and each particle contains many polymer chains (Rao and Geckeler, 2011). Generally, the conventional polymerization method is used for monomers of low water solubility while it employs water-soluble sur-factant and initiator. The monomer is emulsified in the nonsolvent with the help of surfactant molecules. The initiation of the reaction takes place when a monomer molecule is dissolved in the continuous phase and collides with an initiator molecule that may be an ion or a free radical. Polymerization can also be induced by high-energy radiation, including γ-radiation, ultraviolet, or strong visible light by converting the monomer molecule into an initiating radical. Polymerization initiation by adding initiator molecules is the most widely accepted mechanism (Antonietti and Landfester, 2002; Asua, 2002). The formation of NPs can take place before or after the termination of the polymerization reaction (Kreuter, 1982). Polybutylcyanoacrylate (Couvreur et al., 1979), polyethylcyanoacrylate (El-Samaligy et al., 1986), polystyrene (Zhang et al., 2004), polymethylmethacrylate (Cheng et al., 2006; Costa et al., 2009), and polyvinylcarbazole (Su-Jung et al., 2009) NPs were produced by the emulsion polymerization method. The majority of poly(alkylcyanoacrylate) NPs are obtained through anionic polymerization of the corresponding monomer. The type of surfactant molecules employed in the polymeriza-tion have a great impact on the particle size. Polymeric NPs of 50 nm were obtained by employing the nonionic surfactant, Brij 35, whereas the addition of an anionic surfactant led to the increase in size of approximately 300 nm (Vranckx et al., 1996).

10.3.2.1.2 Surfactant-Free Emulsion Polymerization

In spite of being the most commonly used method, conventional emul-sion polymerization suffers from a drawback that it requires addition of sur-factants that need to be removed from the final product, which is a hard, exhaustive, time-consuming, and costly process. Hearn et al. (1985) stud-ied the kinetics of surfactant-free emulsion polymerization of styrene. The emulsifier-free system is more commonly used for vinyl or acryl monomers. In this method, a water-soluble initiator (i.e., KPS, potassium persulfate) is used and formed NPs are stabilized either by ionizable initiators or by ionic comonomers. Micellar-like nucleation (Landfester, 2001) and homogeneous nucleation (Chern et al., 1998) are the two main mechanisms that have been proposed for emulsion polymerization without an emulsifier. The distinc-tion between the two is based on the aqueous solubility of the monomer. Homogeneous nucleation is important in surfactant-free emulsion polymer-ization (Song and Poehlein, 1990). It is the most commonly applied method when monomers are sufficiently soluble in the continuous phase (Kreuter, 1994).

An et al. (2006) prepared polymethyl methacrylic acid (PMMA) NPs by microwave irradiation-induced polymerization and reported the increment in particle size from 103 to 215 nm when the concentration of the monomer was increased from 0.1 to 0.3 mol/L (An et al., 2006). Feng (2004) employed laponite clay to stabilize the emulsions of methyl methacrylic acid (MMA) dispersed in distilled water for the preparation of PMMA particles. The effect of concentration of the stabilizing agent (sodium thiosulfate) on particle size was studied by Cui et al. (2007), and particles in the range of 263.4–172.5 nm were obtained. While Kim et al. (2009) studied the effect of various continuous phases, such as octanol, benzene, and ethyl acetate, NPs of an average size of 60 nm were produced with water and octanol. The above-mentioned studies revealed that monomer, stabilizer and costabilizers concentration, and types of continuous phase affect the particle size. Surfactant-free emulsion polymerization technique has come into sight as a simple ecofriendly process but with the disadvantage of high polydispersity index (Zhang et al., 2001).

10.3.2.2 Miniemulsion Polymerization

Miniemulsion polymerization has recently emerged as a method for the development of polymeric NPs. It differs from emulsion polymerization as it employs the costabilizers of low molecular weight and high shear to reach a steady state while the rest is similar. The method includes water, mixture of monomers, costabilizer, surfactant, and initiator. In this method, surfactants are used in small quantity and the formed miniemulsion has an interfacial tension higher than zero.

Various costabilizers and initiator in combinations have been used for the preparation of polymeric NPs by this method. The combination of sodium lauryl sulfate/dodecyl mercaptan, sodium lauryl sulfate/hexadecane, and Span 80 and Tween 80 have been employed for the preparation of PMMA, poly(*n*-butylacrylate) NPs, and polyacrylic acid NPs, respectively. The polymerization is initiated by free radicals, and the type of radical initiator greatly influenced the particle size. Water-soluble initiators, such as ammonium persulfate, led to the development of microparticles; however, particles turn into nanoparticles with a diameter between 80 and 150 nm when lipophilic radical initiators, such as azobisisobutyronitrile, were employed (Kriwet et al., 1998).

10.3.2.3 Microemulsion Polymerization

Microemulsion polymerization is a new and effective method and shows the similarity with emulsion polymerization as both methods produce colloidal particles of high molecular mass, however, they differ kinetically. Emulsion polymerization exhibits three reaction rate intervals, whereas only two are detected in microemulsion polymerization. Both particle size and the average number of chains per particle are considerably smaller in microemulsion polymerization (Rao and Geckeler, 2011). In contrast to miniemulsion polymerization, it requires high surfactant concentration and acquires an interfacial tension at the o/w interface close to zero.

Typically, water-soluble initiator is added to the aqueous phase of a thermo-dynamically stable microemulsion that contains swollen micelles. Initially, polymerization starts in some thermodynamically stable and spontane-ously formed droplets and then proceeds to other microdroplets. In the later stage, the osmotic and elastic factors of the chains destabilize the frag-ile microemulsions and typically lead to an increase in the particle size, the formation of empty micelles, and secondary nucleation. Very small latexes, 5–50 nm in size, coexist with a majority of empty micelles in the final prod-uct (Rao and Geckeler, 2011).

Several research groups successfully developed the polymeric NPs employ-ing the microemulsion polymerization technique. Macias et al. (1995) devel-oped particles of a copolymer of MMA and *N*-methylolacrylamide (NMA) using sodium bis-sulfosuccinate as surfactant and studied the effects of ini-tiator type and concentration of functional monomer on the reaction kinet-ics. In a similar way, Sosa et al. (2000) also used sodium bis-sulfosuccinate to stabilize vinyl acetate microemulsions and achieved particles smaller than 40 nm in size at a concentration of 1% sodium bis-sulfosuccinate and 3% of vinyl acetate. The types of initiator and its concentration, surfactant, mono-mer, and reaction temperature are the main factors that affect the micro-emulsion polymerization kinetics and the properties of NPs.

10.3.2.4 Interfacial Polymerization

Interfacial polymerization is one of the well-known methods that have been used for the preparation of polymeric NPs (Wu et al., 2009). Polymerization takes place at the interface of two immiscible liquids via reaction between two monomers that affects the NP formation (Karode et al., 1998). Monomers are dissolved in their respective phases, that is, dispersed and continuous phase. Dispersed phase is emulsified into the continuous phase, which is commonly water. The monomer diffuses out at the interface and polym-erizes. This method is essentially applied to very rapid reactions such as the reaction between acid chloride and amide. It may lead to the forma-tion of monolithic matrix-type (nanospheres) or reservoir-type (nanocap-sules) carrier that depends upon the solubility of the formed polymer in the monomer droplet. If the formed polymer is soluble in the droplet, the formation of a matrix-type system occurs and vice versa. The degree of polymerization depends on various factors such as monomer reactivity, monomer concentration, vesicle composition, and temperature of the sys-tem. By varying the above-mentioned factors, NPs of desired size can be achieved. Interfacial cross-linking reactions have also been employed for the preparation of hollow polymeric NPs (Torini et al., 2005), oil-containing (Khoury-Fallouh et al., 1986), and water-containing NPs (Watnasirichaikul et al., 2000). This technique is relatively simple, which makes it a preferred technique in many fields, ranging from encapsulation to preparation of polymers.

10.4 Conclusion

The objective of this chapter is to review the various methods used for the development of polymeric NPs. The development of NPs involves selection of the appropriate method, suitable building-block material, and stabilizers to achieve the desired properties in accordance with the demands of applications. Fundamental knowledge about the techniques used in the preparation of polymeric NPs is yet to be understood as the role of various process variables that affect the particle size, size distribution, and morphology is not fully clear. Various methods of preparing polymeric NPs have their own benefits and drawbacks, though supercritical fluid technology appears to be at the forefront, being seen as a green technology and the most promising candidate for the mass production of solvent-free polymeric NPs. Future research work needs to be more focused on the development of novel techniques that could have precise control over particle size and its morphology as they have strong bearing over properties and applications of these fascinating particles.

Abbreviations

CO_2	Carbon dioxide
FITC	Fluorescein isothiocyanate
HP	Hydroxypropyl
HTCC	N-(2-hydroxyl) propyl-3-trimethyl ammonium chitosan chloride
KPS	Potassium persulfate
Pc	Critical pressure
PEG	Polyethylene glycol
PLA	Poly(lactic acid)
PLGA	Poly(lactic-co-glycolic acid)
PMMA	Poly methyl methacrylic acid
PNIPAAm-PLA	Poly(N-isopropylacrylamide-DL-lactide)
PTHrP	Parathyroid hormone-related protein
PVA	Poly vinyl alcohol
RESOLV	Rapid expansion of supercritical solution into liquid solvent
RESS	Rapid expansion of critical solution
SAS	Supercritical antisolvent
SC	Supercritical
SDS	Sodium dodecyl sulfate
Tc	Critical temperature
THF	Tetrahydrofuran

References

Adibkia, K., Y. Javadzadeh, S. Dastmalchi, G. Mohammadi, F. K. Niri, and M. Alaei-Beirami. 2011. Naproxen-Eudragit RS100 nanoparticles: Preparation and physicochemical characterization. *Colloids Surf B Biointerfaces* 83(1):155–9.

Agnihotri, S. A., N. N. Mallikarjuna, and T. M. Aminabhavi. 2004. Recent advances on chitosan-based micro- and nanoparticles in drug delivery. *J Control Release* 100(1):5–28.

Agueros, M., L. Ruiz-Gaton, C. Vauthier, K. Bouchemal, S. Espuelas, G. Ponchel, and J. M. Irache. 2009. Combined hydroxypropyl-β-cyclodextrin and poly(anhydride) nanoparticles improve the oral permeability of paclitaxel. *Eur J Pharm Sci* 38(4):405–13.

Ahlin, P., J. Kristl, A. Kristl, and F. Vrecer. 2002. Investigation of polymeric nanoparticles as carriers of enalaprilat for oral administration. *Int J Pharm* 239(1–2):113–20.

Akagi, T., T. Kaneko, T. Kida, and M. Akashi. 2005. Preparation and characterization of biodegradable nanoparticles based on poly(γ-glutamic acid) with L-phenylalanine as a protein carrier. *J Control Release* 108(2–3):226–36.

Alexis, F., J. W. Rhee, J. P. Richie, A. F. Radovic-Moreno, R. Langer, and O. C. Farokhzad. 2008. New frontiers in nanotechnology for cancer treatment. *Urol Oncol-Semin Orig Invest* 26(1):74–85.

Allemann, E., R. Gurny, and E. Doelker. 1992. Preparation of aqueous polymeric nanodispersions by a reversible salting-out process: Influence of process parameters on particle size. *Int J Pharm* 87:247–53.

Al-Shamkhani, A., M. Bhakoo, A. Tuboku-Metzger, and R. Duncan. 1991. Evaluation of the biological properties of alginates and gellan and xanthan gums. In *Proceedings and Program of the International Symposium on Controlled Release of Bioactive Materials*, 1991. United Kingdom: Controlled Release Society.

An, Z., W. Tang, C. J. Hawker, and G. D. Stucky. 2006. One-step microwave preparation of well-defined and functionalized polymeric nanoparticles. *J Am Chem Soc* 128(47):15054–5.

Anton, N., J. P. Benoit, and P. Saulnier. 2008. Design and production of nanoparticles formulated from nanoemulsion templates—a review. *J Control Release* 128(3):185–99.

Antonietti, M. and K. Landfester. 2002. Polyreactions in miniemulsions. *Prog Polym Sci* 27:689–757.

Astete, C. E. and C. M. Sabliov. 2006. Synthesis and characterization of PLGA nanoparticles. *J Biomater Sci-Polym Ed* 17(3):247–89.

Asua, J. M. 2002. Miniemulsion polymerization. *Prog Polym Sci* 27:1283–346.

Asua, J. M. 2004. Emulsion polymerization: From fundamental mechanisms to process developments. *J Polym Sci Polym Chem* 42:1025–41.

Ayano, E., M. Karaki, T. Ishihara, H. Kanazawa, and T. Okano. 2011. Poly (N-isopropylacrylamide)-PLA and PLA blend nanoparticles for temperature-controllable drug release and intracellular uptake. *Colloids Surf B Biointerfaces* 99:67–73

Bajpai, A. K., and J. Choubey. 2006. Design of gelatin nanoparticles as swelling controlled delivery system for chloroquine phosphate. *J Mater Sci Mater Med* 17(4):345–58.

Barrat, G., G. Courraze, C. Couvreur, E. Fattal, R. Gref, D. Labarre, P. Legrand, G. Ponchel, and C. Vauthier. 2000. Polymeric micro- and nanoparticles as drug carriers. In *Polymeric Biomaterials*, ed., S. Dumitriu, pp. 753–781. New York: Marcel Dekker.

Barthelmes, J., G. Perera, J. Hombach, S. Dunnhaupt, and A. Bernkop-Schnurch. 2011. Development of a mucoadhesive nanoparticulate drug delivery system for a targeted drug release in the bladder. *Int J Pharm* 416(1):339–45.

Basaran, E., M. Demirel, B. Sirmagul, and Y. Yazan. 2011. Polymeric cyclosporine-A nanoparticles for ocular application. *J Biomed Nanotechnol* 7(5):714–23.

Behrens, I., A. I. Pena, M. J. Alonso, and T. Kissel. 2002. Comparative uptake studies of bioadhesive and nonbioadhesive nanoparticles in human intestinal cell lines and rats: The effect of mucus on particle adsorption and transport. *Pharm Res* 19(8):1185–93.

Bhardwaj, V., D. D. Ankola, S. C. Gupta, M. Schneider, C. M. Lehr, and M. N. Kumar. 2009. PLGA nanoparticles stabilized with cationic surfactant: Safety studies and application in oral delivery of paclitaxel to treat chemical-induced breast cancer in rat. *Pharm Res* 26(11):2495–503.

Bilati, U., E. Allemann, and E. Doelker. 2003. Sonication parameters for the preparation of biodegradable nanocapsules of controlled size by the double emulsion method. *Pharm Dev Technol* 8(1):1–9.

Boudad, H., P. Legrand, G. Lebas, M. Cheron, D. Duchene, and G. Ponchel. 2001. Combined hydroxypropyl-β-cyclodextrin and poly(alkylcyanoacrylate) nanoparticles intended for oral administration of saquinavir. *Int J Pharm* 218(1–2):113–24.

Budhian, A., S. J. Siegel, and K. I. Winey. 2007. Haloperidol-loaded PLGA nanoparticles: Systematic study of particle size and drug content. *Int J Pharm* 336(2):367–75.

Calvo, P., C. Remunan-Lopez, J. L. Vila-Jato, and M. J. Alonso. 1997. Chitosan and chitosan/ethylene oxide–propylene oxide block copolymer nanoparticles as novel carriers for proteins and vaccines. *Pharm Res* 14(10):1431–6.

Caruthers, S. D., S. A. Wickline, and G. M. Lanza. 2007. Nanotechnological applications in medicine. *Curr Opin Biotechnol* 18(1):26–30.

Chavanpatil, M. D., Y. Patil, and J. Panyam. 2006. Susceptibility of nanoparticle-encapsulated paclitaxel to P-glycoprotein-mediated drug efflux. *Int J Pharm* 320(1–2):150–6.

Chawla, J. S. and M. M. Amiji. 2002. Biodegradable poly(epsilon–caprolactone) nanoparticles for tumor-targeted delivery of tamoxifen. *Int J Pharm* 249(1–2):127–38.

Cheng, X. J., M. Chen, S. X. Zhou, and L. M. Wu. 2006. Preparation of SiO_2/PMMA composite particles via conventional emulsion polymerization. *J Polym Sci Part A—Polym Chem* 44(12):3807–16.

Chern, C. S., Y. C. Liou, and T. J. Chen. 1998. Particle nucleation loci in styrene miniemulsion polymerization using alkyl methacrylates as the reactive cosurfactant. *Macromol Chem Phys* 199:1315–22.

Chernyak, Y., F. Henon, R. B. Harris et al. 2001. Formation of perfluoropolyether coatings by the rapid expansion of percritical solutions (RESS) process Part 1: Experimental results. *Ind Eng Chem Res* 40:6118–26.

Cirstoiu-Hapca, A., F. Buchegger, L. Bossy, M. Kosinski, R. Gurny, and F. Delie. 2009. Nanomedicines for active targeting: Physicochemical characterization of paclitaxel-loaded anti-HER2 immunonanoparticles and *in vitro* functional studies on target cells. *Eur J Pharm Sci* 38(3):230–7.

Costa, C., A. F. Santos, M. Fortuny, P. H. H. Araujo, and C. Sayer. 2009. Kinetic advantages of using microwaves in the emulsion polymerization of MMA. *Mater Sci Eng C—Biomimetic Supramol Syst* 29(2):415–19.

Couvreur, P., B. Kante, M. Roland, P. Guiot, P. Bauduin, and P. Speiser. 1979. Polycyanoacrylate nanocapsules as potential lysosomotropic carriers: Preparation, morphological and sorptive properties. *J Pharm Pharmacol* 31(5):331–2.

Cui, X. J., S. L. Zhong, and H. Y. Wang. 2007. Emulsifier-free core-shell polyacrylate latex nanoparticles containing fluorine and silicon in shell. *Polymer* 48(25):7241–48.

De Jaeghere, F., E. Doelker, and E. Gurny. 1999. Nanoparticles. In *Encyclopedia of Control Drug Delivery*, ed. E. Mathiowitz, pp. 641–664. Wiley, New York.

Desgouilles, S., C. Vauthier., D. Bazile, J. Vacus., J. L. Grossiord., M. Veillard, and P. Couvreur. 2003. The design of nanoparticles obtained by solvent evaporation: A comprehensive study. *Langmuir* 19:9504–10.

Dillen, K., C. Bridts, P. Van der Veken, P. Cos, J. Vandervoort, K. Augustyns, W. Stevens, and A. Ludwig. 2008. Adhesion of PLGA or Eudragit/PLGA nanoparticles to *Staphylococcus* and *Pseudomonas*. *Int J Pharm* 349(1–2):234–40.

Domb A.J., L. Bergelson, and S. Amselem. 1996. Lipospheres for controlled delivery of substances. In *Microencapsulation, Methods and Industrial Applications*, ed., S. Benita, pp. 377–410. New York:Marcel Dekker.

Dong, Y. and S. S. Feng. 2005. Poly(D,L-lactide-*co*-glycolide)/montmorillonite nanoparticles for oral delivery of anticancer drugs. *Biomaterials* 26(30):6068–76.

Donnelly, R. F., D. I. Morrow, F. Fay, C. J. Scott, S. Abdelghany, R. R. Singh, M. J. Garland, and A. D. Woolfson. 2010. Microneedle-mediated intradermal nanoparticle delivery: Potential for enhanced local administration of hydrophobic pre-formed photosensitisers. *Photodiagnosis Photodyn Ther* 7(4):222–31.

Duan, J., H. M. Mansour, Y. Zhang, X. Deng, Y. Chen, J. Wang, Y. Pan, and J. Zhao. 2012. Reversion of multidrug resistance by coencapsulation of doxorubicin and curcumin in chitosan/poly(butyl cyanoacrylate) nanoparticles. *Int J Pharm* 426(1–2):193–201.

Dustgania, A., E. V. Farahania, and I. Mohammad. 2008. Preparation of chitosan nanoparticles loaded by dexamethasone sodium phosphate. *Iran J Pharm Res* 4(2):111–14.

Elnaggar, Y. S., M. A. El-Massik, and O. Y. Abdallah. 2011. Fabrication, appraisal, and transdermal permeation of sildenafil citrate-loaded nanostructured lipid carriers versus solid lipid nanoparticles. *Int J Nanomedicine* 6:3195–205.

El-Samaligy, M. S., P. Rohdewald, and H. A. Mahmoud. 1986. Polyalkyl cyanoacrylate nanocapsules. *J Pharm Pharmacol* 38(3):216–8.

Esmaeili, F., F. Atyabi, and R. Dinarvand. 2008. Preparation and characterization of estradiol-loaded PLGA nanoparticles using homogenization–solvent diffusion method. *DARU* 16(4):196–202.

Esmaeili, F., M. Hosseini-Nasr, M. Rad-Malekshahi, N. Samadi, F. Atyabi, and R. Dinarvand. 2007. Preparation and antibacterial activity evaluation of rifampicin-loaded polylactide-*co*-glycolide nanoparticles. *Nanomedicine* 3(2):161–7.

Feng, S. S. 2004. Nanoparticles of biodegradable polymers for new-concept chemotherapy. *Expert Rev Med Devices* 1(1):115–25.

Fessi, H., F. Puisieux, J. P. Devissaguet, N. Ammoury, and S. Benita. 1989. Nanocapsule formation by interfacial polymer deposition following solvent displacement. *Int J Pharm* 55:1–4.

Fontana, M. C., K. Coradini, A. R. Pohlmann, S. S. Guterres, and R. C. Beck. 2010. Nanocapsules prepared from amorphous polyesters: Effect on the physicochemical characteristics, drug release, and photostability. *J Nanosci Nanotechnol* 10(5):3091–9.

Giovino, C., I. Ayensu, J. Tetteh, and J. S. Boateng. 2012. Development and characterisation of chitosan films impregnated with insulin loaded PEG-*b*-PLA nanoparticles (NPs): A potential approach for buccal delivery of macromolecules. *Int J Pharm* 428(1–2):143–51.

Guan, M., Y. Zhou, Q. L. Zhu, Y. Liu, Y. Y. Bei, X. N. Zhang, and Q. Zhang. 2012. *N*-trimethyl chitosan nanoparticle-encapsulated lactosyl-norcantharidin for liver cancer therapy with high targeting efficacy. *Nanomedicine* 8(7):1172–81

Gupta, H., M. Aqil, R. K. Khar, A. Ali, A. Bhatnagar, and G. Mittal. 2010. Sparfloxacin-loaded PLGA nanoparticles for sustained ocular drug delivery. *Nanomedicine–Nanotechnol Biol Med* 6(2):324–33.

Gupta, M. and S. P. Vyas. 2012. Development, characterization and *in vivo* assessment of effective lipidic nanoparticles for dermal delivery of fluconazole against cutaneous candidiasis. *Chem Phys Lipids* 65(4):454–61.

Hans, M. L. and A. M. Lowman. 2002. Biodegradable nanoparticles for drug delivery and targeting. *Curr Opin Solid St Mater Sci* 6:319–27.

Hearn, J., M. C. Wilkinson, A. R. Goodall, and M. Chainey. 1985. Kinetics of the surfactant-free emulsion polymerization of styrene: The post nucleation stage. *J Polym Sci Polym Chem Ed* 23:1869–83.

Hornig, S. and T. Heinze. 2008. Efficient approach to design stable water-dispersible nanoparticles of hydrophobic cellulose esters. *Biomacromolecules* 9(5):1487–92.

Jain, S. K., Y. Gupta, L. Ramalingam, A. Jain, P. Khare, and D. Bhargava. 2010. Lactose-conjugated PLGA nanoparticles for enhanced delivery of rifampicin to the lung for effective treatment of pulmonary tuberculosis. *PDA J Pharm Sci Technol* 64(3):278–87.

Jain, A. K., N. K. Swarnakar, M. Das, C. Godugu, R. P. Singh, P. R. Rao, and S. Jain. 2011. Augmented anticancer efficacy of doxorubicin-loaded polymeric nanoparticles after oral administration in a breast cancer induced animal model. *Mol Pharm* 8(4):1140–51.

Jaiswal, J., S. K. Gupta, and J. Kreuter. 2004. Preparation of biodegradable cyclosporine nanoparticles by high-pressure emulsification–solvent evaporation process. *J Control Release* 96(1):169–78.

Jeon, S. Y., J. S. Park, H. N. Yang, D. G. Woo, and K. H. Park. 2012. Codelivery of SOX9 genes and anti-Cbfa-1 siRNA coated onto PLGA nanoparticles for chondrogenesis of human MSCs. *Biomaterials* 33(17):4413–23.

Jeong, Y. I., H. S. Na, D. H. Seo, D. G. Kim, H. C. Lee, M. K. Jang, S. K. Na, S. H. Roh, S. I. Kim, and J. W. Nah. 2008. Ciprofloxacin-encapsulated poly(DL-lactide-*co*-glycolide) nanoparticles and its antibacterial activity. *Int J Pharm* 352(1–2): 317–23.

Jin, C., L. Bai, H. Wu, J. Liu, G. Guo, and J. Chen. 2008. Paclitaxel-loaded poly(D,L-lactide-*co*-glycolide) nanoparticles for radiotherapy in hypoxic human tumor cells *in vitro*. *Cancer Biol Ther* 7(6):911–6.

Jin, C., L. Bai, H. Wu, W. Song, G. Guo, and K. Dou. 2009. Cytotoxicity of paclitaxel incorporated in PLGA nanoparticles on hypoxic human tumor cells. *Pharm Res* 26(7):1776–84.

Jin, C., L. Bai, H. Wu, F. Tian, and G. Guo. 2007. Radiosensitization of paclitaxel, etanidazole and paclitaxel+etanidazole nanoparticles on hypoxic human tumor cells *in vitro*. *Biomaterials* 28(25):3724–30.

Jung, J. and M. Perrut. 2001. Particle design using supercritical fluids: Literature and patent survey. *J Supercritical Fluids* 20(3):179–219.

Kalaria, D. R., G. Sharma, V. Beniwal, and M. N. Ravi Kumar. 2009. Design of biodegradable nanoparticles for oral delivery of doxorubicin: *In vivo* pharmacokinetics and toxicity studies in rats. *Pharm Res* 26(3):492–501.

Karode, S. K., S. S. Kulkarni, A. K. Suresh, and R. A. Mashelkar. 1998. New insights into kinetics and thermodynamics of interfacial polymerization. *Chem Eng Sci* 53:2649–63.

Kashi, T. S., S. Eskandarion, M. Esfandyari-Manesh, S. M. Marashi, N. Samadi, S. M. Fatemi, F. Atyabi, S. Eshraghi, and R. Dinarvand. 2012. Improved drug loading and antibacterial activity of minocycline-loaded PLGA nanoparticles prepared by solid/oil/water ion pairing method. *Int J Nanomedicine* 7:221–34.

Keawchaoon, L. and R. Yoksan. 2011. Preparation, characterization and *in vitro* release study of carvacrol-loaded chitosan nanoparticles. *Colloids Surf B Biointerfaces* 84(1):163–71.

Keck, C., S. Kobierski, R. Mauludin, and R. H. Muller. 2008. Second generation of drug nanocrystals for delivery of poorly soluble drugs: Smart crystals technology. *Eur J Pharma Biopharmaceut* 62:3–16.

Khoury-Fallouh, A. N., L. Roblot-Treupe, H. Fessi, J. P. Devissaguet, and F. Puisieux. 1986. Development of a new process for the manufacture of poly isobutylcyanoacrylate nanocapsules. *Int J Pharm* 28:125–36.

Kim, S. W., H. G. Cho, and C. R. Park. 2009. Fabrication of unagglomerated polypyrrole nanospheres with controlled sizes from a surfactant-free emulsion system. *Langmuir* 25(16):9030–36.

Kim, J. H., Y. S. Kim, S. Kim, J. H. Park, K. Kim, K. Choi, H. Chung, S. Y. Jeong, R. W. Park, I. S. Kim, and I. C. Kwon. 2006. Hydrophobically modified glycol chitosan nanoparticles as carriers for paclitaxel. *J Control Release* 111(1–2):228–34.

Kim I. S., S. K. Lee., Y. M. Park., Y. B. Lee., S. C. Shin., K. C. Lee., and I. J. Oh. 2005. Physicochemical characterization of poly (L-lactic acid) and poly (D, L-lactide-co-glycolide) nanoparticles with polyethylenimine as gene delivery carrier. *Int J Pharm* 298:255–62.

Kommareddy, S., S. B. Tiwari, and M. M. Amiji. 2005. Long-circulating polymeric nanovectors for tumor-selective gene delivery. *Technol Cancer Res Treat* 4(6):615–25.

Konan, Y. N., R. Gurny, and E. Allemann. 2002. Preparation and characterization of sterile and freeze-dried sub-200 nm nanoparticles. *Int J Pharm* 233:239–52.

Kreuter, J. 1982. The mechanism of termination in heterogeneous polymerization. *J Polym Sci Polym Lett Ed* 20:543–5.

Kreuter, J. 1994. Drug targeting with nanoparticles. *Eur J Drug Metab Pharmacokinet* 19(3):253–6.

Kristl, J., E. Allémann, and R. Gurny. 1996. Formulation and evaluation of zinc–phthalocyanine loaded poly(D,L-lactic acid) nanoparticles. *Acta Pharm* 46:1–12.

Kriwet, B., E. Walter, and T. Kissel. 1998. Synthesis of bioadhesive poly(acrylic acid) nano- and microparticles using an inverse emulsion polymerization method for the entrapment of hydrophilic drug candidates. *J Control Release* 56(1–3):149–58.

Kwon, H. Y., J. Y. Lee, S. W. Choi, Y. S. Jang, and J. H. Kim. 2001. Preparation of PLGA nanoparticles containing estrogen by emulsification–diffusion method. *Colloids Surfaces A—Physicochem Eng Asp* 182(1–3):123–30.

Lamprecht, A., N. Ubrich, H. Yamamoto, U. Schafer, H. Takeuchi, C. M. Lehr, P. Maincent, and Y. Kawashima. 2001. Design of rolipram-loaded nanoparticles: Comparison of two preparation methods. *J Control Release* 71(3):297–306.

Landfester, K. 2001. Polyreactions in miniemulsions. *Macromol Rapid Commun* 22:896–936.

Langer, K., C. Coester, C. Weber, H. von Briesen, and J. Kreuter. 2000. Preparation of avidin-labeled protein nanoparticles as carriers for biotinylated peptide nucleic acid. *Eur J Pharm Biopharm* 49(3):303–7.

La-Van, D., T. McGuire, and R. Langer. 2003. Small-scale system for *in vivo* drug delivery. *Nat Biotechnol* 21:1184–91.

Lee, J., E. C. Cho, and K. Cho. 2004. Incorporation and release behavior of hydrophobic drug in functionalized poly(D,L-lactide)-block-poly(ethylene oxide) micelles. *J Control Release* 94(2–3):323–35.

Lee, M. and S. W. Kim. 2005. Polyethylene glycol-conjugated copolymers for plasmid DNA delivery. *Pharm Res* 22(1):1–10.

Lemoine, D. and V. Preat. 1998. Polymeric nanoparticles as delivery system for Influenza virus glycoproteins. *J Control Release* 54:15–27.

Leroux, J.C., E. Allemann, F. De Jaeghere, E. Doelker, and R. Gurny. 1996. Biodegradable nanoparticles from sustained release formulations to improved site specific drug delivery. *J Control Release* 39:339–50.

Liang, J., F. Li, Y. Fang, W. Yang, X. An, L. Zhao, Z. Xin, L. Cao, and Q. Hu. 2011. Synthesis, characterization and cytotoxicity studies of chitosan-coated tea polyphenols nanoparticles. *Colloids Surf B Biointerfaces* 82(2):297–301.

Lim, K. T., G. H. Subban, H. S. Hwang, J. T. Kim, C. S. Ju, and K. P. Johnston. 2005. Novel semiconducting polymer particles by supercritical fluid process. *Macromol Rapid Commun* 26(22):1779–83.

Liu, M. X., J. Dong, Y. J. Yang, X. L. Yang, and H. B. Xu. 2004. Preparation and toxicity of triptolide-loaded poly (D,L-lactic acid) nanoparticles. *Yao Xue Xue Bao* 39(7):556–60.

Liu, J., Z. Qiu, S. Wang, L. Zhou, and S. Zhang. 2010. A modified double-emulsion method for the preparation of daunorubicin-loaded polymeric nanoparticle with enhanced *in vitro* antitumor activity. *Biomed Mater* 5(6):065002.

Lourenco, C., M. Teixeira, S. Simoes, and R. Gaspar. 1996. Steric stabilization of nanoparticles: Size and surface properties. *Int J Pharm* 138(1): 1–12.

Macias, E. R., L. A. Rodriguez-Guadarrama, B. A. Cisneros, A. Castaneda, E. Mendizabal, and J. E. Puig. 1995. Microemulsion polymerization of methyl methacrylate with the functional monomer N-methylolacrylamide. *Colloid Surface A* 103:119–26.

Mahor, S., E. Collin, B. C. Dash, and A. Pandit. 2011. Controlled release of plasmid DNA from hyaluronan nanoparticles. *Curr Drug Deliv* 8(4):354–62.

Meziani, M. J., P. Pathak, W. Wang, T. Desai, A. Patil, and Y. P. Sun. 2005. Polymeric nanofibers from rapid expansion of supercritical solution. *Ind Eng Chem Res* 44(13):4594–98.

Miao, L. F., J. Yang, C. L. Huang, C. X. Song, Y. J. Zeng, L. F. Chen, and W. L. Zhu. 2008. Rapamycin-loaded poly (lactic-*co*-glycolic) acid nanoparticles for intraarterial local drug delivery: Preparation, characterization, and *in vitro/in vivo* release. *Zhongguo Yi Xue Ke Xue Yuan Xue Bao* 30(4):491–7.

Michael, J. K., J. D. Abraham, and C. V. Michael. 2009. Attenuation of kindles seizures by intranasal delivery of neuropeptide-loaded nanoparticles. *Neurotherapeutics* 6(2):359–71.

Mishra, B., B. B. Patel, and S. Tiwari. 2010. Colloidal nanocarriers: A review on formulation technology, types and applications toward targeted drug delivery. *Nanomedicine* 6(1):9–24.

Moinard-Checot, D., Y. Chevalier, S. Briancon, H. Fessi, and S. Guinebretiere. 2006. Nanoparticles for drug delivery: Review of the formulation and process difficulties illustrated by the emulsion–diffusion process. *J Nanosci Nanotechnol* 6(9–10):2664–81.

Motwani, S. K., S. Chopra, S. Talegaonkar, K. Kohli, F. J. Ahmad, and R. K. Khar. 2008. Chitosan–sodium alginate nanoparticles as submicroscopic reservoirs for ocular delivery: Formulation, optimisation and *in vitro* characterisation. *Eur J Pharm Biopharm* 68(3):513–25.

Mu, L. and S. S. Feng. 2003. A novel controlled release formulation for the anticancer drug paclitaxel (taxol): PLGA nanoparticles containing vitamin E TPGS. *J Control Release* 86(1):33–48.

Murakami, H., M. Kobayashi, H. Takeuchi, and Y. Kawashima. 1999. Preparation of poly(DL-lactide-*co*-glycolide) nanoparticles by modified spontaneous emulsification solvent diffusion method. *Int J Pharm* 187(2):143–52.

Musumeci, T., C. A. Ventura, I. Giannone, B. Ruozi, L. Montenegro, R. Pignatello, and G. Puglisi. 2006. PLA/PLGA nanoparticles for sustained release of docetaxel. *Int J Pharm* 325(1–2):172–9.

Musyanovych, A., J. Schmitz-Wienke, V. Mailander, P. Walther, and K. Landfester. 2008. Preparation of biodegradable polymer nanoparticles by miniemulsion technique and their cell interactions. *Macromol Biosci* 8(2):127–39.

Muthu, M. S. and S. Singh. 2009. Poly(D, L-lactide) nanosuspensions of risperidone for parenteral delivery: Formulation and *in vitro* evaluation. *Curr Drug Deliv* 6(1):62–8.

Na, K., K. H. Lee, D. H. Lee, and Y. H. Bae. 2006. Biodegradable thermosensitive nanoparticles from poly(L-lactic acid)/poly(ethylene glycol) alternating multiblock copolymer for potential anticancer drug carrier. *Eur J Pharm Sci* 27(2–3):115–22.

Niwa, T., H. Takeuchi., T. Hino, N. Kunou, and Y. Kawashima. 1993. Preparations of biodegradable nanospheres of water-soluble and insoluble drugs with D, L-lactide/glycolide copolymer by a novel spontaneous emulsification solvent diffusion method and the drug release behavior. *J Control Rel* 25:89–98.

Oh, I., K. Lee, H. Y. Kwon, Y. B. Lee, S. C. Shin, C. S. Cho, and C. K. Kim. 1999. Release of adriamycin from poly(γ-benzyl-L-glutamate)/poly(ethylene oxide) nanoparticles. *Int J Pharm* 181(1):107–15.

Pangburn S. H., P. V. Tresony, and J. Heller. 1984. In: Partially deacetylated chitin: Its uses in self regulated drug delivery systems. In *Chitin, Chitosan and Related Enzyme*, ed., J.P. Louise, pp. 3–20. New York: Academic Press.

Panyam, J., D. Williams, A. Dash, D. Leslie-Pelecky, and V. Labhasetwar. 2004. Solid-state solubility influences encapsulation and release of hydrophobic drugs from PLGA/PLA nanoparticles. *J Pharm Sci* 93:1804–14.

Pinon-Segundo, E., A. Ganem-Quintanar, V. Alonso-Perez, and D. Quintanar-Guerrero. 2005. Preparation and characterization of triclosan nanoparticles for periodontal treatment. *Int J Pharm* 294(1–2):217–32.

Plapied, L., G. Vandermeulen, B. Vroman, V. Preat, and A. des Rieux. 2010. Bioadhesive nanoparticles of fungal chitosan for oral DNA delivery. *Int J Pharm* 398(1–2):210–8.

Prabha, S., W. Z. Zhou, J. Panyam, and V. Labhasetwar. 2002. Size-dependency of nanoparticle-mediated gene transfection: Studies with fractionated nanoparticles. *Int J Pharm* 244(1–2):105–15.

Qi, J., Y. Lu, and W. Wu. 2012. Absorption, disposition and pharmacokinetics of solid lipid nanoparticles. *Curr Drug Metab* 13(4):418–28.

Quellec, P., R. Gref, E. Dellacherie, F. Sommer, M. D. Tran, and M. J. Alonso. 1999. Protein encapsulation within poly(ethylene glycol)-coated nanospheres. II. Controlled release properties. *J Biomed Mater Res* 47(3):388–95.

Quintanar-Guerrero, D., E. Allémann, H. Fessi, and E. Doelker. 1998. Preparation techniques and mechanisms of formation of biodegradable nanoparticles from preformed polymers. *Drug Dev Ind Pharm* 24:113–28.

Quintanar-Guerrero, D., H. Fessi, E. Allemann, and E. Doekler. 1996. Influence of stabilizing agents and preparative variables on the formation of poly(D,L-lactic acid) nanoparticles by an emulsification–diffusion technique. *Int J Pharm* 143(2):133–41.

Rafati, H., A. G. A. Coombes, J. Adler, J. Holland, and S. S. Davis. 1997. Protein-loaded poly(DL-lactide-*co*-glycolide) microparticles for oral administration: Formulation, structural and release characteristics. *J Control Release* 43(1):89–102.

Rao, J. P. and K. E. Geckeler. 2011. Polymer nanoparticles: Preparation techniques and size-control parameters. *Prog Polym Sci* 36(7):887–913.

Reverchon, E. and R. Adami. 2006. Nanomaterials and supercritical fluids. *J Supercritical Fluids* 37:1–22.

Ricci, M., P. Blasi, S. Giovagnoli, L. Perioli, C. Vescovi, and C. Rossi. 2004. Leucinostatin-A loaded nanospheres: Characterization and *in vivo* toxicity and efficacy evaluation. *Int J Pharm* 275(1–2):61–72.

Saboktakin, M. R., R. M. Tabatabaie, A. Maharramov, and M. A. Ramazanov. 2011. Development and *in vitro* evaluation of thiolated chitosan—Poly(methacrylic acid) nanoparticles as a local mucoadhesive delivery system. *Int J Biol Macromol* 48(3):403–7.

Sashmal, S., S. Mukherjee, S. Ray, R. S. Thakur, L. K. Ghosh, and B. K. Gupta. 2007. Design and optimization of NSAID loaded nanoparticles. *Pak J Pharm Sci* 20(2):157–62.

Saxena, V., M. Sadoqi, and J. Shao. 2004. Indocyanine green-loaded biodegradable nanoparticles: Preparation, physicochemical characterization and *in vitro* release. *Int J Pharm* 278(2):293–301.

Schlicher, E. J. A. M., N. S. Postma, J. Zuidema, H. Talsma, and W. E. Hennink. 1997. Preparation and characterisation of poly(D,L-lactic-*co*-glycolic acid) microspheres containing desferrioxamine. *Int J Pharm* 153:235–45.

Scholes, P. D., A. G. Coombes, L. Illum, S. S. Davis, M. Vert, and M. C. Davies. 1993. The preparation of sub-200 nm poly(lactide-*co*-glycolide) microspheres for site-specific drug delivery. *J Control Release* 25:145–53.

Sengel-Türk, C. T., C. Hascicek, A. L. Dogan, G. Esendagli, D. Guc, and N. Gonul. 2012. Preparation and *in vitro* evaluation of meloxicam-loaded PLGA nanoparticles on HT-29 human colon adenocarcinoma cells. *Drug Dev Ind Pharm* 38(9):1107–16.

Seo, S. A., G. Khang, J. M. Rhee, J. Kim, and H. B. Lee. 2003. Study on *in vitro* release patterns of fentanyl-loaded PLGA microspheres. *J Microencapsul* 20(5):569–79.

Shahnaz, G., A. Vetter, J. Barthelmes, D. Rahmat, F. Laffleur, J. Iqbal, G. Perera, W. Schlocker, S. Dunnhaput, P. Augustijns, and A. Bernkop-Schnurch. 2012. Thiolated chitosan nanoparticles for the nasal administration of leuprolide: Bioavailability and pharmacokinetic characterization. *Int J Pharm* 428(1-2):164–70.

Shrivastava, S. 2008. Nanofabrication for drug delivery and tissue engineering. *Dig J Nanomater Bios* 3:257–63.

Singh, K. H. and U. A. Shinde. 2010. Development and evaluation of novel polymeric nanoparticles of brimonidine tartrate. *Curr Drug Deliv* 7(3):244–51.

Singh, K. H. and U. A. Shinde. 2011. Chitosan nanoparticles for controlled delivery of brimonidine tartrate to the ocular membrane. *Pharmazie* 66(8):594–9.

Song, Z. and G. W. Poehlein. 1990. Kinetics of emulsifier-free emulsion polymerization of styrene. *J Polym Sci Polym Chem* 28:2359–92.

Song, X., Y. Zhao, S. Hou, F. Xu, R. Zhao, J. He, Z. Cai, Y. Li, and Q. Chen. 2008. Dual agents loaded PLGA nanoparticles: Systematic study of particle size and drug entrapment efficiency. *Eur J Pharm Biopharm* 69(2):445–53.

Song, X., Y. Zhao, W. Wu, Y. Bi, Z. Cai, Q. Chen, Y. Li, and S. Hou. 2008. PLGA nanoparticles simultaneously loaded with vincristine sulfate and verapamil hydrochloride: Systematic study of particle size and drug entrapment efficiency. *Int J Pharm* 350(1–2):320–9.

Sosa, N., E. A. Zaragoza, R. G. Lopez, R. D. Peralta, I. Katime, F. Becerra, E. Mendizabal, and J. E. Puig. 2000. Unusual free radical polymerization of vinyl acetate in anionic microemulsion media. *Langmuir* 16(8):3612–19.

Su-Jung, Y., H. Chun, L. Mi-Sun, and N. Kim. 2009. Preparation of poly(N-vinyl-carbazole) (PVK) nanoparticles by emulsion polymerization and PVK hollow particles. *Synth Met* 159:518–22.

Sun, S., N. Liang, Y. Kawashima, D. Xia, and F. Cui. 2011. Hydrophobic ion pairing of an insulin–sodium deoxycholate complex for oral delivery of insulin. *Int J Nanomedicine* 6:3049–56.

Sun, Y. P., M. J. Meziani, P. Pathak, and L. Qu. 2005. Polymeric nanoparticles from rapid expansion of supercritical fluid solution. *Chemistry* 11(5):1366–73.

Thickett, S. C. and R. G. Gilbert. 2007. Emulsion polymerization: State of the art in kinetics and mechanisms. *Polymer* 48(24):6965–91.

Thote, A. J. and R. B. Gupta. 2005. Formation of nanoparticles of a hydrophilic drug using supercritical carbon dioxide and microencapsulation for sustained release. *Nanomedicine: Nanotech Biol Med* 1:85–90.

Torini, L., J. F. Argillier, and N. Zydowicz. 2005. Interfacial polycondensation encapsulation in miniemulsion. *Macromolecules* 38(8):3225–36.

Ungaro, F., I. d'Angelo, C. Coletta, R. d'Emmanuele di Villa Bianca, R. Sorrentino, B. Perfetto, M. A. Tufano, A. Miro, M. I. La Rotonda, and F. Quaglia. 2012. Dry powders based on PLGA nanoparticles for pulmonary delivery of antibiotics: Modulation of encapsulation efficiency, release rate and lung deposition pattern by hydrophilic polymers. *J Control Release* 157(1):149–59.

Vauthier, C. and K. Bouchemal. 2009. Methods for the preparation and manufacture of polymeric nanoparticles. *Pharm Res* 26(5):1025–58.

Vega, E., M. A. Egea, O. Valls, M. Espina, and M. L. Garcia. 2006. Flurbiprofen loaded biodegradable nanoparticles for ophthalmic administration. *J Pharm Sci* 95(11):2393–405.

Ven, H. V., J. Vandervoort, W. Weyenberg, S. Apers, and A. Ludwig. 2012. Mixture designs in the optimisation of PLGA nanoparticles: Influence of organic phase composition on β-aescin encapsulation. *J Microencapsul* 29(2):115–25.

Verheul, R. J., B. Slutter, S. M. Bal, J. A. Bouwstra, W. Jiskoot, and W. E. Hennink. 2011. Covalently stabilized trimethyl chitosan–hyaluronic acid nanoparticles for nasal and intradermal vaccination. *J Control Release* 156(1):46–52.

Vranckx, H., M. Demoustier, and M. Deleers. 1996. A new nanocapsule formulation with hydrophilic core: Application to the oral administration of *Salmon calcitonin* in rats. *J Pharm Pharmacol* 42:345–7.

Watnasirichaikul, S., N. M. Davies, T. Rades, and I. G. Tucker. 2000. Preparation of biodegradable insulin nanocapsules from biocompatible microemulsions. *Pharm Res* 17:684–9.

Wu, M., E. Dellacherie, A. Durand, and E. Marie. 2009. Poly(*n*-butyl cyanoacrylate) nanoparticles via miniemulsion polymerization. 2. PEG-based surfactants. *Colloids Surf B Biointerfaces* 69(1):147–51.

Xu, J., J. H. Zhao, Y. Liu, N. P. Feng, and Y. T. Zhang. 2012. RGD-modified poly(D,L-lactic acid) nanoparticles enhance tumor targeting of oridonin. *Int J Nanomedicine* 7:211–9.

Yang, A., L. Yang, W. Liu, Z. Li, H. Xu, and X. Yang. 2007. Tumor necrosis factor α-blocking peptide loaded PEG-PLGA nanoparticles: Preparation and *in vitro* evaluation. *Int J Pharm* 331(1):123–32.

Yin, Y., D. Chen, M. Qiao, X. Wei, and H. Hu. 2007. Lectin-conjugated PLGA nanoparticles loaded with thymopentin: *Ex vivo* bioadhesion and *in vivo* biodistribution. *J Control Release* 123(1):27–38.

Yousefpour, P., F. Atyabi, E. V. Farahani, R. Sakhtianchi, and R. Dinarvand. 2011. Polyanionic carbohydrate doxorubicin–dextran nanocomplex as a delivery system for anticancer drugs: *In vitro* analysis and evaluations. *Int J Nanomedicine* 6:1487–96.

Zahoor, A., S. Sharma, and G. K. Khuller. 2005. Inhalable alginate nanoparticles as antitubercular drug carriers against experimental tuberculosis. *Int J Antimicrob Agents* 26(4):298–303.

Zambaux, M. F., F. Bonneaux, R. Gref, P. Maincent, E. Dellacherie, M. J. Alonso, P. Labrude, and C. Vigneron. 1998. Influence of experimental parameters on the characteristics of poly(lactic acid) nanoparticles prepared by a double emulsion method. *J Control Release* 50(1–3):31–40.

Zhang, J. Z., Y. Cao, and Y. H. He. 2004. Ultrasonically irradiated emulsion polymerization of styrene in the presence of a polymeric surfactant. *J Appl Polym Sci* 94(2):763–8.

Zhang, Z. and S. S. Feng. 2006. Self-assembled nanoparticles of poly(lactide)—Vitamin E TPGS copolymers for oral chemotherapy. *Int J Pharm* 324(2):191–8.

Zhang, H. Z., F. P. Gao, L. R. Liu, X. M. Li, Z. M. Zhou, X. D. Yang, and Q. Q. Zhang. 2009. Pullulan acetate nanoparticles prepared by solvent diffusion method for epirubicin chemotherapy. *Colloids Surf B Biointerfaces* 71(1):19–26.

Zhang, Z., D. W. Grijpma, and J. Feijen. 2006. Poly(trimethylene carbonate) and monomethoxy poly(ethylene glycol)-block-poly(trimethylene carbonate) nanoparticles for the controlled release of dexamethasone. *J Control Release* 111(3):263–70.

Zhang, G., A. Niu, S. Peng, M. Jiang, Y. Tu, M. Li, and C. Wu. 2001. Formation of novel polymeric nanoparticles. *Acc Chem Res* 34(3):249–56.

Zhang, Q., Z. Shen, and T. Nagai. 2001. Prolonged hypoglycemic effect of insulin-loaded polybutylcyanoacrylate nanoparticles after pulmonary administration to normal rats. *Int J Pharm* 218(1–2):75–80.

Zhao, S. H., X. T. Wu, W. C. Guo, Y. M. Du, L. Yu, and J. Tang. 2010. *N*-(2-hydroxyl) propyl-3-trimethyl ammonium chitosan chloride nanoparticle as a novel delivery system for parathyroid hormone-related protein 1–34. *Int J Pharm* 393(1–2): 268–72.

Zweers, M. L., D. W. Grijpma, G. H. Engbers, and J. Feijen. 2003. The preparation of monodisperse biodegradable polyester nanoparticles with a controlled size. *J Biomed Mater Res B Appl Biomater* 66(2):559–66.

11

Nanoparticles for Ocular Drug Delivery

Jaleh Barar and Yadollah Omidi

CONTENTS

11.1 Introduction 288
11.2 Biological Membranes and Barriers of the Eye 289
    11.2.1 Tear Film 290
    11.2.2 Corneal Route and Barrier 290
    11.2.3 Noncorneal Route: Conjunctiva and Sclera 293
    11.2.4 Blood–Aqueous Barrier 295
    11.2.5 Retina and BRB 295
11.3 Ocular Drug-Delivery Mechanisms 298
    11.3.1 Simple Passive Transport 298
    11.3.2 Carrier-Mediated Transport 298
    11.3.3 Ocular Transport Machineries 299
    11.3.4 Endocytosis and Transcytosis 300
    11.3.5 Topical Absorption of Ocular Drug 301
11.4 Ocular Pharmacotherapy 301
    11.4.1 Conventional Pharmacotherapy of Ocular Diseases 302
    11.4.2 Ocular Nanopharmaceuticals 303
    11.4.3 Liposomal Nanomedicines 305
    11.4.4 Niosomes 311
    11.4.5 Polymer-Based Ocular Nanomedicines 311
    11.4.6 Dendrimeric Nanostructures for Ocular Drug Delivery 317
    11.4.7 Quantum Dots 318
    11.4.8 Gold NPs 319
    11.4.9 Cubosomes 319
    11.4.10 Nanosuspensions 320
    11.4.11 Ocular Nanogenomedicines 321
    11.4.12 Bioavailability of Ocular Nanomedicines 322
11.5 Final Remarks on Ocular Nanomedicines 324
References 325

11.1 Introduction

The physiological characteristics of the eye show unique structural and functional properties. The structure of the eye is composed of the retinal-lined fibrovascular sphere enclosing the aqueous humor, the lens, and the vitreous body (McCaa 1982). The eye is a transparent tissue, which is necessary for normal vision. To attain a clear and normal vision, the communication between the anterior and posterior parts of the eye should be kept in a highly controlled manner. The tight cellular barrier restricts particles to traverse inward/outward of the eye segments, in which various static barriers (different layers of the cornea, sclera, and the retina including blood–aqueous barrier [BAB] and blood–retinal barrier [BRB]), dynamic barriers (choroidal and conjunctival blood flow, lymphatic clearance, and tear dilution), and efflux pumps in conjunction control such transportation. As a result, the unique barrier functions in the eye pose a significant challenge for delivery of a drug alone or in a dosage form, especially to the posterior segment (Gaudana et al. 2010). Figure 11.1 is a schematic illustration of the structure of the eye and the presence of major functional barriers, namely the corneal–epithelial barrier, BAB, and BRB. Despite architectural commonalities among biological barriers, permeability of various substances across BRB and BAB compared with the blood–brain barrier (BBB) in rats has demonstrated significant differences. Lipophilic substances were shown to have high permeabilities across BBB and BRB, in which their retinal uptake index (RUI) values were also markedly higher than the brain uptake index (BUI) values. It seems there is a linear relationship between permeability and log $D_{7.4}$, while efflux transport machineries play important roles in the absorption of ocular drugs from the circulating blood after systemic administration (Toda et al. 2011).

From the drug-delivery point of view, these barriers are considered as a foremost challenge for medicaments targeting ocular site that has attracted many scientists for circumvention of such barriers by evolved novel drug-delivery systems (DDS).

Over the past two decades, nanoparticles (NPs) have received a great deal of attention for drug delivery and targeting because these DDS can accomplish many prerequisite criteria required for therapeutics. The nano-scaled macromolecular particulates appear to provide a platform for optimized delivery of designated drugs into the eye. In general, ocular nanomedicines fall into a size range of 50–250 nm. Therapeutic NPs are either macromolecular active drug or simply implies to the materials used as a drug carrier for dissolving, entrapping, or encapsulating active drug, or attaching/adsorbing the active materials.

Nanomedicine application in ocular drug delivery and targeting is becoming increasingly important, since this new era of DDS, fulfills all the required criteria for successful therapy by not only facilitating the drug penetration and retention, but also providing a controlled and targeted mean for delivery. Utilization of nanotechnology generates a very promising tactic for ocular delivery of poorly soluble drugs, peptides and proteins, and gene-based medications.

11.2 Biological Membranes and Barriers of the Eye

Optimal ocular function is maintained by restrictive biological barriers and membranes. The schematic representation of the eye structure is illustrated in Figure 11.1. While the topical administration of drugs as eyedrops is the most acceptable and applicable method, the fraction of the drug absorbed into the ophthalmic tissue is very small due to lacrimal drainage and systemic absorption. Drug entry into the anterior chamber occurs via the passage through different barriers and membranes that can selectively control

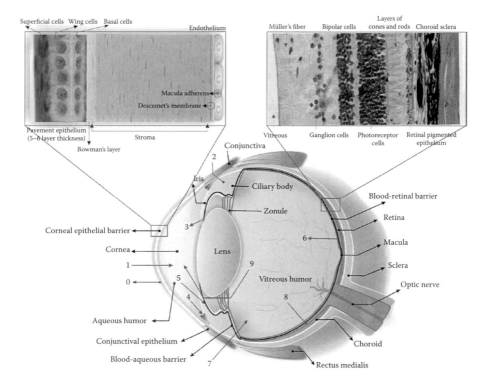

FIGURE 11.1

Schematic illustration of the structure of the eye and presence of major functional barriers. Tear film is the first physiologic impediment against installed topical pharmaceuticals (0). Topical drugs are to cross the cornea to reach the anterior chamber of the eye (1). Hydrophilic drugs and macromolecules are delivered through the conjunctival/scleral route (2). After systemic administration, small compounds are able to penetrate from the iris blood vessels into the anterior chamber (3). The administered pharmaceuticals are prone to be carried away from the anterior chamber either by aqueous humor outflow (4) or by venous blood flow after diffusing across the iris surface (5). To reach vitreous, systemically administered drugs must cross the retinal pigment epithelia (RPE) and the retinal capillary endothelia (RCE), which are the main retinal barriers (6). Ocular drugs can be reached to the vitreous by intravitreal injection (7). Drugs can be removed from the vitreous away through the BRB (8) and/or diffusion into the anterior chamber (9). Left and right panels represent cellular architecture of cornea and retina, respectively.

their traverse. An ideal DDS should be able to cross the endothelial/epithe-lial membranous barrier. Basically the cornea and conjunctiva are consid-ered to play the main role in drug absorption into the ophthalmic target site. However, other biological membranous structures selectively intrude drug access via epithelial and/or endothelial tight junctional constituents. A brief overview of the ocular biological structure and functionality is provided in the following sections.

11.2.1 Tear Film

Tear film is a liquid layer bathing the most anterior refractive surface of the eye and its normal volume and composition is a characteristic of the healthy eye (Montes-Mico 2007). This film, is composed of three distinct layers, lipo-philic layer, glycoprotein-rich layer, and aqueous layer which are secreted and regulated by meibomian glands, lacrimal glands, and goblet cells of the conjunctival epithelium, respectively (Dartt 2004, McCaa 1982). This smooth liquid layer perfectly polishes and protects the corneal surface from infection and possible injury and also reduces the surface friction during eye move-ment and blinking. Tear film is a buffered (pH of 7.2–7.5) aqueous solution with a turnover rate of 15–30% per minute. This relatively fast turnover rate causes drug loss within 15–30 s after application by constant tear flow which results in low bioavailability of topical eye preparations. Tear film complex is vital for the maintenance of eye health, thus novel DDS should effectively circumvent this highly regulated optimal composition. In this regard, gel-forming systems are introduced as a novel topical DDS. The bioavailability of gels directly depends on their formulation constituent but the longer ocu-lar surface contact time is resulted in increased bioavailability as compared to the solutions. For example, Gelrite™ used in the formulation of Timoptic-XEI, results in bleb formation that physically slows the drainage of timolol while other gelling agents may only increase the viscosity (Shedden et al. 2001). Prolonged pharmacological response has been achieved using muco-adhesive (Ludwig 2005) and thermo-sensitive *in situ* gel-forming DDS (Cao et al. 2007). More recently, a nanoemulsion of dorzolamide is formulated as *in situ* gel-forming delivery system with enhanced ocular bioavailability (Ammar et al. 2010). It should be noted that gel-forming ophthalmic solutions may decrease functional visual activity and increase ocular higher-order aberration, but these effects are less and shorter than the ointment formula-tions (Yamamoto et al. 2011).

11.2.2 Corneal Route and Barrier

The cornea is an important barrier that protects the intraocular tissues by limiting the traverse of exogenous substances. In fact, the cornea imposes this role by both mechanical and chemical barrier properties. The human cornea is a clear and avascular structure composed of five distinctive layers:

(i) corneal epithelium which rests on a basement membrane supported by (ii) Bowman's layer; (iii) corneal stroma (substantia propria) which mainly consists of collagen lamellae and supported by (iv) Descemet's membrane and finally (v) supporting endothelial cell layer (Fischbarg 2006, Sunkara and Kompella 2003). Figure 11.2 represents the cornea and corneal cellular organization of various transport-limiting layers as well as its carrier-mediated transport machineries.

Corneal epithelium has a thickness of about 55.8 ± 3.3 µm (Schmoll et al. 2012) and is formed by a thin multicellular layers, including superficial, wing, and basal cells that are morphologically maintained by several cell–cell and cell–substrate interactions. They originate from corneoscleral limbus, and

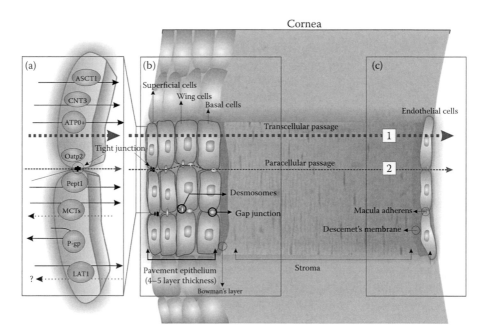

FIGURE 11.2
Corneal cellular organization and transporters. The outer superficial epithelial cells (maximized in panel a) form the tight junctional impediments, which attached to several layers of avascular epithelial cells (b) and biomembranes with a layer of endothelial cells (c) that form the cornea. Topical drug trafficking into the anterior chamber is achieved through transcellular pathway (1), while the outer superficial epithelial cells restrictively control paracellular transportation (2). The inner endothelial cells (c) display macula adherens and are more permeable. Corneal transport machineries (a) selectively controls corneal inward/outward transportation. ASCT, Na+-dependent small neutral amino acid transporter (L-alanine); MCTs, onocarboxylate transporters (lactate, pyruvates, and ketones); CNT3, concentrative nucleoside transporter 3 (thymidine); Oatp2, organic anion transporting polypeptides 2 (unknown); LAT1, large neutral amino acids transporter (L-phenylalanine); P-gp, P-glycoprotein (verpamil and fluorescein); ATB0+, concentrative amino acids transporter (carnitine, valacyclovir, and valganciclovir); Pept1, proton-coupled oligopeptide transporter (POT) di/tripeptide transporter 1 (valacyclovir, valganciclovir, glycylsarcosine, and cephalexin).

then migrate toward the anterior surface of the corneal epithelium where morphologically they become flattened. The corneal epithelium entails a high resistance of the cornea and selectively controls the transport of exogenous materials from apical, basolateral membranes, and also the paracellular pathway (Marshall and Klyce 1983). Cellular junctional proteins such as Cludin-1, Ocludin, zonula occludens (ZO-1 and ZO-2), and desmosomes are distributed in the corneal epithelium (Imayasu et al. 2008, Yi et al. 2000), forming a continuous seal around the epithelial cells, thereby preventing the passage of polar drug molecules into the cornea.

The Bowman's layer (1.87 ± 2.5 µm) (Schmoll et al. 2012) is located between the superficial cells and the stroma and constitutes 85–90% of the corneal mass (Hornof et al. 2005). This layer in fact is a modified and acellular part of the stroma, which has an elastic structure regulating the corneal shape and is mainly composed of strong collagen fibers with a highly hydrophilic nature and is mainly considered as a diffusional barrier (Hornof et al. 2005). Corneal stroma (or substantia propria) is a thick layer (about 90% of the corneal thickness) and mainly composed of hydrated collagen fibrils and functions as a barrier to highly lipophilic drugs. Descemet's membrane is a transparent, highly elastic, and homogenous layer covering the inner surface of the cornea. It provides basement structure for the corneal endothelium and mainly is composed of type IV collagen and laminin. The corneal endothelial monolayer (4–6 µm thick) is formed by hexagonally shaped cells lying on the inner/posterior surface of the cornea facing the anterior chamber of the eye. The abundance of endothelial intracellular organelles (i.e., mitochondria, endoplasmic reticulum, Golgi apparatus, and free ribosomes) and a large nucleus imply metabolic and secretory activity. The corneal endothelia actively govern the transport process across the posterior surface of the cornea and are the main regulators of corneal transparency and hydration. In fact, the corneal endothelial cells display a polarized structure and function, so the distribution of certain transport systems is different in basolateral and apical membranes. The corneal endothelia cells are interdigitated by various junctional complexes (e.g., zonola occludens, macular, and macula adherents), lacking desmosomes (as opposed to corneal epithelia). In addition, the presence of gap junctional complexes results in a leaky barrier to aqueous humor. The leakiness of the corneal endothelia correlates well with the low (20–60 Ω cm^2) transendothelial electrical resistance (Fischbarg et al. 2006), while capillary endothelial cell membranes often display significantly higher bioelectrical resistances as reported for brain microvasculature endothelial cells (>1500 Ω cm^2) (Omidi et al. 2003a, Smith et al. 2007). Although the cornea endothelium is leaky, it is the site of the major active ion and fluid transport mechanisms that maintain constant corneal thickness. Drug molecules traverse across the cornea mainly via passive diffusion although carrier-/receptor-mediated transport systems may also be involved. The partitioning and diffusion potentials of pharmaceuticals within the cellular lipid bilayers are the main driving forces, regardless of the poor bioavailability (<5%)

of the topically used drugs even for small lipophilic molecules (Kyyronen and Urtti 1990). As for many cellular organizations, drug penetration across the cornea into the eye mainly depends on the physicochemical properties of the compound, including octanol–water partition coefficient, molecular weight, solubility, and ionization state. Generally, lipophilic drugs penetrate faster and to a greater extent through the cornea as compared with hydrophilic drugs; furthermore, the greater the molecular size, the less the rate of paracellular permeation. The permeability across corneal epithelia is greater for drugs with higher distribution coefficient. While the permeability of the endothelial layer of the cornea was shown to depend on both distribution coefficient and molecular size; that is, both lipophilic pathway across cells (related to the distribution coefficient) and hydrophilic pathway between cells (related to the molecular size) are involved. Since the endothelium is not a uniquely rate-limiting barrier, it is not considered as a pivotal corneal barrier for drug substances (Prausnitz and Noonan 1998). Considering the corneal impediment, locally administered drugs diffuse into the aqueous humor and anterior uvea, but they are less likely to acquire the desired therapeutic concentration in the retina and vitreous (Duvvuri et al. 2003). Nevertheless, novel nanotechnology-based approaches appear to provide a promising platform for such implementation, for example, the efficiency of polymeric nanostructures (e.g., PLGA or poly-epsilon-caprolacton) has been verified for intraocular targeting of NSAIDs (Valls et al. 2008). Further, the conjunctiva and sclera can provide anterior routes for new potential biotech drugs and macromolecules such as protein and peptide drugs and gene medicines (Barar et al. 2008, Cai et al. 2008).

11.2.3 Noncorneal Route: Conjunctiva and Sclera

The noncorneal route, the so-called conjunctival/scleral pathway, is a competing and parallel route of absorption, which is a minor absorption pathway compared to the corneal route, but for a few compounds its contribution is significant.

The conjunctiva is a mucous transparent membrane, covering the anterior surface of the sclera and lining the inner surface of the eyelids continuously with the cornea. This layer is composed of three membranous structures: (i) the palpebral conjunctiva, the most adhering segment that covers the posterior surface of the eyelids; (ii) the bulbar conjunctiva, coating the anterior part of the eyeball; and (iii) the fornix as a transition part that forms the junction between the eyelid posterior and the eyelid. The conjunctival epithelium plays an important role as a protective barrier on the ocular surface, and it contributes to the maintenance of the tear film by the production of mucus glycoproteins. Apical surface of the conjunctiva epithelium contains functional tight junctional structures so it is also considered as a permeability barrier too (Amaral et al. 2005, Yoshida et al. 2009). In rabbits, the paracellular permeation via the conjunctiva and sclera were 15–25 times greater than the cornea and was affected by the molecular size to a lesser extent (Hamalainen et al. 1997a). By displaying the tight junctions on the apical surface, with a bioelectrical resistance of over 1500 Ω cm^2 (Saha et al. 1996), the conjunctival epithelium has a key role in the control of intra-ocular traverse of substances. Pore size and density of the corneal and conjunctival epithelia has been characterized in rabbits; the results show that the epithelia of conjunctiva presents two times larger pore size with 16 times higher pore density than cornea resulting in almost 230 times greater paracellular space. This provide higher permeability and larger absorptive surface area for ocular delivery of macromolecules (Hamalainen et al. 1997a).

A markedly large amount of the administered pharmaceutical is usually carried by the systemic circulation away while crossing the conjunctiva and the remaining drug penetrates across the sclera to reach the posterior parts (i.e., the uveal tract, the retina, the choroid, and the vitreous humor) (Diebold and Calonge 2010, Edelhauser et al. 2010). Various transporters were shown to be expressed in the conjunctival epithelium. Among them, neutral and cationic amino acids transporter (ATB$^{O,+}$), nucleoside transporter (CNT2), and peptide transporter (PepT1) can be exploited for delivery of various substrates (e.g., acyclovir) (Hosoya et al. 2005b). The functional expression of efflux pumps, including P-glycoprotein (P-gp) and multidrug resistance proteins (MRPs) have also been reported (Gaudana et al. 2010, Yang et al. 2007). However, despite the potential importance of endocytotic pathway for drug delivery, specially nanomedicines, the role of caveolae and/or clathrin-mediated transport in the conjunctiva is yet to be fully revealed. For a comprehensive study of the conjunctival transport systems readers are directed to refer to Hosoya et al. (2005a). There are evidences that the uptake of PLGA NPs in primary cultured conjunctiva epithelial cells is most likely mediated by adsorptive endocytosis. Regarding intraocular delivery of NP, profound study of the role of endocytotic pathway is indeed crucial.

The sclera, an opaque, fibrous layer is continuous with the cornea and extends from the limbus. This layer is mainly composed of collagen and elastin fibers and mucopolysaccharides (Chakravarti et al. 2003). The sclera is poorly vascularized and its permeability is about 10 times more than the cornea but half of the conjunctiva (Ahmed 2003). It is supposed that drugs passing through the sclera can enter the posterior part of the eye, that is, uveal tract, retina, choroid, and vitreous humor. The feasibility of scleral route has been exploited for the delivery of therapeutically active biodrugs (Ambati et al. 2000), so this route may be considered as a less invasive method for NP-based formulations in the treatment of a variety of chorioretinal disorders.

The conjunctival/scleral pathway is considered as the main cause of poor bioavailability of drugs entering the eye (Ahmed 2003) and the remaining drug is then subjected to diffusion via sclera. However, drainage loss through blood vessels of the conjunctiva can greatly impact the conjunctival/scleral pathway. Therefore, this noncorneal route is considered to be nonproductive for most of the ophthalmic drugs, but it should be evoked that the conjuncti-val epithelium is the most viable route for the ocular delivery of peptides and oligonucleotides (Hamalainen et al. 1997b, Schoenwald et al. 1997).

11.2.4 Blood–Aqueous Barrier

BAB is formed in the anterior part of the eye and is structurally comprised of the iris/ciliary blood vessels' endothelium and the nonpigmented ciliary epithelium (Freddo 2001) (Figure 11.1). The tight junctional complexes are displayed in these cells and impede the unspecific traverse of solutes into the intraocular milieu and maintain the transparency and chemical compo-sition of ocular fluids (Freddo 2001). Evaluation of barrier properties of BAB revealed that although iris blood vessels are very tight, the ciliary capillaries are fenestrated and allow penetration of low level of plasma proteins into the aqueous humor (Schlingemann et al. 1998). Various physiological/pathologi-cal conditions such as inflammation may disrupt the integrity of this barrier causing the unlimited drug distribution to the anterior chamber (Urtti 2006). The traverse of substances from the aqueous humor into systemic circulation through the iris microvasculature endothelia implies that it is less restricted. Hence, the drugs dissolved in the aqueous humor can easily penetrate the anterior surface of the iris and absorbed by the iris pigments; thereafter, they are washed from the anterior chamber away by passage into the iris blood vessels (Urtti 2006). The small and lipophilic drugs were shown to enter the uveal blood circulation via the BAB, from where they are eliminated more rapidly than larger and more hydrophilic drugs, which are eliminated by aqueous humor turnover only (Toda et al. 2011). Drug transport from the anterior segment to the posterior segment cannot be considered as an appli-cable strategy, due to the continuous drainage of the aqueous humor (i.e., a turnover of 2.0–3.0 mL/min). Accordingly, the locally used ophthalmic therapies fail to provide an efficient pharmacological effect in the posterior segment (e.g., the retina and the vitreous). The novel therapeutic strategies like intravitreal injections and subconjunctival implants also seem to grant only limited success (Mitra et al. 2006b).

11.2.5 Retina and BRB

Retina is a thin layer formed from neural cells and glial cells (i.e., Müller cells, astrocytes, microglial cells, and oligodendroglial cells) covering the inner wall of the eye (la Cour and Ehinger 2006). The outer part of the ret-ina is composed of a single layer of pigmented cuboidal epithelial cells, the so-called retinal pigment epithelium (RPE) (la Cour and Ehinger 2006) as presented in Figure 11.3. RPE is situated between the neural retina and the choroid and have several functions such as maintenance of the BRB prop-erties and composition of sub-retinal fluid and phagocytosis. Targeting the retina (as for diseases such as proliferative vitreo retinopathy, diabetic

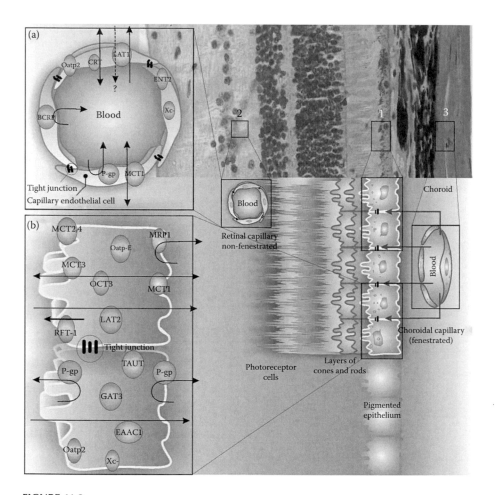

FIGURE 11.3
Retinal cellular organization, barriers and transporters. The outer layer of retinal pigmented epithelium (1) and the inner layer retinal capillary endothelial cells (2) display tight junctions, but not the choroidal capillary endothelial cells (3). Retinal endothelia (a) and epithelia (b) have carrier-mediated transporters. MCTs, monocarboxylate transporters (lactate, pyruvates, and ketones); EAAC, glutamate transporter; ENT2, equilibrium nucleoside transporter 2 (thymidine); Oatp2, organic anion transporting polypeptides 2; LAT1, large neutral amino acids transporter (L-phenylalanine); P-gp, P-glycoprotein (verpamil and vincristin); MRP, multidrug resistance proteins; BCRP, breast cancer–related protein; CRT, creatine transporter; GAT3, GABA transporter; OCT, organic cation transporter; RFT, reduced folate/thiamine transporter; Xc-, glutamate/cysteine exchange transporter; TAUT, taurine transporter.

retinopathy, and age-related macular degeneration [AMD]) is a challenging issue due to the presence of multiple barriers. However, the subretinal route of drug injection allows direct administration of the drug to the RPE and since the RPE cells display phagocytic properties, the particulate DDS such as NPs, may provide a higher intracellular drug level. Hayashi et al.

have shown that IgG adsorbed to the surface of gold NPs can be successfully delivered into photoreceptor cells and RPE (Hayashi et al. 2009).

BRB is located in the posterior segment of the eye and is formed by two types of the endothelial cells in the inner and outer parts, namely the retinal capillary endothelial (RCE) cells and RPE cells, respectively. The inner BRB, RCE cells, cover the lumen of retinal capillaries separating the retina from circulating agents and comprises the microvascular endothelium which lines these vessels. This layer possesses intercellular tight junctional complexes (Gardner et al. 1999), which maintain retina–environment balance. Figure 11.3 demonstrates the retina, retinal cellular organization, and carrier-mediated transport machineries of RPE and RCE cells. Specialized transport processes within the RPE, along with the robust barrier restrictiveness of RPE, control the traverse of nutrients/compounds selectively, at which only selected nutrients are exchanged between the choroid and the retina (Macha and Mitra 2003, Mitra et al. 2006a). Despite the permeation of lipophilic compounds across RCE cells, it is very restricted for the traverse of proteins and small hydrophilic substances (Sunkara and Kompella 2003). In fact, barrier functionality of RCE is similar to that of BBB, while evidence of ultrastructural study reveals the presence of high-density interendothelial junction and endothelial vesicles (Stewart and Tuor 1994). However, existence of high number of pericytes in retinal cells may act as a compensatory line to lower the permeability.

Outer BRB play a central role in retinal physiology and function by regulating the movement of the solutes and nutrients from choroid to the subretinal space. In addition to forming the outer-retinal barrier layer, RPE cells, have many other specialized functions such as supporting the photoreceptors, synthesis of enzymes, growth factors and pigments and regulating the immune reactivity of the retina (Hornof et al. 2005).

BRB is considered as a major obstacle for drug delivery to the retina and the vitreous humor. The systemic route of drug administration is basically constrained by restricted permeation across BRB, and intravitreal administration is associated with some other issues (i.e., patient incompliance and adverse consequence). Regarding optimal drug delivery, development of robust/ideal DDS for targeting of retinal tissue and vitreous has attracted many researchers (Duvvuri et al. 2003). Substantial delivery and sufficient pharmacological effects of drugs within the vitreous and the retina necessitate systemic or intravitreal drug administration. A systemic application, via oral or intravenous administration, requires high doses of the drug since blood flow and restrictive functionality of the BRB allow only a very small fraction of the drug to reach the posterior segment (Hosoya et al. 2011). Taking advantage of the expression of various transport systems and receptors in the cell membrane, targeting such machineries may be considered as a suitable strategy to enhance the poor bioavailability and to overcome the poor permeability concerns. The potent ability of nanomedicines, as a tailor-based system can be simply achieved by engineering their surface, size, structure, and shape. This provides both passive and active targeted DDS.

11.3 Ocular Drug-Delivery Mechanisms

To enter the cellular interior, any compound needs to cross biological membranes and barriers. Cell membrane imposes a barrier functionality to restrict the free traverse of particles/solutes via lipid bilayer. However, the necessary compounds are shuttled into target site via passive/active pathways by employing various transport machineries, that is, carrier-mediated or endocytosis/transcytosis mechanisms.

11.3.1 Simple Passive Transport

Passive transport across the virtually all cell membranes is nonspecific and requires no energy. Molecules such as dissolved gases (e.g., O_2 and CO_2), small uncharged molecules and hydrophobic substances traverse the phospholipid bilayer in a direct proportion of their concentration gradient. Furthermore, lipid solubility and partitionation in the membranous lipid bed is a key factor in determination of the diffusion extent and rate of hydrophobic molecules. On the other hand, facilitated transport (carrier-mediated diffusion) is employed for the transport of vital ions or glucose in their concentration gradient direction in a higher rate compared to simple passive diffusion. For instance, it is well known that nearly all ocular tissues comprise transport machineries for the regulation of intracellular pH, that is, Na^+/H^+ and Cl^-/HCO_3^- exchanger and Na^+/HCO_3^+ symporter (Jentsch et al. 1986a,b).

11.3.2 Carrier-Mediated Transport

There exist a number of uni/bidirectional influx/efflux transporters that assist in the essential nutrient supply of the cells such as glucose transporters (e.g., Glut1), amino acid transporters (LAT1 and LAT2), peptide transporters (Pepts), and monocarboxylate transporters (MCTs) (Omidi and Gumbleton 2005).

The glucose transporter expression and functionality have been extensively studied; Kaulen and coworkers confirmed the widespread localization of this transporter in ciliary body, iris, retinal and in some species in the trabecular meshwork and lens (Kaulen et al. 1991). The Glut-1 is expressed in all of the endothelial and epithelial barriers of the eye (Kumagai et al. 1994); further its colocalization with occluding and ZO-1 in mouse blood ocular barrier has been revealed (Tserentsoodol et al. 1998). LAT1 expression and functionality has been extensively studied in other tissues, for example, brain capillary endothelial cells (Omidi et al. 2008a), but not characterized in the ocular bio-membranes. However, distribution and role of cationic amino acid transporters (CATs) in ocular tissue have been studied (Jager et al. 2009); CAT1 and CAT2 (but not CAT3) are expressed in ocular surface as well as lacrimal apparatus that are differently regulated in various pathophysiological conditions. Ocular membrane transporters possess a main challenge for xenobiotic delivery and targeting of the eye and have been discussed broadly; readers are directed to see Dey et al. (2003).

11.3.3 Ocular Transport Machineries

Cell membranes impose a barrier to the free movement of molecules through a membranous lipid bilayer and associated transport machineries. A solute, based upon molecular properties, is transported across the cell membranes by passive diffusion and/or carrier/receptor-mediated transport (Omidi and Gumbleton 2005). Nearly most of the ocular tissue displays Na^+/H^+ exchanger, Na^+/HCO_3^- symporter, and Cl^-/HCO_3^- exchanger that are involved in the regulation of intracellular pH (Jentsch et al. 1986a). The Na^+/H^+ exchanger is present at the basolateral membranes of both epithelial and endothelial cells, while Na^+/HCO_3^- transporter is predominantly localized at the basolateral side of the corneal endothelium and is faintly expressed in the corneal epithelium. This implies that the distribution pattern of these transporters at the apical and basolateral membrane varies depending upon the cellular needs and physiologic functions.

The influx and efflux transport machineries are functionally expressed in the main membranous barriers of the eye, that is, the cornea; the conjunctiva, the iris–ciliary body, and the retina (see Figure 11.3). The unidirectional/bidirectional influx transporters such as monocarboxylate transporters (MCTs), glucose transporters (e.g., Glut1), amino acid transporters (LAT1 and LAT2), and PepT1 supply essential nutrient requirements of the cells. The LAT1 transporter of the brain capillary endothelial cells functions bidirectionally with greater efflux activity (Omidi et al. 2008a). However, its functional directionality in the corneal/retinal barriers is yet to be fully investigated and so are most of the carrier-mediated transporters in the eye.

In the ATP-binding cassette (ABC) superfamily, the P-gp and MRPs play a key role in the unidirectional efflux of substances (Senthilkumari et al. 2008). The human and rabbit corneal epithelia were shown to significantly express P-gp and MRPs (Karla et al. 2007). Similarly, these efflux pumps have been identified in different tissues of the eye, such as the RCE cells, the retinal pigmented epithelial cells, the ciliary nonpigmented epithelium, the conjunctival epithelial cells, and the iris and ciliary endothelial cells. On grounds of the current knowledge about the functional expression of efflux transporters in ocular tissues, useful modification of drug-delivery strategies is expected in order to increase ocular bioavailability and to harness ophthalmic diseases in a more efficient way (Gaudana et al. 2010, Thrimawithana et al. 2011).

Specialized receptors exist at the ocular barriers to control the passage of xenobiotics. The endocytosis pathway via clathrin-coated and/or caveolae (noncoated/smooth) vesicles are accounted for ocular receptor-mediated transports. The expression of clathrin and the integral protein of the caveolae domain (caveolin-1) as the main routes for internalization of macromolecules have been reported (Contreras-Ruiz et al. 2011, Delgado et al. 2012). Using cultured human retinal pigment epithelial cells (ARPE-19) and a mouse model, Mo et al. reported the involvement of caveolae-mediated endocytosis pathways in the uptake of albumin NPs containing Cu/Zn superoxide dismutase gene (Mo et al. 2007). However, Qaddoumi et al. showed that the endocytosis of the poly(lactic-*co*-glycolic) acid (PLGA) NPs in primary cultured rabbit conjunctival epithelial cells occurs mostly independently of clathrin- and caveolin-1-mediated pathways, despite the transcriptome and protein expression of clathrin (Qaddoumi et al. 2003). Further, the transport of albumin in the rabbit lens epithelial cells revealed the involvement of a transcellular transport mechanism, employing both clathrin- and caveolae-mediated endocytosis/transcytosis pathways (Sabah et al. 2007). Expression of insulin and insulin-like growth factor (IGF)-1 receptors (Ainscough et al. 2009, Rocha et al. 2002) along with transferrin receptor (Kompella et al. 2006) in the ocular cells infer intricacy and ambiguity of macromolecular transportation in the eye, which yet to be fully understood.

11.3.4 Endocytosis and Transcytosis

Receptors are mainly involved in endocytosis or transcytosis of compounds, which contribute to some degree of specificity or selectivity. Clatrin-mediated vesicular uptake is more scrutinized and accounts for most of the receptor-mediated delivery, though caveolae route or other unidentified pathways are not negligible. The existed literature clearly reveals that clathrin (Bando et al. 2007, Dey et al. 2003) and the main structural and functional protein of caveolea, caveolin-1 (Cenedella et al. 2006, Kuehn et al. 2011, Perdue and Yan 2006), are both expressed in various ocular cells, however their functionality is open for further examination. In an examination of clathrin and caveolin-1, Qaddoumi et al. reported the lack of caveolin-1 expression in rabbit conjuctival epithelial primary cells, despite its expression in epithelium of the cornea and trachea. Interestingly they showed clathrin-independent endocytosis of PLGA NPs, despite morphologic evidence for the expression of clathrin protein (Qaddoumi et al. 2003). Recently, the internalization of chitosan-alginate NPs containing carboplatin has been studied in a model of retinoblastoma cell line, Y79; exhibiting a key role for clathrin-mediated endocytosis (Parveen et al. 2010). On the contrary, in a more recent study of hyaluronic acid-chitosan NPs as a vehicle for a model plasmid DNA delivery, two different ocular cells were investigated. The results confirmed caveolae was the dominant mechanism of uptake engaging hyaluronan receptor in both conjunctiva and cornea epithelial cell lines (Contreras-Ruiz et al. 2011).

Mo and coworkers also showed the evidence of caveolae-mediated delivery of NPs of Cu, Zn superoxidase gene formulated using human serum albumin in the human retinal pigment epithelial (Mo et al. 2007). Mounted evidence reveals direct modulatory role of albumin in the internalization by means of caveolae invaginations (Moriyama et al. 2011, Pelkmans and Helenius 2002, Schubert et al. 2001, Tiruppathi et al. 2004), hence this strategy seems to trigger intracellular transport of therapeutic agents.

Utilizing such an approach, rapid, and efficient delivery of intact NPs into and/or across cornea and conjunctiva, an *ex vivo* bovine eye model has been reported, where the surface of NPs were conjugated to the known ligands of cell surface receptors (i.e., a luteinizing hormone-releasing hormone agonist or transferrin) in order to overcome the barrier properties of the corneal epithelium (Kompella et al. 2006).

11.3.5 Topical Absorption of Ocular Drug

Corneal and/or noncorneal routes are the main approaches for the local drug therapy of the eye. However, it should be noted that in the eye cul-de-sac, the medications are subjected to some physiological/biological barriers. First, the administered pharmaceuticals may be carried away by the lacrimal fluids. Second, inevitable systemic absorption occurs through the conjunctival sac as well as the nasal cavity. The corneal route represents the main absorption path for most of the ophthalmic therapeutics. However, corneal absorption is also considered to be a rate-limiting process due to the presence of the corneal epithelium. The second path involves penetration across the conjunctiva and sclera into the intraocular tissues; however, this path appears to be less productive due to the presence of the local capillary beds that remove the drug from target sites to the general circulation. Despite this drawback, poor corneal permeability compounds such as timolol maleate, gentamicin, and prostaglandin PGF_2 α were shown to reach the intraocular section through diffusion across the conjunctiva and sclera. Thus, the absorption mechanism depends mostly on the physiochemical characteristics of the compounds and the biological membranes and barriers of the target tissue; the reader is directed to see Davies 2000, Koevary 2003, Wilson 2004.

11.4 Ocular Pharmacotherapy

The mechanisms such as reflex blinking, lacrimation, tear turnover, and drainage impose absorption problem to the topically applied ophthalmic drugs, resulting in poor absorption of the administered pharmaceuticals and rapid removal of foreign substances from the eye surface. Thus, to maintain a therapeutic drug level in the tear film or at the site of action, repeated instillations of eyedrops are inevitable. However, such frequent use of medications can induce inadvertent consequences due to exposure of highly concentrated drug solutions to the ocular tissues, hence resulting in undesired side effects at the ocular surface. While conventional pharmaceuticals are often associated with such predictable bioimpacts, advanced pharmaceuticals may provide better corollaries with high patient's compliance. Thus, here, we intend to provide an overview on the conventional and advanced pharmaceuticals used for eye diseases.

11.4.1 Conventional Pharmacotherapy of Ocular Diseases

Conventional pharmaceuticals (e.g., eye drops, gels, creams, and ointments) are widely used for the treatment of some eye diseases. In general, the lower is the solubility of a drug in the vehicle, the higher is the chemical potential and the more readily is the drug partitioning into the release medium. Thus, various ocular pharmaceuticals (viscous gel, cream, or ointment) have been designed to release the drugs basically through diffusion and partitioning. Delivery of macromolecules can be more sustained in hydrogels compare to small drug molecule such as pilocarpine and the design of sustained-release dosage forms is largely dependent upon physicochemical properties of drugs and biological site of application. The ophthalmic formulations usually contain high concentrations of their active ingredients because of the relatively poor penetration of the topical use. Therefore, the conventional dosage forms may elicit toxic effects in ocular cells/tissues. To attain successful treatment outcomes, in particular for drugs such as antibiotics, the repeated injections of drugs into the intraocular tissues appear to be indispensable even though it may inevitably increase the risk of retinal detachment or hemorrhage. In the case endophthalmitis, for example, the intravitreal injections of antibiotics along with the adjunctive i.v. injection of antibiotics may be beneficial although the effectiveness of the adjunctive i.v. injection of antibiotics appeared to be skeptical because of restrictive blockage of BRB, and also unembellished systemic toxicity may limit such use. Further, no ideal antibiotic exists for intravitreal use with a broad spectrum of action and a long half-life in the vitreous yet with no/minimal toxicity on the eye (Ashton 2006). It has been reported that the topical pharmacotherapy of the eye may be significantly influenced by some factors such as the drainage of the instilled solution, lacrimation and tear turnover, metabolism, tear evaporation, nonproductive absorption, limited corneal area and poor corneal permeability, and binding by lacrimal proteins (Mitra et al. 2006a). Therefore, sufficient corneal penetration and prolonged contact time with the corneal tissue is of essence for effective and successful ocular drug absorption. To increase drug absorption in the eye, various modalities have been investigated, including: sustained-release formulations such as biodegradable implants (Lee et al. 2010), device DDS (e.g., collagen shields, iontophoresis, and pumps iontophoresis) (Eljarrat-Binstock et al. 2008, Friedberg et al. 1991), prodrugs such as acyclovir dipeptide esters (Anand et al. 2006, Jwala et al. 2011), ion pair formation (Higashiyama et al. 2006), bioadhesives, and mucoadhesives (Kaur and Smitha 2002).

In addition to topical pharmacotherapy, ocular diseases in posterior segments (retinal pathologies such as fungal and bacterial endophthalmitis, viral retinitis, and proliferative vitreal retinopathies) require systemic administration. Nevertheless, systemic pharmacotherapy of the eye is often attributed with limited success mainly because of the excellent BRB restrictiveness excluding the organ from systemic circulation (Barar et al. 2008) and selectively control the inward and outward travers by transport machineries (Tomi and Hosoya 2010). For example, foscarnet sodium or ganciclovir is used to treat cytomegalovirus (CMV) retinitis and endophthalmitis as intravenous or intravitreal injections, while intravitreal injection liposomal formulation of foscarnet appeared to show better pharmacokinetics (Claro et al. 2009). In short, the intravitreal injection of ophthalmologic drugs seems to be the only beneficial treatment of the posterior segment infections/diseases, nevertheless it may also associate with some concerns such as patient noncompliance and endophthalmitis, cataract, astigmatism, and retinal detachment (Shah et al. 2010, Thrimawithana et al. 2011). To circumvent these complications, intravitreal implants have been developed (Fialho et al. 2008, Ghosh et al. 2002, Mruthyunjaya et al. 2006), even though the scleral implants (Schepens and Acosta 1991) and subconjunctival implants (Peng et al. 2011) may attribute with somewhat limited success, mainly because of the repeated need for surgical intervention associated with the presence of a foreign device within the eye.

For noninvasive intraocular delivery, some major considerations should be taken into account, including: (1) safe passage of a drug across the cornea to reach the site of the action, (2) prolong duration of drug action within the target site to minimize the frequency of drug administration, (3) specific targeting of the desired biomarkers to localize the desired pharmacodynamic action with minimal impacts on nonspecific tissues, and (4) effective evading from BAB. While most of the currently used medications for the treatment of the ocular diseases (e.g., glaucoma, conjunctivitis, keratitis, and uveitis) were shown to have bioavailability problems (Mitra et al. 2006a), novel advanced technologies are deemed to favor ocular pharmacotherapy. The ocular DDS have so far been improved by development of prodrugs, use of penetration enhancers, and advancement of novel pharmaceuticals (Sultana et al. 2011, Vandervoort and Ludwig 2007). Of these, multifunctional multimodal nanomedicines appear to be the mainstay platform for advanced medicines. Thus, we will discuss this approach in more detail.

11.4.2 Ocular Nanopharmaceuticals

Circumventing the clearance mechanisms of the eye, nanoformulations possess capability of longer exposure time at the ocular surface resulting

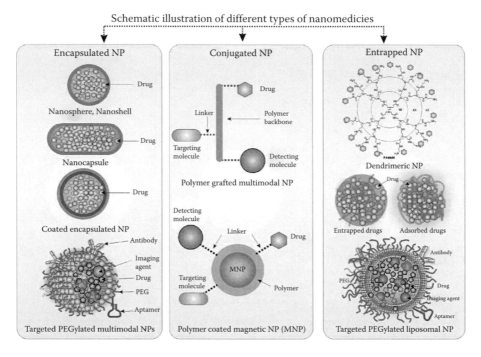

FIGURE 11.4
Schematic illustration of polymer- and lipid-based nanoformulations.

in increased drug concentration and decreased dose and frequency of pharmacotherapy. Figure 11.4 represents schematic illustration of various kinds of nanoformulations.

These nanoformulations can be used for intraocular drug delivery in a controlled manner to reduce the number of injections required and target the site of action with the drug, leading to a decrease in the dose as well as adverse reactions. Despite these benefits, cost-effectiveness and some other problems (e.g., formulation stability, particle size, and control of drug release) are considered as major issues for large-scale production of sterile nanoformulations.

Recently, indomethacin-loaded chitosan (CS) NPs have been produced using modified ionic gelation of the polymer with tripolyphosphate, in which NPs displayed regular well-identified spherical shapes (~280 nm with zeta potential of +17 mV) with 84.8% loading efficiency. Slight initial burst release during the first hour followed by slow and gradual indomethacin release of 76% during a 24-hour period have been revealed during *in vitro* studies (Badawi et al. 2008). Various polymers have been used for construction of polymeric NPs for ocular delivery. PLGA, poly(alkylcyanoacrylate) (PACA), and poly-e-caprolactone (PCL) have been exploited to formulate polymeric nanosuspensions containing anti-inflammatory agents (diclofenac), which were used in rabbit eyes with no sign of irritation or damaging effects to ocular tissues (Agnihotri and Vavia 2009). Also, mucoadhesive microdiscs have been engineered by emulsification methodology with PLGA as a core material and, in some cases, polyethylene glycol (PEG) as a mucoadhesion promoter resulting in enhanced preocular residence time (Choy et al. 2008).

Modified-release liposomal nanoformulations for ocular delivery seem to confer an excellent constitution for increased drug consistency, enhance direct delivery, minimize intraocular toxicity, and controlled ocular delivery by preventing the drug metabolism from the enzymes present at the tear/corneal epithelial surface (Diebold et al. 2007). These are literally examples of unarmed simple nanoformulations that can be grafted with targeting and imaging devices.

The nanostructures are often prone to elimination by reticuloendothelial system (RES) which can predominantly limit the clinical efficacy of systemically administered nanomedicines. RES elimination is largely dependent upon the anatomy and size of NPs, so that NPs >250 nm can be physically trapped by the fenestrations in the spleen while NPs <70 nm can be accumulated in the liver. Thus, NPs in a range of 70–200 nm are able to stay in blood stream for a longer period (Shan et al. 2009). These NPs are predisposed to opsonization, a process that leads the foreign particulate to be covered by opsonins and seen by phagocytic cells (Moghimi and Szebeni 2003, Owens and Peppas 2006). To avoid this phenomenon, NPs are PEGylated. But, regardless of being PEGylated, a 250 nm PEGylated NP can be cleared from the blood stream much more rapidly than a 70 nm PEGylated NP. It is the same for nonstealth NPs, even though size is very important that is, a 250 nm non-PEGylated or PEGylated NP can be removed much faster than a 70 nm PEGylated NP.

11.4.3 Liposomal Nanomedicines

The vesicular lipid bilayers are basically defined as "liposomes," which can contain one or more aqueous compartments. Upon the number of bilayers, these lipid-based globular structures can be categorized into multilamellar and unilamellar vesicles. Drugs, based on their solubility characteristics, can be entrapped in the lipid bilayers or the aqueous compartment. Liposome's size ranges between 10 and 1000 nm and the terminology is devoted to its vesicular lipid bilayer structures, containing of one or more compartment, that is, unilamellar vesicles (ULVs; <0.5 μm) and multilamellar vesicles (MLVs; >0.5 μm), respectively (Fenwick and Cullis 2008). Figure 11.5 represents schematic illustration of various liposomal formulations.

The ULVs are further categorized by their size into small unilamellar vesicles (SUVs; ~20 to ~200 nm), large unilamellar vesicles (LUVs; ~200 nm to ~1 μm) and giant unilamellar vesicles (GUVs; >1 μm) (Mishra et al. 2011). For preparation of nanoliposomes, various methods (e.g., sonication, extrusion, microfluidization, solvent evaporation and combinations of these techniques) have been used (Mozafari 2010). In solvent evaporation method, briefly lipophilic compounds are dissolved in chloroform: methanol mixture which is

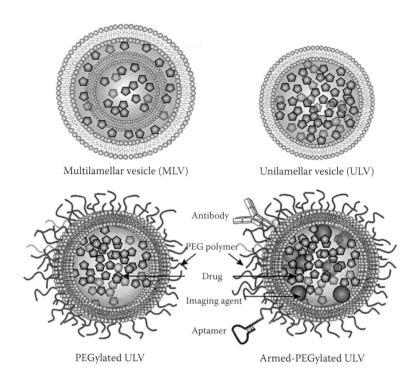

Multilamellar vesicle (MLV)   Unilamellar vesicle (ULV)

Antibody

PEG polymer

Drug

Imaging agent

Aptamer

PEGylated ULV   Armed-PEGylated ULV

FIGURE 11.5
Schematic illustration of various liposomal formulations.

then heated to form a lipid film using a rotor-evaporator at 60°C under vacuum to remove solvent residuals. The lipid film is then hydrated and extruded through polycarbonate filters with designated pore size, then sonicated to get nanosized liposomes. These nanoliposomes can be lyophilized to be kept for longer periods. Nanoliposomes (NLs) were first developed to encapsulate small conventional therapeutic drugs, in which the earliest attempts involved the passive entrapment of drugs resulted in the rapid production of stable, homogeneous populations of LUVs (~100 nm).

Liposomes are constructed by amphiphilic molecules assembling an aqueous core enclosed by a lipid bilayer. Their diversity provides enormous characteristic versatility being very attractive DDS. Furthermore, liposome resistance to thermodynamic perturbation that may happen during administration along with their stability in suspension formulations potentiate their application as a fascinating delivery vehicle over other DDS such as micellar DDS (Mishra et al. 2011). Among various DDS, NLs have widely been investigated because they present: (1) tunable size, (2) controllability on composition of liposome by exploiting various modified/bioactive lipids (e.g., thiolated lipids, fluorescent lipids, themo/pH sensitive lipids), (3) longer blood circulation through coating with polyethylene glycol (PEG), monosialoganglioside or phosphatidylinositol, for example, the STEALTH® (ALZA) liposomes that are PEGylated, (4) controlled-release profile in target site, (5) bioconjugation possibility with targeting or imaging agents (Figure 11.5), and (6) biocompatibility and significantly diminished side effects.

Liposomes are able to overcome limited permeation of poorly absorbed medicines through generating close contact with corneal and conjunctival epithelial cells, resulting in improved residence time that facilitates drug delivery to the anterior eye segment. On the other hand, successful delivery of designated drugs into the posterior segment by means of NLs is largely dependent upon: (1) enhanced intraviteral half-life, and (2) robust strategies to specifically target the target site (Mishra et al. 2011).

PEGylated and targeting device armed NLs have shown greater clinical outcomes in the posterior segment of the eye. Table 11.1 represents selected

TABLE 11.1

Selected Liposomal Nanoformulations Used as Ocular DDS

Formulation	Application	Main Findings	Reference
Ganciclovir (GCV) liposomal formulation	Two compartmental pharmacokinetic studies in albino rabbits	Higher biodistribution GCV in sclera, cornea, iris, lens, and vitreous humor	Shen and Tu (2007)
Ciprofloxacin liposomes dispersed in hydrogel	Transcorneal permeation	Greater transcorneal permeation and improved bioavailability in the rabbits eyes	Hosny (2010a)
Minocycline nanoliposomes (NLs)	Streptozotocin-induced diabetic retinopathy in Sprague Dawley rat	Successful delivery of drugs to retina by subconjunctival injection minocycline NLs	Kaiser et al. (2013)
Pigment epithelium-derived factor (PEDF) immunonaoliposomes (INLs)	Choroidal neovascularization (CNV)	Substantial inhibition of CNV by PEDF encapsulated NLs combined with ultrasonic exposure in CNV models of BN rats	Li et al. (2010)
C6-ceramide NLs	Corneal inflammation	Significant inhibition of corneal inflammation without undesired side effects in mice of corneal inflammation	Sun et al. (2008)
Bevacizumab (Avastin) NLs	Intravitreal delivery of Avastin to retina	Prolonged residency of bevacizumab NLs in the vitreous of rabbits	Abrishami et al. (2009)
Latanoprost NLs	Glaucoma	Long-term sustained delivery of latanoprost (90 days) in the rabbit eyes	Natarajan et al. (2012)
Edaravone loaded liposomes	Light-induced retinal damage (LRD)	Significant prevention of LRD in mice	Shimazaki et al. (2011)

examples of liposomal formulations for ocular applications. Once administered, NLs can come into intimate contact with corneal and conjunctival epithelial cells and facilitate the drug absorption process. Accordingly, improved ocular absorption was shown for cyclosporine A from liposomes incorporated into collagen shields (Pleyer et al. 1994), and acyclovir-containing liposomes (Law et al. 2000). NLs are not usually taken up by healthy tissue as is the free drug because the normal tissues in corneal/noncorneal routes are continuous with nonfenestrated endothelium and tight endothelial junctions that prevent the extravasation of small liposomal carriers. The basal tissues also inhibit the extravasation of macromolecules. Based upon the disease/dugs used, the NLs can be used for active targeting of designated markers resulting in preferential accumulation of encapsulated drugs within the sites of disease.

The corneal permeation of liposomal formulations depends mainly on two factors of size and charge, which occur in the order of $SUV^+ > MLV^- > SUV^-$ $> SUV > MLV > $ free drug. Besides, the physicochemical property of a drug can expressively affect the transcorneal flux of the liposomal formulation. While, the positively charged NLs display better corneal permeation than the neutral and negatively charged ones; they are also able to induce intrinsic gene expression changes leading to activation of cell death program (Omidi et al. 2008b, 2005, 2003b). In terms of injectable formulations, it should be stated that the positively charged NLs are susceptible to RES elimination process. Neutral liposomes can evade the elimination by RES, nevertheless they show higher self-aggregation tendency. PEGylated NLs with average size of 100 nm are less predisposed to opsonization and thus exhibiting significantly longer circulation time in blood (Lian and Ho 2001). Drug release from liposomal systems is dependent on the concentration of the drug in the liposome. Thus, in the case of long-term treatment, the high concentration of drugs encapsulated in liposomal carriers may cause inevitable problems such as vitreous clouding. Nonetheless, in the case of endophthalmitis, such adverse reactions can be compromised. Sometimes, liposome entrapment can decrease the efficacy of drugs as reported for amphotericin B in a rabbit model with fungal (*Candida albicans*) endophthalmitis (Barza et al. 1985).

As it is evident from the literatures, many advancements have been made in liposome formulation and variety of techniques have been developed for better drug protection (see Table 11.1), long (>6 h) circulation lifetime and elevated drug retention (Fenske et al. 2008). A single intravitreal injection of vasoactive intestinal peptide (VIP) loaded in rhodamine-conjugated liposomes (VIP-Rh-Lip) in Lewis rats with experimental autoimmune uveoretinitis (EAU) was reported to result in macrophages expressed transforming growth factor-beta2, low levels of major histocompatibility complex class II, and nitric oxide synthase-2 in VIP-Rh-Lip-treated eyes in which the intraocular levels of interleukin (IL)-2, interferon-gamma, IL-17, IL-4, GRO/KC, and CCL5 were reduced with increased IL-13 (Camelo et al. 2009). The elimination of liposomes from the vitreous occurs via a diffusional process through the anterior chamber, where SUVs and LUVs show half-life of 10 and 20 days, respectively (Barza et al. 1987). NLs have also been successfully exploited for the delivery of biotechnological drugs such as proteins-, peptides-, and gene-based therapies (plasmid-DNA containing desired genes, antisense oligonucleotides and small interference RNA, SiRNA). For example, *in vivo* efficacy of vasoactive intestinal peptide after ocular administration of liposome preparations alone (Camelo et al. 2009) or within hyaluronic acid gel (Lajavardi et al. 2009) has been approved in endotoxin and autoimmune induced uveitis, respectively. Subconjunctival injection of liposome-encapsulated tissue plasminogen activator (tPA) appeared to be effective on the absorption rate of subconjunctival hemorrhages in rabbits, showing enhanced subconjunctival hemorrhages absorption, especially during the early stages with minimal systemic and ocular absorption (Han et al. 2011). Recently, liposomal latanoprost has been formulated using egg-phosphatidylcholine and administered as a single subconjunctival injection to the rabbits to control glaucoma (Natarajan et al. 2012). Slow and sustained release characteristics (60% release in 14 days) of the *in vitro* experiments were well correlated with *in vivo* results, showing significantly lowered intraocular pressure (IOP) for up to 90 days as compared with daily administration of topical latanoprost with no signs of inflammation. In 2010, Zhang et al. reported that intravitreal injection of liposomal tacrolimus (FK506), which is an immunosuppressive drug, in Lewis rats with experimental autoimmune uveoretinitis (EAU) can highly effectively suppress the process of EAU without any side effect on retinal function or systemic cellular immunity (Zhang et al. 2010).

So far, a few liposomal formulations have been approved by FDA. Liposomal amphotericin B, as an eye drop dosage form, was shown to display better penetration and longer shelf life in ambient temperature for the favor of hospitalized patients' drug administration (Morand et al. 2007). It was primarily prepared to lower the toxicity (fourfold lower toxicity), but was also administrated intravitreally in monkey (Barza et al. 1985) and subconjunctically in rabbits (Kaji et al. 2009). An intravenous dosage form of liposomal amphotericin B (AmBisone®, Fujisawa Pharmaceutical Company, Ltd.), which was approved by FDA in 1997, is used as antifungal and antiprotozoan therapy. It displays more efficacy as reported for treatment of *Fusarium* keratitis in different stages of infection in a human subject case study performed more recently (Touvron et al. 2009). Subconjunctival injection of liposomal amphotericin B has been proved to be the best choice of treatment for mycotic keratitis (Kaji et al. 2009). Furthermore, Visudyne® is a liposomal DDS (approved in 2000, Novartis Pharmaceutical Inc.), formulated using cationic liposome and drug verteporfin, which is the first line effective choice for photodynamic therapy of subfoveal choroidal neovascularization, pathological myopia or presumed ocular histoplasmosis syndrome (Keam et al. 2003). There exist many evidences for the effectiveness of ocular delivery of liposomal formulations compared to their conventional counterparts. Of these, we could highlight superior transcorneal permeation of liposomal diclofenac formulated by low-molecular-weight chitosan (Li, Zhuang et al. 2009), ganciclovir consisting of phosphatidylcholine (Shen and Tu 2007), gatifloxacin hydrogel formulation formulated using phosphatidylcholine and cholesterol (Hosny 2010b), demeclocycline (Afouna et al. 2005).

Cationic lipids (CLs), extensively utilized as nonviral gene delivery systems, have also gained many attention for efficient treatment of ophthalmic disease. Solid lipid nanoparticles (SLNs) were used for topical ocular delivery of tobramycin (TOB). Topical administration of TOB-SLNs (~100 nm diameter) containing 0.3% w/v TOB in rabbits resulted in significantly higher TOB bioavailability in the aqueous humor (Cavalli et al. 2002). More recently, SLNs methazolamide (MTA) as an antiglaucoma agent was formulated using modified emulsion-solvent evaporation method to evaluate their potential in glaucoma (Li et al. 2011). Based upon the pharmacodynamic analysis, these researchers found that MTA-SLNs had higher therapeutic efficacy, later occurrence of maximum action, and more prolonged effect than drug solution and commercial product. Cyclosporin A (CsA) encapsulating SLNs have successfully been used in rabbit and sheep eyes (Basaran et al. 2010, Gokce et al. 2009). Due to the better characteristics such as smaller particle size (248.00 +/− 0.33 nm) with narrow size distribution (PI = 0.25 +/− 0.00) and high zeta potential (50.30 +/− 0.78 mV), SLNs was able to deliver the CsA to both aqueous and vitreous humor without any inter-individual variance.

A major drawback of liposomal system for application is the possible toxicity driven from either drug or the liposomal vehicle. The level of toxicity from liposomal preparations is influenced by size, lipid composition as well as their pharmacokinetic performance. One of the most important applications of liposomes is enhancing therapeutic efficiency by improving the pharmacokinetic profile, and therefore they offer a convenient way of sustained drug release from a relatively inert depot and tend to decrease the risk of toxicity associated with high dose of drug (Mishra et al. 2011, Szoka et al. 1987). Nonetheless, the long-term impacts of liposomal injections in the eye are not well known (Hsu 2007). For instance, intravitreal injection of liposomes is shown to impair vitreous clarity (Peyman et al. 1987), that can be of concern specially when long-term treatment is required with high dose of encapsulated drug. The effect of composition and size of liposomes on the LD50 of amphotericin B has been studied by Francis C. Szoka and coworkers (Szoka et al. 1987). They reported that presence of cholesterol and as well as increased size of liposomes reduced the lethality in mice; however *in vitro*, noncholesterol containing liposomes were less toxic. It may be anticipated that SUV generally would be less toxic than LMLV preparations due to a reduction in the rate of transfer of the drug from the liposome into cellular membranes but not to a major redistribution of the drug in the organs of the body tissues (Barza et al. 1987).

11.4.4 Niosomes

Vesicular structures of nonionic surfactants are called "niosomes" that is similar to liposomal structures. Various types of surfactants have been shown to form niosomal vesicles, which possess same encapsulation capacity as liposomes. Niosomes can entrap both hydrophilic and hydrophobic solutes. They are mainly composed of nonionic surfactants (e.g., alkyl ethers, alkyl esters, alkyl amides, fatty acid and amino acid compounds), cholesterol (to improve the rigidity), and charged molecules (to increase stability of niosomes by electrostatic repulsion) (Azeem et al. 2009, Rajera et al. 2011). For example, to reduce the intraocular pressure (IOP) in patients with glaucoma, niosomal formulations of acetazolamide (a carbonic anhydrase inhibitor with low solubility and low permeability coefficient) were prepared and coated with Carbopol to grant a bioadhesive effect. Upon application in male albino rabbits, the pharmacodynamic studies showed 33% fall in IOP with the developed formulation for 6 h after instillation while the peak concentration of drug absorbed in the aqueous humor from the niosomal formulations was significantly higher. High drug concentration 20 min after instillation indicated higher penetration of drugs through niosomal formulations (Aggarwal et al. 2007). Similarly, to improve the characteristic signs of diabetic keratopathy (e.g., impaired corneal sensation and delayed wound repair), niosomal formulations of naltrexone (NTX) have recently been formulated using charged lipids (e.g., dicetyl phosphate, stearyl amine) and surfactants (e.g., poly-24-oxyethylene cholesteryl ether, and sodium cholate). Based upon *ex vivo* transcorneal permeation studies using excised cow corneas, the niosomal formulations were found to enhance NTX corneal permeability without imposing any irritant impacts (Abdelkader et al. 2011).

11.4.5 Polymer-Based Ocular Nanomedicines

The unique structural flexibility of polymers (e.g., shape, size, physical state and surface) has revolutionized the field of DDS (Pillai and Panchagnula 2001). Polymers as the most adaptable class of materials are extensively used for drug formulations from both synthetic and natural sources. Polymeric nanoparticles (PNPs) with a size range of 10 to 1000 nm display great potential as colloidal DDS. PNPs are mainly formulated using emulsion and solvent evaporation technique or nanoprecipitation to incorporate the bioactive compounds, while chemical conjugation/grafting is also used for multimodal/multifunctional PNPs (Figure 11.4). Based on biological behavior of polymers, PNPs can be divided into biodegradable and nonbiodegradable NPs. Having shown substantial biocompatibility, the biodegradable PNPs offer many advantages over nonbiodegradable systems, including reduced host response, biotransformation and clearance by the body (Omidi and Davaran 2011). Nonetheless, biodegradable PNPs are predisposed to biological destruction in a time-dependent manner, which can occur through the

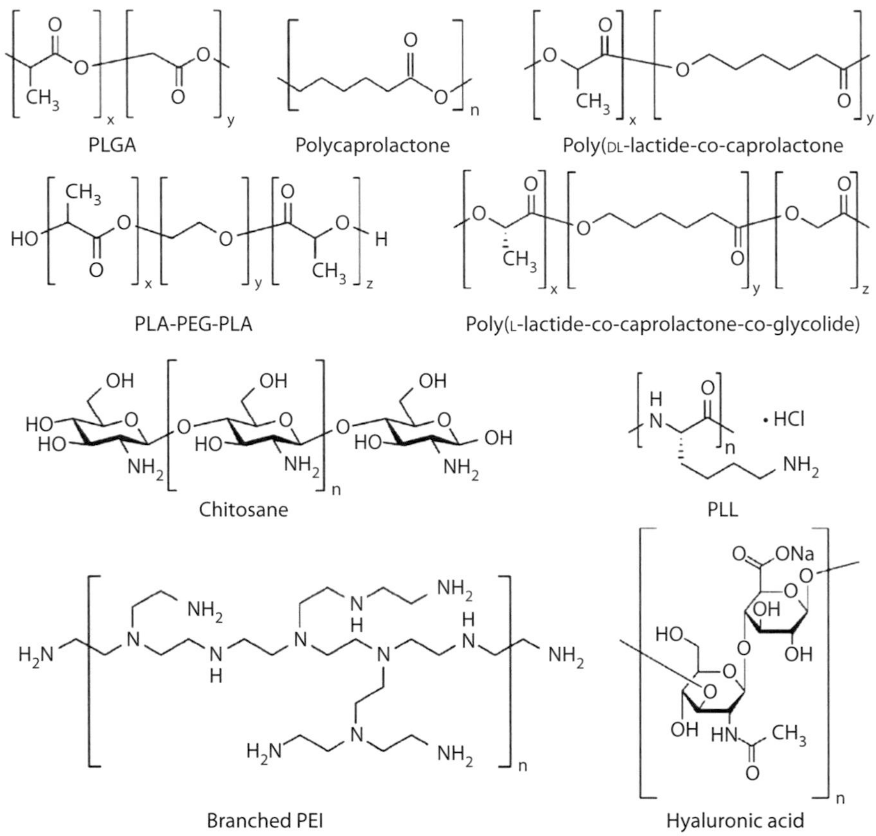

FIGURE 11.6
Molecular structures of selected polymers used for ocular drug/gene delivery. PLGA, poly(lactic-*co*-glycolic acid); PLA-PEG-PLA, polylactide-block-poly(ethylene glycol)-block-polylactide; PLL, poly(L-lysine); PEI, poly(ethyleneimine).

different mechanisms, that is, (1) cleavage of the cross-linked or water-soluble backbone in the three-dimensional network of soluble macromolecules, (2) hydrolysis, ionization, or protonation of pendant groups in water-insoluble molecules, and (3) hydrolytic cleavage of labile bonds in the polymer backbone of high-molecular-weight water-insoluble macromolecules (Kimura and Ogura 2001). Figure 11.6 and Table 11.2, respectively, show the molecular structures of some selected polymers used for ocular drug delivery and their applications in ophthalmology.

Among polymeric formulations, bioadhesive polymers provide a robust backbone for topical DDS by retrieving the contact time between drug compound and corneal tissue (du Toit et al. 2011). In addition, bioadhesive polymers have been exploited to improve the pharmacokinetic properties of ocular nanopharmaceuticals and inserts. For example, in a study, piroxicam

TABLE 11.2

Selected Polymeric Nanoformulations Used as Ocular DDS

Polymer	Nanomedicine	Application and Findings	Reference
Poly-epsilon-caprolactone	Nanosphere	Substantial delivery of cyclosporine A by hyaluronic acid coated poly-epsilon-caprolactone nanospheres into the cornea of rabbits	Yenice et al. (2008)
Polyester	Nanocapsule	Successful topical delivery of cyclosporin A into ocular tissues in rabbits	Calvo et al. (1996)
Eudragit RS100	Nanosuspension	Substantial inhibition of endotoxin-induced uveitis by topical delivery of piroxicam and methylprednisolone acetate in rabbits	Adibkia et al. (2007a,b)
Eudragit RL100	Nanoparticle	Significant ophthalmic delivery of cloricromene in rabbits	Bucolo et al. (2004)
Hyaluronan-chitosan polymers	Nanoparticle	Gene transportation across the ocular mucosa and transfection of ocular tissue in rabbits	de la Fuente et al. (2008)
PLGA and PLGL	Nanoparticle	Profound delivery of diclofenac sodium with no irritant effects on cornea, iris, and conjunctiva in rabbits	Agnihotri and Vavia (2009)
Dendrimer	Nanoparticle	Light-induced photochemical internalization-mediated gene delivery using packaged DNA enveloped in a dendrimeric photosensitizer	Nishiyama et al. (2005)
Chitosan	Nanoparticle	Successful delivery and sustained-release of brimonidine tartrate in rabbits	Singh and Shinde (2011)
MPEG-hexPLA	Nanomicelles	CsA nanomicelles corneal administration with significantly higher cornea transparency and lower edema after 7 and 13 days of the surgery, and reduced neovascularization in rats	Tommaso et al. (2012)

Note: PLGA, poly(lactide-*co*-glycolide); PLGL, poly(lactide-*co*-glycolide-leucine); MPEG-hexPLA, methoxy poly(ethylene) glycol-hexylsubstituted poly(lactides) copolymers.

was formulated using different polymers, and formulations with better adhesion properties (containing 0.5% carbopol and 1% HPMC) showed improved availability and drug release profile (Gilhotra et al. 2009).

Among other polymers extensively used in nanomedicines, are poly lactic acid (PLA), poly glycolic acid (PGA) and their copolymer PLGA. In the body, they are subjected to degradation through hydrolysis of ester backbone and elimination as carbon dioxide and water via a distinct pathway; as a result, they show great potential both *in vitro* and *in vivo.*

Anatomically, the inner and outer BRB separate the retina and the vitreous from the systemic circulation. This segregation result in decreased reciprocal traverse of molecules between them. Using PNPs, we are able to improve drug permeation, to control the release rate of a designated drug, and to target designated cellular biomarkers (Sahoo et al. 2008). In fact, because of the anatomical architectural hallmarks of the eye, topical dosage forms are the most used medications even though they are often subjected to drainage from the ocular surface resulting in low bioavailability. While the fluid-based pharmaceuticals fail to reach the posterior segments and ocular barriers make ocular drug delivery to the posterior segment a challenging issue, implementation of PNPs may be beneficial to ophthalmic diseases in many ways. Importance of ocular application of PNPs (in particular the biodegradable ones) can be eminent if one notes side effects of ocular pharmacotherapy via intravitreal injection. Such inadvertent adverse reactions were reported for the treatment of AMD with the antivascular endothelial growth factor (VEGF) therapies, that are, pegaptanib (Macugen®), ranibizumab (Lucentis®), and bevacizumab (Avastin®) (Ng et al. 2006, Abrishami et al. 2009, El Sanharawi et al. 2010). Although systemic administrations are deemed to be a suitable approach, it shows limited applicability solely for some pharmaceuticals that possess appropriate physicochemical and biopharmaceutical characteristics. The systemic administration are associated with repetitive use resulting in poor patient compliance, difficulty of insertion in the case of ocular inserts, and being invasive when injected/implanted that is also associated with some tissue damage.

It should be highlighted that the utility of PNPs are largely dependent upon (1) lipophilic-hydrophilic characteristics of PNPs, (2) the biodegradation rate of PNP, and (3) the retention efficiency in the precorneal pocket (Kothuri et al. 2003). Thus, to attain the maximal effects of PNPs in the precorneal pocket, bioadhesive properties of PNPS favors ocular pharmacotherapy through enhancing the retention time of NPs in the ocular cul-de-sac, and thus reducing their fast elimination. Targeted modified (e.g., PEGylated) PNPs may also be administered intravenously and reach the target sites via blood stream (Sanders et al. 2007). Angiogenesis plays a pivotal role in some ocular diseases (e.g., diabetic retinopathy, central retinal vein occlusion, choroidal neovascularization (CNV), and intraocular solid tumors) (Rajappa et al. 2010), therefore targeted therapy of ocular vasculature may provide a great treatment modality. This notion requires exploitation of specific biomarkers within the ocular tissue to be able to accommodate designated drugs in desired ocular sites by means of PNPs. It should be noted that no lymph system is presented in the retinal microenvironment; hence therapy of retinal diseases attributed with neovascularization (e.g., wet AMD) can be similar to the strategies used for therapy of solid tumors. This explicitly indicates that PNPs will provide enhanced permeability and retention (EPR) effects. Once coupled with homing device, PNPs can be accumulated in target sites. In short, these facts further highlight the biological impacts on required pharmacotherapy to achieve enhanced drug permeation, controlled release of drugs, and targeted pharmacotherapy through specific targeting ocular specific markers by means of ocular nanomedicines. In fact, polymer-based encapsulation of drugs can protect sensitive compounds from biodegradation resulting in prolonged/controlled release profile. Thus, PNPs may confer better controlling tools for various chronic ocular diseases. For example, in the case of chronic CMV retinitis, intravitreal delivery of ganciclovir (GCV) as a preferred strategy demands a safe vehicle with controlled release profile. Given 13-hour half-life, otherwise, frequent injections of GCV will be inevitable to preserve the therapeutic level of GCV in vitreous. It should be emphasized that repetitive injections may associate with inadvertent side effects such as cataract development, retinal detachment, and endophthalmitis, while PNPs can overcome such difficulties (Sahoo et al. 2008). Likewise, the nano-scaled colloidal carrier system "Piloplex®" consisting of pilocarpine, ionically bound to poly(methyl) methacrylate-*co*-acrylic, has been considered as an effective modality in glaucoma patients with twice-daily instillations. Although erodible PNPs are superior to nonbiodegradable ones, in part due to less harm on tissue, they last shorter because of biodegradation. Thus, in some cases, it is unavoidable to use synthetic non-biodegradable PNPs. We have successfully exploited Eudragit PNPs to formulate sustained-release nanosuspensions of piroxicam and methylprednisolone acetate (MPA), which showed effective impacts on controlling the endotoxin-induced uveitis in rabbits (Adibkia et al. 2007a,b).

It should be stated that biodegradable PNPs are prone to erosion/biotransformation in a time-dependent manner, in part by mechanisms such as: (1) cleavage of the cross-linked or water-soluble backbone, (2) hydrolysis, (3) ionization, (4) protonation of pendant groups in the water-insoluble macromolecules, and (5) hydrolytic cleavage of labile bonds in the polymer backbone high-molecular-weight water-insoluble macromolecules. Therefore, depend upon final aim of a designated PNP formulation, the size and type of polymers can be modified to get the desired pattern of drug release as well as longevity of drugs in ocular tissue (Kimura and Ogura 2001).

To improve the poor ocular bioavailability, recently PLGA NPs (180–190 nm with zeta potential of −22 mV) of sparfloxacin were formulated and showed an extended drug release profile that obeyed the Peppas kinetic model. Gamma scintigraphy analysis for precorneal residence time resulted in good retention over the entire precorneal area for PLGA-SF NPs, which cleared from the corneal region at a very slow rate unlike SF that cleared very rapidly and reached the systemic circulation through the nasolacrimal drainage system (Gupta et al. 2010). Besides, to enhance cellular integration and promote retinal repopulation, PLGA NPs (containing matrix metalloproteinase 2 (MMP2)) were cotransplanted with retinal progenitor cells (RPCs) to the subretinal space of adult retinal degenerative Rho-/- mice. Significant increases in the number of cells migrating beyond the barrier into the degenerative retina were observed while no changes in the differentiation characteristics of RPCs were seen (Yao et al. 2011). As a result, it can be deduced that cotransplantation of MMP2-PLGA NPs with RPCs may provide an effective strategy for retinal repair. This also infers biodegradable PNPs impacts on ocular tissue engineering. Likewise, the poly-L-lysine-coated PLGA microspheres containing retinoic acid (RA) was used as a matrix to culture pluripotent P19 embryonic carcinoma cells resulting in differentiation of P19 cells into neural cells (Nojehdehian et al. 2009).

In a study, the neuroprotective effects of small pigment epithelium-derived factor (PEDF) peptides injected intravitreally as free peptides or delivered in PLGA NPs were examined in retinal ischemic injury in C57/BL6 mice. Although the injection of PEDF peptide (alone or as PLGA-based nanospheres) showed protective effects, the PLGA-PEDF nanospheres displayed significantly longer-term protection of the retinal ganglion cell layer with no noticeable side effects for 7 days (Li et al. 2006).

Implementation of PNPs using PLGA NPs to study the efficacy of pSEC. shRNA.VEGF- in the sustained regression of murine corneal neovascularization (KNV) resulted in significant regression in the mean fractional areas of KNV ($0.125 +/- 0.042$; 12.5%, $p < 0.01$). This simply indicates that PNPs can be used as effective nontoxic nanocarriers for gene therapy to suppress ocular neovascularization (Qazi et al. 2012). A higher decrease of the sodium arachidonate–induced inflammation was reported by using PLGA NPs containing flurbiprofen in the rabbit eye after topical instillation, which indicates usefulness of biodegradable PNPs for the inhibition of ocular inflammation (Vega et al. 2006). Similarly, intravitreal injections of PLA micro/nanospheres containing 1% adriamycin/doxorubicin were reported to grant a sustained release kinetic for at least 2 weeks. Despite being considered as a safe carrier, using DNA microarray technology, we examined the genocompatibility of PLGA NPs and witnessed less changes in gene expression in comparison with the synthetic polymers such as PAMAM dendrimers (Omidi and Davaran 2011).

Other biodegradable PNPs were shown to have similar potentials in ocular drug delivery and targeting. For example, chitosan (CS) is a polycationic biodegradable polymer with low immunogenicity (Alves and Mano 2008). This positively charged natural carbohydrate polymer is an attractive candidate for many medical applications such as gene/drug delivery. CS interacts with polyanionic surface of ocular mucosa which is an adhesive phenomenon for many nanotechnology-based formulations such as gels, inserts, and colloidal medicines (Wadhwa et al. 2009). In an interesting investigation, animals were treated with CS NPs loaded with cyclosporin A, whose significantly higher corneal and conjunctival accumulation provided better treatment outcomes (de Campos et al. 2001). In the same way, it has been shown that the amounts of fluorescent NPs (formulated using CS) were significantly higher in the cornea and the conjunctiva where CS NPs were detected even after 24 h (de Campos et al. 2004). Despite the fact that CS is approved as a safe substance for wound dressing by FDA, the safety of all additional conjugations and residuals should be taken into account (Kean and Thanou 2010). Its combination with other polymers such as PLGA and hyaluronic acid (HA) provide unique NPs. For example, through ionotropic gelation technique, CS and HA

NPs (100–235 nm and zeta-potential of −30 to +28 mV) were formulated and loaded with a model plasmid. These PNPs were able to be internalized by endocytosis mediated via hyaluronan receptor CD44 and provide high transfection levels (de la Fuente et al. 2008). Similarly, to determine internalization pathways in cornea-derived and conjunctiva-derived cells, CS-HA nanoparticles were shown to be internalized via the active transport mechanism mediated by hyaluronan receptors through a caveolin-dependent endocytic pathway (Contreras-Ruiz et al. 2011). Such findings further support the potential use of CS-HA NPs to deliver designated drugs/genetic materials to the ocular cells. Of note, ocular tissues have a negative charge and thus positively charged PNPs are able to bestow a prolonged contact time between the drug and the tissue, resulting in enhanced absorption and mucoadhesion. Owing to efficient binding and penetration into conjunctival and corneal epithelia, CS NPs appear to be a promising DDS for ocular diseases.

11.4.6 Dendrimeric Nanostructures for Ocular Drug Delivery

In 1984, first dendrimer was established and named Starburst™ polyamidoamine (PAMAM) dendrimer based upon its dendritic architecture. They are consisted of concentric and geometrically progressive layers that are created via radial amplification from a single initiator core molecule containing either three or four reactive sites such as ammonia or ethylene diamine (Tomalia et al. 1984). As shown in Figure 11.7, architecturally, they are nanostructural macromolecules with three dimensions (Loutsch et al. 2003).

These nanostructures provide globular nanosystems of 1–100 nm depending on the molecular weight and number of generations. Its surface ultimately determines the structure's interactions with its environment, as a result of which drugs/genes can be incorporated with and released in a controlled manner (Vandervoort and Ludwig 2007). The surface of dendrimers can be modified or decorated by designated functional groups such as small molecules and macromolecules (e.g., DNA, antibodies, and proteins). These nanostructures have been implanted as ocular DDS with promising corollaries. For example, to inhibit laser-induced CNV, lipophilic amino-acid dendrimer was successfully used to deliver an anti-VEGF oligonucleotide (ODN) into the eyes of rats with results of CNV inhibition for 4–6 months (Marano et al. 2005). In addition, ternary complexes were shown to significantly enhance transgene expression *in vitro*, so that the subconjuvctival injection of the ternary complex followed by laser irradiation resulted in specific transgene expression only in the laser-irradiated site (Nishiyama et al. 2005).

Further, polypropyleneimine octaamine dendrimers cross-linked with collagen were reported to support human corneal epithelial cell growth and adhesion without imposing toxic impacts. Such 3D nanostructures, hence, can be used as appropriate scaffolds for corneal tissue engineering (Duan and Sheardown 2006). Recently, complex of puerarin and PAMAM

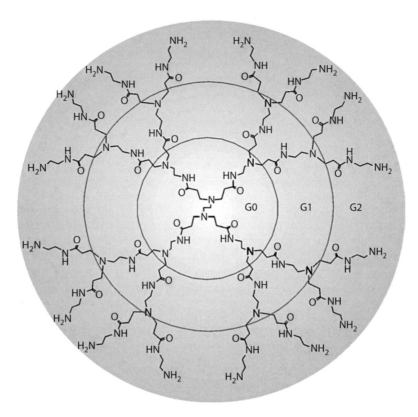

FIGURE 11.7
Polyamidoamine (PAMAM) dendrimer (G0, generation 0; G1, generation 1; G2, generation 2).

dendrimers were prepared and evaluated as an ocular DDS looking at the corneal permeation and ocular residence time in rabbits. The results showed that the puerarin-dendrimer complexes were able to produce longer ocular residence times in rabbits with no damages to the epithelium or endothelium (Yao et al. 2010). More recently, nano-scaled dendrimer hydrogels (DH) made from ultraviolet-cured polyamidoamine dendrimer and tethered with PEG-acrylate chains were found to be mucoadhesive to mucin particles and nontoxic to human corneal epithelial cells, showing increased timolol maleate uptake in bovine corneal epithelium, stroma, and endothelium (Holden et al. 2012). These applications of nanostructured dendrimers bring on some other research horizons that will certainly advance the ocular drug delivery and targeting.

11.4.7 Quantum Dots

Quantum dot (QD) semiconductors are the most studied nanocrystals used as an imaging agent in the formulation of cancer nanomedicine and theranostics because of possessing superior fluorescent properties (Tan et al. 2011). Once excited by a laser beam, the QDs can emit fluorescent light based on their size, while the band gap energy determines the energy and hence color. The QD fluorescent light is inversely proportional to the size of the QD, that is the smaller the size the bluer the emission. The optical spectra of various QDs appear to be different, which is largely dependent on architecture of a cadmium selenide (CdSe)/zinc sulfide (ZnS) QDs resulting in emission spectra of monodispersed CdSe/ZnS QDs with diameters from 2 to 6 nm. QDs have been used in ophthalmology to investigate the tear film dynamic multilayered structure. While efforts to understand such dynamics have been limited by the techniques and biomarkers used, QDs (indium phosphide-gallium (InP/Ga) QDs) showed great potential to monitor the dynamics of the tear film layers *in vivo* without the drawbacks of previously used methodologies (Khanal and Millar 2010). Using QDs, a distinct three-layered tear film was found as (1) an inner mucin layer attached to the epithelial cells, (2) a fluid aqueous layer, and (3) an outer viscoelastic lipid layer. Also, QDs have successfully been used to trace lymphatic drainage from the mouse eye (Tam et al. 2011).

11.4.8 Gold NPs

Gold NPs (GNPs) have been used as delivery and imaging systems even though it has not fully studied for its application(s) in the eye. However, recently, GNPs have been examined for subretinal delivery of immunoglobulin G (IgG) adsorbed onto GNPs in the rabbit retina. In this approach, electrostatically adsorbed IgG onto GNPs were injected into the subretinal space of rabbit eyes and followed up for 3 months by examination of fundus photographs, immunohistochemistry against goat IgG, and transmission electron microscopy (TEM). It was found that GNPs can locate within the outer segments and in the lysosomes in the RPE without any apparent cytotoxicity of the RPE. This clearly indicates that GNPs can successfully deliver the IgG into photoreceptor cells and RPE, as a result GNPs might be an alternative drug-delivery method to photoreceptors and RPE (Hayashi et al. 2009).

11.4.9 Cubosomes

Cubosomes, as cubic phase NPs, are self-assembled liquid crystalline NPs, whose unique structure (based on intermingles oil and water molecules) makes them as nanoporous system that can be used as delivery system. In a study, to improve dexamethasone (DEX) preocular retention and enhanced ocular bioavailability, cubosomes were used as ocular DDS (Gan et al. 2010). By fragmenting a cubic crystalline phase of monoolein and water in the presence of stabilizer Poloxamer 407, DEX cubosome particles were produced and showed significantly higher apparent permeability coefficient as compared with that of Dex-Na phosphate eye drops. While the retention of cubosomes was significantly longer than that of solution and carbopol gel, *in vivo* pharmacokinetics evaluations indicated a marked increase in DEX administered in cubosomes. Similarly, to reduce ocular irritancy and improve bioavailability, flurbiprofen (FB) was loaded to cubosomes (150 nm) and successfully administered in rabbits' eyes. While the histological examinations showed no adverse impacts on the integrity of the cornea, FB cubosomes resulted in significant reduction of irritation, indicating excellent ocular tolerance (Han et al. 2010). In short, it appears that cubosomes can be considered as a promising nanosystem for effective ocular drug delivery.

11.4.10 Nanosuspensions

Formulation of poorly water-soluble drugs is considered as a big challenge, which becomes more intense for class III insoluble drugs that are poorly soluble in both aqueous and organic media, and drugs with a log P value of 2. These compounds tend to show an erratic absorption profile with highly variable bioavailability as their clinical impacts are (1) dissolution-rate limited and (2) affected by fed/fasted state of the patient. Thus, various strategies (e.g., micronization, cosolvents solubilization, permeation enhancers) used to tackle the formulation challenges resulted in limited successes. Nanosuspensions can resolve such dilemma providing better characteristics on particles size distribution, morphology, zeta potential, saturation solubility and dissolution velocity as well as *in vivo* biological performance (Patravale et al. 2004). Various approaches have been undertaken to produce nanosuspensions including formulations using NPs.

Among various drugs used in ophthalmic diseases, steroidal and nonsteroidal anti-inflammatory drugs (NSAIDs) are routinely used in ocular surgeries. However, they are often associated with undesired side effects. Localized therapy of ocular inflammation by these pharmaceuticals needs to be optimized since most ocular diseases are classically treated with topical eyedrops, which usually require the frequent utilization of highly concentrated solutions. To tackle this, using Eudragit®RS100 polymer, we have previously formulated nanosuspensions of piroxicam and methylprednisolone acetate, used in rabbits with endotoxin-induced uveitis. Having used these nanosuspensions, we significantly controlled the endotoxin-induced uveitis (Adibkia et al. 2007a,b). Figure 11.8 represents piroxicam nanosuspensions that were successfully used for controlling the endotoxin-induced uveitis.

Given that the Eudragit®RS100 possesses an appropriate stability and size distribution characteristics together with its positive surface charge (30 mV), this polymer is considered as a suitable ocular DDS (Pignatello et al. 2002). Using this polymer, cloricromene (a coumarine derivative with antithrombotic and anti-ischemic activities) NPs (80 nm) were formulated with zeta potential values of +27.3 mV. Once applied to rabbit eyes, they showed no sign of toxicity or irritation to ocular tissues while showing great *in vivo* performance (Bucolo et al. 2004).

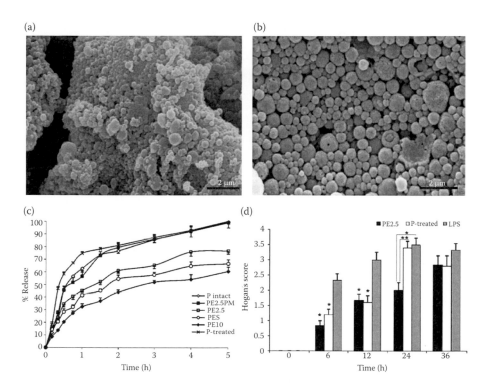

FIGURE 11.8
Piroxicam nanosuspensions used to control endotoxin-induced uveitis in rabbits. (a) Piroxicam:Eudragit RS100 (PE) nanoparticles (NPs). (b) Eudragit RS100 NPs alone. (c) Release profile of piroxicam from nanosuspensions. (d) Hogan's score for treated eyes with piroxicam microsuspension and piroxicam:Eudragit RS100 NPs. P-intact, untreated intact piroxicam; P-treated, treated piroxicam; PE2.5, piroxicam: ERS NPs (1:2.5 ratio); PM, physical mixture. LPS, lipopolysaccharide. (Data were adapted with permission from Adibkia, K. et al. 2007b. *J Drug Target* 15: 407–416.)

Recently, PLGA and poly(lactide-*co*-glycolide-leucine) loaded with diclofenac sodium were formulated as nanosuspension, which showed no irritant effect on cornea, iris, and conjunctiva for as long as 24 h after application (Agnihotri and Vavia 2009). Hydrocortisone (HC) nanosuspensions (300 nm) were formulated by means of microfluidic nanoprecipitation applied to the albino rabbits' eyes, and the ocular bioavailability was evaluated. It was found that nanosuspension were significantly increased the bioavailability (Ali et al. 2011).

11.4.11 Ocular Nanogenomedicines

Owing to the unique architecture of the eye, nanogenomedicines can be explicitly delivered. Thus far, ocular pathologies have been tackled with

26 gene therapy trials (out of 1786 gene therapy clinical trials) focusing on various conditions such as retinitis pigmentosa, glaucoma, diabetic macular edema, and AMD (http://www.wiley.co.uk/genmed/clinical/). While proof-of-concept for vector-based gene therapies has been established in several experimental models of human ocular diseases, it is expected that futuristic nanogenomedicines will be more effective therapeutics because combined genome-based technologies can be exploited to engineer multimodal molecular Trojan horses to suppress/stimulate bunch of dysregulated gene markers (Ali 2012, Li et al. 2011). Of the genomedicines, short interfering RNA (siRNA) technology appeared to be the most plausible system with remarkable preclinical/clinical potential. Viral and nonviral vectors (even combination of both) have been used for the delivery of designated genes to the selected cells/tissue. Of these, nonviral vectors were shown to exert the maximal gene transfer capacity as NPs (the so-called nanogenomedicines). For example, CS-HA NPs (100–235 nm and zeta-potential of −30-+28 mV) were used for the delivery of genes to the cornea and conjunctiva using model plasmid pEGFP or pbeta-gal in human corneal epithelial and normal human conjunctival cells. It was found that HA-CS NPs were able to provide high transfection levels without affecting cell viability (de la Fuente et al. 2008).

Table 11.3 represents the latest ocular gene therapy clinical trials. It should be evoked that fomivirsen (Vitaraven®, Isis Pharmaceuticals, Inc. 1998) is the first FDA approved antisense drug and prescribed for the treatment of cytomegalovirus infections that is administered as intraocular injection. Particular attention has been devoted to the CK30-PEG compacted DNA NPs that have been successfully tested in the eye, lung, and brain (Badawi et al. 2008).

Ocular nanogenomedicines are in their infancies and it will be expanded toward targeting other genes involved in the eye diseases. To avoid immunogenic responses, it is anticipated that viral vectors will be engineered as NPs coated with stimuli responsive polymers/lipids to be activated in the site of action.

11.4.12 Bioavailability of Ocular Nanomedicines

Most of nano-scaled DDS undergo cellular uptake into ocular tissues, mainly via endocytosis. Although the uptake percentage of the total doses of NPs and their contribution to overall ocular drug bioavailability is not clear, the up-taken NPs are subjected to biological transformations at cellular levels (Barar and Omidi 2011). Besides, all ophthalmic drugs are prone to metabolism, which is performed by functional expression of various enzymes involved in a variety of stages of drug metabolism and detoxification (Duvvuri et al. 2004). These metabolizing machineries of the eye are primarily expressed in various tissues (e.g., the retina-choroid), which appear to play an important role in ocular homeostasis by preventing the

TABLE 11.3

Ocular Nanogenomedicines in Clinical Trials

Indication	Phase	Vector	Gene(s)
Age related macular degeneration (AMD)	Phase I/II	Adeno-associated virus	sFLT01
AMD	Phase I	Adeno-associated virus	Platelet-derived growth factor (PDGF)
AMD		Lentivirus	Endostatin angiostatin
AMD	Phase I/II	Lentivirus	siRNA for vascular endothelial growth factor (C and 5)
AMD	Phase II	—	siRNA against vascular endothelial growth factor receptor-1 (Sirna-27)
Diabetic macular edema (DME)	Phase II	—	siRNA against C and 5
Lebers congenital amaurosis (LCA)	Phase I	Adeno-associated virus	hRPE65
Choroideraemia	Phase I	Adeno-associated virus	Rab escort protein 1 (REP1)
Superficial corneal opacity	Phase I/II	Reterovirus	dnG1 Cyclin
Retinitis pigmentosa	Phase I	Naked/plasmid DNA	Ciliary neurotrophic factor (CNTF)
Glaucoma	Phase I	Adenovirus	p21 WAF-1/Cip1
Retinal RPE65 mutations	Phase I	Adeno-associated virus	RPE65
Macular degeneration	Phase II	Naked/plasmid DNA	CNTF
Retinitis pigmentosa	Phase II	Naked/plasmid DNA	CNTF
Leber congenital (RPE65 mutations)	Phase III	Adeno-associated virus	RPE65
Stargardt's macular degeneration (SMD)	Phase I/II	Lentivirus	Retina-specific ABC transporter (ABCR)

Source: From http://www.abedia.com/wiley/.

entry of xenobiotics into, and/or eliminating xenobiotics from the ocular tissues. Various cytochrome P450 (CYP) enzymes have been identified in ocular tissues, including CYPs 1A, 1B1, 2B, 2C, 2J, 3A, 4B1, 39A1, and NADPH reductase (Attar et al. 2005). Ocular nanomedicines are deemed to circumvent such metabolizing impacts and improve the ocular bioavailability. For example, a single topical instillation of acyclovir-PLA nanospheres in rabbits provided a prolonged high concentration in aqueous humor (Giannavola et al. 2003). Similarly, enhanced bioavailability was reported for the topical use of NPs of amikacin-poly(butyl cyanoacrylate) (PBCA), acyclovir-poly(ethyl cyanoacrylate), betaxolol-poly(isobutyl cyanoacrylate), cloricromene-ERL, cyclophosphamide-PBCA, hydrocortisone-BSA, ibuprofen-ERS/ERL, metipranolol-PIBCA/PCL, and progesterone-PBCA; for more details, readers are referred to Bu et al. 2007.

11.5 Final Remarks on Ocular Nanomedicines

Permeation of small drugs across BAB and BRB vary based on their physicochemical characteristics and impacts of these biological membranes and barriers. Traditionally, most of ophthalmic drugs are delivered to the eye via aqueous vehicles. However, the aqueous vehicles exhibit poor ocular bioavailability, in part because of rapid drainage and lacrimation. Thus far, pharmacotherapy of the eye has been significantly improved through implementation of advanced DDS. To improve the ophthalmic delivery of poor water soluble drugs, many approaches have been used including: hydrogels, microparticles, NPs, and liposomal formulations. Of these DDS, nanoformulations have raised promising potential for efficient ocular delivery in particular to the posterior segment of the eye that demands safe drug delivery to the retina, the choroid, or the ciliary body. However, regarding ocular drug therapy, we have witnessed the application of a few advanced therapeutics such as Visudyne® from Novartis Pharma AG (Bakri and Kaiser 2004), Macugen® from Eyetech Pharmaceuticals/Pfizer (Ng et al. 2006) and Retaane® (Alcon Inc.) administered as a single periocular injection every six months (Ni and Hui 2009). It is expected, in close proximity, to face with clinical application of bunch of ocular nanomedicines as multimodal noninvasive ocular DDS. The central goal of these advanced modalities is to provide an efficient and safe delivery to the specific ocular cells/tissue, wherein they should show longer residency. To some extent, this is achievable by ocular nanomedicines through bioadhesive systems such as CS-HA NPs as natural biopolymers. Such bioadhesive nanosystems can maximize ocular drug absorption by prolonging the drug residence time in the cornea and the conjunctiva, while minimizing precorneal drug loss. Ideally, for long-term use, these bioadhesive nanosystems should be nontoxic and represent site specificity with minimal immunogenicity and maximal bioavailability through enhancing absorption (particularly for protein/peptide-based macromolecules) or inhibiting the metabolizing enzymes. Finally, it should be stated that not all attempts to apply *de novo* nanotechnology approaches in biomedical sciences have met with the same success as those cited here in this chapter, and sometimes, these novel technologies tools provoke a great deal of challenges and hurdles. In fact, nanopharmaceuticals tend to function not in the same predictive ways that routinely used small molecules act. They may interact with biomolecules of the target cells/tissue and impose undesired biological impacts at molecular levels as a particular genomic, proteomic, or metabolomics signature. They may reprogram the genomic/

epigenomic pattern of diseased/benign cells, which should be taken into consideration before their clinical translations.

References

Abdelkader, H., Ismail, S., Kamal, A., and Alany, R. G. 2011. Design and evaluation of controlled-release niosomes and discomes for naltrexone hydrochloride ocular delivery. *J Pharm Sci* 100: 1833–1846.

Abrishami, M., Zarei-Ghanavati, S., Soroush, D. et al. 2009. Preparation, characterization, and *in vivo* evaluation of nanoliposomes-encapsulated bevacizumab (avastin) for intravitreal administration. *Retina* 29: 699–703.

Adibkia, K., Omidi, Y., Siahi, M. R. et al. 2007a. Inhibition of endotoxin-induced uveitis by methylprednisolone acetate nanosuspension in rabbits. *J Ocul Pharmacol Ther* 23: 421–432.

Adibkia, K., Siahi Shadbad, M. R., Nokhodchi, A. et al. 2007b. Piroxicam nanoparticles for ocular delivery: Physicochemical characterization and implementation in endotoxin-induced uveitis. *J Drug Target* 15: 407–416.

Afouna, M. I., Khattab, I. S., and Reddy, I. K. 2005. Preparation and characterization of demeclocycline liposomal formulations and assessment of their intraocular pressure-lowering effects. *Cutan Ocul Toxicol* 24: 111–124.

Aggarwal, D., Pal, D., Mitra, A. K., and Kaur, I. P. 2007. Study of the extent of ocular absorption of acetazolamide from a developed niosomal formulation, by microdialysis sampling of aqueous humor. *Int J Pharm* 338: 21–26.

Agnihotri, S. M. and Vavia, P. R. 2009. Diclofenac-loaded biopolymeric nanosuspensions for ophthalmic application. *Nanomedicine* 5: 90–95.

Ahmed, I. 2003. The noncorneal route in ocular drug delivery. In *Ophthalmic Drug Delivery Systems*, ed. A. K. Mitra, 335–363. New York: Marcel Dekker.

Ainscough, S. L., Feigl, B., Malda, J., and Harkin, D. G. 2009. Discovery and characterization of IGFBP-mediated endocytosis in the human retinal pigment epithelial cell line ARPE-19. *Exp Eye Res* 89: 629–637.

Ali, H. S., York, P., Ali, A. M., and Blagden, N. 2011. Hydrocortisone nanosuspensions for ophthalmic delivery: A comparative study between microfluidic nanoprecipitation and wet milling. *J Control Release* 149: 175–181.

Ali, R. R. 2012. Ocular gene therapy: Introduction to the special issue. *Gene Ther* 19: 119–120.

Alves, N. M. and Mano, J. F. 2008. Chitosan derivatives obtained by chemical modifications for biomedical and environmental applications. *Int J Biol Macromol* 43: 401–414.

Amaral, J., Fariss, R. N., Campos, M. M. et al. 2005. Transscleral-RPE permeability of PEDF and ovalbumin proteins: Implications for subconjunctival protein delivery. *Invest Ophthalmol Vis Sci* 46: 4383–4392.

Ambati, J., Gragoudas, E. S., Miller, J. W. et al. 2000. Transscleral delivery of bioactive protein to the choroid and retina. *Invest Ophthalmol Vis Sci* 41: 1186–1191.

Ammar, H. O., Salama, H. A., Ghorab, M., and Mahmoud, A. A. 2010. Development of dorzolamide hydrochloride *in situ* gel nanoemulsion for ocular delivery. *Drug Dev Ind Pharm* 36: 1330–1339.

Anand, B. S., Katragadda, S., Gunda, S., and Mitra, A. K. 2006. *In vivo* ocular pharmacokinetics of acyclovir dipeptide ester prodrugs by microdialysis in rabbits. *Mol Pharm* 3: 431–440.

Ashton, P. 2006. Retinal drug delivery. In *Intraocular Drug Delivery*, ed. G. J. Jaffe, P. Ashton, and P. A. Pearson, 1–25. New York: Taylor & Francis Group, LLC.

Attar, M., Shen, J., Ling, K. H., and Tang-Liu, D. 2005. Ophthalmic drug delivery considerations at the cellular level: Drug-metabolising enzymes and transporters. *Expert Opin Drug Deliv* 2: 891–908.

Azeem, A., Anwer, M. K., and Talegaonkar, S. 2009. Niosomes in sustained and targeted drug delivery: Some recent advances. *J Drug Target* 17: 671–689.

Badawi, A. A., El-Laithy, H. M., El Qidra, R. K., El, M. H., and El, D. M. 2008. Chitosan based nanocarriers for indomethacin ocular delivery. *Arch Pharm Res* 31: 1040–1049.

Bakri, S. J. and Kaiser, P. K. 2004. Verteporfin ocular photodynamic therapy. *Expert Opin Pharmacother* 5: 195–203.

Bando, H., Shadrach, K. G., Rayborn, M. E., Crabb, J. W., and Hollyfield, J. G. 2007. Clathrin and adaptin accumulation in drusen, Bruch's membrane and choroid in AMD and non-AMD donor eyes. *Exp Eye Res* 84: 135–142.

Barar, J., Javadzadeh, A. R., and Omidi, Y. 2008. Ocular novel drug delivery: Impacts of membranes and barriers. *Expert Opin Drug Deliv* 5: 567–581.

Barar, J. and Omidi, Y. 2011. Cellular trafficking and subcellular interactions of cationic gene delivery nanomaterials. *J Pharm Nut Sci* 1: 68–81.

Barza, M., Baum, J., Tremblay, C., Szoka, F., and D'amico, D. J. 1985. Ocular toxicity of intravitreally injected liposomal amphotericin B in rhesus monkeys. *Am J Ophthalmol* 100: 259–263.

Barza, M., Stuart, M., and Szoka, F., Jr. 1987. Effect of size and lipid composition on the pharmacokinetics of intravitreal liposomes. *Invest Ophthalmol Vis Sci* 28: 893–900.

Basaran, E., Demirel, M., Sirmagul, B., and Yazan, Y. 2010. Cyclosporine-A incorporated cationic solid lipid nanoparticles for ocular delivery. *J Microencapsul* 27: 37–47.

Bu, H. Z., Gukasyan, H. J., Goulet, L. et al. 2007. Ocular disposition, pharmacokinetics, efficacy and safety of nanoparticle-formulated ophthalmic drugs. *Curr Drug Metab* 8: 91–107.

Bucolo, C., Maltese, A., Maugeri, F. et al. 2004. Eudragit RL100 nanoparticle system for the ophthalmic delivery of cloricromene. *J Pharm Pharmacol* 56: 841–846.

Cai, X., Conley, S., and Naash, M. 2008. Nanoparticle applications in ocular gene therapy. *Vision Res* 48: 319–324.

Calvo, P., Sanchez, A., Martinez, J. et al. 1996. Polyester nanocapsules as new topical ocular delivery systems for cyclosporin A. *Pharm Res* 13: 311–315.

Camelo, S., Lajavardi, L., Bochot, A. et al. 2009. Protective effect of intravitreal injection of vasoactive intestinal peptide-loaded liposomes on experimental autoimmune uveoretinitis. *J Ocul Pharmacol Ther* 25: 9–21.

Cao, Y., Zhang, C., Shen, W. et al. 2007. Poly(N-isopropylacrylamide)-chitosan as thermosensitive *in situ* gel-forming system for ocular drug delivery. *J Control Release* 120: 186–194.

Cavalli, R., Gasco, M. R., Chetoni, P., Burgalassi, S., and Saettone, M. F. 2002. Solid lipid nanoparticles (SLN) as ocular delivery system for tobramycin. *Int J Pharm* 238: 241–245.

Cenedella, R. J., Neely, A. R., and Sexton, P. 2006. Multiple forms of 22 kDa caveolin-1 alpha present in bovine lens cells could reflect variable palmitoylation. *Exp Eye Res* 82: 229–235.

Chakravarti, S., Paul, J., Roberts, L. et al. 2003. Ocular and scleral alterations in gene-targeted lumican-fibromodulin double-null mice. *Invest Ophthalmol Vis Sci* 44: 2422–2432.

Choy, Y. B., Park, J. H., McCarey, B. E., Edelhauser, H. F., and Prausnitz, M. R. 2008. Mucoadhesive microdiscs engineered for ophthalmic drug delivery: Effect of particle geometry and formulation on preocular residence time. *Invest Ophthalmol Vis Sci* 49: 4808–4815.

Claro, C., Ruiz, R., Cordero, E. et al. 2009. Determination and pharmacokinetic profile of liposomal foscarnet in rabbit ocular tissues after intravitreal administration. *Exp Eye Res* 88: 528–534.

Contreras-Ruiz, L., de la Fuente, M., Parraga, J. E. et al. 2011. Intracellular trafficking of hyaluronic acid-chitosan oligomer-based nanoparticles in cultured human ocular surface cells. *Mol Vis* 17: 279–290.

Dartt, D. A. 2004. Control of mucin production by ocular surface epithelial cells. *Exp Eye Res* 78: 173–185.

Davies, N. M. 2000. Biopharmaceutical considerations in topical ocular drug delivery. *Clin Exp Pharmacol Physiol* 27: 558–562.

de Campos, A. M., Diebold, Y., Carvalho, E. L., Sanchez, A., and Alonso, M. J. 2004. Chitosan nanoparticles as new ocular drug delivery systems: *In vitro* stability, *in vivo* fate, and cellular toxicity. *Pharm Res* 21: 803–810.

de Campos, A. M., Sanchez, A., and Alonso, M. J. 2001. Chitosan nanoparticles: A new vehicle for the improvement of the delivery of drugs to the ocular surface. Application to cyclosporin A. *Int J Pharm* 224: 159–168.

de la Fuente, M., Seijo, B., and Alonso, M. J. 2008. Novel hyaluronic acid-chitosan nanoparticles for ocular gene therapy. *Invest Ophthalmol Vis Sci* 49: 2016–2024.

Delgado, D., Del Pozo-Rodriguez, A., Solinis, M. A. et al. 2012. Dextran and prot-amine-based solid lipid nanoparticles as potential vectors for the treatment of x-linked juvenile retinoschisis. *Hum Gene Ther* 23: 345–55.

Dey, S., Anand, B. S., Patel, J., and Mitra, A. K. 2003. Transporters/receptors in the anterior chamber: Pathways to explore ocular drug delivery strategies. *Expert Opin Biol Ther* 3: 23–44.

Diebold, Y. and Calonge, M. 2010. Applications of nanoparticles in ophthalmology. *Prog Retin Eye Res* 29: 596–609.

Diebold, Y., Jarrin, M., Saez, V. et al. 2007. Ocular drug delivery by liposome-chitosan nanoparticle complexes (LCS-NP). *Biomaterials* 28: 1553–1564.

du Toit, L. C., Pillay, V., Choonara, Y. E., Govender, T., and Carmichael, T. 2011. Ocular drug delivery—a look towards nanobioadhesives. *Expert Opin Drug Deliv* 8: 71–94.

Duan, X. and Sheardown, H. 2006. Dendrimer crosslinked collagen as a corneal tissue engineering scaffold: Mechanical properties and corneal epithelial cell interactions. *Biomaterials* 27: 4608–4617.

Duvvuri, S., Majumdar, S., and Mitra, A. K. 2003. Drug delivery to the retina: Challenges and opportunities. *Expert Opin Biol Ther* 3: 45–56.

Duvvuri, S., Majumdar, S., and Mitra, A. K. 2004. Role of metabolism in ocular drug delivery. *Curr Drug Metab* 5: 507–515.

Edelhauser, H. F., Rowe-Rendleman, C. L., Robinson, M. R. et al. 2010. Ophthalmic drug delivery systems for the treatment of retinal diseases: Basic research to clinical applications. *Invest Ophthalmol Vis Sci* 51: 5403–5420.

El Sanharawi, M., Kowalczuk, L., Touchard, E. et al. 2010. Protein delivery for retinal diseases: From basic considerations to clinical applications. *Prog Retin Eye Res* 29: 443–465.

Eljarrat-Binstock, E., Orucov, F., Aldouby, Y., Frucht-Pery, J., and Domb, A. J. 2008. Charged nanoparticles delivery to the eye using hydrogel iontophoresis. *J Control Release* 126: 156–161.

Fenske, D. B., Chonn, A., and Cullis, P. R. 2008. Liposomal nanomedicines: An emerging field. *Toxicol Pathol* 36: 21–29.

Fenwick, B. W. and Cullis, P. R. 2008. Liposomal nanomedicines. *Expert Opin Drug Deliv* 5: 25–44.

Fialho, S. L., Behar-Cohen, F., and Silva-Cunha, A. 2008. Dexamethasone-loaded poly(epsilon-caprolactone) intravitreal implants: A pilot study. *Eur J Pharm Biopharm* 68: 637–646.

Fischbarg, J. 2006. *The Biology of the Eye*. Amsterdam: Elsevier Science.

Fischbarg, J., Diecke, F. P., Iserovich, P., and Rubashkin, A. 2006. The role of the tight junction in paracellular fluid transport across corneal endothelium. Electro-osmosis as a driving force. *J Membr Biol* 210: 117–130.

Freddo, T. F. 2001. Shifting the paradigm of the blood-aqueous barrier. *Exp Eye Res* 73: 581–592.

Friedberg, M. L., Pleyer, U., and Mondino, B. J. 1991. Device drug delivery to the eye. Collagen shields, iontophoresis, and pumps. *Ophthalmology* 98: 725–732.

Gan, L., Han, S., Shen, J. et al. 2010. Self-assembled liquid crystalline nanoparticles as a novel ophthalmic delivery system for dexamethasone: Improving preocular retention and ocular bioavailability. *Int J Pharm* 396: 179–187.

Gardner, T. W., Antonetti, D. A., Barber, A. J., Lieth, E., and Tarbell, J. A. 1999. The molecular structure and function of the inner blood-retinal barrier. Penn State Retina Research Group. *Doc Ophthalmol* 97: 229–237.

Gaudana, R., Ananthula, H. K., Parenky, A., and Mitra, A. K. 2010. Ocular drug delivery. *AAPS J* 12: 348–360.

Ghosh, F., Hansson, L. J., Bynke, G., and Bekassy, A. N. 2002. Intravitreal sustained-release ganciclovir implants for severe bilateral cytomegalovirus retinitis after stem cell transplantation. *Acta Ophthalmol Scand* 80: 101–104.

Giannavola, C., Bucolo, C., Maltese, A. et al. 2003. Influence of preparation conditions on acyclovir-loaded poly-D,L-lactic acid nanospheres and effect of PEG coating on ocular drug bioavailability. *Pharm Res* 20: 584–590.

Gilhotra, R. M., Gilhotra, N., and Mishra, D. N. 2009. Piroxicam bioadhesive ocular inserts: Physicochemical characterization and evaluation in prostaglandin-induced inflammation. *Curr Eye Res* 34: 1065–1073.

Gokce, E. H., Sandri, G., Egrilmez, S. et al. 2009. Cyclosporine a-loaded solid lipid nanoparticles: Ocular tolerance and *in vivo* drug release in rabbit eyes. *Curr Eye Res* 34: 996–1003.

Gupta, H., Aqil, M., Khar, R. K. et al. 2010. Sparfloxacin-loaded PLGA nanoparticles for sustained ocular drug delivery. *Nanomedicine* 6: 324–333.

Hamalainen, K. M., Kananen, K., Auriola, S., Kontturi, K., and Urtti, A. 1997. Characterization of paracellular and aqueous penetration routes in cornea, conjunctiva, and sclera. *Invest Ophthalmol Vis Sci* 38: 627–634.

Han, S. B., Baek, S. H., Park, J. S. et al. 2011. Effect of subconjunctivally injected liposome-encapsulated tissue plasminogen activator on the absorption rate of subconjunctival hemorrhages in rabbits. *Cornea* 30: 1455–1460.

Han, S., Shen, J. Q., Gan, Y. et al. 2010. Novel vehicle based on cubosomes for ophthalmic delivery of flurbiprofen with low irritancy and high bioavailability. *Acta Pharmacol Sin* 31: 990–998.

Hayashi, A., Naseri, A., Pennesi, M. E., and De Juan, E., Jr. 2009. Subretinal delivery of immunoglobulin G with gold nanoparticles in the rabbit eye. *Jpn J Ophthalmol* 53: 249–256.

Higashiyama, M., Tajika, T., Inada, K., and Ohtori, A. 2006. Improvement of the ocular bioavailability of carteolol by ion pair. *J Ocul Pharmacol Ther* 22: 333–339.

Holden, C. A., Tyagi, P., Thakur, A. et al. 2012. Polyamidoamine dendrimer hydrogel for enhanced delivery of antiglaucoma drugs. *Nanomedicine* 8:776–783.

Hornof, M., Toropainen, E., and Urtti, A. 2005. Cell culture models of the ocular barriers. *Eur J Pharm Biopharm* 60: 207–225.

Hosny, K. M. 2010a. Ciprofloxacin as ocular liposomal hydrogel. *AAPS PharmSciTech* 11: 241–246.

Hosny, K. M. 2010b. Optimization of gatifloxacin liposomal hydrogel for enhanced transcorneal permeation. *J Liposome Res* 20: 31–37.

Hosoya, K., Lee, V. H., and Kim, K. J. 2005a. Roles of the conjunctiva in ocular drug delivery: A review of conjunctival transport mechanisms and their regulation. *Eur J Pharm Biopharm: Off J Arbeitsgemeinschaft Fur Pharmazeutische Verfahrenstechnik e.V* 60: 227–240.

Hosoya, K., Lee, V. H., and Kim, K. J. 2005b. Roles of the conjunctiva in ocular drug delivery: A review of conjunctival transport mechanisms and their regulation. *Eur J Pharm Biopharm* 60: 227–240.

Hosoya, K., Tomi, M., and Tachikawa, M. 2011. Strategies for therapy of retinal diseases using systemic drug delivery: Relevance of transporters at the blood-retinal barrier. *Expert Opin Drug Deliv* 8: 1571–1587.

Hsu, J. 2007. Drug delivery methods for posterior segment disease. *Curr Opin Ophthalmol* 18: 235–239.

Imayasu, M., Shiraishi, A., Ohashi, Y., Shimada, S., and Cavanagh, H. D. 2008. Effects of multipurpose solutions on corneal epithelial tight junctions. *Eye Contact Lens* 34: 50–55.

Jager, K., Bonisch, U., Risch, M., Worlitzsch, D., and Paulsen, F. 2009. Detection and regulation of cationic amino acid transporters in healthy and diseased ocular surface. *Invest Ophthalmol Vis Sci* 50: 1112–1121.

Jentsch, T. J., Janicke, I., Sorgenfrei, D., Keller, S. K., and Wiederholt, M. 1986a. The regulation of intracellular pH in monkey kidney epithelial cells (BSC-1). Roles of Na+/H+ antiport, Na+-HCO3(-)-(NaCO3-) symport, and Cl-/HCO3- exchange. *J Biol Chem* 261: 12120–12127.

Jentsch, T. J., Schwartz, P., Schill, B. S. et al. 1986b. Kinetic properties of the sodium bicarbonate (carbonate) symport in monkey kidney epithelial cells (BSC-1). Interactions between Na+, HCO-3, and pH. *J Biol Chem* 261: 10673–10679.

Jwala, J., Boddu, S. H., Shah, S. et al. 2011. Ocular sustained release nanoparticles containing stereoisomeric dipeptide prodrugs of acyclovir. *J Ocul Pharmacol Ther* 27: 163–172.

Kaiser, J. M., Imai, H., Haakenson, J. K. et al. 2013. Nanoliposomal minocycline for ocular drug delivery. *Nanomedicine* 9: 130–140.

Kaji, Y., Yamamoto, E., Hiraoka, T., and Oshika, T. 2009. Toxicities and pharmaco-kinetics of subconjunctival injection of liposomal amphotericin B. *Graefes Arch Clin Exp Ophthalmol* 247: 549–553.

Karla, P. K., Pal, D., and Mitra, A. K. 2007. Molecular evidence and functional expression of multidrug resistance associated protein (MRP) in rabbit corneal epithelial cells. *Exp Eye Res* 84: 53–60.

Kaulen, P., Kahle, G., Keller, K., and Wollensak, J. 1991. Autoradiographic mapping of the glucose transporter with cytochalasin B in the mammalian eye. *Invest Ophthalmol Vis Sci* 32: 1903–1911.

Kaur, I. P. and Smitha, R. 2002. Penetration enhancers and ocular bioadhesives: Two new avenues for ophthalmic drug delivery. *Drug Dev Ind Pharm* 28: 353–369.

Keam, S. J., Scott, L. J., and Curran, M. P. 2003. Verteporfin: A review of its use in the management of subfoveal choroidal neovascularisation. *Drugs* 63: 2521–2554.

Kean, T. and Thanou, M. 2010. Biodegradation, biodistribution and toxicity of chitosan. *Adv Drug Deliv Rev* 62: 3–11.

Khanal, S. and Millar, T. J. 2010. Nanoscale phase dynamics of the normal tear film. *Nanomedicine* 6: 707–713.

Kimura, H. and Ogura, Y. 2001. Biodegradable polymers for ocular drug delivery. *Ophthalmologica* 215: 143–155.

Koevary, S. B. 2003. Pharmacokinetics of topical ocular drug delivery: Potential uses for the treatment of diseases of the posterior segment and beyond. *Curr Drug Metab* 4: 213–222.

Kompella, U. B., Sundaram, S., Raghava, S., and Escobar, E. R. 2006. Luteinizing hormone-releasing hormone agonist and transferrin functionalizations enhance nanoparticle delivery in a novel bovine ex vivo eye model. *Mol Vis* 12: 1185–1198.

Kothuri, M. K., Pinnamaneni, S., Das, N. G., and Das, S. K. 2003. Microparticles and nanoparticles in ocular drug delivery. In *Ophthalmic Drug Delivery Systems*, ed. A. K. Mitra, 437–466. New York: Marcel Dekker, Inc.

Kuehn, M. H., Wang, K., Roos, B. et al. 2011. Chromosome 7q31 POAG locus: Ocular expression of caveolins and lack of association with POAG in a US cohort. *Mol Vis* 17: 430–435.

Kumagai, A. K., Glasgow, B. J., and Pardridge, W. M. 1994. GLUT1 glucose transporter expression in the diabetic and nondiabetic human eye. *Invest Ophthalmol Vis Sci* 35: 2887–2894.

Kyyronen, K. and Urtti, A. 1990. Improved ocular: Systemic absorption ratio of timolol by viscous vehicle and phenylephrine. *Invest Ophthalmol Vis Sci* 31: 1827–1833.

la Cour, M. and Ehinger, B. 2006. The Reina. In *Advances in Organ Biology: The Biology of the Eye*, ed. E. Edward Bittar, 195–254. Netherlands: Elsevier.

Lajavardi, L., Camelo, S., Agnely, F. et al. 2009. New formulation of vasoactive intestinal peptide using liposomes in hyaluronic acid gel for uveitis. *J Control Release* 139: 22–30.

Law, S. L., Huang, K. J., and Chiang, C. H. 2000. Acyclovir-containing liposomes for potential ocular delivery. Corneal penetration and absorption. *J Control Release* 63: 135–140.

Lee, S. S., Hughes, P., Ross, A. D., and Robinson, M. R. 2010. Biodegradable implants for sustained drug release in the eye. *Pharm Res* 27: 2043–2053.

Li, R., Jiang, S., Liu, D. et al. 2011. A potential new therapeutic system for glaucoma: Solid lipid nanoparticles containing methazolamide. *J Microencapsul* 28: 134–141.

Li, H., Tran, V. V., Hu, Y. et al. 2006. A PEDF N-terminal peptide protects the retina from ischemic injury when delivered in PLGA nanospheres. *Exp Eye Res* 83: 824–833.

Li, T., Zhang, M., Han, Y. et al. 2010. Targeting therapy of choroidal neovascularization by use of polypeptide- and PEDF-loaded immunoliposomes under ultrasound exposure. *J Huazhong Univ Sci Technolog Med Sci* 30: 798–803.

Li, N., Zhuang, C., Wang, M. et al. 2009. Liposome coated with low molecular weight chitosan and its potential use in ocular drug delivery. *International Journal of Pharmaceutics* 379: 131–138.

Lian, T. and Ho, R. J. 2001. Trends and developments in liposome drug delivery systems. *J Pharm Sci* 90: 667–680.

Loutsch, J. M., Ong, D., and Hill, J. M. 2003. Dendrimers: An innovative and enhanced ocular drug delivery system. In *Ophthalmic Drug Delivery Systems*, ed. A. K. Mitra, 467–492. New York: Marcel Dekker, Inc.

Ludwig, A. 2005. The use of mucoadhesive polymers in ocular drug delivery. *Adv Drug Deliv Rev* 57: 1595–1639.

Macha, S. and Mitra, A. K. 2003. Overview of ocular drug delivery. In *Ophthalmic Drug Delivery Systems*, ed. A. K. Mitra, 1–12. New York: Marcel Dekker, Inc.

Marano, R. J., Toth, I., Wimmer, N., Brankov, M., and Rakoczy, P. E. 2005. Dendrimer delivery of an anti-VEGF oligonucleotide into the eye: A long-term study into inhibition of laser-induced CNV, distribution, uptake and toxicity. *Gene Ther* 12: 1544–1550.

Marshall, W. S. and Klyce, S. D. 1983. Cellular and paracellular pathway resistances in the "tight" Cl- -secreting epithelium of rabbit cornea. *J Membr Biol* 73: 275–282.

McCaa, C. S. 1982. The eye and visual nervous system: Anatomy, physiology and toxicology. *Environ Health Perspect* 44: 1–8.

Mishra, G. P., Bagui, M., Tamboli, V., and Mitra, A. K. 2011. Recent applications of liposomes in ophthalmic drug delivery. *J Drug Deliv* 2011: 863734.

Mitra, A. K., Anand, B. S., and Duvvuri, S. 2006a. Drug delivery to the eye. In *The Biology of Eye*, ed. J. Fischbarg, 307–351. New York: Academic Press.

Mitra, A. P., Lin, H., Datar, R. H., and Cote, R. J. 2006b. Molecular biology of bladder cancer: Prognostic and clinical implications. *Clin Genitourin Cancer* 5: 67–77.

Mo, Y., Barnett, M. E., Takemoto, D., Davidson, H., and Kompella, U. B. 2007. Human serum albumin nanoparticles for efficient delivery of Cu, Zn superoxide dismutase gene. *Mol Vis* 13: 746–757.

Moghimi, S. M. and Szebeni, J. 2003. Stealth liposomes and long circulating nanoparticles: Critical issues in pharmacokinetics, opsonization and protein-binding properties. *Prog Lipid Res* 42: 463–478.

Montes-Mico, R. 2007. Role of the tear film in the optical quality of the human eye. *J Cataract Refract Surg* 33: 1631–1635.

Morand, K., Bartoletti, A. C., Bochot, A. et al. 2007. Liposomal amphotericin B eye drops to treat fungal keratitis: Physico-chemical and formulation stability. *Int J Pharm* 344: 150–153.

Moriyama, T., Tsuruta, Y., Shimizu, A. et al. 2011. The significance of caveolae in the glomeruli in glomerular disease. *J Clin Pathol* 64: 504–509.

Mozafari, M. R. 2010. Nanoliposomes: Preparation and analysis. *Methods Mol Biol* 605: 29–50.

Mruthyunjaya, P., Khalatbari, D., Yang, P. et al. 2006. Efficacy of low-release-rate fluocinolone acetonide intravitreal implants to treat experimental uveitis. *Arch Ophthalmol* 124: 1012–1018.

Natarajan, J. V., Ang, M., Darwitan, A. et al. 2012. Nanomedicine for glaucoma: Liposomes provide sustained release of latanoprost in the eye. *Int J Nanomedicine* 7: 123–131.

Ng, E. W., Shima, D. T., Calias, P. et al. 2006. Pegaptanib, a targeted anti-VEGF aptamer for ocular vascular disease. *Nat Rev Drug Discov* 5: 123–132.

Ni, Z. and Hui, P. 2009. Emerging pharmacologic therapies for wet age-related macular degeneration. *Ophthalmologica* 223: 401–410.

Nishiyama, N., Iriyama, A., Jang, W. D. et al. 2005. Light-induced gene transfer from packaged DNA enveloped in a dendrimeric photosensitizer. *Nat Mater* 4: 934–941.

Nojehdehian, H., Moztarzadeh, F., Baharvand, H., Nazarian, H., and Tahriri, M. 2009. Preparation and surface characterization of poly-L-lysine-coated PLGA microsphere scaffolds containing retinoic acid for nerve tissue engineering: *In vitro* study. *Colloids Surf B Biointerfaces* 73: 23–29.

Omidi, Y., Barar, J., Ahmadian, S., Heidari, H. R., and Gumbleton, M. 2008a. Characterization and astrocytic modulation of system L transporters in brain microvasculature endothelial cells. *Cell Biochem Funct* 26: 381–391.

Omidi, Y., Barar, J., and Akhtar, S. 2005. Toxicogenomics of cationic lipid-based vectors for gene therapy: Impact of microarray technology. *Curr Drug Deliv* 2: 429–441.

Omidi, Y., Barar, J., Heidari, H. R. et al. 2008b. Microarray analysis of the toxicogenomics and the genotoxic potential of a cationic lipid-based gene delivery nanosystem in human alveolar epithelial a549 cells. *Toxicol Mech Methods* 18: 369–378.

Omidi, Y., Campbell, L., Barar, J. et al. 2003a. Evaluation of the immortalised mouse brain capillary endothelial cell line, b.End3, as an *in vitro* blood-brain barrier model for drug uptake and transport studies. *Brain Res* 990: 95–112.

Omidi, Y. and Davaran, S. 2011. Impacts of biodegradable polymers: Towards biomedical applications. In *A Handbook of Applied Biopolymer Technology: Synthesis, Degradation and Applications*, ed. S. K. Sharma, A. Mudhoo, and J. H. Clark, 388–418. London: Royal Society of Chemistry.

Omidi, Y. and Gumbleton, M. 2005. Biological membranes and barriers. In *Biomaterials for Delivery and Targeting of Proteins Nucleic Acids*, ed. R. I. Mahato, 232–274. New York: CRC Press.

Omidi, Y., Hollins, A. J., Benboubetra, M. et al. 2003b. Toxicogenomics of non-viral vectors for gene therapy: A microarray study of lipofectin- and oligofectamine-induced gene expression changes in human epithelial cells. *J Drug Target* 11: 311–323.

Owens, D. E., 3rd and Peppas, N. A. 2006. Opsonization, biodistribution, and pharmacokinetics of polymeric nanoparticles. *Int J Pharm* 307: 93–102.

Parveen, S., Mitra, M., Krishnakumar, S., and Sahoo, S. K. 2010. Enhanced antiproliferative activity of carboplatin-loaded chitosan-alginate nanoparticles in a retinoblastoma cell line. *Acta Biomater* 6: 3120–3131.

Patravale, V. B., Date, A. A., and Kulkarni, R. M. 2004. Nanosuspensions: A promising drug delivery strategy. *J Pharm Pharmacol* 56: 827–840.

Pelkmans, L. and Helenius, A. 2002. Endocytosis via caveolae. *Traffic* 3: 311–320.

Peng, Y., Ang, M., Foo, S. et al. 2011. Biocompatibility and biodegradation studies of subconjunctival implants in rabbit eyes. *PLoS One* 6: e22507.

Perdue, N. and Yan, Q. 2006. Caveolin-1 is up-regulated in transdifferentiated lens epithelial cells but minimal in normal human and murine lenses. *Exp Eye Res* 83: 1154–1161.

Peyman, G. A., Khoobehi, B., Tawakol, M. et al. 1987. Intravitreal injection of liposome-encapsulated ganciclovir in a rabbit model. *Retina* 7: 227–229.

Pignatello, R., Bucolo, C., and Puglisi, G. 2002. Ocular tolerability of Eudragit RS100 and RL100 nanosuspensions as carriers for ophthalmic controlled drug delivery. *J Pharm Sci* 91: 2636–2641.

Pillai, O. and Panchagnula, R. 2001. Polymers in drug delivery. *Curr Opin Chem Biol* 5: 447–451.

Pleyer, U., Elkins, B., Ruckert, D. et al. 1994. Ocular absorption of cyclosporine A from liposomes incorporated into collagen shields. *Curr Eye Res* 13: 177–181.

Prausnitz, M. R. and Noonan, J. S. 1998. Permeability of cornea, sclera, and conjunctiva: A literature analysis for drug delivery to the eye. *J Pharm Sci* 87: 1479–1488.

Qaddoumi, M. G., Gukasyan, H. J., Davda, J. et al. 2003. Clathrin and caveolin-1 expression in primary pigmented rabbit conjunctival epithelial cells: Role in PLGA nanoparticle endocytosis. *Mol Vis* 9: 559–568.

Qazi, Y., Stagg, B., Singh, N. et al. 2012. Nanoparticle-mediated delivery of shRNA. VEGF-A plasmids regresses corneal neovascularization. *Invest Ophthalmol Vis Sci* 53: 2837–2844.

Rajappa, M., Saxena, P., and Kaur, J. 2010. Ocular angiogenesis: Mechanisms and recent advances in therapy. *Adv Clin Chem* 50: 103–121.

Rajera, R., Nagpal, K., Singh, S. K., and Mishra, D. N. 2011. Niosomes: A controlled and novel drug delivery system. *Biol Pharm Bull* 34: 945–953.

Rocha, E. M., Cunha, D. A., Carneiro, E. M. et al. 2002. Insulin, insulin receptor and insulin-like growth factor-I receptor on the human ocular surface. *Adv Exp Med Biol* 506: 607–610.

Sabah, J. R., Schultz, B. D., Brown, Z. W. et al. 2007. Transcytotic passage of albumin through lens epithelial cells. *Invest Ophthalmol Vis Sci* 48: 1237–1244.

Saha, P., Kim, K. J., and Lee, V. H. 1996. A primary culture model of rabbit conjunctival epithelial cells exhibiting tight barrier properties. *Curr Eye Res* 15: 1163–1169.

Sahoo, S. K., Dilnawaz, F., and Krishnakumar, S. 2008. Nanotechnology in ocular drug delivery. *Drug Discov Today* 13: 144–151.

Sanders, N. N., Peeters, L., Lentacker, I., Demeester, J., and De Smedt, S. C. 2007. Wanted and unwanted properties of surface PEGylated nucleic acid nanoparticles in ocular gene transfer. *J Control Release* 122: 226–235.

Schepens, C. L. and Acosta, F. 1991. Scleral implants: An historical perspective. *Surv Ophthalmol* 35: 447–453.

Schlingemann, R. O., Hofman, P., Klooster, J. et al. 1998. Ciliary muscle capillaries have blood-tissue barrier characteristics. *Exp Eye Res* 66: 747–754.

Schmoll, T., Unterhuber, A., Kolbitsch, C. et al. 2012. Precise thickness measurements of bowman's layer, epithelium, and tear film. *Optom Vis Sci* 89: E795–802.

Schoenwald, R. D., Deshpande, G. S., Rethwisch, D. G., and Barfknecht, C. F. 1997. Penetration into the anterior chamber via the conjunctival/scleral pathway. *J Ocul Pharmacol Ther* 13: 41–59.

Schubert, W., Frank, P. G., Razani, B. et al. 2001. Caveolae-deficient endothelial cells show defects in the uptake and transport of albumin in vivo. *J Biol Chem* 276: 48619–48622.

Senthilkumari, S., Velpandian, T., Biswas, N. R., Sonali, N., and Ghose, S. 2008. Evaluation of the impact of P-glycoprotein (P-gp) drug efflux transporter blockade on the systemic and ocular disposition of P-gp substrate. *J Ocul Pharmacol Ther* 24: 290–300.

Shah, S. S., Denham, L. V., Elison, J. R. et al. 2010. Drug delivery to the posterior segment of the eye for pharmacologic therapy. *Expert Rev Ophthalmol* 5: 75–93.

Shan, X., Yuan, Y., Liu, C. et al. 2009. Influence of PEG chain on the complement activation suppression and longevity *in vivo* prolongation of the PCL biomedical nanoparticles. *Biomed Microdevices* 11: 1187–1194.

Shedden, A. H., Laurence, J., Barrish, A., and Olah, T. V. 2001. Plasma timolol concentrations of timolol maleate: Timolol gel-forming solution (TIMOPTIC-XE) once daily versus timolol maleate ophthalmic solution twice daily. *Doc Ophthalmol* 103: 73–79.

Shen, Y. and Tu, J. 2007. Preparation and ocular pharmacokinetics of ganciclovir liposomes. *AAPS J* 9: E371–377.

Shimazaki, H., Hironaka, K., Fujisawa, T. et al. 2011. Edaravone-loaded liposome eyedrops protect against light-induced retinal damage in mice. *Invest Ophthalmol Vis Sci* 52: 7289–7297.

Singh, K. H. and Shinde, U. A. 2011. Chitosan nanoparticles for controlled delivery of brimonidine tartrate to the ocular membrane. *Die Pharmazie* 66: 594–599.

Smith, M., Omidi, Y., and Gumbleton, M. 2007. Primary porcine brain microvascular endothelial cells: Biochemical and functional characterisation as a model for drug transport and targeting. *J Drug Target* 15: 253–268.

Stewart, P. A. and Tuor, U. I. 1994. Blood-eye barriers in the rat: Correlation of ultrastructure with function. *J Comp Neurol* 340: 566–576.

Sultana, Y., Maurya, D. P., Iqbal, Z., and Aqil, M. 2011. Nanotechnology in ocular delivery: Current and future directions. *Drugs Today (Barc)* 47: 441–455.

Sun, Y., Fox, T., Adhikary, G., Kester, M., and Pearlman, E. 2008. Inhibition of corneal inflammation by liposomal delivery of short-chain, C-6 ceramide. *J Leukoc Biol* 83: 1512–1521.

Sunkara, G. and Kompella, U. B. 2003. Membrane transport processes in the eye. In *Ophthalmic Drug Delivery Systems*, ed. A. K. Mitra, 13–58. New York: Marcel Dekker, Inc.

Szoka, F. C., Jr., Milholland, D., and Barza, M. 1987. Effect of lipid composition and liposome size on toxicity and *in vitro* fungicidal activity of liposome-intercalated amphotericin B. *Antimicrob Agents Chemother* 31: 421–429.

Tam, A. L., Gupta, N., Zhang, Z., and Yucel, Y. H. 2011. Quantum dots trace lymphatic drainage from the mouse eye. *Nanotechnology* 22: 425101.

Tan, A., Yildirimer, L., Rajadas, J. et al. 2011. Quantum dots and carbon nanotubes in oncology: A review on emerging theranostic applications in nanomedicine. *Nanomedicine (Lond)* 6: 1101–1114.

Thrimawithana, T. R., Young, S., Bunt, C. R., Green, C., and Alany, R. G. 2011. Drug delivery to the posterior segment of the eye. *Drug Discov Today* 16: 270–277.

Tiruppathi, C., Naqvi, T., Wu, Y. et al. 2004. Albumin mediates the transcytosis of myeloperoxidase by means of caveolae in endothelial cells. *Proc Natl Acad Sci USA* 101: 7699–7704.

Toda, R., Kawazu, K., Oyabu, M., Miyazaki, T., and Kiuchi, Y. 2011. Comparison of drug permeabilities across the blood-retinal barrier, blood-aqueous humor barrier, and blood-brain barrier. *J Pharm Sci* 100: 3904–3911.

Tomalia, D. A., Baker, H., Dewald, J. et al. 1984. New class of polymers: Starburst-dendritic macromolecules. *Polym J* 17: 117–132.

Tomi, M. and Hosoya, K. 2010. The role of blood-ocular barrier transporters in retinal drug disposition: An overview. *Expert Opin Drug Metab Toxicol* 6: 1111–1124.

Tommaso, C. D., Bourges, J. L., Valamanesh, F. et al. 2012. Novel micelle carriers for cyclosporin A topical ocular delivery: *In vivo* cornea penetration, ocular distribution and efficacy studies. *Eur J Pharm Biopharm* 81: 257–264.

Touvron, G., Denis, D., Doat, M. et al. 2009. Successful treatment of resistant Fusarium solani keratitis with liposomal amphotericin B. *J Fr Ophtalmol* 32: 721–726.

Tserentsoodol, N., Shin, B. C., Suzuki, T., and Takata, K. 1998. Colocalization of tight junction proteins, occludin and ZO-1, and glucose transporter GLUT1 in cells of the blood-ocular barrier in the mouse eye. *Histochem Cell Biol* 110: 543–551.

Urtti, A. 2006. Challenges and obstacles of ocular pharmacokinetics and drug delivery. *Adv Drug Deliv Rev* 58: 1131–1135.

Valls, R., Vega, E., Garcia, M. L., Egea, M. A., and Valls, J. O. 2008. Transcorneal permeation in a corneal device of non-steroidal anti-inflammatory drugs in drug delivery systems. *Open Med Chem J* 2: 66–71.

Vandervoort, J. and Ludwig, A. 2007. Ocular drug delivery: Nanomedicine applications. *Nanomedicine (Lond)* 2: 11–21.

Vega, E., Egea, M. A., Valls, O., Espina, M., and Garcia, M. L. 2006. Flurbiprofen loaded biodegradable nanoparticles for ophtalmic administration. *J Pharm Sci* 95: 2393–2405.

Wadhwa, S., Paliwal, R., Paliwal, S. R., and Vyas, S. P. 2009. Chitosan and its role in ocular therapeutics. *Mini Rev Med Chem* 9: 1639–1647.

Wilson, C. G. 2004. Topical drug delivery in the eye. *Exp Eye Res* 78: 737–743.

Yamamoto, T., Hiraoka, T., and Oshika, T. 2011. Time course of changes in functional visual acuity and ocular wavefront aberration after instillation of ofloxacin gel-forming ophthalmic solution. *Nihon Ganka Gakkai Zasshi* 115: 1094–1100.

Yang, J. J., Ann, D. K., Kannan, R., and Lee, V. H. 2007. Multidrug resistance protein 1 (MRP1) in rabbit conjunctival epithelial cells: Its effect on drug efflux and its regulation by adenoviral infection. *Pharm Res* 24: 1490–1500.

Yao, W., Sun, K., Mu, H. et al. 2010. Preparation and characterization of puerarin-dendrimer complexes as an ocular drug delivery system. *Drug Dev Ind Pharm* 36: 1027–1035.

Yao, J., Tucker, B. A., Zhang, X. et al. 2011. Robust cell integration from co-transplantation of biodegradable MMP2-PLGA microspheres with retinal progenitor cells. *Biomaterials* 32: 1041–1050.

Yenice, I., Mocan, M. C., Palaska, E. et al. 2008. Hyaluronic acid coated poly-epsilon-caprolactone nanospheres deliver high concentrations of cyclosporine A into the cornea. *Exp Eye Res* 87: 162–167.

Yi, X., Wang, Y., and Yu, F. S. 2000. Corneal epithelial tight junctions and their response to lipopolysaccharide challenge. *Invest Ophthalmol Vis Sci* 41: 4093–4100.

Yoshida, Y., Ban, Y., and Kinoshita, S. 2009. Tight junction transmembrane protein claudin subtype expression and distribution in human corneal and conjunctival epithelium. *Invest Ophthalmol Vis Sci* 50: 2103–2108.

Zhang, R., He, R., Qian, J. et al. 2010. Treatment of experimental autoimmune uveoretinitis with intravitreal injection of tacrolimus (FK506) encapsulated in liposomes. *Invest Ophthalmol Vis Sci* 51: 3575–3582.

12

Toxicology of Nanoparticles

Siva K. Nalabotu and Eric R. Blough

CONTENTS

12.1 Introduction to Nanotechnology 337
12.2 Unique Properties and Applications of Nanomaterials 339
12.3 Toxicity of Nanomaterials 340
    12.3.1 Factors Responsible for the Nanomaterial Toxicity 341
    12.3.2 Routes of Exposure to ENPs 341
    12.3.3 Respiratory Route of Exposure 341
    12.3.4 Ingestion Route of Exposure 342
    12.3.5 Dermal Route of Exposure 343
    12.3.6 Drug-Delivery Route of Exposure 343
12.4 Cellular Effects of the ENPs 343
    12.4.1 Cellular Uptake of ENPs 343
12.5 Mechanisms of NP Toxicity 344
    12.5.1 Oxidative Stress: Reactive Oxygen Species 345
    12.5.2 Mechanisms of ROS Production and Apoptosis 345
    12.5.3 Mitochondrial Pathway of Apoptosis 346
    12.5.4 ENPs-Induced Inflammation 347
    12.5.5 ENPs-Induced Genotoxicity and Carcinogenesis 347
    12.5.6 ENPs-Induced Reproductive and Developmental Toxicity 348
12.6 Regulatory Efforts 348
References 349

12.1 Introduction to Nanotechnology

Recently, there has been an increased usage of the terms "nanotechnology," "nanomaterials," and "nanoparticles." The entire world is looking at "nanotechnology" since it has excellent beneficial effects in various stages of human life. Henceforth, the scientific community, including academia, industry, and various regulatory bodies have been investing a lot of money, time, and resources to develop various types of nanoproducts through innovative ideas to meet cost effective, less harmful, and more beneficial, less volume consumption, and as an alternative to the existing products.

Nanotechnology research receives tremendous funding both from public and private sectors. It has been estimated that the investments in nanotechnology industry increased from $13 billion in 2004 to $50 billion in 2006 and it is estimated to reach $2.6 trillion dollars in 2014 [1,2]. The National Science Foundation has proposed that the worldwide market consumption size of nanoparticles (NPs) would be $1 trillion between 2010 and 2015 [2]. Among these, the pharmaceutical industry consumption alone would be about $180 billion between 2010 and 2015 [3].

Nanotechnology can be defined as the design, synthesis, and application of materials and devices whose size and shape have been engineered at the nanoscale (1–100 nm). Materials that have structural components less than 1 µm in at least one dimension are called as nanomaterials. Particles with at least one dimension less than 1 µm and potentially as small as atomic and molecular length scales (~0.2 nm) are defined as NPs [4,5]. There are two types of NPs: (1) naturally occurring NPs (e.g., produced naturally in volcanoes, forest fires, or as combustion by-products), and (2) engineered nanoparticles (ENPs), deliberately developed to be used in application (e.g., carbon black, fumed silica, titanium dioxide (TiO_2), iron oxide (FeO_x), quantum dots (QDs), fullerenes, and carbon nanotubes (CNTs)) [4,5].

While various types of NPs are available in nature, recent advancement in this technology is to develop and produce different types of ENPs. ENPs (less frequently also "manufactured nanoparticles") are produced manually to have specific properties or a specific composition [4]. Although, more than 100s of the ENPs are available today, the Organization for Economic Co-operation and Development (OECD) has formed a committee called Working Party on Manufactured Nanomaterials (WPMN). This committee has identified 14 most beneficial ENPs to evaluate their characteristics and its applicability as well as safety [6,7]. On priority basis, the following ENPs are considered for evaluation:

- Fullerenes (C60)
- Single-walled carbon nanotubes (SWCNTs)
- Multi-walled carbon nanotubes (MWCNTs)
- Silver NPs
- Iron NPs
- Carbon black
- Titanium dioxide
- Aluminum oxide
- Cerium oxide
- Zinc oxide
- Silicon dioxide
- Polystyrene dendrimers
- Nano clays

The above-mentioned ENPs have extraordinary properties and applications in various sectors. In addition to that, there is lot of scope to use these materials in various additional sectors.

12.2 Unique Properties and Applications of Nanomaterials

Nanomaterials have unique properties, which make them to behave differently from their bulk counterparts. The unique properties of the nanomaterials are because of their surface and quantum effects [4,8]. These effects give the nanomaterials their high reactivity as well as different optical, electrical, and magnetic properties [9]. Nanoscale materials have increased surface area-to-volume ratio, which make them highly reactive. Regarding its increased reactivity, we can use these materials for various applications. For example, the ratio of surface area-to-volume ratio is 1000 times higher for a particle with 60 nm size than the particles with 60 μm diameter. Therefore, the reactivity of the NP is approximately 1000-fold higher than the micrometer particle [4].

As quantum effects start to dominate at the nanoscale, nanoscale materials have enhanced mechanical, photonic, optical, electrical, and paramagnetic properties [4]. For example, normally, gold is yellow in color, however, at the nanoscale level, it appears in different colors such as red, blue, and green based on the size of the NPs [10,11] (Figure 12.1). Some NPs such as super paramagnetic iron oxide (SPIONs) and gold NPs can be used as efficient imaging agents for disease diagnosis and treatment as it has enhanced optical properties at the nanoscale level [11,12].

Regarding the unique properties and extensive applications of NPs in various fields, it has been estimated that more than 800 nanoproducts are being manufactured by 322 companies all over the world [13]. These products have

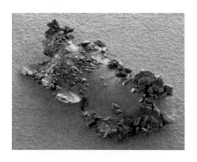
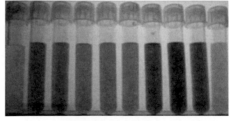

Different sizes of colloidal gold particles

2   5   6   12   16   18   24   60   90 150 nm

FIGURE 12.1
(**See color insert.**) Alteration in the optical properties of gold NPs as a function of size of the NPs. (From Erik C.D. et al. *Chem Soc Rev*, 2012, **41**(7), 274–79. http://www.ansci.wisc.edu/facstaff/ Faculty/pages/albrecht/albrecht_web/Programs/microscopy/colloid.html.)

been used at various domains for different applications such as electronics (chips, screens), energy (production, catalysis, and storage), materials (lubricants, abrasives, paints, tires, and sportswear), consumer products (clothes, goggles, skin lotions, and sun screens), automotive, soil/water remediation (pollution absorption, water filtering, and disinfection), pesticides, chemicals, and pharmaceutical industries [2,4,5,14,15]. Apart from these applications, tremendous research is ongoing to utilize these nanomaterials in food products (additives, packaging), medical imaging, and drug-delivery systems [16–19]. It is worthy of mention that the future of human kind is going to be influenced by nanoproducts at each and every stage of life. Even though, they have tremendous applications in various sectors, there are increasing concerns over exposure to NPs as there are increased reports about the toxicity of nanomaterials.

12.3 Toxicity of Nanomaterials

Although organisms including animals and human beings have been exposed to various naturally occurring nanomaterials and NPs throughout evolution, the risk of exposure to engineered nanomaterials has increased recently more due to the increased industrialization [5]. To meet the industrial needs and its applications, there is a huge demand to make various nanomaterials in bulk by various companies. Owing to its huge production, usage and disposal will lead to a high potential threat to the ecosystem and the environment. Although, several hundred nanomaterials are available in the natural environment, toxicologists and regulatory agencies are worried about the ENPs and its exposure. The ENPs are the most important source of exposure to the environment as they can enter from the manufacturing industries and spread in the environment. These materials can easily enter living systems through various routes such as inhalation, ingestions, and absorption through the skin [20–23]. It is also possible that ENPs can enter the food cycle through contamination of food and water that are close to the manufacturing industries [18,24]. Another possibility to accumulate these ENPs on the surface is during production, utilization, disposal, and recycling [24].

Even though several reports have been published on the toxicity of nanomaterials on animal models, one of the case study recently reported in *European Respiratory Journal* about the environmental risk and health issues of human beings when they were exposed to nanomaterials [25]. The report is: "Seven women, who worked in a paint industry for 5–13 months in China, had severe respiratory stress and shortness of breath. Due to these complaints, they were admitted to Beijing Chaoyang Hospital, Beijing, China. When the pathological examination of the patients' lungs was done, they found nonspecific pulmonary inflammation, pulmonary fibrosis, and foreign-body granulomas of the pleura. In addition to the above examination, TEM analysis also confirmed the presence of round polyacrylate NPs ~30 nm in diameter in the cytoplasm, karyoplasm of pulmonary epithelium—mesothelial cells, and in chest fluid. Based on these clinical observations and analysis, the authors concluded that long-term exposure to polyacrylate NPs could result in serious damage to the human lungs." To our knowledge, this is the first clinical report that spoke about human toxicity due to nanomaterials and explains to the scientific community around the world about possible toxicity of ENPs to humans.

12.3.1 Factors Responsible for the Nanomaterial Toxicity

Nanomaterials have unique and special properties which make them useful for various applications, at the same time, these properties make them to be toxic to various organ systems [5,26]. Here, the authors discuss the factors that are responsible for the toxicity of nanomaterials. One of the factors is the size which influences the charge and surface chemistry of the NP [14,27]. Second, when the materials reach the nanoscale, they often display different chemical and electronic properties/reactivity and can have toxicological properties that differ from their bulk materials [5,28]. Owing to their small size, they can easily penetrate into subcellular components of the cells and cause toxicological effects in those organs [5,29,30].

The shape of the NP also plays a vital role to determine the toxicity [27]. NPs have different shapes such as spherical, needle-like, tubes, platelets, and so on. In general, ENPs that are rod or needle shaped are more toxic than the ones that are round in shape. One study was conducted on 0.9 nm single-walled carbon nanotubes (rods) versus fullerenes (spheres). The result from this study revealed that nanotubes are more toxic than the fullerenes as the shape of the NP has influence on the absorption and deposition of NPs in various organ systems [31–33]. A number of studies have shown that both physical and chemical factors are important determinants to the toxicity of NPs and along with the changes in the size, shape, other physicochemical properties (agglomeration state, crystal structure, chemical composition, surface area, and surface chemistry, surface charge, etc.) of a NP can result in adverse effects [9,26].

12.3.2 Routes of Exposure to ENPs

As mentioned earlier, the main source of NPs to enter the ecosystem is from ENPs. ENPs are being released into the environment from the manufacturing industries. The main routes of exposure of ENPs into the organism are through inhalation, ingestion, drug delivery, and through the dermal route [4,5] (Figure 12.2).

12.3.3 Respiratory Route of Exposure

Once the nanomaterials are inhaled by the respiratory route, they either get phagocytized by the alveolar macrophages or get lodged in the lungs by

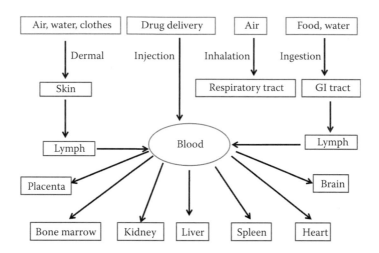

FIGURE 12.2
Routes of exposure to ENPs. (Modified from Oberdorster, G., E. Oberdorster, and J. Oberdorster, *Environ Health Perspect*, 2005. **113**(7): 823–39.)

diffusing through the epithelial cells of the lungs [5]. Once these nanomaterials are lodged in the lungs, through transcytosis they can move across the epithelia of the respiratory tract into the interstitium and reach the blood either through circulation or via the lymphatic system [4,5]. They can also easily reach various organs such as the liver, kidney, spleen, heart, the brain, and bone marrow [5,34–36]. Research studies have been conducted using copper, nickel, gold, and manganese oxide NPs. Results from these studies show that these particles enter the nervous system through the endings of the sensory nerve fibers that are embedded in the airway epithelia [37–41]. Apart from the systemic route of entry, the ENPs have also entered the brain by crossing the blood–brain barrier [39]. Further, there are some studies which show that the ENPs can even travel to the embryos through the placenta [42]. However, NPs which enter into the respiratory system through inhalation can be cleared either by physical or chemical process [4,5,43]. The physical processes of elimination are by absorption and diffusion or by binding to proteins, and other subcellular structures and eventually may be cleared into the blood and lymphatic circulation [43]. Chemical process of elimination depends on the local extracellular and intracellular conditions [44,45].

12.3.4 Ingestion Route of Exposure

Another major route of exposure of ENPs is through ingestion. ENPs can enter the digestive tract through oral ingestion by consuming contaminated food and water near the manufacturing industries or the ENPs that have been cleared through respiratory clearance pathways such as mucociliary escalator mechanism [34,43,46]. Once the nanomaterials are taken up by the gut, they can be either absorbed by the small intestine and enter into the blood stream or they can be eliminated without any absorption [47]. Most of the studies conducted on the oral route of exposure have shown that most of the ENPs passed through the digestive tract and are eliminated through feces [48,49]. On the other hand, when the nanomaterials are absorbed by the small intestine, they can also reach crucial organs such as the liver, kidney, spleen, heart, and the brain through systemic circulation [48,49].

12.3.5 Dermal Route of Exposure

The most important route of exposure of ENPs is through the skin. NPs such as zinc oxide, nanosilver, and titanium dioxide are being used in cosmetic industry to make sunscreen lotions poses as a potential source of exposure through the skin [50,51]. Even though the skin has a highly protective layer of epidermis, some NPs have shown to penetrate through the epidermis into the dermis that has a rich supply of blood and lymph macrophages, lymph vessels, and sensory nerve endings [50,52,53]. Some of the studies have also shown that the NPs can reach the regional lymph nodes of the skin through circulation and accumulate in the lymph nodes [54].

12.3.6 Drug-Delivery Route of Exposure

Research has been going on to assess the best route of delivery of ENPs as drug molecules. ENPs have shown to have excellent beneficial effects in medical applications, including disease diagnosis, imaging, and the treatment of various disease conditions [55]. Some ENPs such as iron oxide NPs, gold NPs, and magnetic NPs show more beneficial effects in imaging and in the treatment of cancer cells. Another promising ENP is cerium oxide NPs which are being used as antioxidants to treat various medical conditions such as cardiovascular disease, neuronal injury, and radiation-induced tissue damage [55–59].

12.4 Cellular Effects of the ENPs

12.4.1 Cellular Uptake of ENPs

Once ENPs reach various organs through circulation, they can enter various cells more easily through different mechanisms. The possible mechanisms for entry of ENPs into cells include: endocytosis (phagocytosis or pinocytosis), membrane penetration, or passive diffusion through transmembrane channels [5]. The transmembrane passage of ENPs depends on certain characteristics of compounds such as the physicochemical properties of particles (including chemical composition, size, shape, and agglomeration status), type of cells under which they are exposed (professional phagocytes

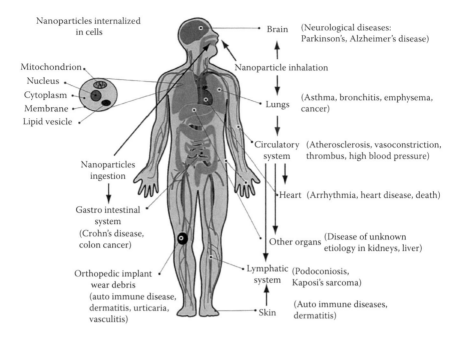

FIGURE 12.3
Various effects of the ENPs after they interact with the cellular and subcellular components in various organ systems in the human body, as studied from the epidemiological *in vitro* and *in vivo* studies. (From Buzea, C., Pacheco, II, and K. Robbie, *Biointerphases*, 2007. **2**(4): MR17–71. With permission.)

vs. nonprofessional phagocytes), serum components, and surfactants [4]. As soon as the ENPs are taken up by the organs can be seen in various locations of the cell, such as in the outer cell membrane [60], the cytoplasm [60], mitochondria [61], lipid vesicles [62], nuclear membrane [63], or within the nucleus [64,65]. For example, when C60 molecules have entered into the cells they can be visualized in the nuclear membrane, and inside the nucleus [65]. The ENPs can damage the organelles or the DNA, or cause cell death depending on their location inside the cells. The cellular effects induced by NPs also depend on the route of exposure, target organ, and the composition of the NPs [5,26,66]. NPs have been shown to induce various diseases in the organism. Figure 12.3 shows the possible NP-mediated diseases after they interact with various subcellular components in various organs.

12.5 Mechanisms of NP Toxicity

ENPs can induce various adverse effects through different cellular and molecular mechanisms such as oxidative stress, induction of inflammation, genetic damage, inhibition of cell division, and eventually leads to cell death, the cell death can be either by necrotic or apoptotic [67–70]. Here, authors would like to explain in detail about the mechanisms of the toxicity induced by various NPs.

12.5.1 Oxidative Stress: Reactive Oxygen Species

Recent evidence from mammalian systems suggested that oxidative stress is an important mechanism owing to the toxicity of the ENPs [68,71]. Oxidative stress can be caused either by depletion of antioxidants or increased production of ROS or reactive nitrogen species (RNS). Most of the studies in different systems suggested that oxidative stress with the consequent generation of ROS can serve as a common mediator for ENPs-induced toxicity. ROS include: superoxide anion ($O^{2-\bullet}$), peroxide ($O_2^{-2\bullet}$), hydroxyl radical ($^\bullet OH$), and singlet oxygen ($^1O_2$), an excited form of oxygen. Oxygen-derived radicals are generated constantly as part of normal aerobic life. A prominent feature of ROS is that they have extremely high chemical reactivity, which explains not only their normal biological activities, but how they inflict damage on cells. When they are produced in excess, they have more toxic effects on the cells as they can damage proteins, lipids, and DNA, and thereby cause death of cells. One of the best-known toxic effects of oxygen radicals is damage to cellular membranes (plasma, mitochondrial, and endomembrane systems), which is initiated by a process known as lipid peroxidation.

Several *in vitro* studies on the toxicity of ENPs have shown generation of ROS, for example, by TiO_2 [72], CeO_2 [73], and CNTs [74]. On the other hand, some authors have found that ENPs, for example, CeO_2, may also have protective effects against oxidative stress [58,59]. This apparent dichotomy underlines the need for research on NP–cell interactions and mechanistic aspects of ENP metabolism in organisms and specific cells. Many ENPs are photochemically active in the sense that they generate excited electrons when exposed to light (e.g., TiO_2, ZnO, SiO_2, fullerenes). In the presence of oxygen, these electrons can form superoxide radicals by direct electron transfer [75].

12.5.2 Mechanisms of ROS Production and Apoptosis

There are different mechanisms to produce ROS in the cell. ENPs follow one of the following mechanisms to produce ROS. ROS can be generated directly from the surface of particles when both oxidants and free radicals are present on the surface of the particles [76–78]. Some NPs have shown to activate inflammatory cells such as alveolar macrophages and neutrophils, which in turn results in the production of ROS and RNS [78–80]. ENPs such as TiO_2, ZnO, CeO_2, and silver NPs are shown to deposit on the cellular surface or inside the subcellular organelles and also shown to induce oxidative stress signaling cascade that eventually results in the oxidative stress in the cell [4]. Mitochondria are one of the major target organelles for NP-induced oxidative stress. When the ENPs deposit in the mitochondria, they are shown to damage the structure and function of the mitochondria [81]. NPs of various sizes and chemical compositions are shown to preferentially localize in the mitochondria, induce major structural damage, and contribute to oxidative stress [61]. Treatment of rat liver cell line with silver NPs resulted in membrane damage, reduced glutathione levels, and increase in ROS production, indicating an influence of NPs on the respiratory chain [82].

Mitochondria are the major sites of ROS production in the cell. ROS are known to affect mitochondrial membrane potential and trigger a series of mitochondrial associated events, including apoptosis. High level of ROS in the mitochondria can result in free radical attack of membrane phospholipids, proceeding mitochondrial membrane depolarization. Mitochondrial depolarization, considered as irreversible steps in the apoptotic process, can trigger a cascade of caspases. During oxidative phosphorylation, some of these electrons occasionally escape from the electron transport chain and are accepted by molecular oxygen to form extremely reactive superoxide anion radical ($O^{2-\bullet}$), which gets further converted into hydrogen peroxide (H_2O_2) and in turn may be fully reduced to water or partially reduced to hydroxyl radical ($OH^\bullet$), one of the strongest oxidants in nature [81]. ENPs can increase the rate of superoxide anion production, either by blocking the electron transport or by accepting an electron from a respiratory carrier and transferring it to molecular oxygen without inhibiting the respiratory chain [76,83]. Deposition of ENPs in the mitochondria can alter its normal functioning by disrupting the electron transport chain, ultimately resulting in the production of ROS.

12.5.3 Mitochondrial Pathway of Apoptosis

Apart from affecting the cellular proteins, lipids, and DNA, ROS have a very crucial role in inducing apoptosis in the mitochondria. When there is increased oxidative stress in the cell, it may either result in the apoptosis or necrosis of the cell, depending on the extent of oxidative stress. Apoptotic pathway has been the major mechanism of cellular death due to the ENPs-induced toxicity. Among the apoptotic pathways, mitochondrial pathway has been the major pathway to study the toxicological effects of ENPs. The generation of ROS, changes in mitochondrial membrane potential, and caspase-3 activation are known to be major elements of the mitochondrial pathway of apoptosis. ROS is predominately produced in the mitochondria, then leading to the free radical attack of membrane phospholipids and loss of mitochondria membrane potential, which leads to an increase of cytochrome c release from damaged mitochondria activation of caspases and then resulting in apoptosis.

Mitochondria is a major subcellular compartment where the Bcl-2 family members interact with each other or exert their function independently. The Bcl-2 family of proteins include proteins that can either inhibit (Bcl-2, Bcl-xL, etc.) or favor (Bax, Bak, Bad, etc.) apoptosis. Bcl-2 is an antiapoptotic protein which is predominately present in the mitochondria. Bcl-2 prevents apoptosis by suppressing oxyradical-mediated membrane damage and stabilizing mitochondrial membrane potential. The proapoptotic protein Bax regulates the mitochondrial pathway by triggering the release of apoptotic factors such as cytochrome c into the cytosol where it binds to APAF-1 and causes formation of a complex. This complex binds to procaspases-9 and results in the formation of *apoptosome*. The apoptosome cleaves the procaspases-9 into its active fragments and the active caspase-9 fragments causes the cleavage of the effector caspase, procaspase-3 into its active fragments. The active caspase-3 causes the cleavage of the nuclear proteins and cytosolic proteins that result in the apoptotic death of the cell [83–86].

12.5.4 ENPs-Induced Inflammation

Inflammation is the protective mechanism of the organism against adverse reactions induced by foreign chemicals or organisms. If there is a limited inflammation in the organism, it has a protective role in general, but when it extends beyond a certain point, the inflammation can cause disease in the organism. ENPs like fullerenes, CNTs, silver NPs, and TiO_2 NPs have shown to increase the production of inflammatory mediators or cytokines into the circulation and thereby have shown to cause increased oxidative stress, hypersensitive reactions, allergic response, or granulomas in the target organs [30,67,87,88]. ENPs have shown to activate transcription factor nuclear factor kappa B, which then translocates to nucleus and then known to induce pro-inflammatory genes such as TNF-α, IL-8, IL-2, and IL-6 that result in increased inflammation and eventually causes inflammation-mediated oxidative stress [89,90].

12.5.5 ENPs-Induced Genotoxicity and Carcinogenesis

Genotoxic effects of conventional particles are driven by two mechanisms—direct genotoxicity and indirect (inflammatory processes mediated) genotoxicity. NPs may act via either of these pathways since they may cause inflammation and they can also enter cells and cause oxidative stress. There is some evidence that the small size may allow NPs to penetrate into sub-cellular compartments that normally exclude environmental particles, like the mitochondria and nucleus. The presence of nanomaterials in both mitochondria and the nucleus opens the possibility for oxidative stress-mediated indirect genotoxicity, and direct interaction of NPs with DNA and histones [68,91]. ENPs have shown to deposit in the nucleus and cause acetylation of the histones and finally alter the DNA structure and function [92,93]. ENPs can also produce free radicals and inflammatory mediators in the cell that indirectly damages the DNA or they can interfere with the cell division process by directly interacting with the nucleosomes, microtubules, and actin filaments [91,94]. ENPs like silver, TiO_2, and ZnO that are important constituents of sunscreen lotions have shown to induce tumors and granulomas in various organs by altering the DNA repair, or inducing DNA damage or activating p53 and proteins related to cell division process [95,96].

12.5.6 ENPs-Induced Reproductive and Developmental Toxicity

As mentioned earlier, the ENPs can reach almost every part of the body. When it reaches the reproductive organs, they can damage the reproductive cells and thereby cause infertility in the organism. Silver NPs have already shown to induce cytotoxicity of the male germ cell lines of the mouse [97]. In another study, reports also evidenced that silver NPs could cause genotoxicity and cytotoxicity effects in mouse testicular cells [98]. Other NPs called carbon black has shown to induce kidney toxicity in the offspring of the dams when they were exposed to carbon black NPs [99]. Some of the ENPs study reports have shown to reach the placenta and induce developmental defects in the newborn. ENPs such as silica and TiO_2 have been found in the fetal brain and liver after crossing the placenta in mice and thereby reduced the size of the fetus [100].

12.6 Regulatory Efforts

Reports from various studies conducted worldwide on the toxicological evaluation of ENPs have shown that they can induce different toxicological effects on various organs through different mechanisms. Therefore, it is an urgent need to have proper regulation protocol/procedure to assess the exposure levels and risk of individual nanomaterials in and around the manufacturing industries as well as in the environment.

All over the world, various regulatory agencies such as SCENIHR, Scientific Committee on Emerging and Newly Identified Health Risks; EFSA, European Food Safety Authority; and CEN, European Committee for Standardization and international organizations like OECD and ISO) have been trying to develop, validate, and standardize various common protocols/procedures to demonstrate how to use, dispose of various nanomaterials, and what are the possible harmful effects of individual nanomaterials and its concentration on human and the environment [101]. One of the major limitations for regulatory agencies to assess the risk factor of individual nanomaterials is the lack of proper classifications of various nanomaterials. Therefore, it seems to be the biggest challenge for policy makers. For example, silver NPs comes under the chemical category but it has been used longer for various other applications such as coating for washing machines now washing machines come under the classification as "devices" rather than "chemicals." Therefore, there is a chance to escape from the common regulatory classifications [4]. Recently, the USEPA has taken initiatives to classify silver NPs as pesticides because it is being used as antimicrobial agents [102], and also taking possible steps to ban the silver NPs. Usually, the implementation of current laws and regulations for nanotoxicology are limited because of the inadequate knowledge on the properties and applications of nanomaterials [103].

To develop, validate, and standardize various harmonized protocols/procedures and implement these protocols in the area of nanotechnology is the only possible way to ensure a sustainable development and prevent negative impacts on public health and the environment. Various steps have been taken by regulatory agencies to define characteristics of NPs to make them as comprehensive useful materials in everyday human life without having any adverse effects on the public health. Safe technology is always the best one for the growth and progress of the world and hoping for the less concerned nanotechnology products to take part in human life. We foresee a future with better-informed, and hopefully more cautious manipulation of engineered nanomaterials, as well as the development of laws and policies for safely managing all aspects of nanomaterial manufacturing, industrial and commercial use, and recycling.

References

1. NANOtechnology: Untold promise, unknown risk. *Consum Rep*, 2007. **72**(7): 40–5.
2. Hobson, D.W., Commercialization of nanotechnology. *Wiley Interdiscip Rev Nanomed Nanobiotechnol*, 2009. **1**(2): 189–202.
3. Kibble, A., Pharma 2020—An economist conference shaping the future of the pharmaceuticals industry. *IDrugs*, 2008. **11**(5): 331–3.
4. Buzea, C., Pacheco, II, and K. Robbie, Nanomaterials and nanoparticles: Sources and toxicity. *Biointerphases*, 2007. **2**(4): MR17–71.
5. Oberdorster, G., E. Oberdorster, and J. Oberdorster, Nanotoxicology: An emerging discipline evolving from studies of ultrafine particles. *Environ Health Perspect*, 2005. **113**(7): 823–39.
6. Simonelli, F. et al., Cyclotron production of radioactive CeO(2) nanoparticles and their application for *in vitro* uptake studies. *IEEE Trans Nanobiosci*, 2011. **10**(1): 44–50.
7. Environment Directorate, O.F.E.C.-O.A.D., Working party on manufactured nanomaterials: List of manufactured nanomaterials and list of endpoints for

phase one of the OECD Testing Programme. ENV/JM/MONO(2008)13/REV, 2008.

8. Singh, S. and H.S. Nalwa, Nanotechnology and health safety—Toxicity and risk assessments of nanostructured materials on human health. *J Nanosci Nanotechnol*, 2007. **7**(9): 3048–70.

9. Kumar, V. et al., Evaluating the toxicity of selected types of nanochemicals. *Rev Environ Contam Toxicol*, 2012. **215**: 39–121.

10. Jennings, T. and G. Strouse, Past, present, and future of gold nanoparticles. *Adv Exp Med Biol*, 2007. **620**: 34–47.

11. Dreaden, E.C. et al., The golden age: Gold nanoparticles for biomedicine. *Chem Soc Rev*, 2011. **41**(7): 2740–79.

12. Islam, T. and M.G. Harisinghani, Overview of nanoparticle use in cancer imaging. *Cancer Biomark*, 2009. **5**(2): 61–7.

13. Fiorino, D.J., Voluntary initiatives, regulation, and nanotechnology oversight charting a path. Woodrow Wilson International Center for Scholars; Project on Emerging Nanotechnologies. 2010.

14. Malsch, D.H.A.I., Hazards and risks of engineered nanoparticles for the environment and human health. *Sustainability*, 2009. **1**(2071–1050): 1161–94.

15. Hofmann-Amtenbrink, M., H. Hofmann, and X. Montet, Superparamagnetic nanoparticles—A tool for early diagnostics. *Swiss Med Wkly*, 2010. **140**: w13081.

16. Islam, T. and L. Josephson, Current state and future applications of active targeting in malignancies using superparamagnetic iron oxide nanoparticles. *Cancer Biomark*, 2009. **5**(2): 99–107.

17. Bhaskar, S. et al., Multifunctional nanocarriers for diagnostics, drug delivery and targeted treatment across blood–brain barrier: Perspectives on tracking and neuroimaging. *Part Fibre Toxicol*, 2010. **7**: 3.

18. Tiede, K. et al., Detection and characterization of engineered nanoparticles in food and the environment. *Food Addit Contam Part A Chem Anal Control Expo Risk Assess*, 2008. **25**(7): 795–821.

19. Morris, V.J., Emerging roles of engineered nanomaterials in the food industry. *Trends Biotechnol*, 2011. **29**(10): 509–16.

20. Gottschalk, F. and B. Nowack, The release of engineered nanomaterials to the environment. *J Environ Monit*, 2011. **13**(5): 1145–55.

21. Bernhardt, E.S. et al., An ecological perspective on nanomaterial impacts in the environment. *J Environ Qual*, 2010. **39**(6): 1954–65.

22. Cassee, F.R. et al., Exposure, health and ecological effects review of engineered nanoscale cerium and cerium oxide associated with its use as a fuel additive. *Crit Rev Toxicol*, 2011. **41**(3): 213–29.

23. Woskie, S., Workplace practices for engineered nanomaterial manufacturers. *Wiley Interdiscip Rev Nanomed Nanobiotechnol*, 2010. **2**(6): 685–92.

24. Petosa, A.R. et al., Aggregation and deposition of engineered nanomaterials in aquatic environments: Role of physicochemical interactions. *Environ Sci Technol*, 2010. **44**(17): 6532–49.

25. Ren, H. and X. Huang, Polyacrylate nanoparticles: Toxicity or new nanomedicine? *Eur Respir J*, 2010. **36**(1): 218–21.

26. Warheit, D.B. et al., Health effects related to nanoparticle exposures: Environmental, health and safety considerations for assessing hazards and risks. *Pharmacol Ther*, 2008. **120**(1): 35–42.

27. Yang, H. et al., Comparative study of cytotoxicity, oxidative stress and genotoxicity induced by four typical nanomaterials: The role of particle size, shape and composition. *J Appl Toxicol*, 2009. **29**(1): 69–78.

28. Bystrzejewska-Piotrowska, G., J. Golimowski, and P.L. Urban, Nanoparticles: Their potential toxicity, waste and environmental management. *Waste Manage*, 2009. **29**(9): 2587–95.

29. Khlebtsov, N. and L. Dykman, Biodistribution and toxicity of engineered gold nanoparticles: A review of *in vitro* and *in vivo* studies. *Chem Soc Rev*, 2011. **40**(3): 1647–71.

30. Trickler, W.J. et al., Silver nanoparticle induced blood–brain barrier inflammation and increased permeability in primary rat brain microvessel endothelial cells. *Toxicol Sci*, 2010. **118**(1): 160–70.

31. Simon-Deckers, A. et al., Size-, composition- and shape-dependent toxicological impact of metal oxide nanoparticles and carbon nanotubes toward bacteria. *Environ Sci Technol*, 2009. **43**(21): 8423–9.

32. Lam, C.W. et al., A review of carbon nanotube toxicity and assessment of potential occupational and environmental health risks. *Crit Rev Toxicol*, 2006. **36**(3): 189–217.

33. Jia, G. et al., Cytotoxicity of carbon nanomaterials: Single-wall nanotube, multi-wall nanotube, and fullerene. *Environ Sci Technol*, 2005. **39**(5): 1378–83.

34. Kreyling, W.G., S. Hirn, and C. Schleh, Nanoparticles in the lung. *Nat Biotechnol*, 2010. **28**(12): 1275–6.

35. Geiser, M. and W.G. Kreyling, Deposition and biokinetics of inhaled nanoparticles. *Part Fibre Toxicol*, 2010. **7**: 2.

36. Sadauskas, E. et al., Biodistribution of gold nanoparticles in mouse lung following intratracheal instillation. *Chem Cent J*, 2009. **3**: 16.

37. Tjalve, H. et al., Uptake of manganese and cadmium from the nasal mucosa into the central nervous system via olfactory pathways in rats. *Pharmacol Toxicol*, 1996. **79**(6): 347–56.

38. Elder, A. et al., Translocation of inhaled ultrafine manganese oxide particles to the central nervous system. *Environ Health Perspect*, 2006. **114**(8): 1172–8.

39. Sharma, H.S. and A. Sharma, Nanoparticles aggravate heat stress induced cognitive deficits, blood–brain barrier disruption, edema formation and brain pathology. *Prog Brain Res*, 2007. **162**: 245–73.

40. Oberdorster, G. et al., Translocation of inhaled ultrafine particles to the brain. *Inhal Toxicol*, 2004. **16**(6–7): 437–45.

41. Tallkvist, J. et al., Transport and subcellular distribution of nickel in the olfactory system of pikes and rats. *Toxicol Sci*, 1998. **43**(2): 196–203.

42. Blum, J.L. et al., Cadmium associated with inhaled cadmium oxide nanoparticles impacts fetal and neonatal development and growth. *Toxicol Sci*, 2012. **126**(2): 478–86.

43. Scheuch, G. et al., Deposition, imaging, and clearance: What remains to be done? *J Aerosol Med Pulm Drug Deliv*, 2010. **23**(Suppl 2): S39–57.

44. Henning, A. et al., Influence of particle size and material properties on mucociliary clearance from the airways. *J Aerosol Med Pulm Drug Deliv*, 2010. **23**(4): 233–41.

45. Geiser, M., Update on macrophage clearance of inhaled micro- and nanoparticles. *J Aerosol Med Pulm Drug Deliv*, 2010. **23**(4): 207–17.

46. Gaiser, B.K. et al., Assessing exposure, uptake and toxicity of silver and cerium dioxide nanoparticles from contaminated environments. *Environ Health*, 2009. **8**(Suppl 1): S2.

47. Kim, Y.S. et al., Twenty-eight-day oral toxicity, genotoxicity, and gender-related tissue distribution of silver nanoparticles in Sprague–Dawley rats. *Inhal Toxicol*, 2008. **20**(6): 575–83.
48. Nefzger, M. et al., Distribution and elimination of polymethyl methacrylate nanoparticles after peroral administration to rats. *J Pharm Sci*, 1984. **73**(9): 1309–11.
49. Zhao, C.M. and W.X. Wang, Biokinetic uptake and efflux of silver nanoparticles in *Daphnia magna. Environ Sci Technol*, 2010. **44**(19): 7699–704.
50. Smijs, T.G. and J.A. Bouwstra, Focus on skin as a possible port of entry for solid nanoparticles and the toxicological impact. *J Biomed Nanotechnol*, 2010. **6**(5): 469–84.
51. Nohynek, G.J. et al., Safety assessment of personal care products/cosmetics and their ingredients. *Toxicol Appl Pharmacol*, 2010. **243**(2): 239–59.
52. Simko, M. and M.O. Mattsson, Risks from accidental exposures to engineered nanoparticles and neurological health effects: A critical review. *Part Fibre Toxicol*, 2010. **7**: 42.
53. Wu, J. et al., Toxicity and penetration of TiO_2 nanoparticles in hairless mice and porcine skin after subchronic dermal exposure. *Toxicol Lett*, 2009. **191**(1): 1–8.
54. Borm, P.J. et al., The potential risks of nanomaterials: A review carried out for ECETOC. *Part Fibre Toxicol*, 2006. **3**: 11.
55. Yang, K. et al., Quantum dot-based visual *in vivo* imaging for oral squamous cell carcinoma in mice. *Oral Oncol*, 2010. **46**(12): 864–8.
56. Minelli, C., S.B. Lowe, and M.M. Stevens, Engineering nanocomposite materials for cancer therapy. *Small*, 2010. **6**(21): 2336–57.
57. Ting, G. et al., Nanotargeted radionuclides for cancer nuclear imaging and internal radiotherapy. *J Biomed Biotechnol*, 2010. **9**(5): 37–54
58. Colon, J. et al., Protection from radiation-induced pneumonitis using cerium oxide nanoparticles. *Nanomedicine*, 2009. **5**(2): 225–31.
59. Niu, J. et al., Cardioprotective effects of cerium oxide nanoparticles in a transgenic murine model of cardiomyopathy. *Cardiovasc Res*, 2007. **73**(3): 549–59.
60. Stefani, D., D. Wardman, and T. Lambert, The implosion of the Calgary General Hospital: Ambient air quality issues. *J Air Waste Manage Assoc*, 2005. **55**(1): 52–9.
61. Xia, T. et al., Comparison of the abilities of ambient and manufactured nanoparticles to induce cellular toxicity according to an oxidative stress paradigm. *Nano Lett*, 2006. **6**(8): 1794–807.
62. Berton, M. et al., Uptake of oligonucleotide-loaded nanoparticles in prostatic cancer cells and their intracellular localization. *Eur J Pharm Biopharm*, 1999. **47**(2): 119–23.
63. Chawla, J.S. and M.M. Amiji, Cellular uptake and concentrations of tamoxifen upon administration in poly(epsilon-caprolactone) nanoparticles. *AAPS PharmSci*, 2003. **5**(1): E3.
64. Rouse, R.L. et al., Soot nanoparticles promote biotransformation, oxidative stress, and inflammation in murine lungs. *Am J Respir Cell Mol Biol*, 2008. **39**(2): 198–207.
65. Porter, A.E. et al., Uptake of C60 by human monocyte macrophages, its localization and implications for toxicity: Studied by high resolution electron microscopy and electron tomography. *Acta Biomater*, 2006. **2**(4): 409–19.
66. Drescher, D. et al., Toxicity of amorphous silica nanoparticles on eukaryotic cell model is determined by particle agglomeration and serum protein adsorption effects. *Anal Bioanal Chem*, 2011. **400**(5): 1367–73.
67. Stone, V., H. Johnston, and M.J. Clift, Air pollution, ultrafine and nanoparticle toxicology: Cellular and molecular interactions. *IEEE Trans Nanobiosci*, 2007. **6**(4): 331–40.

68. Li, N., T. Xia, and A.E. Nel, The role of oxidative stress in ambient particulate matter-induced lung diseases and its implications in the toxicity of engineered nanoparticles. *Free Radic Biol Med*, 2008. **44**(9): 1689–99.

69. Ju-Nam, Y. and J.R. Lead, Manufactured nanoparticles: An overview of their chemistry, interactions and potential environmental implications. *Sci Total Environ*, 2008. **400**(1–3): 396–414.

70. Johnston, H.J. et al., A review of the *in vivo* and *in vitro* toxicity of silver and gold particulates: Particle attributes and biological mechanisms responsible for the observed toxicity. *Crit Rev Toxicol*, 2010. **40**(4): 328–46.

71. Mocan, T. et al., Implications of oxidative stress mechanisms in toxicity of nanoparticles (review). *Acta Physiol Hung*, 2010. **97**(3): 247–55.

72. Xiong, D. et al., Effects of nano-scale TiO_2, ZnO and their bulk counterparts on zebrafish: Acute toxicity, oxidative stress and oxidative damage. *Sci Total Environ*, 2011. **409**(8): 1444–52.

73. Eom, H.J. and J. Choi, Oxidative stress of CeO_2 nanoparticles via p38-Nrf-2 signaling pathway in human bronchial epithelial cell, Beas-2B. *Toxicol Lett*, 2009. **187**(2): 77–83.

74. Clichici, S. et al., Blood oxidative stress generation after intraperitoneal administration of functionalized single-walled carbon nanotubes in rats. *Acta Physiol Hung*, 2011. **98**(2): 231–41.

75. Kumar, A. et al., Engineered ZnO and TiO(2) nanoparticles induce oxidative stress and DNA damage leading to reduced viability of *Escherichia coli*. *Free Radic Biol Med*, 2011. **51**(10): 1872–81.

76. Yamakoshi, Y. et al., Active oxygen species generated from photoexcited fullerene (C60) as potential medicines: O2-* versus 1O2. *J Am Chem Soc*, 2003. **125**(42): 12803–9.

77. Hotze, E.M. et al., Mechanisms of photochemistry and reactive oxygen production by fullerene suspensions in water. *Environ Sci Technol*, 2008. **42**(11): 4175–80.

78. Zhang, Z. et al., On the interactions of free radicals with gold nanoparticles. *J Am Chem Soc*, 2003. **125**(26): 7959–63.

79. Lee, H.M. et al., Nanoparticles up-regulate tumor necrosis factor-alpha and CXCL8 via reactive oxygen species and mitogen-activated protein kinase activation. *Toxicol Appl Pharmacol*, 2009. **238**(2): 160–9.

80. Kennedy, I.M., D. Wilson, and A.I. Barakat, Uptake and inflammatory effects of nanoparticles in a human vascular endothelial cell line. *Res Rep Health Eff Inst*, 2009. **136**: 3–32.

81. Boonstra, J. and J.A. Post, Molecular events associated with reactive oxygen species and cell cycle progression in mammalian cells. *Gene*, 2004. **337**: 1–13.

82. Hussain, S.M. et al., *In vitro* toxicity of nanoparticles in BRL 3A rat liver cells. *Toxicol In Vitro*, 2005. **19**(7): 975–83.

83. Turrens, J.F., Mitochondrial formation of reactive oxygen species. *J Physiol*, 2003. **552**(Pt 2): 335–44.

84. Lenaz, G., The mitochondrial production of reactive oxygen species: Mechanisms and implications in human pathology. *IUBMB Life*, 2001. **52**(3–5): 159–64.

85. Kakarla, S.K. et al., Chronic acetaminophen attenuates age-associated increases in cardiac ROS and apoptosis in the Fischer Brown Norway rat. *Basic Res Cardiol*, 2010. **105**(4): 535–44.

86. Asano, S. et al., Aging influences multiple indices of oxidative stress in the heart of the Fischer 344/NNia x Brown Norway/BiNia rat. *Redox Rep*, 2007. **12**(4): 167–80.

87. Morimoto, Y. and I. Tanaka, Effects of nanoparticles on humans. *Sangyo Eiseigaku Zasshi*, 2008. **50**(2): 37–48.
88. Nielsen, G.D. et al., *In vivo* biology and toxicology of fullerenes and their derivatives. *Basic Clin Pharmacol Toxicol*, 2008. **103**(3): 197–208.
89. Marano, F. et al., Nanoparticles: Molecular targets and cell signalling. *Arch Toxicol*, 2011. **85**(7): 733–41.
90. Park, E.J. et al., Carbon fullerenes (C60s) can induce inflammatory responses in the lung of mice. *Toxicol Appl Pharmacol*, 2010. **244**(2): 226–33.
91. Trouiller, B. et al., Titanium dioxide nanoparticles induce DNA damage and genetic instability *in vivo* in mice. *Cancer Res*, 2009. **69**(22): 8784–9.
92. Khalil, W.K. et al., Genotoxicity evaluation of nanomaterials: DNA damage, micronuclei, and 8-hydroxy-2-deoxyguanosine induced by magnetic doped CdSe quantum dots in male mice. *Chem Res Toxicol*, 2011. **24**(5): 640–50.
93. Choi, A.O. et al., Quantum dot-induced epigenetic and genotoxic changes in human breast cancer cells. *J Mol Med (Berl)*, 2008. **86**(3): 291–302.
94. Folkmann, J.K. et al., Oxidatively damaged DNA in rats exposed by oral gavage to C60 fullerenes and single-walled carbon nanotubes. *Environ Health Perspect*, 2009. **117**(5): 703–8.
95. Mroz, R.M. et al., Nanoparticle-driven DNA damage mimics irradiation-related carcinogenesis pathways. *Eur Respir J*, 2008. **31**(2): 241–51.
96. Loden, M. et al., Sunscreen use: Controversies, challenges and regulatory aspects. *Br J Dermatol*, 2011. **165**(2): 255–62.
97. Braydich-Stolle, L. et al., *In vitro* cytotoxicity of nanoparticles in mammalian germline stem cells. *Toxicol Sci*, 2005. **88**(2): 412–9.
98. Asare, N. et al., Cytotoxic and genotoxic effects of silver nanoparticles in testicular cells. *Toxicology*, 2012. **291**(1–3): 65–72.
99. Umezawa, M. et al., Maternal exposure to carbon black nanoparticle increases collagen type VIII expression in the kidney of offspring. *J Toxicol Sci*, 2011. **36**(4): 461–8.
100. Yamashita, K. et al., Silica and titanium dioxide nanoparticles cause pregnancy complications in mice. *Nat Nanotechnol*, 2011. **6**(5): 321–8.
101. Norwegian Pollution Control Authority. Environmental fate and ecotoxicity of engineered nanoparticles. Report no. TA 2304/2007. Eds.: E.J. Joner, T. Hartnik and C.E. Amundsen. Bioforsk, Ås. 64 pp. 2008.
102. Henig, R.M., Our silver-coated future. *In Onearth*, 2007. **29**(3): 22–29.
103. Franco, A. et al., Limits and prospects of the "incremental approach" and the European legislation on the management of risks related to nanomaterials. *Regul Toxicol Pharmacol*, 2007. **48**(2), 171–83.
104. Erik, C.D. et al., The golden age: Gold nanoparticles for biomedicine. *Chem Soc Rev*, 2012, **41**(7), 2740–79.

13

Animal and Cellular Models for Use in Nanoparticles Safety Study

Kevin M. Rice and Eric R. Blough

CONTENTS

13.1 Introduction 355
13.2 Nanomaterial Characterization 356
    13.2.1 Key Physicochemical Characteristics 358
    13.2.2 Dose Metrics 360
    13.2.3 Characterization Prioritization 361
    13.2.4 Analysis Methods 363
13.3 Models of Ecotoxicity 364
    13.3.1 Alternative Nonanimal Methods 368
        13.3.1.1 Plants Models 372
        13.3.1.2 *In Vitro* Models 375
        13.3.1.3 *In Vitro* Testing Methods 384
13.4 Treatment Options for Nanotoxicity 399
13.5 Conclusion 399
References 400

13.1 Introduction

As we begin this chapter on nanosafety and the use of animals and cell culture in determining safety strategies, we must first understand the environmental culture surrounding nanotechnology and the industrial variables that have brought us to this point in time. In the fall of 2009, a meeting was held in Triangle Park, North Carolina with representatives including industrial scientists, university researchers, government regulators, and consumer advocates examining the known safety data concerning nanoscale titanium dioxide. One of the participants, a Connecticut toxicologist from the Yale School of Public Health and the University of Connecticut School of Community Medicine, Dr. Gary Ginsburg stated, "The horse has already left the barn, it's already out there. In this case the environment is the Guinea pig. All we can do at this point is really try to do a good job of seeing what is getting into the human ecology" (Kaplan, 2010). From this viewpoint, we have an understanding that nanosafety is lagging far behind the cutting-edge development of nano-technology and its associated science. The fast-growing world of engineered nanoparticles, nanocomposite materials, and nanoapplications far surpasses our understanding regarding nanosafety of engineered nanomaterials (ENM). It is important to note that some nanoparticles were in use as far back as the 1950s only became common in household products in the 1990s (Kaplan, 2010). Even with more than 20 years of commercially available products containing nanoparticles and ENM, we have no idea of the true environmental, biologi-cal, or global effects of nanoparticles. A warning bell has been sounded and agencies both in Europe and in America have began to implement strategies to better evaluate ENM safety but we are decades behind in the development of standardized and approved models and screening protocols to evaluate nano-safety. Ideally, we must also remember that any safety or toxicological evalu-ation of ENMs must be accompanied by a detailed characterization of all the physicochemical properties of the specific ENM under evaluation (Zuin et al., 2007).

Because naturally occurring forms of nanoparticles exist, characterization of ENMs, nanoscale by-products of chemical and natural processes, and natu-rally occurring nanomaterials is of great importance. Each nanomaterial has its own unique ecological and biological responses due to the wide variety of properties among nanomaterials. This requires that extensive characterization, classification, and individualized studies for each nanomaterial be performed.

Within the current body of literature regarding ENMs, there exists a wide array of results regarding the effects of ENMs. This is primarily due to the broad range of methods and approaches used to reach these conclusions. The need for standardized tests and screening methods for ENM evaluation is greatly needed to eradicate these inconsistencies. Determining the toxic effects of ENMs requires better comparisons and conclusions to be drawn from ENM toxicological evaluation. New and improved standards for toxico-logical screening are needed as the field of nanotoxicology continues to grow.

As we approach the area of nanosafety, we must first examine the variables associated with nanomaterials. This will provide clarity of the complexity associated with assessing nanosafety as well as understanding the needs and requirements for various models to investigate the numerous variables associated with nanosafety. We will then examine these variables within the context of ecotoxicity, and *in vivo* and *in vitro* testing models for nanotoxicity.

13.2 Nanomaterial Characterization

The desirable properties of nanomaterials are largely dependent upon their nanoscale properties. These unique characteristics differentiate them from other solid, liquid, and gaseous materials. It is strongly predicted that these physicochemical parameters are the principal elements in their biological activity and subsequent beneficial or toxic effects. Although these physicochemical properties hold much promise in regard to the potential application of nanomaterials, they may also possess detrimental qualities and are not usually considered when conducting toxicity screening studies. Some studies, although limited in number, have indicated that careful consideration is needed with regard to nanomaterial characterization while evaluating the biological activity of nanomaterials (Brown et al., 2001; Donaldson et al., 2000; Oberdorster, 2000; Sayes et al., 2004; Shvedova et al., 2003; Warheit et al., 2004). The nanomaterial characterization required to obtain appropriate toxicological screening is expected to be as complex and diverse as the various characteristics of the nanomaterials themselves.

A full understanding regarding the potential significance of all the nanomaterial characteristics and the mechanistic association with toxicity is yet to be developed. Until such associations are developed, it is necessary that all potentially significant nanomaterial characteristics be measured. Sufficient information should be collected to allow for retrospective interpretation of collected data; this is of vital importance as the field and discipline of nanotoxicity is in its infancy. The development of new findings and better understanding of the mechanisms of nanomaterial toxicity will allow for better retrospective interpretation of present nanomaterial toxicity screening studies. This concept imposes a great challenge to nanotoxicological research; developing a screening strategy that requires the collection of every characterization criteria is clearly impractical. Research has therefore begun to categorize these characterization criteria into essential, desirable, and of interest (Oberdorster et al., 2005a). To add more complexity to the evaluation of these characterization criteria, the context of exposure must also be evaluated. The point along the life cycle of the nanomaterial may alter its properties or characteristics. If the exposure occurred within a manufacturing setting, then the assessment would need to reflect the characterization criteria at that moment in time. This provides multiple time points at which a nanomaterial can be evaluated during manufacturing, as produced or supplied, over a period of storage (changes during shelf life), various avenues of human exposure, after exposure (reflecting biological changes), or as administered (if prepared for pharmacological of consumer-based product), just to name a few. For each of these toxicity screening points, exposure route and dose characterization against physical metrics are of great importance.

Of greatest importance with regard to nanomaterial safety and their potential hazardous properties is the direct risk to humans. The overall impact of the potential risk to human health is largely associated with the probability of exposure, extent of the exposure, route of entry, and the behavior associated with their nanostructure within the body (Figure 13.1).

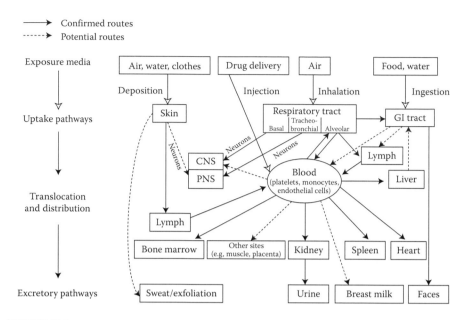

FIGURE 13.1
Biokinetics of nanosized particles. While many uptake and translocation routes have been demonstrated, others still are hypothetical and need to be investigated. Largely unknown are translocation rates as well as accumulation and retention in critical target sites and their underlying mechanisms. These as well as potential adverse effects will be largely dependent on the physicochemical characteristics of the surface and core of nanosized particles. Both qualitative and quantitative changes in nanosized particles' biokinetics in a diseased or compromised organism also need to be considered. (Reprinted with permission from Oberdorster, G. et al., 2005a. Principles for characterizing the potential human health effects from exposure to nanomaterials: Elements of a screening strategy. *Part Fibre Toxicol*, 2, 8. Copyright 2005 American Chemical Society.)

As stated earlier, the physicochemical characteristics of the nanomaterials will provide the greatest insight into the potential adverse effects of nanomaterial exposure.

13.2.1 Key Physicochemical Characteristics

Perhaps the closest analogy to nanomaterials with regard to a substance that is not fully characterized by mass and chemical composition alone is that of fiber particles. The key parameters of fibrous particle pathogenicity are dimension, durability, and dose (the three D's). The diameter of the fiber is inversely proportional to the depth at which the fiber penetrates into the lung. The chemistry of fibers affects its biopersistence and durability (Oberdorster et al., 2005a). Fiber length can stimulate inflammatory mediator release from macrophages and the quantity of alkali can affect the durability (Searl, 1994). Other studies have indicated that surface area and the surface area activity play a role in the carcinogenic or toxic effect of inhaled particles (Fubini, 1997; Oberdorster et al., 1994). Reactive oxygen species and free radical formation have been shown to be directly linked to particle surface characteristics and in the development of cancer and fibrosis (Fubini, 1997).

The nanoscopic size of nanomaterials may provide a great deal of potential application but also opens up a wide range of potential toxicological possibilities. The extreme increase in surface-to-volume ratio when compared to bulk material, the nanoscale structure, structure-dependent electron configuration, in addition to size are capable of giving nanomaterials a range of unusual properties. The minute size of these particles allows nanoparticles to easily enter the respiratory tract and deposit to distal regions of the lung. On the cellular level, nanoparticles may readily translocate to various parts of the body, and may penetrate between or through cells or pass directly into the cell through the cell membrane. The possibility of inhaled nanoparticle translocation to tissues, organs, and the nervous system has been suggested by a few reports (Kreyling et al., 2002; Oberdorster et al., 2004; Semmler et al., 2004).

The determining factor of nanomaterial toxicity may not rest completely upon the particle size. The total surface area and the overall number of particles present may play as critical a role in determining nanomaterial toxicity as size alone. Because of the size of the nanomaterials, a greater proportion of the atoms/molecules can be found at the surface as opposed to internalized within the material. This is a result of the increase in the surface area of nanomaterials when compared with the bulk product; as size decreases, the surface area per unit mass increases. The biological reactivity of a nanomaterial can be linked to the increase of particle surface energy resulting from the large surface-to-volume ratio of a nanomaterial.

Plates, tubes, spheres, cubes, needles, and so on are just a few of the variety of shapes known to occur within nanoscale materials. It is not yet known how the shape of a nanomaterial affects the potential for toxicity. The kinetics of absorption and deposition within the body may also be affected by the shape of the nanomaterial.

The composition of nanomaterials provides unique properties concerning the reactivity of the nanomaterial. Chemical composition such as biomolecules, compound polymers, metal/metal oxides, and compound are all variables which should be considered with regards to factors associated with toxicity. In some instances, these substance classes can be combined to form even more complex structures of core–shells. The biological effect of a nanomaterial will be modified according to its reactive groups, particle surface, and surface chemistry. The agglomeration or aggregation of nanomaterials under ambient conditions can produce a variety of forms, such as spherical structures, chains, dendritic structures, or a number of other possibilities. Surface derivatization or coating strategies have been employed by many to stabilize nanomaterials to maintain the individual particle characteristics. These and other such modifications alter the surface of the nanomaterial, and such surface modification can significantly alter the distribution of the material throughout the body. The biological effect of the nanomaterial has also been demonstrated to be changed when various coating strategies have been used (Araujo et al., 1999; Kirchner et al., 2001).

When conducting a toxicological assessment of a nanomaterial, the following physicochemical properties have been recommended for evaluating any test material (Oberdorster et al., 2005a):

- Size distribution
- Agglomeration state
- Shape
- Crystal structure
- Chemical composition—including spatially averaged (bulk) and spatially resolved heterogeneous composition
- Surface area
- Surface chemistry
- Surface charge
- Porosity

13.2.2 Dose Metrics

Careful consideration should be given to the metrics to be used to quantify the dose within any toxicity screening study. Quantitative interpretation of the data can only be achieved through the use of well-characterized materials using a physical metric to measure the dose. The various physicochemical characteristics associated with nanomaterials provide a wide range of potential variables that may elicit a toxicological response; however, the use of a physical metric such as *mass, surface area*, or *particle number* is most widely accepted. The selection of the appropriate dose metric is largely dependent on the anticipated response and the parameters hypothesized to be closely associated with the theorized outcome; however, the metric that can be the most accurately measured is also a suitable alternative. Sufficient information should be collected to derive dose measurements according to all three primary physical metrics. If appropriate measurements of particle size distribution are collected or the relationship between nanomaterial mass, surface area, and particles size is known, the possibility to derive these dose metrics may exist. It must also be noted that within the confines of the experimental setup, all care must taken to document preparation and conditions of administered nanomaterials. For instance, a liquid medium preparation of nanomaterials for techniques such as pharyngeal aspiration or intratracheal instillation should have full characterization of the mass, surface area, and particle number of the nanomaterials being administered within the context of the delivery vector and the nature and amount of the material within the suspension.

Inhalation studies pose a great deal of complication with regard to nanomaterial assessment. The need to measure dose over time is one additional challenge present in inhalation studies. Also, the use of off-line mass concentration, aerosol size distribution, off-line surface area measurements, and particle number concentration adds a wide range of complexities. Toxicological models associated with inhalation studies provide a great deal of insight into exposure limits of nanomaterials, and a detailed review of the methods associated with the testing is available in a review by Oberdörster et al. (2005b).

13.2.3 Characterization Prioritization

Three specific criteria must be considered when developing recommendations for the characterization of nanomaterials for toxicity screening studies: the exposure setting being evaluated, the importance of measuring a specific parameter within the context of the exposure setting, and the feasibility of performing the needed measurement of the given parameter within the exposure context. Table 13.1 presents the off-line material characterization recommendation for nanomaterial toxicity screening.

It is recommended that all information be recorded regarding agglomeration state, storage, preparation, production, and heterogeneity. In addition, processing and production information needs to be recorded to enable the replication of testing and retrospective interpretation of toxicity data. Because physicochemical changes can occur over time, it is essential that all information be documented for storage conditions and time, which include atmosphere composition, exposure to light, humidity, and temperature. A demonstrated time course with respect to physicochemical stability would also be needed to provide insight into toxicological changes of stored nanomaterials or for the purpose of product shelf-life evaluation. If the product is altered in some way during the storage or shipment, or through environmental changes, this may produce alterations in the nanomaterial that change the toxicity, alter the effectiveness of pharmaceutical application or render the nanomaterial functionless. For the purpose of disposal of nanomaterial waste, understanding the effect of time on the physicochemical properties and associated toxicology of nanomaterials is vitally important. Understanding if and when a nanomaterial becomes inert and poses no ecotoxicological or toxicological threat is crucial not only for disposal but also for litigation in the event of a potential spill or manufacturer liability. When nanomaterials are prepared in a heterogeneous mixture, information regarding relative abundance of the different components within the mixture, as well as information regarding specific delivery mechanisms as they apply to the different components, and if associations in the bulk materials are maintained in the administered materials, need to be recorded.

The biological activity of a nanomaterial may be significantly affected by postadministrative alterations to the nanomaterials such as changes in

TABLE 13.1

Recommendations on Material Characterization

Characterization (Off-Line)	Human Exposure	Toxicity Screening Studies		
		Supplied Material	Administered Material	Material *In Vivo/In Vitro*
Size distribution (primary particles)	E (Combine with agglomeration state)	E	D	D
Shape	E	E	O	O
Surface area	D	E	D	O
Composition	E	E	O	O
Surface chemistry	D	E	D	D/O
Surface contamination	D	N	D	N
Surface charge— suspension/solution	O	E	E	O
Surface charge—powder (use bio-fluid surrogate)	O	E	N	O
Crystal structure	O	E	O	O
Particle physicochemical structure	E	E	D	D
Agglomeration state	E	N	E	D
Porosity	D	D	N	N
Method of production	E	E	—	—
Preparation process	—	—	E	—
Heterogeneity	D	E	E	D
Prior storage of material	E	E	E	—
Concentration	E	—	E	D

Source: Adapted with permission from Oberdorster, G. et al., 2005a. *Part Fibre Toxicol*, 2, 8. Copyright 2005 BioMed Central.

Note: E: These characterizations are considered to be essential.

D: These characterizations are considered to provide valuable information, but are not recommended as essential due to constraints associated with complexity, cost, and availability.

O: These characterizations are considered to provide valuable but nonessential information.

N: These characterizations are not considered to be of significant value to screening studies.

agglomeration state. Primary, secondary, and tertiary changes at different structural scales due to agglomeration state should be documented. The primary structural-scale agglomeration state reflects the lowest level of particle structure as seen at the primary particle level. The secondary-scale agglomeration state reflects the self-assembled structures resulting from primary particle agglomerates. The tertiary-scale agglomeration state reflects the assembly of secondary structures. The mechanisms for the formation of these various agglomeration states can provide important insight into the potential toxicity or alteration in function as a result of agglomerate formation. Identification of the binding forces responsible for the formation of these agglomerates should be noted such as van der Waals forces, electrostatic interaction, or sintered bonds. The examination of nanomaterial agglomeration or deagglomeration should be evaluated within various liquid media. This is of importance with regard to pharmaceutical preparation or application as well as *in vitro/in vivo* and various toxicological screening that involves a wide range of solutions. For instance, the introduction of a well-characterized nanomaterial solution into a biological system via intravenous injection, upon administration the nanomaterials may change in agglomeration or physicochemical properties within the context of the blood.

Alteration in the physicochemical properties of nanoparticles can also occur within the confines of their application. Depending on the end-product application, the nanomaterial can be exposed to a wide variety of environmental factors, for instance, a nanomaterial coating on a product that will be exposed to direct sunlight, or changes in elements of weather can produce an unknown alteration in the nanomaterial-based coating, which may result in a breakdown of the coat and release of nanomaterials from their intended application into a novel exposure route. Any alteration in the physicochemical properties of these end-application products would alter its toxicological profile. Irrespective of the end-product application or the unknown possibilities of toxicological exposure, it must be noted that the potential benefits the field of nanomaterials possess are great. With this in mind, as the field of nanosafety/nanotoxicology progresses, care must be taken not to terminate the advancement of this field but to put in place the best foundation upon which to evaluate both *a novo* and retrospectively the safety concerns as well as the potential beneficial properties of the burgeoning number of nanomaterials. This can best be done by careful consideration and documentation of all material characteristics.

The highest priority of material characterization is at the level of administration, followed by characterization after *in vitro* or *in vivo* administration, and complemented by characterization as produced or supplied. Table 13.1 reflects recommended characterizations in both feasibility and hierarchy with regard to making measurements within the respective contexts.

13.2.4 Analysis Methods

Table 13.1 presents a list of nanomaterial properties and the developmental and established analytical techniques available for nanomaterial characterization. Toxicity screening studies have a wide range of available techniques to choose from with regard to nanomaterial characterization; a list of these techniques can be found in Table 13.2 and are listed as they are related to the nanomaterial characteristics of interest. Additional information regarding the various techniques can be found in a wide variety of sources. It must be noted that some of these techniques are suited only for certain preparation, class, or form of nanomaterials. To understand the appropriate method to use to obtain the characteristic of interest, it is best to contact someone who has an expertise in the particular technique required to obtain this information. Even the best instrument if not properly utilized will not generate the quality or appropriate type of data desired. With regard to nanomaterial, knowledge and understanding of the equipment and technique are even more important due to the nanoscopic nature of the material of interest. Preparation of samples and the conditions for the examination of the nanomaterials for a specific technique may in itself alter the nanomaterials or not be suited for the sample conditions in which they have been prepared. For instance, the use of a scanning electron microscope is not suited for the examination of a nanoparticle suspended within a solution. In these cases, methods must be implemented to prepare the sample in a way compatible with the method employed.

13.3 Models of Ecotoxicity

When considering the safety issues associated with ENM, we must be aware of the various routes of potential exposure. Figure 13.2 provides a general schematic of some of these various routes of exposure. From production, transport, storage, end user, to disposal, the potential for ENMs to pose safety risk exists. At each point along the existence of the ENM life cycle, there is a potential for various organisms to come in contact with or be exposed to the ENM. To date, no true model has been developed to assess the potential exposure or safety limits of ENMs throughout their life cycle. Once ENMs are released into the atmosphere, these atmospheric ENMs may settle on the soil or water. Water that has been contaminated by ENMs, such as in oceans, lakes, or rivers, may vaporize and carry into the air these ENMs and then redistribute these ENMs to various ecosystems for potential exposure to a myriad of organisms. ENMs from contaminated soil or contaminated water have the potential to enter the food chain through plant and livestock, resulting in bioaccumulation and biomagnification within various food sources currently used for human consumption. However, many of these potential exposure mechanisms have yet to be investigated.

Nanosafety has become a major concern worldwide, and ecotoxicity, the identification of chemical hazard to the environment, is one area of

TABLE 13.2

Applicability of a Range of Analytical Techniques for Providing Specific Physicochemical Information on Engineered Nanomaterials in the Context of Toxicity Screening Studies

Physicochemical characteristic	Analytical Technique														
	Transmission Electron Microscopy (TEM)	Scanning Electron Microscopy (SEM)	X-Ray Diffraction (XRD)	X-Ray Photon Spectroscopy (XPS)	Auger Spectroscopy (AES)	Secondary Ion Mass Spectrometry (SIMS)	Scanning Probe Microscopy (SPM)	Dynamic Light Scattering (DLS)	Zeta potential	Size Exclusion Chromatography	Analytical Ultracentrifugation	Differential Mobility Analysis (DMA)	Isothermal Adsorption (e.g., BET)	Spectroscopic Techniques (UV–vis, IR, Raman, NMR)	Elemental Analysis (e.g., ICP-MS/AA, etc.)
Size distribution	▲						●	●		●	●	●			
Size (primary particles)	●	●	●												
Shape	▲	●					●	✓				✓			
Surface area	●	◇					◇	◇				✓	●		
Composition	●	●		●	●	▲					◇				▲
Surface chemistry	✓	✓		●		✓	✓		◇					●	
Surface contamination				●	●		✓							✓	
Surface charge–suspension/solution									▲						
Surface charge–powder (use bio-fluid surrogate)									▲					✓	

continued

TABLE 13.2 (continued)

Applicability of a Range of Analytical Techniques for Providing Specific Physicochemical Information on Engineered Nanomaterials in the Context of Toxicity Screening Studies

	Analytical Technique														
	Transmission Electron Microscopy (TEM)	Scanning Electron Microscopy (SEM)	X-Ray Diffraction (XRD)	X-Ray Photon Spectroscopy (XPS)	Auger Spectroscopy (AES)	Secondary Ion Mass Spectrometry (SIMS)	Scanning Probe Microscopy	Dynamic Light Scattering (DLS)	Zeta potential	Size Exclusion Chromatography	Analytical Ultracentrifugation	Differential Mobility Analysis (DMA)	Isothermal Adsorption (e.g., BET)	Spectroscopic Techniques (UV–vis, IR, Raman, NMR)	Elemental Analysis (e.g., ICP-MS/AA, etc.)
Crystal structure	•	◊	▲												
Particle physicochemical structure	▲	•	✓			✓					✓				
Agglomeration state	▲	•					•	✓		✓	✓	•	•		
Porosity	◊						◊						•		
Heterogeneity	▲	•												✓	

Source: Adapted with permission from Oberdorster, G. et al., 2005a. *Part Fibre Toxicol*, 2, 8. Copyright 2005 BioMed Central.)

Note: Other applicable techniques are available that have not been listed.

▲, Highly applicable;

•, Capable of providing information in some cases;

✓, Capable of providing information in some cases, with validation from more accurate/applicable techniques;

◊, Capable of providing qualitative or semiquantitative information.

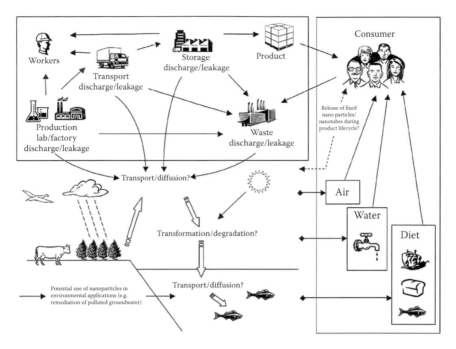

FIGURE 13.2
Potential routes of exposure to ENMs. (Royal Society. 2004. *Nanoscience and Nanotechnologies: Opportunities and Uncertainties.* London, p. 109.)

growing concern with regard to ENMs. Europe has taken the lead with regard to policy and regulatory requirements with regard to ENMs. Upon the release of an assessment on "Nanoscience and Nanotechnologies: Opportunities and Uncertainties" by the Royal Society and Royal Academy of Engineering in 2004 (Royal Society, 2004), many regulatory concepts were developed, including the evaluation of nanosized chemicals within the registration, evaluation, authorization, and restriction of chemicals (REACH) risk assessment procedures established by the European Parliament in 2006 (Parliament, 2006a,b). These regulations required that chemicals be evaluated for ecotoxicology against a base set of organisms, which include (1) an algal species, (2) an aquatic invertebrate, and (3) fish. Of particular interest to ENMs, the Royal Society indicated that nanomaterials be regulated as new chemicals (Royal Society, 2004).

To date, few ENMs have been evaluated according to the REACH risk assessment, and most studies that have been published have not reported the findings in traditional ecotoxicological endpoints. Although limited records exist for REACH-approved assessment, a growing body of publications exists with regard to ecotoxicological animal models.

13.3.1 Alternative Nonanimal Methods

Although the European Centre for the Validation of Alternative Methods (ECVAM) has not validated any nonanimal method for ecotoxicty testing (ECVAM 2011), there is a growing concern that the number of fish needed to conduct the required ecotoxicity studies will be large and that a reduction strategy may be needed to minimize the number of animals needed or at least prescreen ENMs for toxicity ranges to limit the animal requirements to sufficiently, scientifically, ethically, and economically meet the testing needs for ENMs. There is growing list of both *in vitro* and *in silico* approaches that have been proposed to replace or supplement *in vivo* aquatic toxicity, which include:

- Bacterial cell assays, based on luminescent reporter genes
- Fish cell-based cytotoxicity assays
- Fish cell-based assays with toxicological endpoints
- Mammalian cell assays with cytotoxicological or alternative end points
- Fish embryo assays/embryo survival and/or pathophysiological changes
- *In vitro* endocrine disruptor assays
- Genomic microarrays (toxicogenomics)
- Quantitative structural–activity relationship ((Q)SAR) and other computational programs
- Incorporating the above assays into test batteries and/or tiered testing schemes

Although these nonanimal models have not been approved by any regulatory agency, and although there is a lack of studies directly geared toward the efficacy of these models with regard to ecotoxicological assessment of ENMs, there is a growing body of data that provide some insight into the effect of ENMs on various organisms found within an ecological setting. A list of organisms that have been used to evaluate ENM toxicity can be found in Table 13.3. Although there is no standardization of reporting, and none of these studies meets the regulatory requirements of any governmental regulatory body, it is of importance to note that most of these organisms can be found at the lowest tier of an ecological food chain. With this information in mind, the consideration must be made regarding the ecological impact changes in these lower organisms would have if environmental exposure occurred.

If the ENMs produce toxic effects, this would result in an elimination of these organisms from the food chain, which could potentially escalate upwards into the elimination of higher organisms due to reduced food supply. If exposure to ENMs produced a genetic alteration within the lower organisms depending upon the type of mutation, a new species could emerge,

TABLE 13.3

Ecotoxicity

Common Name	Species	Reference
African clawed frog	*Xenopus laevis*	Mouchet et al. (2008)
Algae (microalgae)	*Pseudokirchneriella subcapitata*	Fouqueray et al. (2012), McLaughlin and Bonzongo (2012), Gao et al. (2011), Van Hoecke et al. (2008, 2009, 2011a, 2011b), Kennedy et al. (2010), Rodea-Palomares et al. (2011), Hartmann et al. (2010), Naha et al. (2009a), Bouldin et al. (2008), Aruoja et al. (2009), Franklin et al. (2007), Baun et al. (2008b), Warheit et al. (2007)
Amphipod crustacean	*Hyalella azteca*	Stanley et al. (2010)
Amphipod crustacean	*Leptocheirus plumulosus*	Kennedy et al. (2008)
Beavertail fairy shrimp	*Thamnocephalus platyurus*	Manusadzianas et al. (2012), Patra et al. (2011), Blinova et al. (2010), Naha et al. (2009a, 2009b), Van Hoecke et al. (2009), Heinlaan et al. (2008), Blaise et al. (2008)
California blackworm	*Lumbriculus variegatus*	Pakarinen et al. (2011), Poda et al. (2011), Stanley et al. (2010)
Carp (gold fish)	*Carassius auratus*	Handy et al. (2010), Zhu et al. (2008b, 2008c), Dodd and Jha (2009), Reeves et al. (2008), Sinyakov et al. (2006)
Ciliate protozoan	*Tetrahymena thermophila*	Mortimer et al. (2010, 2011), Werlin et al. (2011), Blinova et al. (2010)
Common carp	*Cyprinus carpio*	Handy et al. (2011), Hao and Chen (2012), Liu et al. (2012a), Zhao et al. (2011), Gaiser et al. (2012), Letts et al. (2011), Hao et al. (2009), Shinohara et al. (2009), Sun et al. (2009), Zhang et al. (2006, 2007)
Earthworm (dendras)	*Eisenia ventena*	Hooper et al. (2011), Scott-Fordsmand et al. (2008)
Earthworm (red wiggler)	*Eisenia foetida*	Canas et al. (2011), Coleman et al. (2010), Coutris et al. (2012), Gomes et al. (2012a, 2012b), Hayashi et al. (2012), Heckmann et al. (2011), Hooper et al. (2011), Johnson et al. (2011), Lapied et al. (2010, 2011), Li and Alvarez (2011), Li et al. (2010a, 2011a), Oughton et al. (2008), Pakarinen et al. (2011), Poda et al. (2011), Scott-Fordsmand et al. (2008), Shoults-Wilson et al. (2011a, 2011b), Unrine et al. (2010a, 2010b), van der Ploeg et al. (2011), Verma et al. (2011)
Estuarine meiobenthic copepod	*Amphiascus tenuiremis*	Ferguson et al. (2008), Templeton et al. (2006)
European perch	*Perca fluviatilis*	Handy et al. (2011), Bilberg et al. (2010, 2011)

continued

TABLE 13.3 (continued)

Ecotoxicity

Common Name	Species	Reference
Facultative anaerobic Gram-positive bacterium	*Staphylococcus aureus*	Yan et al. (2011)
Flathead minnow	*Pimephales promelas*	Handy et al. (2011), Zhu et al. (2006), Christen and Fent (2012), Jovanovic et al. (2011a, 2011b), Kennedy et al. (2010), Laban et al. (2010)
Fresh water green algae (pond scum, green weed)	*Desmodesmus subspicatus*	Hund-Rinke and Simon (2006)
Freshwater flea	*Daphnia magna*	Handy et al. (2011), Adams et al. (2006), Allen et al. (2010), Alloy and Roberts (2011), Bang et al. (2011), Baun et al. (2008a, 2008b), Blinova et al. (2010), Brausch et al. (2010, 2011), Dabrunz et al. (2011), Fan et al. (2011), Fang et al. (2011), Fouqueray et al. (2012), Gaiser et al. (2011, 2012), Heinlaan et al. (2008), (2011), Hund-Rinke and Simon (2006), Jackson et al. (2009), Kennedy et al. (2010), Kim et al. (2010a, 2010c, 2010d, 2011), Lee et al. (2009, 2010, 2012), Li et al. (2010b), Lovern and Klaper (2006), Lovern et al. (2007), Mendonca et al. (2011), Naha et al. (2009a, 2009b), Pace et al. (2010), Petersen et al. (2011), Poynton et al. (2011), Romer et al. (2011), Seda et al. (2012), Seitz et al. (2012), Spohn et al. (2009), Tan et al. (2012), Tao et al. (2009), Van Hoecke et al. (2009), Warheit et al. (2007), Wiench et al. (2009), Yang et al. (2010), Zahir and Rahuman (2012), Zaldivar and Baraibar (2011), Zhao and Wang (2010, 2011a, 2011b), Zhu et al. (2006, 2010a)
Freshwater hydroid	*Hydra attenuate*	Blaise et al. (2008)
Gram-negative bacteria	*Escherichia coli*	Yan et al. (2011), Jarmila and Vavrikova (2011), Robbens et al. (2010)*reviews only over 800 articles
Gram-negative bacterium	*Pseudomonas putida*	Beloqui et al. (2009), Bunge et al. (2010), Fabrega et al. (2009), Fang et al. (2007), Gajjar et al. (2009), Li et al. (2011c), Meerburg et al. (2012), Rotaru et al. (2012)
Gram-positive bacterium (Group B streptococcus or GBS)	*Streptococcus agalactiae*	Yan et al. (2011), Huang et al. (2008)

TABLE 13.3 (continued)

Ecotoxicity

Common Name	Species	Reference
Gram-positive bacterium	*Bacillus subtilus*	Fang et al. (2007)
Gram-positive bacterium (spore forming)	*Bacillus megaterium*	Culha et al. (2008), Fu et al. (2005), Kahraman et al. (2007a, 2007b), Karmakar et al. (2010), Lin et al. (2009c), Mishra et al. (2011), Saravanan et al. (2011), Smith et al. (2011)
Green algae	*Chlamydomonas reinhardtii*	Domingos et al. (2011), Lubick (2008), Navarro et al. (2008b), Perreault et al. (2012a, 2012b), Petit et al. (2010), Saison et al. (2010), Wang et al. (2008), Yang et al. (2012)
Green algae (microalgae)	*Chlorella kessleri*	Fujiwara et al. (2008)
Japanese killifish	*Oryzius latipes*	Handy et al. (2011), Chae et al. (2009), Chen et al. (2011), Hu et al. (2010), Kashiwada 2006, Kim et al. (2010b, 2011), Lee et al. (2011), Li et al. (2008, 2009), Manabe et al. (2011), Paterson et al. (2011), Perkel (2011), Wise et al. (2010), Wu et al. (2010), Zhu et al. (2010b)
Largemouth bass	*Micropterus salmoides*	Handy et al. (2011), Oberdorster (2004)
Photobacterium	*Vibrio fischeri*	Arce et al. (2012), Blaise et al. (2008), Doshi et al. (2008), Heinlaan et al. (2008), Lopes et al. (2012), Mortimer et al. (2008), Naha et al. (2009a, 2009b), Navalon et al. (2011), Pereira et al. (2011), Perreault et al. (2012a), Velzeboer et al. (2008)
Prokaryotic unicellular protozoan	*Stylonychia mytilus*	Zhao et al. (2005)
Rainbow trout	*Oncorhynchus mykiss*	Handy et al. (2011), Adomako et al. (2012), Blaise et al. (2008), Blaser et al. (2008), Farkas et al. (2010, 2011), Federici et al. (2007), Fraser et al. (2011), Gagne et al. (2010), Hildebrand et al. (2010), Hondroulis et al. (2010), Johnston et al. (2010), Kuhnel et al. (2009), Ramsden et al. (2009), Scown et al. (2009, 2010), Sekar et al. (2011), Sharma (2009), Thomas et al. (2011), Vevers and Jha (2008), Warheit et al. (2007)
Salamander	*Ambystoma mexicanum*	Mouchet et al. (2008)
Saltwater minnow	*Fundulus heteroclitus*	Blickley and McClellan-Green (2008)
Spionid worm	*Streblospio benedicti*	Ferguson et al. (2008)
Turkey tail mushroom	*Trametes versicolor*	Bokare et al. (2010), Gitsov et al. (2008), Hu et al. (2009, 2007), Liu et al. (2011), Pedroza et al. (2007), Schreiner et al. (2009), Shah et al. (2010)

continued

TABLE 13.3   (continued)

Ecotoxicity

Common Name	Species	Reference
Water flea	*Ceriodaphnia dubia*	Bouldin et al. (2008), Gao et al. (2011), Hu et al. (2012), Ingle et al. (2008), Li et al. (2011b), McLaughlin and Bonzongo (2012), Wang et al. (2011a, 2011b), Zahir and Rahuman (2012)
Water flea	*Daphnia pulex*	Griffitt et al. (2008), Klaper et al. (2009)
Woodlouse	*Porcellio scaber*	Jemec et al. (2008), Novak et al. (2012), Pipan-Tkalec et al. (2010), Valant et al. (2009, 2012)
Wrinkled crust mushroom	*Philebia tremellosa*	Schreiner et al. (2009)
Zebrafish	*Danio renio*	Handy et al. (2011), Henry et al. (2007), Hu et al. (2011), Liu et al. (2012b), Bilberg et al. (2012), Asharani et al. (2011), Xia et al. (2011), Fent et al. (2010), Ispas et al. (2009), Bar-Ilan et al. (2009), Asharani et al. (2008)

a drug resistance could occur, or a more virulent strain could develop. The possibility also exists that there may be no detrimental effect on the lower organisms but the ENMs may bioaccumulate or biotransform to produce a toxic effect on higher organisms. The limited knowledge of how ENMs affect various ecosystems only highlights the need for increased research efforts with regard to the ecotoxicity of ENMs. Although most of this is speculative, there have been reports that nanoparticles in algae and tobacco are transmitted to the next trophic level (Judy et al., 2011; Navarro et al., 2008a).

Although this chapter is focused on the safety aspects of ENMs, it is of importance to note that even though there is a limited body of data regarding the ecosafety aspects of ENMs, the body of data regarding the potential beneficial effects of ENMs is just as limited. For instance, the potential exists for agricultural application of ENMs that may provide great potential for environmental safety. If existing pesticides could be produced into nanoparticles with improved effectiveness that would reduce the quantity needed to produce the same effect, this would be a great improvement provided the biodegradation of the ENM pesticide was sufficient to eliminate consumer exposure. All in all, the field of ENM ecological science is greatly limited and our understanding regarding ENMs with the environment has yet to catch up with the rate of ENM development.

13.3.1.1 Plants Models

When considering nanosafety, we do not readily think of the effect nanoparticles may have on plants. Essential and nonessential elements can be absorbed by plants from their environment (Ke et al., 2007). These elements can be both toxic and beneficial and once stored in plants will be transferred to plant consumers (Rico et al., 2011). This ability for plants to absorb elements from their environment was exploited by researchers from Stanford in 2003. Gardea-Torresdey and colleagues found that alfalfa plants were able to take up gold or silver from solid media and produce gold or silver nanoparticles, respectively (Gardea-Torresdey et al., 2002, 2003). The mechanism responsible for uptake of environmental elements is believed to be capable of absorbing nanomaterials (NMs) (Rico et al., 2011). Naturally occurring NMs have been present in the environment throughout the entire evolutionary development of plants. But, as the rate of the production of ENMs increases, the probability of plan exposure to ENMs greatly increases. The effect ENMs have on plants and their associated food chains are unknown (Darlington et al., 2009; Pidgeon et al., 2009).

For the most part, the botanical concerns of ENMs have largely been unaddressed. Plant physiologists are yet to evaluate the effect ENMs have on fundamental processes such as planned nutrition, plant hormone function, seed germination, environmental stress physiology, photosynthesis, nastic movements, tropisms, respiration, photomorphogenesis, photoperiodism, stomata function and transpiration, and dormancy. The majority of data currently available regarding ENMs primarily evaluate the effects of the class of ENMs known as nanoparticles (NP) on plant physiology and focuses on germination stage and cell cultures. To date, a variety of plants have been investigated to evaluate the potential of NP uptake; a list of these plants can be found in Table 13.4; however, no conclusive data have emerged regarding the mechanism of nanoparticle uptake, translocation, accumulation, or biotransformation. The next section deals with the current mechanisms of nanoparticle uptake.

13.3.1.1.1 *Nanoparticle Uptake into Plants*

In addition to the species of plant, the various physicochemical characteristics of nanomaterials play a critical role in the mechanism of uptake, translocation, and accumulation of the nanomaterials. Figure 13.3 provides a pictorial representation of a model plant and the various proposed mechanisms of uptake, biotransformation, and translocation of nanomaterials (Chen et al., 2010; Lee et al., 2008a; Parsons et al., 2010). To date, limited data exist regarding plant and nanomaterial interaction (Rico et al., 2011).

Once the particles have been taken into the plant, the potential exist for nanomaterial/plant cell interaction there are several proposed avenues of plant cell/nanomaterial uptake. Figure 13.4 details these proposed routes of entry, which include endocytosis, binding to organic chemicals in the environmental media, creating new pores, binding to carrier proteins, through ion channels, or through aquaporins (Rico et al., 2011). Subsequent transport into plants may also occur through root exudates of complex formation with membrane transporters (Kurepa et al., 2010a; Watanabe et al., 2008) (Figure 13.4). Transportation of nanomaterials that have been taken up by the cell

TABLE 13.4

To Date Plant Physiology and Toxicology Have Been Studied in the Plants Listed Below

Common Name	Species	Reference
Alfalfa	*Medicago sativa*	Lopez-Moreno et al. (2010b), Gardea-Torresdey et al. (2002, 2003), Bali et al. (2010), Harris and Bali (2008)
Barley	*Hordeum vulgare*	El-Temsah and Joner (2012)
Cabbage	*Brassica oleracea*	Canas et al. (2008)
Carrot	*Daucus carota*	Canas et al. (2008)
Corn	*Zea mays*	Lin and Xing (2007), Barrena et al. (2009), Asli and Neumann (2009), Lopez-Moreno et al. (2010b), Birbaum et al. (2010), Răcuciu and Creangă (2009)
Cottonwood	*Populus deltoids*	Ma and Wang (2010)
Cucumber	*Cucumis sativus*	Lin and Xing (2007), Barrena et al. (2009), Canas et al. (2008)
Flax	*Linum usitatissimum* L.	El-Temsah and Joner (2012)
Hazel nut	*Corylus avella*	
Lettuce	*Lactuca sativa*	Lin and Xing (2007), Barrena et al. (2009), Canas et al. (2008), Shah and Belozerova (2009)
Lima bean	*Phaseolus limensis*	Zhu et al. (2008a)
Indian rhododendron	*Melastoma malabathricum*	Watanabe et al. (2008)
Mesquite	*Prosopis* sp.	Parsons et al. (2010)
Mouse-ear cress	*Arabisopsis thaliana*	Kurepa et al. (2010b), Madrid and Friedman (2010), Rondeau-Mouro et al. (2008)
Mungbean	*Phaseolus radiate*	Lee et al. (2008)
Mustard greens	*Brassica juncea*	Haverkamp and Marshall (2009), Harris and Bali (2008)
Onion	*Allium cepa*	Chen et al. (2010), Whitby and Quirke (2007), Canas et al. (2008), Kumari et al. (2009), Ghosh et al. (2010), Babu et al. (2008)
Pumpkin	*Cucurbita mixta*	Zhu et al. (2008a), Wang et al. (2011c), Corredor et al. (2009)
Radish	*Raphanus sativus*	Lin and Xing (2007), Barrena et al. (2009)
Rape	*Brassica napus*	Lin and Xing (2007), Barrena et al. (2009)
Red kidney beans	*Phaseolus vulgaris*	Doshi et al. (2008b)
Rice	*Oryza* sp.	Madrid and Friedman (2010), Tan and Fugetsu (2007), Tan et al. (2009), Lin et al. (2009a, 2009b)
Ryegrass	*Lolium* sp.	Lin and Xing (2007, 2008), Doshi et al. (2008), El-Temsah and Joner (2012)
Soybean	*Glycine max*	Lopez-Moreno et al. (2010a, 2010b), Lu et al. (2002)
Spinach	*Spinacia olerace*	Zheng et al. (2005), Hong et al. (2005), Gao et al. (2006), Yang et al. (2007), Linglan et al. (2008)
Tobacco	*Nicotiana tabacum*	Parsons et al. (2010), Judy et al. (2011)
Tomatoes	*Lycopersicon esculentum*	Khodakovskaya et al. (2009), Canas et al. (2008), Lopez-Moreno et al. (2010b)
Wheat	*Triticum aetivum*	Lee et al. (2008), Wild and Jones, (2009)
Zucchini	*Cucurbita pepo*	Stampoulis et al. (2009)

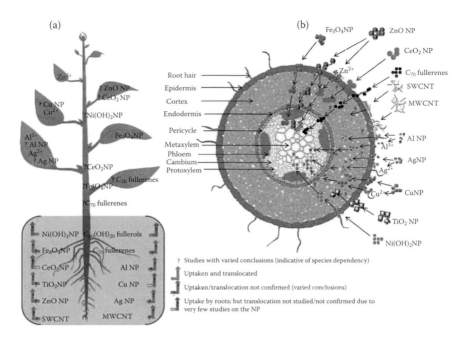

FIGURE 13.3
Uptake, translocation, and biotransformation pathway of various nanoparticles in a plant system: (a) plant showing the selective uptake and translocation of nanoparticles; (b) transverse section of the root absorption zone showing the differential nanoparticle interaction on exposure. (Adapted with permission from Rico, C. M. et al. 2011. Interaction of nanoparticles with edible plants and their possible implications in the food chain. *J Agric Food Chem*, 59, 3485–98. Copyright 2011 American Chemical Society.)

can occur through symplastical or apoplastical transport or from cell to cell through plasmodesmata. The mechanisms remain to be explored as to why only some plant species readily take up nanomaterials.

13.3.1.2 In Vitro Models

One of the most significant challenges facing the manufacturing, research, and regulatory communities is the development of testing strategies to characterize the hazardous potential of the burgeoning number of ENMs. The essential element of all proposed tiered approaches for toxicity assessment of nanomaterials include *in vitro* studies. This is a carryover from the utilization of *in vitro* studies in the research paradigms for chemicals, pharmaceuticals, and consumer products, into fine and ultrafine particulates.

One of the most attractive characteristics of *in vitro* models for toxicological evaluation of ENMs is their ability to be developed into a high-throughput system for rapid and cost-effective screening of ENMs hazards. Despite the use of various *in vitro* models within a wide range of fields for toxicological assessment, little attention has been given to the critical evaluation of the

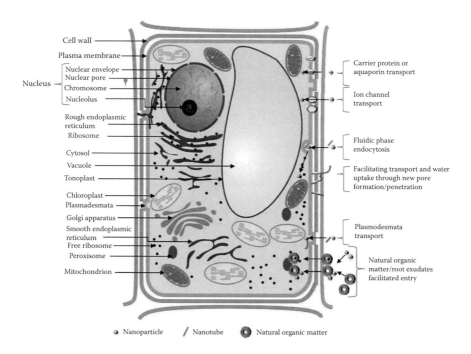

Cell wall

Plasma membrane

Nucleus
Nuclear envelope
Nuclear pore
Chromosome
Nucleolus

Rough endoplasmic reticulum
Ribosome

Cytosol

Vacuole

Tonoplast

Chloroplast
Plasmadesmata

Golgi apparatus
Smooth endoplasmic reticulum
Free ribosome
Peroxisome

Mitochondrion

Carrier protein or aquaporin transport

Ion channel transport

Fluidic phase endocytosis

Facilitating transport and water uptake through new pore formation/penetration

Plasmodesmata transport

Natural organic matter/root exudates facilitated entry

Nanoparticle   Nanotube   Natural organic matter

FIGURE 13.4

Probable modes of cellular uptake of the nanoparticles in a plant cell. (Adapted with permission from Rico, C. M. et al. 2011. Interaction of nanoparticles with edible plants and their possible implications in the food chain. *J Agric Food Chem*, 59, 3485–98. Copyright 2011 American Chemical Society.)

suitability of *in vitro* systems with regard to particle dosimetry and particle/ solution dynamics. Because ENMs within *in vitro* models remain insoluble, additional considerations must be made with regard to particle/solution dynamics. For instance, in an ideal setting, ENMs should be evenly dispersed throughout the culture media and maintain their individual particle characteristics; however, in most situations, particles can aggregate, settle, or diffuse differently within each *in vitro* model and in accordance to a wide range of particle characteristics that include surface physicochemistry, size, shape, density, zeta potential, and charge. Owing to the dynamics and complexity associated with ENMs in an *in vitro* system, it is expected that true cellular exposure may be significantly affected, and data generated without better defining the myriad of factors associated with ENMs within *in vitro* models may be less comparable across particle types and *in vitro* models (i.e., adherent vs. nonadherent culturing methods).

Although various cell types have been utilized in evaluating the toxicity of ENMs, there is a great need to develop a better understanding of dose response assessment to ENMs, as well as particle/solution dynamics and media interaction within these *in vitro* model systems. Teeguarden et al.

proposed the development of a new paradigm for particles dosimetry within *in vitro* models in their 2006 review (Teeguarden et al., 2007). This new paradigm of *in vitro* dosimetry of particles and ENMs focuses on the cellular dose rather than the exposure. Teequarden's paradigm is a shift away from classical *in vitro* toxicological assessment which assumes the test compound is dissolved within the solution.

Particle/solution dynamics play a vital role in the processes and factors controlling cellular dosage of ENMs. The potential for ENMs to agglomerate, diffuse, settle, and change surface charge/chemistry over time in solution will affect the nature of the particles and alter their transport into cells. The various properties of the particles and the solution play a critical role in the particles fait within an *in vitro* system. The size of the particles in addition to charge, surface chemistry, shape, and density will alter the sedimentation and diffusion rate, agglomeration, and various additional variables all of which are affected by the presence of proteins, viscosity, and density of the media solution used within the *in vitro* system. Each parameter introduces a contributing factor to the amount of ENMs the cell experiences. Because the nature of these variables adds complexity to the experimental design, the evaluation of the dose of ENMs the cell is exposed to is of critical importance when considering the toxic effects of ENMs. For instance, if an ENM remains suspended in solution during a toxicological assessment using an adherent cell line, the toxic exposure limit may be greatly overestimated; however, if the ENMs settle out rapidly, the cell will experience a large and rapid exposure to the ENMs and the toxic effect will be seen at a lower concentration.

In classical chemical dosimetry, two dimensions are considered for *in vitro* assessment of toxicity: time and duration. However, with ENMs, the nanoparticle dosimetry deals not only with time and amount but also with particle characterization. To complicate things even further, time and dosage become multifactorial as we mentioned above. The rate of particle settlement affects the timing of the cellular response (Figure 13.5). If an assessment of a specific ENM was to be performed in which the particle settled out of solution at a slow rate, the exposure time before initial cellular response would be delayed based on the settling rate.

13.3.1.2.1 In Vitro Dosimetry Metrics Considerations

As we have laid the foundation, it is becoming apparent that there are multiple levels at which ENM exposure can be defined within an *in vitro* experiment. At each of these levels, the specificity concerning site and mode of action may vary. The administered dose to the culture media reflects the most nonspecific level of ENMs dosage, while the apparent particle exposure at the level of cell or culture flask surface provides a more accurate representation of potential cultured cell exposure. The most specific of these levels is that of cellular dose or the amount of ENMs taken up by the cells (Figure 13.6). Even with the complexity associated with determining which

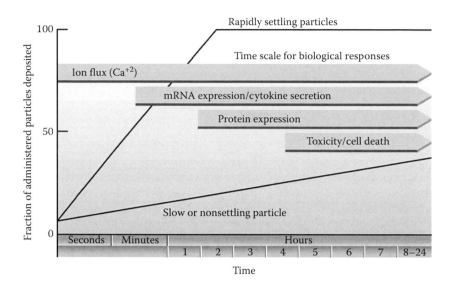

FIGURE 13.5
Illustration of the influence of particle transport rate on cellular dose *in vitro* as a function of time overlaid with the time scale for common measures of biological response. Both the rate and extent of transport of nanoparticles vary with settling and diffusion rate and can differ significantly for test materials within the time frame of typical *in vitro* experiments. For instance, monodisperse 100-nm gold nanoparticles will settle completely in less than 1.5 h from media 1–2 mm deep. (Adapted with permission from Teeguarden, J. G. et al. 2007. Particokinetics *in vitro*: Dosimetry considerations for *in vitro* nanoparticle toxicity assessments. *Toxicol Sci, 95,* 300–12. Copyright 2006 Oxford University Press.)

level is best to use for evaluating toxic or potential safety issues associated with ENMs, there still exist three nonspecific metrics that affect dose, which include number of particles (concentration), surface area of the particles, and the nominal media mass. These principal concepts are derived from the proposed metrics for evaluating *in vitro* dose–response assessments (Braydich-Stolle et al., 2005; Fubini et al., 2004; Gurr et al., 2005; Hussain et al., 2005; Oberdorster et al., 2005a; Sayes et al., 2006; Stringer et al., 1996).

The calculation of these metrics is relatively easy and based on the material characteristics according to the following equations (Teeguarden et al., 2007):

$$\text{Surface area concentration} = \frac{\text{mass concentration}}{\text{particle density}} \times \frac{6}{d} \qquad (13.1)$$

$$\text{Surface area concentration} = \#\,\text{concentration} \times \pi d^2 \qquad (13.2)$$

$$\#\,\text{concentration} = \frac{\text{mass concentration}}{\text{particle density}} \times \frac{6}{\pi d^2} \qquad (13.3)$$

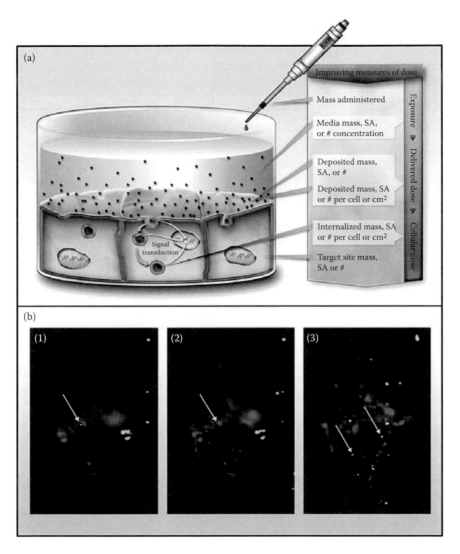

FIGURE 13.6
(See color insert.) Dose for nanoparticles *in vitro* increases in specificity and relevancy as dose measures move from administered amount to amount delivered to cells or internalized by cells (a) SA, surface area; #, particle number. (b) Images of an alveolar epithelial cell (C10), grown in culture and exposed to fluorescence-tagged 500-nm amorphous silica particles, demonstrate the principles shown in (a). The cell membrane is marked (red) by a membrane-specific fluorescent marker (wheat germ agglutinin), which was also internalized over time as an integral part of endocytotic vesicles. (b.1) Illustrates delivered dose: a silica particle (green) on the apical surface of the cell. The particle is no longer visible as the focal plane moves into the interior of the cell (b.2). Silica particles taken up into the cell are observed as the focal plane moves farther into the interior of the cell (b.3). (Adapted with permission from Teeguarden, J. G. et al. 2007. Particokinetics *in vitro*: Dosimetry considerations for *in vitro* nanoparticle toxicity assessments. *Toxicol Sci*, 95, 300–12. Copyright 2006. Oxford University Press.)

$$\# concentration = \frac{surface\ area\ concentration}{\pi d^2} \qquad (13.4)$$

Within these equations, the particles are assumed to be spherical. # indicates the number of particles, *particle density* is expressed in g/cm³, *d* is the diameter of a particle in cm, *mass concentration* is the mass of the particles per mL of media g/mL, and *surface area concentration* is the total surface area of the particle within the media cm²/mL.

These dosimetry considerations provide us with three levels of specificity for evaluating ENM dosing within an *in vitro* system: exposure, deliverable dose, and cellular dose. Within each of these levels, the particle dosage can be represented by the three metrics calculated from the above equations: mass concentration, surface area concentration, and particle number concentration. From a toxicological standpoint, the levels and metric assessment of exposure above the level of deliverable dose poorly reflect the effect ENMs have on cellular response. The cells can only respond to ENMs to which they come in contact; therefore, the ENMs that remain suspended in the media do not affect or elicit a cellular response. With this in mind, it is easy to understand that evaluating these metrics at the level of delivered dose will better reflect the true toxicological effect of the ENMs as opposed to the total mass administered to the culture or the *nominal media concentration* (particle mass to media volume ratio). This level of delivered dose can be compared to dose delivered per surface area of cells in culture and has the potential to be directly scalable and comparable to *in vivo* studies. However, a better assessment of cellular response to ENM dosage appears within the level of cellular dose or the dose the cell internalizes. At this level, the particle size and cellular uptake come into consideration as well as various other particle-dependent variables. This level of cellular dosage provides great insight into the mechanistic understanding of ENMs toxicity and their mode of action within the cell but is difficult to measure in practice.

13.3.1.2.2 Particokinetics

To better understand the level of deliverable dose, we must take into consideration the variables that take part in particle/solution dynamics. Teeguarden et al. (2007) defined these variables as particokinetics. Particokinetics represent the solution dynamics of particles that impact on the transport of ENMs to cells within an *in vitro* system. These variables are associated with the characteristics of the particles, properties of the media, and the processes responsible for particle/solution dynamics. Particokinetics can be organized into three board groups of factors that affect diffusion, gravitational settling, and agglomeration. Understanding the variables that contribute to the development of the *in vitro* delivery dose will provide insight into the cellular dosage level, but presents multiple limitations with regard to quantification.

Within the solution, the passive movement of particles known as diffusion typically occurs through the spontaneous shift of particles from areas of high chemical potential to that of low chemical potential. Particle uptake by cells can propagate a change in concentration gradient along the unstirred layer immediately above the cells, disrupting the potential of an equilibrium state. Because this process is gradient driven, the presence of equilibrium state would indicate the absence of diffusion-mediated transport. Because particle size is one of the primary factors associated with particle diffusion, other particles and media characteristics have little effect on the diffusion rate. The rate of diffusion can be calculated using the diffusion coefficient (D, cm^2/s) in accordance with Fick's law:

$$D = \frac{RT}{N6\pi\mu d} \tag{13.5}$$

where
  R = gas constant (8.314 J/K/mol)
  T = temperature (K)
  N = Avogadro's number (6.0221415×10^{23} mol^{-1})
  μ = solution viscosity (kg/m/s)
  d = particle diameter (m)

The diffusion coefficient operates in accordance with the Stokes–Einstein relation and is an inverse function of particle size. Utilizing the following equations (Bergqvist et al., 1987; Einstein, 1905)

$$t = \frac{<r^2>}{2D} \tag{13.6}$$

$$\text{root mean squared distance} = <r^2>$$

The time for a given particle to travel over a defined distance can be calculated. Because the diffusion coefficient is inversely proportional to particle size and the time required to travel a given distance via diffusional transport is a function of the diffusion coefficient, as the particle size increases, the distance traveled by the particle over a given time decreases proportionally to the particle size. Simply said, the larger the particle, the slower the particle moves by diffusion. To illustrate this point, a 1-nm particle can travel a distance of 1 cm in a day, whereas a 1000-nm particle would take ~3 years to travel the same distance (Teeguarden et al., 2007).

As particle size increases, the principal deliverer mechanism for particles to the surface of the culture flask and subsequently interaction with the adherent cells is the mechanism of gravitational settling. Three forces are responsible for the rate of gravitational settling: buoyancy, drag, and gravity.

The mass, size, density, and volume of the particle in addition to the density and viscosity of the media contribute to the rate of settling. Stoke's law allows us to calculate the terminal settling velocity of particles in solution (Teeguarden et al., 2007):

$$v_{sed} = \frac{2g(\rho_p - \rho_m)d^2}{9\mu} \tag{13.7}$$

where
  g = gravitational acceleration
  ρ_p and ρ_m = particle and media density
  d = particle diameter
  μ = viscosity of the media

It is to be noted that with increased particle size, gravitational settling increases. As with diffusion, this mathematical model of particokinetics is based on a spherical particle and would need to be modified to apply to ENMs bearing alternative shapes. In addition, it must be noted that environmental factors within the media may influence the function of gravitational settling within an *in vitro* system. For instance, protein–particle interaction can affect the gravitational settling.

With these potential environmental associated changes in particokinetics, we come to the final factor regarding delivery dose, which is agglomeration or the clumping of single particles into groups of particles. These particle agglomerations affect the particle gravitational settling. The factors associated with agglomeration are varied and should be addressed on a particle by particle as well as an *in vitro* by *in vitro* model bases.

Even with this complex approach, some conclusions can be drawn to better design and apply toxicological assessment of ENMs. Figure 13.7 provides a generalized representation of the concept of delivered dose to particle size in the context of the various contributing factors associated with particokinetics. Even within the context of Figure 13.7, it must be recognized that the time required for diffusion and gravitational settling are not addressed. Figure 13.7, represents the point at which the particokinetics within the *in vitro* system reaches completion. As shown in Figure 13.5, the time component remains a critical variable in the assessment of cellular response to ENMs exposure/dosing.

In addition, depending upon which metric is used to evaluate toxicity, the interpretation of the data may provide a varied degree of inaccuracy. This is the reason why proper characterization of nanomaterials is critical and retrospective analysis of data is necessary for proper understanding regarding newly discovered understanding regarding nanomaterial properties. For instance, the use of a metric of mass may provide mixed results regarding the toxicological profile of a nanomaterial. If a nanoparticle of three distinct sizes is evaluated to interrogate its toxicity, you may obtain three distinct

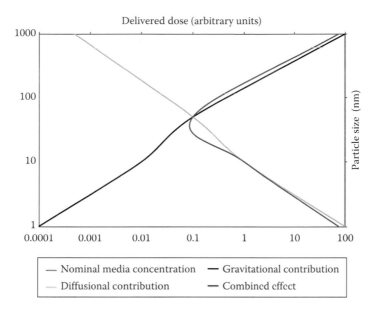

FIGURE 13.7
(See color insert.) Generalized representation of the particokinetic contribution to delivered dose within an *in vitro* system. As particle size increases, the contribution of diffusion to delivered dose decreases while the contribution of gravitational settling increases. It is estimated that at about 50 nm, the effective contribution of diffusion and gravitational settling are near equilibrium.

toxicological profiles, each based on varying degrees of mass. The slope of response may be similar but the true factor regarding the toxicological property of each may be masked. The use of the metric of surface area may provide better understanding regarding the true toxicological properties of the nanomaterial in question. In such a hypothetical case, the surface area profile of all three sizes may overlay perfectly to reveal the characteristic directly responsible for the toxicity of this nanomaterial.

This simplistic example may not fully express the complexity of the interplay with respect to the myriad of variable and characteristic associate with nanomaterials and the possible interactions and contribution of each of these components to the true toxicology of nanomaterials. To this end, it is vitally important that all care be taken in fully characterizing all nanomaterials for toxicological testing.

In addressing the metric of *mass contribution*, particle *surface area concentration* and *particle number concentration*, we must take into consideration that each of these metric provides an alternative aspect with regard to exposure limits. The contribution, complexity, and appropriate use of these metric are yet to be validated and each metric contributed greatly to the overall understanding of the ENMs toxicological profile. A more detailed review of these metrics has been addressed by Teeguarden et al. (2007).

13.3.1.3 *In Vitro* Testing Methods

Exposure to nanomaterials can occur through various routes. In this section, we will address the toxicological assessment of nanomaterial from the four main routes of exposure: injection, inhalation, ingestion, and deposition. These screening strategies will examine the relevant capability of nanomaterial entry into the body through these routes and the expression of biological activity and translocation upon entry.

As we approach the potential of *in vitro* testing, we must understand the limitation and application of the various toxicological testing methods for nanomaterials, with particular interest in several generic issues:

1. *Expression of dose*: As we have mentioned earlier, the use of a dose metric is critically important when considering toxicity and other responses. In addition, full characterization of the nanomaterial is required for complete analysis and retrospective evaluation.

2. *Control particles*: As we know the use of a positive and negative control is important, especially when viewed in respect to nanomaterials and the uncertainty regarding the appropriate dose metric. All experiments should contain an adequate positive and negative control particle. Allowing a particle of known toxicity to serve as a benchmark will greatly improve the data collection and also serve to validate the experimental methodology. Some proposed benchmark particles included fine TiO_2 as an inert particle or standard crystalline silica (quartz; e.g., Min-U-Sil or DQ12) (Oberdorster et al., 2005a).

3. *Adsorption of proteins by nanoparticles*: The capability of proteins to adsorb onto nanomaterials is one of the consequences of the large surface area of nanoparticles. Adsorption onto key proteins such as fibronectin, TGF-β (Kim et al., 2003), and albumin (Brown et al., 2000) have been reported with various types of nanoparticles. False-negatives may occur within certain test due to the absorption of a key protein to the nanomaterial. This protein would then be removed from the supernatant and produce a confounding endpoint.

4. *Advantages and disadvantages*: *In vivo* studies are costly and require specialized skill, and the practice has been to utilize as much *in vitro* studies and adjunct as possible to offset cost and reduce animal use. *In vitro* studies do provide a less complicated mechanism for evaluating specific biological signaling pathways and provide a higher degree of control of the test conditions. *In vivo* studies are more complex with regard to experimental variables. This is seen in some instances where the effect of the testing is not necessarily due to the site-specific action of the toxicant but may be the result of a proinflammatory effect, or various other systemic influences. With the use of *in vitro* techniques, the isolation of these complement system can occur and provide a more detailed explanation of the

response and the contributing factor associated with the *in vivo* outcome, although dosimetry mismatches, oversimplification, *in vivo*
adverse effects, and lack of involvement of complete inflammatory
response are all inherent problems associated with the validation of
in vitro approaches, which have been well documented.

In addition to the use of various animal models for the toxicological assessment of nanomaterials, various techniques have been developed to decrease
the number of animals required to perform a broad screening of toxic compounds. From evaluations of the literature, nanoparticles have been tested
in a wide range of animals from mice to pigs, but there is no standardized
model or systematic screening regiment established for nanotoxicological
assessment within animal models. To provide a more consistent flow, we
will address the systems independent of the species. In some instances, the
availability of *in vitro* models will be addressed with regard to the route of
exposure. Tables 13.5 and 13.6 provide a list of models of organ and exposure
routes (Oberdorster et al., 2005a).

13.3.1.3.1 Injection

The major promise of nanomedicine is the use of nanomaterials for treatment of disease. Most pharmacological applications of nanomaterials have
two primary routes of administration, injection or ingestion. Within this section, we will look at the major organ systems that may be affected by the
route of injection and the potential models of toxicological evaluation within
these systems. The five major systems that have the potential for direct exposure to injected nanomaterials are the blood, endothelium, spleen, liver,
heart, and kidneys.

13.3.1.3.1.1 Blood   The understanding of how a nanomaterial responds in
the blood is vital to not only its toxicity but also to any beneficial application it may have. Fractionated blood products such as serum with complements, isolated platelets, red blood cells, or leukocytes provide great *in vitro*
models for studies regarding blood nanomaterial interaction within the circulating blood. The evaluation of nanomaterials against relevant endpoints,
including complement activation, production of RNS/ROS, platelet activation, chemokine/cytokine release from leukocytes, and red blood cell interactions are possible through *in vitro* and *in vivo* methods. The potential also
exists for entry into the blood through translocation from another route of
entry (Nemmar et al., 2002; Oberdorster et al., 2002). As mentioned earlier,
the potential also exist for protein particles interactions, the presence of various circulating proteins may alter the nanomaterial, or the potential exist
for these particles to be taken into the circulating cells. These event may
change the functional characteristics of the particles, may cause circulating
cells types to be preferentially exposed resulting in either cell-specific toxicity or beneficial response, may alter the dose metric being used to evaluate

TABLE 13.5

Available *In Vitro* Systems for Portal of Entry Testing

Portal of Entry	Cell/Tissue Type	Effect	Endpoint	Research Gap
Lung	Epithelium	Toxicity	Trypan blue, LDH, apoptosis	
		Inflammation	Gene expression, oxidative stress, signal transduction pathways	
		Translocation	Transfer of nanoparticles across membranes	Translocation process
		Carcinogenesis	Genotoxicity, comet assay, 8OHdG, *hprt* assay, proliferation assay	
	Macrophages	Toxicity	Trypan blue, LDH, apoptosis	
		Chemotaxis	Chemotaxis assay	Recognition/ activation/ phagocytosis process
		Phagocytosis	Particle uptake into cells, cytoskeletal staining	
		Inflammation	Gene expression, oxidative stress, signal transduction pathways	Additional markers?
	Immune cells	Immune response	Cytokine profile, adjuvant effects	Additional markers?
	Endothelium	Inflammation	Adhesion molecules, oxidative stress	Additional markers?
		Coagulation	Von Willebrand factor, tissue factor	
	Fibroblasts	Inflammation	Oxidative stress, cytokine profile, gene expression profile	
		Fibrosis	Collagen synthesis, cell proliferation	
	Lung slices	Inflammation	Oxidative stress, signal transduction pathway, immunohistopathology	
		Translocation	Particles across membranes	Translocation process
		Fibrosis	Collagen synthesis	
Skin	Cell systems (e.g., HEK)	Cytotoxicity inflammation	Cell viability–MTT, neutral red, cytokine profile	
	Flow-through diffusion systems	Absorption		

TABLE 13.5 (continued)

Available *In Vitro* Systems for Portal of Entry Testing

Portal of Entry	Cell/Tissue Type	Effect	Endpoint	Research Gap
	Isolated skin flap model	Absorption, cytotoxicity, inflammation	Glucose utilization, any other markers depending on endpoints (cytokine profiles, histopath, etc.)	
Mucosa	Intestinal epithelium (GI tract)	Cytotoxicity	Cell viability—MTT, neutral red, trypan blue, apoptosis	
		Inflammation	Cytokine profile, oxidative stress, signal transduction pathway	
		Translocation	Permeability assays	
	GALT	Inflammation	Cytokine profile, oxidative stress	
		Immune response	Adjuvant effects	Additional markers?
	Buccal epithelium (oral cavity)	Cytotoxicity	Cell viability—MTT, neutral red, trypan blue, apoptosis	
		Inflammation	Cytokine profile, oxidative stress, signal transduction pathway	
		Translocation	Permeability assays	
	Vaginal epithelium (reproductive system)	Cytotoxicity	Cell viability—MTT, neutral red, trypan blue, apoptosis	
		Inflammation	Cytokine profile, oxidative stress, signal transduction pathway	
		Translocation	Permeability assays	

Source: Adapted with permission from Oberdorster, G. et al. 2005a. *Part Fibre Toxicol*, 2, 8. Copyright 2005 BioMed Central.

toxicity, or may sequester the nanomaterials from being delivered to a potential target system.

13.3.1.3.1.2 Endothelium The vasculature of the body is lined by a thin layer of cells known as the endothelium. This thin layer can be exposed to nanomaterials through injections or alternative routes of entry that are highly vascularized or through translocation of nanomaterials from alternative

TABLE 13.6

Available *In Vitro* Systems for Potential Target Organs

Target Organ	Cell/Tissue Type	Effect	Endpoint	Research Gap
Endothelium	Endothelial cells (e.g., HUV-EC-C)	Cytotoxicity	Cell viability—MTT, neutral red, trypan blue, apoptosis	
		Homeostasis	Oxidative stress, gene expression profile	Additional markers?
		Translocation	Permeability assays	
Blood	Red blood cells, platelets, bone marrow (megakaryocytes)	Inflammation/ immune response	Platelet activation	
			Cytokine/chemokine release from leukocytes	
			Oxidative stress	
			Complement activation	
		RBC/particle interactions		Markers?
Liver	Hepatocytes	Toxicity	Cell viability—MTT, neutral red, trypan blue, apoptosis	
	Kupffer cells	Inflammation	Cytokine profile, oxidative stress, signal transduction pathway, gene expression	
		Coagulation	Von Willebrand factor, tissue factor	
	Isolated perfused liver slices	Translocation, distribution	Histopathology	Translocation process
	Liver slices	Toxicity studies	Cytotoxicity, P450 assay, ATP assays, GSH content	Additional markers? genomics, proteomics?
	Collagen sandwich cultures	Toxicity studies	Cytotoxicity, P450 assay, ATP assays, GSH content	Additional markers? genomics, proteomics?
Spleen	Lymphocytes	Immune response	Cytokine profile	
Central and peripheral nervous system	Neuronal cells	Toxicity	Cytotoxicity—trypan blue, LDH, apoptosis	

TABLE 13.6 (continued)

Available *In Vitro* Systems for Potential Target Organs

Target Organ	Cell/Tissue Type	Effect	Endpoint	Research Gap
		Inflammation	Cytokine profile, oxidative stress, signal transduction pathway, gene expression	
		Translocation	Gene expression, microscopic examination	
	Astroglial, microglial cells	Inflammation	Cytokine profile, oxidative stress, signal transduction pathway, gene expression	
Heart	Cardiomyocytes	Toxicity	Cytotoxicity—trypan blue, LDH, apoptosis	
		Inflammation	Cytokine profile, oxidative stress, signal transduction pathway, gene expression	
		Function	Beat—rhythm testing	
Kidney	Cell (e.g., HK-2, MDCK, LCC-PK1)	Toxicity	Cytotoxicity—trypan blue, LDH apoptosis	
		Inflammation	Cytokine profile, oxidative stress, signal transduction pathway, gene expression	
		Translocation	Permeability assays	Additional markers?
	Kidney slices	Toxicity	Cytotoxicity—trypan blue, LDH, apoptosis	
		Inflammation	Cytokine profile, oxidative stress, signal transduction pathway, gene expression	
		Translocation	Permeability assays	Additional markers?

Source: Adapted with permission from Oberdorster, G. et al. 2005a. *Part Fibre Toxicol,* 2, 8. Copyright 2005 BioMed Central.

routes on entry into the circulation. Homeostasis of the vasculature is affected by alteration in RNS production; by utilizing cultured endothelial cells, the effect of nanomaterials on vascular homeostasis may be elucidated (Fleming and Busse, 1999; Harrison et al., 1991; O'Donnell, 2003). Endothelial cellular effects, blood–brain barrier, and alveolo capillary barrier transport of nanomaterials can potentially be evaluated by the use of *in vitro* cultures.

13.3.1.3.1.3 Spleen   Accumulation of nanomaterials in the spleen may pose severe consequences to the immune systems. The spleen is largely responsible for lymphoid maturation and immune processing. Toxicological effects of nanomaterials within the spleen may culminate in a major immunopathology. To complement and more precisely address the effects of nanomaterials on the spleen, isolated cells from the spleen can be studied *in vitro* to assess nanomaterial affects. Functional aspects such as lymphocyte proliferation and dendritic cell function, markers of lymphoid cell differentiation, and immune responsivity and antigen processing *in vitro* can be utilized as endpoints for toxicological assessment.

13.3.1.3.1.4 Liver   The functional and structural heterogeneity of the liver makes it a very complex organ. Xenobiotics and foreign materials are primarily defended against or biotransformed in the liver. The liver possesses many functions and is composed of many different cell types. The liver has an integral circulatory system consisting of two distinct blood supplies. Necrosis and inflammation are two forms of histological lesions that can be used to characterize liver injury in response to nanomaterial toxicity. The cytochrome P450 metabolic pathway in one of the most common mechanisms for evaluating hepatocellular injury on the molecular level and may be a promising pathway for investigating nanomaterial toxicity. It would be expected due to the link between the liver and the biliary system that nanomaterials may pose an exposure threat to the biliary system. Because the liver excretes materials into the bile, fecal excrement or bile may contain markers for evaluating the effect of nanomaterials on the hepatic and biliary systems. Activation of proapoptotic receptor enzymes, protein synthesis inhibition, alcohol dehydrogenase activation, disruption of calcium homeostasis, and cytochrome P450 activation are all reported mechanisms associated with *in vivo* hepatocellular injury and may be potential endpoints for toxicological assessment of nanomaterial safety. The potential exists to predict toxicity in humans by employing the use of *in vitro* assays utilizing human-derived cells. But we must keep in mind that enzyme function within humans has a considerable amount of variability.

> *Liver slices*: Nanomaterials can be studied utilizing freshly isolated livers slices. Liver slices are a good model due to the fact the slice maintains the normal tissue organization. With the improvement in this technique, the precision of slicing provides a great deal of accuracy and repeatability.

Isolated perfused liver: Detailed characterization of particle distribution within the organ can be obtained through the use of a complicated model of isolated liver perfusion. This system closely mimics the *in vivo* environment of the liver and would be a suitable model for the study of nanomaterial toxicity within the hepatic system.

Primary human hepatocytes: Well-characterized primary human hepatocytes are commercially available for culture studies. In most cases, a full complement of metabolizing enzymes and metabolic profiling has been conducted on these primary cell lines. The demand for liver transplants has increased in recent years as have the availability of human cells.

Collagen sandwich cultures: For several days, the functional and structural integrity of the liver can be maintained through the collagen sandwich culture. This model system allows for the evaluation of aspartate aminotransferase and alanine aminotransferase enzymes release to be monitored due to the fact that the bile canaliculi are well maintained.

Additional *in vitro* systems are available for evaluating hepatic effects of nanomaterial exposure. Changes in CYP450 can be evaluated in isolate hepatocyte studies to assess hepatic metabolism. Live toxicity and function can be evaluated by using whole liver homogenate, liver slices, or subcellular fractions. Identification of metabolite formation can be determined by the use of LC/MS on microsomes. Proteomic and transcriptional profiling can also be areas of interest within these studies. Various endpoints can be utilized within these studies such as ATP content, GSH content, peroxisomal proliferation, covalent protein binding, mitochondrial function, cell detachment, membrane damage, cell morphology, alamar blue metabolism, cell viability, gene and protein expression, and albumin synthesis to name a few. It must be remembered that the nature of *in vitro* assays only provides a window into the individual cell-type response and that genotypic and phenotypic difference do exist with regard to immortalized cell when compared with the organ of interest. As with all *in vitro* studies care must be taken when applying the information gleaned from these studies, the limitation and assumptions must be duly noted with regard to the predictive value of the nanomaterial toxicity as ascertained from such studies (Dambach et al., 2005; Worth and Balls, 2002).

13.3.1.3.1.5 Heart   With injection of nanomaterials, the potential exists for these particles to find their way into the microcirculation of the heart and subsequently into the heart muscle where they may affect cardiac function. Within an *in vivo* model, the effect of nanomaterial toxicity to cardiac function could be assessed by the use of ECG, echocardiography, or an organ *ex vivo* Langendorff preparation. Metabolism, viability, and ionic homeostasis could be evaluated with the use of cultured cardiomyocytes. Specific culturing techniques will produce a rhythmic *in vitro* culture of cardiomyocytes that could be used to evaluate rhythm alteration, specific change in signaling or ionic channel response.

Cardiac slices: Nanomaterials can be studied utilizing freshly isolated heart slices. Heart slices are a good model due to the fact that the slice maintains the normal tissue organization. With the improvement in this technique the precision of slicing provides a great deal of accuracy and repeatability.

Isolated perfused heart (Langendorff): Detailed characterization of particle distribution within the organ can be obtained through the use of a complicated model of isolated heart perfusion. This system closely mimics the *in vivo* environment of the heart and would be a suitable model for the study of nanomaterial toxicity within the heart.

13.3.1.3.1.6 Kidney   Any material entering the blood stream has the potential to be filtered out of the body through the kidney. Because the kidney is the primary filtration system for the body, it is no surprise that nanoparticles can be excreted out of the body by the kidneys. It is believed that particles above 5 nm in size may be unable to pass out of the body through the kidney (Longmire et al., 2008). The use of *in vitro* testing has the potential to throw some light into the largely unknown effect nanomaterials may have on the renal system. Renal tubules penetration and translocation are very important in evaluating the pharmaceutical application of nanomaterials. Important indicators of renal homeostasis including modulation in the release of growth factors, signal transduction response, ion channel flux, cellular viability, and proteinases can act as endpoints for the evaluation of nanomaterial toxicity. The commercially available well-characterized cells derived from isolated proximal nephrons, proximal ducts, glomeruli, or distal tubule/collecting ducts can be used to assess nanomaterial toxicity as well (Raychowdhury et al., 2004; Ryan et al., 1994). In addition, a number of immortalized cell lines are available that can provide a low-cost cytotoxicological testing alternative to kidney slices. The evaluation of cytotoxicity can be performed on the human embryonic kidney cell line HEK-293 (Chou et al., 2003). Toxicological effects of *in vitro* mechanistic of nanomaterials can be conducted using LLC-PK1 cells and MDKK cells (Panneerselvam and Freeze, 1996; Rustom et al., 2003).

Kidney slices: Nanomaterials can be studied utilizing freshly isolated kidney slices. Kidney slices are a good model due to the fact the slice maintains the normal tissue organization. With the improvement in this technique, the precision of slicing provides a great deal of accuracy and repeatability. Oxidative stress, particle translocation, toxicity, and signal transduction responses can all be assessed by use of kidney slices (Ricardo et al., 1994; Vickers et al., 2004).

Isolated perfused kidney: Detailed characterization of particle distribution within the organ can be obtained through the use of a complicated model of isolated kidney perfusion. This system closely mimics the *in vivo* environment of the kidney and would be a suitable model for the study of nanomaterial toxicity within the renal system.

13.3.1.3.2 Inhalation

Some pharmaceutical agents can be delivered through inhalation. With regard to nanomaterials, this route of exposure can be of great interest. The potential of nanoparticles to aerosolize is very great given their size. Exposure to aerosolized nanomaterials can be intentional for the purpose of treatment, accidental in the case of environmental exposure, or chronic in the case of a manufacturing environment. In any case, the toxic effect of an inhaled nanomaterial is of great concern and appropriate measures should be taken to limit exposure and understand the postexposure effects.

13.3.1.3.2.1 Lungs   There are many models in addition to animal inhalation and installation studies that can be utilized *in vitro* to investigate the effect of nanoparticles on lung tissue. Once a particle has entered the respiratory system, it can be deposited in the airway of the alveolar epithelium. It immediately encounters the epithelial lining fluid or mucus within the airway and can be cleared through interaction with macrophages or mucus movement. Additionally, these inhaled nanomaterials may make contact with the immune system, endothelial, and fibroblasts cells by entering the interstitium.

Epithelium: The alveolar region and the conducting airways are lined with epithelium that represents the first barrier to particle deposition. This barrier acts to limit the entrance of materials from the respiratory tract into the body. For this reason, *in vitro* studies utilizing alveolar and bronchial epithelial cells can provide important information regarding nanoparticle effects on the respiratory system. Various cytokine expression (IL-8, MCP-1, etc.) (Fubini et al., 1998; Gilmour et al., 2003), inflammation-related transcription factors such as NF-κB and AP-1 (Schins and Donaldson, 2000; Timblin et al., 1998), and LDH release can all serve as endpoints of nanoparticle toxicity. Nitrosated proteins as a measure of active nitrogen species (Hess et al., 2005), oxidized glutathione as endpoints (Barrett et al., 1999), and dichlorofluorescein (Stringer and Kobzik, 1998) can all be used to evaluate nitrosative and oxidative stress, both of which are proposed mechanisms of cell damage. Pathogenic particles are believed to induce oxidative/nitrosative stress. Glutathione peroxidase and superoxide dismutase are antioxidant genes (Janssen et al., 1993) that can be upregulated in response to oxidative/nitrosative stress and may be potential indicators of nanomaterial toxicity.

Bromo-deoxyuridine incorporation can be used to measure the effect nanomaterials have on cellular proliferation (Quinlan et al., 1995) in addition to a number of other proliferation assays.

8-Hydroxy-deoxyguanosine measurements and COMET assays can be quantified to directly measure genotoxicity, this can act as an endpoint for the potential of cancer (Schins, 2002, Schins et al., 2002). The harmful effects of inhaled nanomaterials may be averted if the epithelium translocation of nanoparticles acts as a decimatory mechanism. Currently, there are few publications that specifically address *in vitro* epithelial particle movement. Understanding the regulation of translocation events is limited and such studies are vitally important in developing a concise understanding or respiratory nanomaterial interaction.

Macrophages: The deposition of particles in the lungs can produce a cellular response primarily driven by macrophages. A variety of assays are available that can provide insight into the mechanism by which nanoparticles affect macrophages. Lactate dehydrogenase release can be used to assess cellular toxicity. The oxidative burst (OB) associated with the phagocytosis of particles (Brown et al., 1998) by macrophages could be investigated. In addition, the release of cytokines (interleukin-6 (IL-6), tumor necrosis factor alpha (TNFα), etc.), activator protein 1 (AP-1) nuclear transfer of inflammation-related transcription factors, nuclear factor kappa B (NF-κB) release are also results of phagocytotic activity of macrophages. A highly toxic superoxide radical, peroxynitrite can be produced in response to an elevation in nitric oxide (NO) production as a result of particle exposure (Chao et al., 1996, Coffey et al., 2002). If NO and OB production is impaired infection could occur due to a reduction in the microbicidal activity, exaggeration of the NO and OB production can induce injury in the epithelial cells. The phagocytic function of the macrophage have been shown to be impaired by the nanomaterial (Renwick et al., 2001).

Fibroblasts: If the nanomaterials are capable of gaining access to the interstitium, then the fibroblasts can be affected. The nanomaterial interaction with the fibroblast can result in at least two critical responses. These responses can produce relevant endpoints that can be tested *in vitro*. Autocrine stimulation of growth factor (platelet-derived growth factor, transforming growth factor beta, etc.), increases in extracellular or fibroblast growth are measurable endpoint as a result of a fibrogenic response. Cytokine/chemokine gene expression is a measurable endpoint to an inflammatory response. The inflammatory or fibrogenic response following nanomaterial fibroblast interaction is largely unknown.

Immune system: If the modulation of dendritic cellular function via entering the interstitium of the nanomaterial or if interaction with lymphocytes occurs because of the nanomaterial, then the possibility exists for an immunopathological event to occur. Immune response due to dendritic and macrophage antigen presentation as a result of the nanomaterial provide endpoints for investigation.

Cocultures: To closely represent the conditions, *in vivo* culture conditions can be modified to contain multiple cell types such as epithelial cells/endothelial cells or epithelial cells/macrophages, in addition to monocultures of lung cells.

Lung slices: As with the liver, kidney, and heart, lung tissue can also be sectioned for nanomaterial toxicological assessment within *in vitro* cultures. This will allow for the exposure of the multiple cell types within the section to the conditions as would occur *in vivo*.

Cell lines versus freshly derived cells: Because most cell lines are of cancer origin or have been immortalized in some way that may affect their native response, the use of freshly derived primary cells is a critical tool to confirm *in vitro* results if possible. For instance, if the endpoint under investigation is cancer, then the use of a cancer cell is inappropriate for this investigation. If a cancer cell line is used in comparison with a noncancer cell, it will insure that the response is not affected by the cancer cell and that the response resembles that which would be seen in a noncancer cell.

Whole heart–lung preparation: In the absence of blood, the heart and lung are perfused with a physiological solution of known ingredients, which can be highly regulated and controlled to maintain tissue viability and proper oxygenation. This Langendorff heart–lung preparation produces an environment to assess nanoparticle behavior and tissue effects under highly controlled conditions. The transport between the lungs and the vasculature can be evaluated through the exsanguinated heart and lung preparation as proper perfusion is maintained (Meiring et al., 2005).

13.3.1.3.2.2 Nervous System   Entry into the nervous system can take place through various exposure routes, including the respiratory tract, blood, and dermal exposure. The method and avenue of translocation of nanomaterials into the nervous system are largely unknown.

Central nervous system: The effect that nanomaterials have on neuronal function can be assessed utilizing *in vitro* systems for study. Ion regulation, metabolic status, apoptosis, effects on the action potential, and ROS/RNS production are potential endpoints for evaluating nanoparticle effects. The involvement of neuronal macrophages known as microglial cells can also be studied in a similar manner to that outlined regarding macrophages in the lungs. The effect of nanomaterials on oligodendrocytes, glial cells, and astrocytes are also of importance to the study of nanomaterial safety.

Peripheral nervous system: A nervous supply is present irrespective of the portal of entry or the target organ. The surface of the body for instance has numerous sensory nerves that could be potentially affected by exposure to nanomaterials. There are a number of ways in which nanomaterials can potentially gain access to, be transported to, or affect these nerves. Using relative endpoints, the effects of nanomaterials can be studied using neuron culture of peripheral nerves (e.g., dorsal root ganglion neurons). Ionic homeostasis, metabolism, and viability can be evaluated *in vitro* for cultured parasympathetic and sympathetic neurons of the autonomic nervous system in response to nanomaterials in culture.

13.3.1.3.3 Ingestion

Many pharmaceuticals are orally delivered and the complexity associated with this route of administration have given rise to various packaging strategies, release kinetic models, and a wide range of additional considerations to administer drug into the body. In addressing this exposure route of nanosafety, these concerns are of importance as well. The movement of nanomaterial through the digestive systems and the various environments these particles encounter through this trek give rise to multiple opportunities for these particles to be altered in some way due to changing exposure conditions thus altering the properties of the nanomaterials original administrate form. Yet again, the need for complete characterization is paramount. Multiple strategies exist for looking at the potential alteration of the nanomaterials as they pass through the acidic environment of the stomach and on into the remaining gastrointestinal systems. At this point, we will only look at the cellular/organ level, not the potential for nanomaterial alteration. It is of importance to note that the potential does exist, and for pharmaceutical applications it must be taken into consideration.

13.3.1.3.3.1 Mucosa   The gastrointestinal tract, vagina, lungs, oral cavity, and nasal cavity are lined with a moist tissue known as the mucosa. This mucosa can be exposed to nanomaterials from various sources but as mentioned earlier the gastrointestinal tract is one of the main routes of pharmacological delivery. This delivery route will produce a significant level of nanomaterial exposure to the GI tract. Studies conducted using 10–500 nm particles delivered via gavage or through oral feeding have examined the efficiency of nanoparticle uptake in the GI tract (Jani et al., 1992, 1994; Powell et al., 2000). In as little as 60 min, these nanoparticles translocated into the circulatory system and were associated this with the gastrointestinal associated lymphatic tissue (GALT) having passed through the mucosal lining and epithelial barrier (Moghimi et al., 2001). Tissue constructs and immortalized cell lines can

be used for *in vitro* studies of intestinal epithelium in addition to *in vivo* studies. Many pharmaceutical studies have used the immortalized cell line of the Caco cells to determine intestinal permeability. This cell line would be useful in investigating the uptake of nanomaterials across the intestinal epithelial barrier (Zhou and Yokel, 2005). Mechanistic understanding of the translocation process and *in vitro* translocation rate studies could be adapted from these studies. Other useful tools for nanoparticle research are the IEC-6 and IEC-18 cell lines. Mechanistic studies of the intestinal epithelial lining have been extensively done in these cells (Kishikawa et al., 2002; Li et al., 1999; Quaroni and Isselbacher, 1981). ROS/RNS and cytokine release and activation of various signaling pathways have been studied in these cells after toxicant exposure (Smith et al., 2005, Urayama et al., 1998). Other mucosal exposure routes are the oral lining and vagina; these portals of exposure may be less significant but at least in one instance the development of a silver nanoparticle for the treatment of yeast infections has been proposed (Monteiro et al., 2012), which could be used to treat both vaginal yeast infection and oral yeast infection (thrush). These treatments would then expose the oral and vaginal mucosa to nanomaterials. Impact and translocation can be studied for these exposure routes through tissue constructs and a variety of cell lines and models (Fichorova and Anderson, 1999; Kubilus et al., 2002, 2004).

13.3.1.3.4 Deposition

Dermal exposure to nanomaterials can occur in various situations, from aerosolized particulates landing on the skin to drug delivery patches containing nanomedicines, not to mention the current market of cosmetic products already utilizing nanoparticles. Irrespective of the mode of exposure, little is known about the toxic limits or the mechanism for nanomaterial uptake.

13.3.1.3.4.1 Skin The integument or skin is the largest organ in the body. It is the primary route of exposure to all environmental factors. During the manufacturing process, environmental release, accidental spill, or intentional applied nanomaterials can and will contact the skin. The nanomaterials have the potential to be lodged within the avascular layer of the epidermis and are not susceptible to removal by phagocytosis (Monteiro-Riviere and Riviere, 1999). The very fact that the skin creates a barrier for protecting the body and maintains a relative biological isolation is very beneficial, but because the lipid domain of this organ system can be exploited as a route of drug delivery, there are a number of concerns regarding nanomaterials. Currently, drugs using lipid nanoparticles and liposomes have been delivered through the lipid domain of the skin. The absorption of large particles of titanium and zinc oxide (compounds found in topical skin products) penetrate the stratum corneum with higher rates of absorption in oils then in water (Lansdown and Taylor, 1997). The ability of nanomaterials to pass through the skin, or to be transported in the presence of oily residues, not to mention the size of the nanomaterials, may be of such finite scope that the skin poses no potential barrier.

The catalytic properties of various nanomaterials could induce a wide range of toxicological effects. If these particles pass through the skin and into the body systemically, these effects could be seen in any major organ system. The ability to decontaminate the skin after exposure becomes a great concern. The two major means of postexposure decontamination dilution and solubilization may be ineffective with regard to nanomaterials. Research is greatly needed to address these and other potential concerns with nanomaterial safety.

The primary route of potential exposure to nanomaterials is the skin; therefore, it is critical that systemic and dermal exposure be investigated to ascertain the effects of a broad range of nanomaterials. Whether accumulation within the dermal tissue following systemically administered nanomaterials and its absorption across the stratum corneum barrier occurs remain unknown with regard to nanomaterials. Nanomaterial could be sequestered within the epidermis. This would result in substantial epidermal keratinocyte exposure. Nanoparticles size could affect the traverse time through the stratum corneum layers; for drug delivery, this would be beneficial if the rate increased compared to the bulk compound, but in cases of toxicology, this rapid uptake could be of great concern.

In vivo starting doses for toxicity testing can be estimated by first conducting *in vitro* testing, this is a good strategy to employ to reduce the number of animals needed, to limit the amount of nanomaterials that need to be disposed of after testing, and to limit the amount of nanomaterials needed especially when the nanomaterials are difficult to obtain in large quantities (Health, 2001). In all *in vitro* systems, at least three or four concentrations with controls should be used. The two essential components of any risk assessment, cutaneous *hazard* after both systemic and topical exposure and systemic *exposure* after topical administration, can be ascertained from data generated from these preliminary tests.

> *Cell culture*: There are various cell types and design platforms that can be used to evaluate nanomaterial toxicity in cell culture. As with all models of cell culture, there are a number of endpoint assays that can be utilized to examine the effects of nanomaterial exposure. The existence of both immortalized cell lines and primary cell lines for the various cell types that compose the integument system makes the investigation of the effect of nanomaterials very plausible. In addition, the use of skin section in culture provides an additional level of testing to complement the *in vitro* cell culture research. In all cases, it must be remembered that data generated from these models only provide a true representation of the *in vivo* effects.

> *Isolated perfused porcine skin flap (IPPSF)*: An ideal model for the study of nanomaterial toxicity and absorption is the IPPSF. Within this model, there is a great deal of control. The dermis and epidermis remain viable and the microcirculation remains intact and functional. The preparation of the skin flap entails surgically removing a

section of the abdomen of a pig while leaving the vasculature intact for the purpose of perfusion. This tissue is then maintained in a culturing chamber to insure tissue viability. The nanomaterials are then applied to the skin and the solution used to perfuse the preparation can be assessed for the presence of nanomaterials (Monteiro-Riviere, 1990; Riviere et al., 1986; Riviere and Monteiro-Riviere, 1991).

Irritation testing using EPISKIN and Epiderm and corrosive testing using Corrositex, commercially available EPISKIN, and rat transcutaneous electrical resistance (TER) can also be used to perform acute *in vitro* toxicity assays. Owing to marked interactions with nanoparticles, the major traditional endpoints of skin toxicity, a colorimetric assay for measuring cellular activity, the MTT assay is largely unpredictive with regard to cell viability when assessing nanoparticle effects.

13.3.1.3.5 *Exposure via Translocation*

In the event of translocation, various target organs at distal sites to the exposure site may be affected. This deposition of nanomaterials presupposes redistribution and translocation of nanoparticles away from the route of exposure such as blood, lungs, skin, or gut. Nanomaterials have the potential to be biotransformed as they make their way to these distal exposure sites, and consideration should be given to potential changes in the characteristics of the nanomaterials and how they may alter the nanomaterial toxicology.

13.4 Treatment Options for Nanotoxicity

To date, no literature exists for treatment option for toxic exposure to nanomaterials. The absence of an antidote or treatment for nanomaterial exposure only exemplifies the need for research in this growing field. Better characterization, well-defined dose metric, proper understanding of nanomaterial disposal, environmental effects of the nanomaterials and environmental and biological transformation of the nanomaterial are critical to provide a foundation upon which the set safety exposure limits and launch effect treatment plans for nanomaterial overdose.

13.5 Conclusion

ENMs possess great potential for developing new and better approaches to pharmaceutical development as well as a myriad of other research and manufacturing fields. However, the limited knowledge of how ENMs affect the ecosystems and biological world can create a great deal of apprehension in regard to the utilization of these ENMs. Although the knowledge is limited and the potential for toxic and beneficial effects of ENMs remains unclear, the best approach to understanding the world of nanomaterials is to develop a systematic approach to investigating the beneficial and detrimental effects. Until this knowledge is developed, the field of nanotechnology will remain limited in it true application growth.

The field of nanotoxicity is growing and the potential exist that in the near future the current limitations regarding our ability to rapidly and systematically assess the toxicity of nanomaterials may become less of a limitation to the screening process. Until then, the best approach to nanosafety is particle characterization and systematic assessment of individual ENM constructs.

References

2011. European Center of Validation of Alternative Methods [Online]. Institute for Health and Consumer Protection. Available: http://ecvam.jrc.it/index.htm [Accessed April 2, 2012].

Adams, L. K., Lyon, D. Y., Mcintosh, A., and Alvarez, P. J. 2006. Comparative toxicity of nano-scale TiO_2, SiO_2 and ZnO water suspensions. *Water Sci Technol*, 54, 327–34.

Adomako, M., ST-Hilaire, S., Zheng, Y., Eley, J., Marcum, R. D., Sealey, W., Donahower, B. C., Lapatra, S., and Sheridan, P. P. 2012. Oral DNA vaccination of rainbow trout, *Oncorhynchus mykiss* (Walbaum), against infectious haematopoietic necrosis virus using PLGA [Poly(D,L-lactic-*co*-glycolic acid)] nanoparticles. *J Fish Dis*, 35, 203–14.

Allen, H. J., Impellitteri, C. A., Macke, D. A., Heckman, J. L., Poynton, H. C., Lazorchak, J. M., Govindaswamy, S., Roose, D. L., and Nadagouda, M. N. 2010. Effects from filtration, capping agents, and presence/absence of food on the toxicity of silver nanoparticles to *Daphnia magna*. *Environ Toxicol Chem*, 29, 2742–50.

Alloy, M. M. and Roberts, A. P. 2011. Effects of suspended multi-walled carbon nanotubes on daphnid growth and reproduction. *Ecotoxicol Environ Saf*, 74, 1839–43.

Araujo, L., Lobenberg, R., and Kreuter, J. 1999. Influence of the surfactant concentration on the body distribution of nanoparticles. *J Drug Target*, 6, 373–85.

Arce, V. B., Bertolotti, S. G., Oliveira, F. J., Airoldi, C., Arques, A., Santos-Juanes, L., Gonzalez, M. C., Cobos, C. J., Allegretti, P. E., and Martire, D. O. 2012. Triplet state of 4-methoxybenzyl alcohol chemisorbed on silica nanoparticles. *Photochem Photobiol Sci*. 11, 1032–40.

Aruoja, V., Dubourguier, H. C., Kasemets, K., and Kahru, A. 2009. Toxicity of nanoparticles of CuO, ZnO and TiO_2 to microalgae *Pseudokirchneriella subcapitata*. *Sci Total Environ*, 407, 1461–8.

Asharani, P. V., Lian Wu, Y., Gong, Z., and Valiyaveettil, S. 2008. Toxicity of silver nanoparticles in zebrafish models. *Nanotechnology*, 19, 255102.

Asharani, P. V., Lianwu, Y., Gong, Z., and Valiyaveettil, S. 2011. Comparison of the toxicity of silver, gold and platinum nanoparticles in developing zebrafish embryos. *Nanotoxicology*, 5, 43–54.

Asli, S. and Neumann, P. M. 2009. Colloidal suspensions of clay or titanium dioxide nanoparticles can inhibit leaf growth and transpiration via physical effects on root water transport. *Plant Cell Environ*, 32, 577–84.

Babu, K., Deepa, M., Shankar, S. G., and Rai, S. 2008. Effect of nano-silver on cell division and mitotic chromosomes: A prefatory siren. *Internet J Nanotechnol*, 2. Available: http://www.ispub.com/journal/the-internet-journal-of-nanotechnology/volume-2-number-2/effect-of-nano-silver-on-cell-division-and-mitotic-chromosomes-a-prefatory-siren.html#sthash.6oP8mTi8.dpbs

Bali, R., Siegele, R., and Harris, A. 2010. Biogenic Pt uptake and nanoparticle formation in *Medicago sativa* and *Brassica juncea*. *J Nanoparticle Res*, 12, 3087–95.

Bang, S. H., Le, T. H., Lee, S. K., Kim, P., Kim, J. S., and Min, J. 2011. Toxicity assessment of titanium (IV) oxide nanoparticles using *Daphnia magna* (water flea). *Environ Health Toxicol*, 26, e2011002.

Bar-Ilan, O., Albrecht, R. M., Fako, V. E., and Furgeson, D. Y. 2009. Toxicity assessments of multisized gold and silver nanoparticles in zebrafish embryos. *Small*, 5, 1897–910.

Barrena, R., Casals, E., Colon, J., Font, X., Sanchez, A., and Puntes, V. 2009. Evaluation of the ecotoxicity of model nanoparticles. *Chemosphere*, 75, 850–7.

Barrett, E., Johnston, C., Oberdorster, G., and Finkelstein, J. 1999. Silica-induced chemokine expression in alveolar type II cells is mediated by TNF-alpha-induced oxidant stress. *Am J Physiol*, 276, L979–88.

Baun, A., Hartmann, N. B., Grieger, K., and Kusk, K. O. 2008a. Ecotoxicity of engineered nanoparticles to aquatic invertebrates: A brief review and recommendations for future toxicity testing. *Ecotoxicology*, 17, 387–95.

Baun, A., Sorensen, S. N., Rasmussen, R. F., Hartmann, N. B., and Koch, C. B. 2008b. Toxicity and bioaccumulation of xenobiotic organic compounds in the presence of aqueous suspensions of aggregates of nano-C(60). *Aquat Toxicol*, 86, 379–87.

Beloqui, A., Guazzaroni, M. E., Pazos, F., Vieites, J. M., Godoy, M., Golyshina, O. V., Chernikova, T. N. et al. 2009. Reactome array: Forging a link between metabolome and genome. *Science*, 326, 252–7.

Bergqvist, L., Sundberg, R., Rydén, S., and Strand, S.-E. 1987. The "critical colloid dose" in studies of reticuloendothelial function. *J Nucl Med*, 28, 1424–9.

Bilberg, K., Doving, K. B., Beedholm, K., and Baatrup, E. 2011. Silver nanoparticles disrupt olfaction in Crucian carp (*Carassius carassius*) and Eurasian perch (*Perca fluviatilis*). *Aquat Toxicol*, 104, 145–52.

Bilberg, K., Hovgaard, M. B., Besenbacher, F., and Baatrup, E. 2012. *In vivo* toxicity of silver nanoparticles and silver ions in zebrafish (*Danio rerio*). *J Toxicol*, 2012, 293784.

Bilberg, K., Malte, H., Wang, T., and Baatrup, E. 2010. Silver nanoparticles and silver nitrate cause respiratory stress in Eurasian perch (*Perca fluviatilis*). *Aquat Toxicol*, 96, 159–65.

Birbaum, K., Brogioli, R., Schellenberg, M., Martinoia, E., Stark, W. J., Gunther, D., and Limbach, L. K. 2010. No evidence for cerium dioxide nanoparticle translocation in maize plants. *Environ Sci Technol*, 44, 8718–23.

Blaise, C., Gagne, F., Ferard, J. F., and Eullaffroy, P. 2008. Ecotoxicity of selected nano-materials to aquatic organisms. *Environ Toxicol*, 23, 591–8.

Blaser, S. A., Scheringer, M., Macleod, M., and Hungerbuhler, K. 2008. Estimation of cumulative aquatic exposure and risk due to silver: Contribution of nano-functionalized plastics and textiles. *Sci Total Environ*, 390, 396–409.

Blickley, T. M. and McClellan-Green, P. 2008. Toxicity of aqueous fullerene in adult and larval *Fundulus heteroclitus*. *Environ Toxicol Chem*, 27, 1964–71.

Blinova, I., Ivask, A., Heinlaan, M., Mortimer, M., and Kahru, A. 2010. Ecotoxicity of nanoparticles of CuO and ZnO in natural water. *Environ Pollut*, 158, 41–7.

Bokare, V., Murugesan, K., Kim, Y. M., Jeon, J. R., Kim, E. J., and Chang, Y. S. 2010. Degradation of triclosan by an integrated nano-bio redox process. *Bioresour Technol*, 101, 6354–60.

Bouldin, J. L., Ingle, T. M., Sengupta, A., Alexander, R., Hannigan, R. E., and Buchanan, R. A. 2008. Aqueous toxicity and food chain transfer of Quantum DOTs in fresh-water algae and *Ceriodaphnia dubia*. *Environ Toxicol Chem*, 27, 1958–63.

Brausch, K. A., Anderson, T. A., Smith, P. N., and Maul, J. D. 2010. Effects of function-alized fullerenes on bifenthrin and tribufos toxicity to *Daphnia magna*: Survival, reproduction, and growth rate. *Environ Toxicol Chem*, 29, 2600–6.

Brausch, K. A., Anderson, T. A., Smith, P. N., and Maul, J. D. 2011. The effect of fuller-enes and functionalized fullerenes on *Daphnia magna* phototaxis and swimming behavior. *Environ Toxicol Chem*, 30, 878–84.

Braydich-Stolle, L., Hussain, S., Schlager, J. J., and Hofmann, M.-C. 2005. *In vitro* cyto-toxicity of nanoparticles in mammalian germline stem cells. *Toxicol Sci*, 88, 412–19.

Brown, D., Roberts, N., and Donaldson, K. 1998. Effect of coating with lung lining fluid on the ability of fibres to produce a respiratory burst in rat alveolar macro-phages. *Toxicol In Vitro*, 12, 15–24.

Brown, D., Stone, V., Findlay, P., Macnee, W., and Donaldson, K. 2000. Increased inflam-mation and intracellular calcium caused by ultrafine carbon black is independent of transition metals or other soluble components. *Occup Environ Med*, 57, 685–91.

Brown, D., Wilson, M., Macnee, W., Stone, V., and Donaldson, K. 2001. Size-dependent proinflammatory effects of ultrafine polystyrene particles: A role for surface area and oxidative stress in the enhanced activity of ultrafines. *Toxicol Appl Pharmacol*, 175, 191–199.

Bunge, M., Sobjerg, L. S., Rotaru, A. E., Gauthier, D., Lindhardt, A. T., Hause, G., Finster, K., Kingshott, P., Skrydstrup, T., and Meyer, R. L. 2010. Formation of palladium(0) nanoparticles at microbial surfaces. *Biotechnol Bioeng*, 107, 206–15.

Canas, J. E., Long, M., Nations, S., Vadan, R., Dai, L., Luo, M., Ambikapathi, R., Lee, E. H., and Olszyk, D. 2008. Effects of functionalized and nonfunctional-ized single-walled carbon nanotubes on root elongation of select crop species. *Nanomater Environ*, 27, 1922–31.

Canas, J. E., Qi, B., Li, S., Maul, J. D., Cox, S. B., Das, S., and Green, M. J. 2011. Acute and reproductive toxicity of nano-sized metal oxides (ZnO and TiO) to earth-worms (*Eisenia fetida*). *J Environ Monit*, 13, 3351–7.

Chae, Y. J., Pham, C. H., Lee, J., Bae, E., Yi, J., and Gu, M. B. 2009. Evaluation of the toxic impact of silver nanoparticles on Japanese medaka (*Oryzias latipes*). *Aquat Toxicol*, 94, 320–7.

Chao, C., Park, S., and Aust, A. 1996. Participation of nitric-oxide and iron in the oxidation of DNA in asbestos-treated human lung epithelial-cells. *Arch Biochem Biophys*, 326, 152–7.

Chen, P. J., Su, C. H., Tseng, C. Y., Tan, S. W., and Cheng, C. H. 2011. Toxicity assessments of nanoscale zerovalent iron and its oxidation products in medaka (*Oryzias latipes*) fish. *Mar Pollut Bull*, 63, 339–46.

Chen, R., Ratnikova, T. A., Stone, M. B., Lin, S., Lard, M., Huang, G., Hudson, J. S., and Ke, P. C. 2010. Differential uptake of carbon nanoparticles by plant and Mammalian cells. *Small*, 6, 612–7.

Chou, C., Riviere, J., and Monteiro-Riviere, N. 2003. The cytotoxicity of jet fuel aromatic hydrocarbons and dose-related interleukin-8 release from human epidermal keratinocytes. *Arch Toxicol*, 77, 384–91.

Christen, V. and Fent, K. 2012. Silica nanoparticles and silver-doped silica nanoparticles induce endoplasmatic reticulum stress response and alter cytochrome P4501A activity. *Chemosphere*, 87, 423–34.

Coffey, M., Phare, S., and Peters-Golden, M. 2002. Interaction between nitric oxide, reactive oxygen intermediates, and peroxynitrite in the regulation of 5-lipoxygenase metabolism. *Biochim Biophys Acta*, 1584, 81–90.

Coleman, J. G., Johnson, D. R., Stanley, J. K., Bednar, A. J., Weiss, C. A., Jr., Boyd, R. E., and Steevens, J. A. 2010. Assessing the fate and effects of nano aluminum oxide in the terrestrial earthworm, *Eisenia fetida*. *Environ Toxicol Chem*, 29, 1575–80.

Corredor, E., Testillano, P. S., Coronado, M. J., Gonzalez-Melendi, P., Fernandez-Pacheco, R., Marquina, C., Ibarra, M. R. et al. 2009. Nanoparticle penetration and transport in living pumpkin plants: *In situ* subcellular identification. *BMC Plant Biol*, 9, 45.

Coutris, C., Hertel-Aas, T., Lapied, E., Joner, E. J., and Oughton, D. H. 2012. Bioavailability of cobalt and silver nanoparticles to the earthworm Eisenia fetida. *Nanotoxicology*, 6, 186–95.

Culha, M., Adiguzel, A., Yazici, M. M., Kahraman, M., Sahin, F., and Gulluce, M. 2008. Characterization of thermophilic bacteria using surface-enhanced Raman scattering. *Appl Spectrosc*, 62, 1226–32.

Dabrunz, A., Duester, L., Prasse, C., Seitz, F., Rosenfeldt, R., Schilde, C., Schaumann, G. E., and Schulz, R. 2011. Biological surface coating and molting inhibition as mechanisms of TiO$_2$ nanoparticle toxicity in *Daphnia magna*. *PLoS One*, 6, e20112.

Dambach, D., Andrews, B., and Moulin, F. 2005. New technologies and screening strategies for hepatotoxicity: Use of *in vitro* models. *Toxicol Pathol*, 33, 17–26.

Darlington, T. K., Neigh, A. M., Spencer, M. T., Nguyen, O. T., and Oldenburg, S. J. 2009. Nanoparticle characteristics affecting environmental fate and transport through soil. *Environ Toxicol Chem*, 28, 1191–9.

Dodd, N. J. and Jha, A. N. 2009. Titanium dioxide induced cell damage: A proposed role of the carboxyl radical. *Mutat Res*, 660, 79–82.

Domingos, R. F., Simon, D. F., Hauser, C., and Wilkinson, K. J. 2011. Bioaccumulation and effects of CdTe/CdS quantum dots on *Chlamydomonas reinhardtii*—nanoparticles or the free ions? *Environ Sci Technol*, 45, 7664–9.

Donaldson, K., Stone, V., Gilmour, P., Brown, D., and Macnee, W. 2000. Ultrafine particles: Mechanisms of lung injury. *Phil Trans Roy Soc London Series*, 358, 2741–9.

Doshi, R., Braida, W., Christodoulatos, C., Wazne, M., and O'Connor, G. 2008. Nano-aluminum: Transport through sand columns and environmental effects on plants and soil communities. *Environ Res*, 106, 296–303.

Einstein, A. 1905. Über die von der molekularkinetischen Theorie der Wärme geforderte Bewegung von in ruhenden Flüssigkeiten suspendierten Teilchen. *Annalen der Physik*, 322, 549–60.

El-Temsah, Y. S. and Joner, E. J. 2012. Impact of Fe and Ag nanoparticles on seed germination and differences in bioavailability during exposure in aqueous suspension and soil. *Environ Toxicol*, 27, 42–9.

Fabrega, J., Renshaw, J. C., and Lead, J. R. 2009. Interactions of silver nanoparticles with *Pseudomonas putida* biofilms. *Environ Sci Technol*, 43, 9004–9.

Fan, W., Cui, M., Liu, H., Wang, C., Shi, Z., Tan, C., and Yang, X. 2011. Nano-TiO$_2$ enhances the toxicity of copper in natural water to *Daphnia magna*. *Environ Pollut*, 159, 729–34.

Fang, J., Lyon, D. Y., Wiesner, M. R., Dong, J., and Alvarez, P. J. 2007. Effect of a fullerene water suspension on bacterial phospholipids and membrane phase behavior. *Environ Sci Technol*, 41, 2636–42.

Fang, L., Borggaard, O. K., Holm, P. E., Hansen, H. C., and Cedergreen, N. 2011. Toxicity and uptake of TRI- and dibutyltin in *Daphnia magna* in the absence and presence of nano-charcoal. *Environ Toxicol Chem*, 30, 2553–61.

Farkas, J., Christian, P., Gallego-Urrea, J. A., Roos, N., Hassellov, M., Tollefsen, K. E., and Thomas, K. V. 2011. Uptake and effects of manufactured silver nanoparticles in rainbow trout (*Oncorhynchus mykiss*) gill cells. *Aquat Toxicol*, 101, 117–25.

Farkas, J., Christian, P., Urrea, J. A., Roos, N., Hassellov, M., Tollefsen, K. E., and Thomas, K. V. 2010. Effects of silver and gold nanoparticles on rainbow trout (*Oncorhynchus mykiss*) hepatocytes. *Aquat Toxicol*, 96, 44–52.

Federici, G., Shaw, B. J., and Handy, R. D. 2007. Toxicity of titanium dioxide nanoparticles to rainbow trout (*Oncorhynchus mykiss*): Gill injury, oxidative stress, and other physiological effects. *Aquat Toxicol*, 84, 415–30.

Fent, K., Weisbrod, C. J., Wirth-Heller, A., and Pieles, U. 2010. Assessment of uptake and toxicity of fluorescent silica nanoparticles in zebrafish (*Danio rerio*) early life stages. *Aquat Toxicol*, 100, 218–28.

Ferguson, P. L., Chandler, G. T., Templeton, R. C., Demarco, A., Scrivens, W. A., and Englehart, B. A. 2008. Influence of sediment-amendment with single-walled carbon nanotubes and diesel soot on bioaccumulation of hydrophobic organic contaminants by benthic invertebrates. *Environ Sci Technol*, 42, 3879–85.

Fichorova, R. and Anderson, D. 1999. Differential expression of immunobiological mediators by immortalized human cervical and vaginal epithelial cells. *Biol Reprod*, 60, 508–14.

Fleming, I. and Busse, R. 1999. NO: The primary EDRF. *J Mol Cell Cardiol*, 31, 5–14.

Fouqueray, M., Dufils, B., Vollat, B., Chaurand, P., Botta, C., Abacci, K., Labille, J., Rose, J., and Garric, J. 2012. Effects of aged TiO$_2$ nanomaterial from sunscreen on *Daphnia magna* exposed by dietary route. *Environ Pollut*, 163, 55–61.

Franklin, N. M., Rogers, N. J., Apte, S. C., Batley, G. E., Gadd, G. E., and Casey, P. S. 2007. Comparative toxicity of nanoparticulate ZnO, bulk ZnO, and ZnCl2 to a freshwater microalga (Pseudokirchneriella subcapitata): The importance of particle solubility. *Environ Sci Technol*, 41, 8484–90.

Fraser, T. W., Reinardy, H. C., Shaw, B. J., Henry, T. B., and Handy, R. D. 2011. Dietary toxicity of single-walled carbon nanotubes and fullerenes (C60) in rainbow trout (Oncorhynchus mykiss). *Nanotoxicology*, 5, 98–108.

Fu, G., Vary, P. S., and Lin, C. T. 2005. Anatase TiO$_2$ nanocomposites for antimicrobial coatings. *J Phys Chem B*, 109, 8889–98.

Fubini, B. 1997. Surface reactivity in the pathogenic response to particulates. *Environ Health Perspect*, 105, 1013–20.

Fubini, B., Aust, A., Bolton, R., Borm, P., Brunch, J., and Ciapetto, G. 1998. Non-animal tests for evaluating the toxicology of solid xenobiotics. *Atla-Altern Lab Anim,* 26, 579–617.

Fubini, B., Fenoglio, I., Ceschino, R., Ghiazza, M., Martra, G., Tomatis, M., Borm, P., Schins, R., and Bruch, J. 2004. Relationship between the state of the surface of four commercial quartz flours and their biological activity *in vitro* and *in vivo*. *Int J Hyg Environ Health,* 207, 89–104.

Fujiwara, K., Suematsu, H., Kiyomiya, E., Aoki, M., Sato, M., and Moritoki, N. 2008. Size-dependent toxicity of silica nano-particles to *Chlorella kessleri*. *J Environ Sci Health A Tox Hazard Subst Environ Eng,* 43, 1167–73.

Gagne, F., Fortier, M., Yu, L., Osachoff, H. L., Skirrow, R. C., Van Aggelen, G., Gagnon, C., and Fournier, M. 2010. Immunocompetence and alterations in hepatic gene expression in rainbow trout exposed to CdS/CdTe quantum dots. *J Environ Monit,* 12, 1556–65.

Gaiser, B. K., Biswas, A., Rosenkranz, P., Jepson, M. A., Lead, J. R., Stone, V., Tyler, C. R., and Fernandes, T. F. 2011. Effects of silver and cerium dioxide micro- and nano-sized particles on *Daphnia magna*. *J Environ Monit,* 13, 1227–35.

Gaiser, B. K., Fernandes, T. F., Jepson, M. A., Lead, J. R., Tyler, C. R., Baalousha, M., Biswas, A. et al. 2012. Interspecies comparisons on the uptake and toxicity of silver and cerium dioxide nanoparticles. *Environ Toxicol Chem,* 31, 144–54.

Gajjar, P., Pettee, B., Britt, D. W., Huang, W., Johnson, W. P., and Anderson, A. J. 2009. Antimicrobial activities of commercial nanoparticles against an environmental soil microbe, *Pseudomonas putida* KT2440. *J Biol Eng,* 3, 9.

Gao, F., Hong, F., Liu, C., Zheng, L., Su, M., Wu, X., Yang, F., Wu, C., and Yang, P. 2006. Mechanism of nano-anatase TiO_2 on promoting photosynthetic carbon reaction of spinach. *Biol Trace Elem Res,* 111, 239–53.

Gao, J., Wang, Y., Folta, K. M., Krishna, V., Bai, W., Indeglia, P., Georgieva, A., Nakamura, H., Koopman, B., and Moudgil, B. 2011. Polyhydroxy fullerenes (fullerols or fullerenols): Beneficial effects on growth and lifespan in diverse biological models. *PLoS One,* 6, e19976.

Gardea-Torresdey, J. L., Gomez, E., Peralta-Videa, J. R., Parsons, J. G., Troiani, H., and Jose-Yacaman, M. 2003. Alfalfa sprouts: A natural source for the synthesis of silver nanoparticles. *Langmuir,* 19, 1357–61.

Gardea-Torresdey, J. L., Parsons, J. G., Gomez, E., Peralta-Videa, J., Troiani, H. E., Santiago, P., and Yacaman, M. J. 2002. Formation and growth of Au nanoparticles inside live alfalfa plants. *Nano Lett,* 2, 397–401.

Ghosh, M., Bandyopadhyay, M., and Mukherjee, A. 2010. Genotoxicity of titanium dioxide (TiO_2) nanoparticles at two trophic levels: Plant and human lymphocytes. *Chemosphere,* 81, 1253–62.

Gilmour, P., Rahman, I., Donaldson, K., and Macnee, W. 2003. Histone acetylation regulates epithelial IL-8 release mediated by oxidative stress from environmental particles. *Am J Physiol Lung Cell Mol Physiol,* 284, L533–40.

Gitsov, I., Hamzik, J., Ryan, J., Simonyan, A., Nakas, J. P., Omori, S., Krastanov, A., Cohen, T., and Tanenbaum, S. W. 2008. Enzymatic nanoreactors for environmentally benign biotransformations. 1. Formation and catalytic activity of supramolecular complexes of laccase and linear-dendritic block copolymers. *Biomacromolecules,* 9, 804–11.

Gomes, S. I., Novais, S. C., Gravato, C., Guilhermino, L., Scott-Fordsmand, J. J., Soares, A. M., and Amorim, M. J. 2012a. Effect of Cu-nanoparticles versus one Cu-salt:

Analysis of stress biomarkers response in *Enchytraeus albidus* (Oligochaeta). *Nanotoxicology,* 6, 134–43.

Gomes, S. I., Novais, S. C., Scott-Fordsmand, J. J., DE Coen, W., Soares, A. M., and Amorim, M. J. 2012b. Effect of Cu-nanoparticles versus Cu-salt in Enchytraeus albidus (Oligochaeta): Differential gene expression through microarray analysis. *Comp Biochem Physiol C Toxicol Pharmacol,* 155, 219–27.

Griffitt, R. J., Luo, J., Gao, J., Bonzongo, J. C., and Barber, D. S. 2008. Effects of particle composition and species on toxicity of metallic nanomaterials in aquatic organisms. *Environ Toxicol Chem,* 27, 1972–8.

Gurr, J. R., Wang, A. S., Chen, C. H., and Jan, K. Y. 2005. Ultrafine titanium dioxide particles in the absence of photoactivation can induce oxidative damage to human bronchial epithelial cells. *Toxicology,* 213, 66–73.

Handy, R. D., Al-Bairuty, G., Al-Jubory, A., Ramsden, C. S., Boyle, D., Shaw, B. J., and Henry, T. B. 2011. Effects of manufactured nanomaterials on fishes: A target organ and body systems physiology approach. *J Fish Biol,* 79, 821–53.

Hao, L. and Chen, L. 2012. Oxidative stress responses in different organs of carp (*Cyprinus carpio*) with exposure to ZnO nanoparticles. *Ecotoxicol Environ Saf.* 80, 103–10.

Hao, L., Wang, Z., and Xing, B. 2009. Effect of sub-acute exposure to TiO$_2$ nanoparticles on oxidative stress and histopathological changes in Juvenile Carp (*Cyprinus carpio*). *J Environ Sci (China),* 21, 1459–66.

Harris, A. and Bali, R. 2008. On the formation and extent of uptake of silver nanoparticles by live plants. *J Nanoparticle Res,* 10, 691–5.

Harrison, D., Treasure, C., Mugge, A., Dellsperger, K., and Lamping, K. 1991. Hypertension and the coronary circulation. With special attention to endothelial regulation. *Am J Hypertens,* 4, 454S–59S.

Hartmann, N. B., Von DER Kammer, F., Hofmann, T., Baalousha, M., Ottofuelling, S., and Baun, A. 2010. Algal testing of titanium dioxide nanoparticles—testing considerations, inhibitory effects and modification of cadmium bioavailability. *Toxicology,* 269, 190–7.

Haverkamp, R. and Marshall, A. 2009. The mechanism of metal nanoparticle formation in plants: Limits on accumulation. *J Nanoparticle Res,* 11, 1453–63.

Hayashi, Y., Engelmann, P., Foldbjerg, R., Szabo, M., Somogyi, I., Pollak, E., Molnar, L. et al. 2012. Earthworms and humans *in vitro*: Characterizing evolutionarily conserved stress and immune responses to silver nanoparticles. *Environ Sci Technol,* 46, 4166–73

Heckmann, L. H., Hovgaard, M. B., Sutherland, D. S., Autrup, H., Besenbacher, F., and Scott-Fordsmand, J. J. 2011. Limit-test toxicity screening of selected inorganic nanoparticles to the earthworm Eisenia fetida. *Ecotoxicology,* 20, 226–33.

Heinlaan, M., Ivask, A., Blinova, I., Dubourguier, H. C., and Kahru, A. 2008. Toxicity of nanosized and bulk ZnO, CuO and TiO$_2$ to bacteria *Vibrio fischeri* and crustaceans *Daphnia magna* and *Thamnocephalus platyurus*. *Chemosphere,* 71, 1308–16.

Heinlaan, M., Kahru, A., Kasemets, K., Arbeille, B., Prensier, G., and Dubourguier, H. C. 2011. Changes in the *Daphnia magna* midgut upon ingestion of copper oxide nanoparticles: A transmission electron microscopy study. *Water Res,* 45, 179–90.

Henry, T. B., Menn, F. M., Fleming, J. T., Wilgus, J., Compton, R. N., and Sayler, G. S. 2007. Attributing effects of aqueous C60 nano-aggregates to tetrahydrofuran decomposition products in larval zebrafish by assessment of gene expression. *Environ Health Perspect,* 115, 1059–65.

Hess, D., Matsumoto, A., Kim, S., Marshall, H., and Stamler, J. 2005. Protein S-nitrosylation: Purview and parameters. *Nat Rev Mol Cell Biol,* 6, 150–66.

Hildebrand, H., Kuhnel, D., Potthoff, A., Mackenzie, K., Springer, A., and Schirmer, K. 2010. Evaluating the cytotoxicity of palladium/magnetite nano-catalysts intended for wastewater treatment. *Environ Pollut*, 158, 65–73.

Hondroulis, E., Liu, C., and Li, C. Z. 2010. Whole cell based electrical impedance sensing approach for a rapid nanotoxicity assay. *Nanotechnology*, 21, 315103.

Hong, F., Zhou, J., Liu, C., Yang, F., Wu, C., Zheng, L., and Yang, P. 2005. Effect of nano-TiO₂ on photochemical reaction of chloroplasts of spinach. *Biol Trace Elem Res*, 105, 269–79.

Hooper, H. L., Jurkschat, K., Morgan, A. J., Bailey, J., Lawlor, A. J., Spurgeon, D. J., and Svendsen, C. 2011. Comparative chronic toxicity of nanoparticulate and ionic zinc to the earthworm *Eisenia veneta* in a soil matrix. *Environ Int*, 37, 1111–7.

Hu, J., Wang, D., and Wang, J. 2012. Bioaccumulation of Fe2O3(magnetic) nanoparticles in *Ceriodaphnia dubia*. *Environ Pollut*, 162, 216–22.

Hu, X., Liu, J., Zhou, Q., Lu, S., Liu, R., Cui, L., Yin, D., Mayer, P., and Jiang, G. 2010. Bioavailability of organochlorine compounds in aqueous suspensions of fullerene: Evaluated with medaka (Oryzias latipes) and negligible depletion solid-phase microextraction. *Chemosphere*, 80, 693–700.

Hu, X., Wang, P., and Hwang, H. M. 2009. Oxidation of anthracene by immobilized laccase from Trametes versicolor. *Bioresour Technol*, 100, 4963–8.

Hu, X., Zhao, X., and Hwang, H. M. 2007. Comparative study of immobilized Trametes versicolor laccase on nanoparticles and kaolinite. *Chemosphere*, 66, 1618–26.

Hu, Y. L., Qi, W., Han, F., Shao, J. Z., and Gao, J. Q. 2011. Toxicity evaluation of biodegradable chitosan nanoparticles using a zebrafish embryo model. *Int J Nanomed*, 6, 3351–9.

Huang, Z., Zheng, X., Yan, D., Yin, G., Liao, X., Kang, Y., Yao, Y., Huang, D., and Hao, B. 2008. Toxicological effect of ZnO nanoparticles based on bacteria. *Langmuir*, 24, 4140–4.

Hund-Rinke, K. and Simon, M. 2006. Ecotoxic effect of photocatalytic active nanoparticles (TiO₂) on algae and daphnids. *Environ Sci Pollut Res Int*, 13, 225–32.

Hussain, S. M., Hess, K. L., Gearhart, J. M., Geiss, K. T., and Schlager, J. J. 2005. *In vitro* toxicity of nanoparticles in BRL 3A rat liver cells. *Toxicol In Vitro*, 19, 975–83.

Ingle, T. M., Alexander, R., Bouldin, J., and Buchanan, R. A. 2008. Absorption of semiconductor nanocrystals by the aquatic invertebrate Ceriodaphnia dubia. *Bull Environ Contam Toxicol*, 81, 249–52.

Ispas, C., Andreescu, D., Patel, A., Goia, D. V., Andreescu, S., and Wallace, K. N. 2009. Toxicity and developmental defects of different sizes and shape nickel nanoparticles in zebrafish. *Environ Sci Technol*, 43, 6349–56.

Jackson, B. P., Pace, H. E., Lanzirotti, A., Smith, R., and Ranville, J. F. 2009. Synchrotron X-ray 2D and 3D elemental imaging of CdSe/ZnS quantum dot nanoparticles in *Daphnia magna*. *Anal Bioanal Chem*, 394, 911–7.

Jani, P., Florence, A., and Mccarthy, D. 1992. Further histological evidence of the gastrointestinal absorption of polystyrene nanospheres in the rat. *Int J Pharm*, 84, 245–52.

Jani, P., Mccarthy, D., and Florence, A. 1994. Titanium dioxide (rutile) particle uptake from the rat GI tract and translocation to systemic organs after oral administration. *Int J Pharm*, 105, 157–68.

Janssen, Y., Van Houten, B., Borm, P., and Mossman, B. 1993. Cell and tissue responses to oxidative damage. *Lab Invest*, 69, 261–74.

Jarmila, V. and Vavrikova, E. 2011. Chitosan derivatives with antimicrobial, antitumour and antioxidant activities—a review. *Curr Pharm Des*, 17, 3596–607.

Jemec, A., Drobne, D., Remskar, M., Sepcic, K., and Tisler, T. 2008. Effects of ingested nano-sized titanium dioxide on terrestrial isopods (Porcellio scaber). *Environ Toxicol Chem*, 27, 1904–14.

Johnson, A. C., Bowes, M. J., Crossley, A., Jarvie, H. P., Jurkschat, K., Jurgens, M. D., Lawlor, A. J. et al. 2011. An assessment of the fate, behaviour and environmental risk associated with sunscreen TiO nanoparticles in UK field scenarios. *Sci Total Environ*, 409, 2503–10.

Johnston, B. D., Scown, T. M., Moger, J., Cumberland, S. A., Baalousha, M., Linge, K., Van Aerle, R., Jarvis, K., Lead, J. R., and Tyler, C. R. 2010. Bioavailability of nanoscale metal oxides TiO(2), CeO(2), and ZnO to fish. *Environ Sci Technol*, 44, 1144–51.

Jovanovic, B., Anastasova, L., Rowe, E. W., and Palic, D. 2011a. Hydroxylated fullerenes inhibit neutrophil function in fathead minnow (Pimephales promelas Rafinesque, 1820). *Aquat Toxicol*, 101, 474–82.

Jovanovic, B., Anastasova, L., Rowe, E. W., Zhang, Y., Clapp, A. R., and Palic, D. 2011b. Effects of nanosized titanium dioxide on innate immune system of fathead minnow (Pimephales promelas Rafinesque, 1820). *Ecotoxicol Environ Saf*, 74, 675–83.

Judy, J. D., Unrine, J. M., and Bertsch, P. M. 2011. Evidence for biomagnification of gold nanoparticles within a terrestrial food chain. *Environ Sci Technol*, 45, 776–81.

Kahraman, M., Yazici, M. M., Sahin, F., Bayrak, O. F., and Culha, M. 2007a. Reproducible surface-enhanced Raman scattering spectra of bacteria on aggregated silver nanoparticles. *Appl Spectrosc*, 61, 479–85.

Kahraman, M., Yazici, M. M., Sahin, F., and Culha, M. 2007b. Experimental parameters influencing surface-enhanced Raman scattering of bacteria. *J Biomed Opt*, 12, 054015.

Kaplan, S. 2010. EPA: On nanoparticle safety, we know nothing. *The Investigative Fund, Politics Daily*. Available: http://www.theinvestigativefund.org/investigations/envirohealth/1253/epa%3A_on_nanoparticle_safety,_we_know_nothing/

Karmakar, S., Kundu, S., and Kundu, K. 2010. Bioconversion of silver salt into silver nanoparticles using different microorganisms. *Artif Cells Blood Substit Immobil Biotechnol*, 38, 259–66.

Kashiwada, S. 2006. Distribution of nanoparticles in the see-through medaka (Oryzias latipes). *Environ Health Perspect*, 114, 1697–702.

Ke, W., Xiong, Z.-T., Chen, S., and Chen, J. 2007. Effects of copper and mineral nutrition on growth, copper accumulation and mineral element uptake in two Rumex japonicus populations from a copper mine and an uncontaminated field sites. *Environ Exp Bot*, 59, 59–67.

Kennedy, A. J., Hull, M. S., Bednar, A. J., Goss, J. D., Gunter, J. C., Bouldin, J. L., Vikesland, P. J., and Steevens, J. A. 2010. Fractionating nanosilver: Importance for determining toxicity to aquatic test organisms. *Environ Sci Technol*, 44, 9571–7.

Kennedy, A. J., Hull, M. S., Steevens, J. A., Dontsova, K. M., Chappell, M. A., Gunter, J. C., and Weiss, C. A., Jr. 2008. Factors influencing the partitioning and toxicity of nanotubes in the aquatic environment. *Environ Toxicol Chem*, 27, 1932–41.

Khodakovskaya, M., Dervishi, E., Mahmood, M., Xu, Y., Li, Z., Watanabe, F., and Biris, A. S. 2009. Carbon nanotubes are able to penetrate plant seed coat and dramatically affect seed germination and plant growth. *ACS Nano*, 3, 3221–7.

Kim, H., Liu, X., Kobayashi, T., Kohyama, T., Wen, F., and Romberger, D. 2003. Ultrafine carbon black particles inhibit human lung fibroblast-mediated collagen gel contraction. *Am J Respir Cell Mol Biol*, 28, 111–21.

Kim, J., Kim, S., and Lee, S. 2011. Differentiation of the toxicities of silver nanoparticles and silver ions to the Japanese medaka (Oryzias latipes) and the cladoceran *Daphnia magna*. *Nanotoxicology*, 5, 208–14.

Kim, J., Park, Y., Yoon, T. H., Yoon, C. S., and Choi, K. 2010a. Phototoxicity of CdSe/ZnSe quantum dots with surface coatings of 3-mercaptopropionic acid or tri-n-octylphosphine oxide/gum arabic in *Daphnia magna* under environmentally relevant UV-B light. *Aquat Toxicol*, 97, 116–24.

Kim, K. T., Jang, M. H., Kim, J. Y., and Kim, S. D. 2010b. Effect of preparation methods on toxicity of fullerene water suspensions to Japanese medaka embryos. *Sci Total Environ*, 408, 5606–12.

Kim, K. T., Klaine, S. J., Cho, J., Kim, S. H., and Kim, S. D. 2010c. Oxidative stress responses of *Daphnia magna* exposed to TiO(2) nanoparticles according to size fraction. *Sci Total Environ*, 408, 2268–72.

Kim, K. T., Klaine, S. J., Lin, S., Ke, P. C., and Kim, S. D. 2010d. Acute toxicity of a mixture of copper and single-walled carbon nanotubes to *Daphnia magna*. *Environ Toxicol Chem*, 29, 122–6.

Kirchner, C., Liedl, T., Kudera, S., Pellegrino, T., Munoz, J., and Gaub, H. 2001. Cytotoxicity of colloidal CdSe and CdSe/ZnS nanoparticles. *Nano Lett*, 5, 331–38.

Kishikawa, H., Miura, S., Yoshida, H., Hirokawa, M., Nakamizo, H., and Higuchi, H. 2002. Transmural pressure induces IL-6 secretion by intestinal epithelial cells. *Clin Exp Immunol*, 129, 86–91.

Klaper, R., Crago, J., Barr, J., Arndt, D., Setyowati, K., and Chen, J. 2009. Toxicity biomarker expression in daphnids exposed to manufactured nanoparticles: Changes in toxicity with functionalization. *Environ Pollut*, 157, 1152–6.

Kreyling, W., Semmler, M., Erbe, F., Mayer, P., Takenaka, S., and Schulz, H. 2002. Translocation of ultrafine insoluble iridium particles from lung epithelium to extrapulmonary organs is size dependent but very low. *J Toxicol Environ Health A*, 65, 1513–1530.

Kubilus, J., Breyfogle, B., Sheasgreen, J., Hayden, P., Wertz, P., and Dale, B. 2004. Characterization of new buccal and gingival epithelial tissue. MatTek Corporation web page, 1–2. Available: http://www.mattek.com/pages/abstracts/abstractview/article/325-characterization-of-new-buccal-and-gingival-epithelial-tissue-models/

Kubilus, J., Cannon, C., Klausner, M., and Lonardo, E. 2002. Human tissue model for vaginal irritation studies. *Toxicologist*, 66, 378.

Kuhnel, D., Busch, W., Meissner, T., Springer, A., Potthoff, A., Richter, V., Gelinsky, M., Scholz, S., and Schirmer, K. 2009. Agglomeration of tungsten carbide nanoparticles in exposure medium does not prevent uptake and toxicity toward a rainbow trout gill cell line. *Aquat Toxicol*, 93, 91–9.

Kumari, M., Mukherjee, A., and Chandrasekaran, N. 2009. Genotoxicity of silver nanoparticles in *Allium cepa*. *Scie Total Environ*, 407, 5243–5246.

Kurepa, J., Paunesku, T., Vogt, S., Arora, H., Rabatic, B. M., Lu, J., Wanzer, M. B., Woloschak, G. E., and Smalle, J. A. 2010a. Uptake and distribution of ultrasmall anatase TiO2 alizarin red S nanoconjugates in arabidopsis thaliana. *Nano Lett*, 10, 2296–302.

Kurepa, J., Paunesku, T., Vogt, S., Arora, H., Rabatic, B. M., LU, J., Wanzer, M. B., Woloschak, G. E., and Smalle, J. A. 2010b. Uptake and distribution of ultrasmall anatase TiO2 Alizarin red S nanoconjugates in Arabidopsis thaliana. *Nano Lett*, 10, 2296–302.

Laban, G., Nies, L. F., Turco, R. F., Bickham, J. W., and Sepulveda, M. S. 2010. The effects of silver nanoparticles on fathead minnow (Pimephales promelas) embryos. *Ecotoxicology*, 19, 185–95.

Lansdown, A. and Taylor, A. 1997. Zinc and titanium oxides: Promising UV-absorbers but what influences do they have on the intact skin? *Int J Cosmetic Science*, 19, 167–72.

Lapied, E., Moudilou, E., Exbrayat, J. M., Oughton, D. H., and Joner, E. J. 2010. Silver nanoparticle exposure causes apoptotic response in the earthworm Lumbricus terrestris (Oligochaeta). *Nanomedicine (Lond)*, 5, 975–84.

Lapied, E., Nahmani, J. Y., Moudilou, E., Chaurand, P., Labille, J., Rose, J., Exbrayat, J. M., Oughton, D. H., and Joner, E. J. 2011. Ecotoxicological effects of an aged TiO2 nanocomposite measured as apoptosis in the anecic earthworm Lumbricus terrestris after exposure through water, food and soil. *Environ Int*, 37, 1105–10.

Lee, J., Ji, K., Kim, J., Park, C., Lim, K. H., Yoon, T. H., and Choi, K. 2010. Acute toxicity of two CdSe/ZnSe quantum dots with different surface coating in *Daphnia magna* under various light conditions. *Environ Toxicol*, 25, 593–600.

Lee, S. W., Kim, S. M., and Choi, J. 2009. Genotoxicity and ecotoxicity assays using the freshwater crustacean *Daphnia magna* and the larva of the aquatic midge Chironomus riparius to screen the ecological risks of nanoparticle exposure. *Environ Toxicol Pharmacol*, 28, 86–91.

Lee, W. M., An, Y. J., Yoon, H., and Kweon, H. S. 2008. Toxicity and bioavailability of copper nanoparticles to the terrestrial plants mung bean (Phaseolus radiatus) and wheat (Triticum aestivum): Plant agar test for water-insoluble nanoparticles. *Nanomater Environ*, 27, 1915–1921.

Lee, W. M., Ha, S. W., Yang, C. Y., Lee, J. K., and An, Y. J. 2011. Effect of fluorescent silica nanoparticles in embryo and larva of Oryzias latipes: Sonic effect in nanoparticle dispersion. *Chemosphere*, 82, 451–9.

Lee, Y. J., Kim, J., Oh, J., Bae, S., Lee, S., Hong, I. S., and Kim, S. H. 2012. Ion-release kinetics and ecotoxicity effects of silver nanoparticles. *Environ Toxicol Chem*, 31, 155–9.

Letts, R. E., Pereira, T. C., Bogo, M. R., and Monserrat, J. M. 2011. Biologic responses of bacteria communities living at the mucus secretion of common carp (Cyprinus carpio) after exposure to the carbon nanomaterial fullerene (C60). *Arch Environ Contam Toxicol*, 61, 311–7.

Li, D. and Alvarez, P. J. 2011. Avoidance, weight loss, and cocoon production assessment for Eisenia fetida exposed to C in soil. *Environ Toxicol Chem*, 30, 2542–5.

Li, D., Fortner, J. D., Johnson, D. R., Chen, C., Li, Q., and Alvarez, P. J. 2010a. Bioaccumulation of 14C60 by the earthworm Eisenia fetida. *Environ Sci Technol*, 44, 9170–5.

Li, H., Zhang, J., Wang, T., Luo, W., Zhou, Q., and Jiang, G. 2008. Elemental selenium particles at nano-size (Nano-Se) are more toxic to Medaka (Oryzias latipes) as a consequence of hyper-accumulation of selenium: A comparison with sodium selenite. *Aquat Toxicol*, 89, 251–6.

Li, H., Zhou, Q., Wu, Y., Fu, J., Wang, T., and Jiang, G. 2009. Effects of waterborne nano-iron on medaka (Oryzias latipes): Antioxidant enzymatic activity, lipid peroxidation and histopathology. *Ecotoxicol Environ Saf*, 72, 684–92.

Li, L. Z., Zhou, D. M., Peijnenburg, W. J., Van Gestel, C. A., Jin, S. Y., Wang, Y. J., and Wang, P. 2011a. Toxicity of zinc oxide nanoparticles in the earthworm, Eisenia fetida and subcellular fractionation of Zn. *Environ Int*, 37, 1098–104.

Li, M., Czymmek, K. J., and Huang, C. P. 2011b. Responses of Ceriodaphnia dubia to TiO2 and Al2O3 nanoparticles: A dynamic nano-toxicity assessment of energy budget distribution. *J Hazard Mater,* 187, 502–8.

Li, M., Hurren, R., Zastawny, R., Ling, V., and Buick, R. 1999. Regulation and expression of multidrug resistance (MDR) transcripts in the intestinal epithelium. *Br J Cancer,* 80, 1123–31.

Li, M., Pokhrel, S., Jin, X., Madler, L., Damoiseaux, R., and Hoek, E. M. 2011c. Stability, bioavailability, and bacterial toxicity of ZnO and iron-doped ZnO nanoparticles in aquatic media. *Environ Sci Technol,* 45, 755–61.

Li, T., Albee, B., Alemayehu, M., Diaz, R., Ingham, L., Kamal, S., Rodriguez, M., and Bishnoi, S. W. 2010b. Comparative toxicity study of Ag, Au, and Ag-Au bimetallic nanoparticles on *Daphnia magna. Anal Bioanal Chem,* 398, 689–700.

Lin, C., Fugetsu, B., Su, Y., and Watari, F. 2009a. Studies on toxicity of multi-walled carbon nanotubes on Arabidopsis T87 suspension cells. *J Hazard Mater,* 170, 578–583.

Lin, D. and Xing, B. 2007. Phytotoxicity of nanoparticles: Inhibition of seed germination and root growth. *Environ Pollut,* 150, 243–50.

Lin, D. and Xing, B. 2008. Root uptake and phytotoxicity of ZnO nanoparticles. *Environ Sci Technol,* 42, 5580–5.

Lin, S., Reppert, J., Hu, Q., Hudson, J. S., Reid, M. L., Ratnikova, T. A., Rao, A. M., Luo, H., and Ke, P. C. 2009b. Uptake, translocation, and transmission of carbon nanomaterials in rice plants. *Small,* 5, 1128–32.

Lin, Z., Xue, R., Ye, Y., Zheng, J., and Xu, Z. 2009c. A further insight into the biosorption mechanism of Pt(IV) by infrared spectrometry. *BMC Biotechnol,* 9, 62.

Linglan, M., Chao, L., Chunxiang, Q., Sitao, Y., Jie, L., Fengqing, G., and Fashui, H. 2008. Rubisco activase mRNA expression in spinach: Modulation by nanoanatase treatment. *Biol Trace Elem Res,* 122, 168–78.

Liu, J., Niu, J., Yin, L., and Jiang, F. 2011. *In situ* encapsulation of laccase in nanofibers by electrospinning for development of enzyme biosensors for chlorophenol monitoring. *Analyst,* 136, 4802–8.

Liu, Y., Cheng, X. J., Dang, Q. F., Ma, F. K., Chen, X. G., Park, H. J., and Kim, B. K. 2012a. Preparation and evaluation of oleoyl-carboxymethy-chitosan (OCMCS) nanoparticles as oral protein carriers. *J Mater Sci Mater Med,* 23, 375–84.

Liu, Y., Liu, B., Feng, D., Gao, C., Wu, M., He, N., Yang, X., Li, L., and Feng, X. 2012b. A progressive approach on zebrafish toward sensitive evaluation of nanoparticles' toxicity. *Integr Biol (Camb),* 4, 285–91.

Longmire, M., Choyke, P., and Kobayashi, H. 2008. Clearance properties, nano-sized particles and molecules as imaging agents: Physiologic considerations. *Nanomedicine,* 3, 703–17.

Lopes, I., Ribeiro, R., Antunes, F. E., Rocha-Santos, T. A., Rasteiro, M. G., Soares, A. M., Goncalves, F., and Pereira, R. 2012. Toxicity and genotoxicity of organic and inorganic nanoparticles to the bacteria Vibrio fischeri and Salmonella typhimurium. *Ecotoxicology,* 21, 637–48.

Lopez-Moreno, M. L., De La Rosa, G., Hernandez-Viezcas, J. A., Castillo-Michel, H., Botez, C. E., Peralta-Videa, J. R., and Gardea-Torresdey, J. L. 2010a. Evidence of the differential biotransformation and genotoxicity of ZnO and CeO2 nanoparticles on soybean (Glycine max) plants. *Environ Sci Technol,* 44, 7315–20.

Lopez-Moreno, M. L., De La Rosa, G., Hernandez-Viezcas, J. A., Peralta-Videa, J. R., and Gardea-Torresdey, J. L. 2010b. X-ray absorption spectroscopy (XAS) corroboration of the uptake and storage of CeO(2) nanoparticles and assessment of their differential toxicity in four edible plant species. *J Agric Food Chem*, 58, 3689–93.

Lovern, S. B. and Klaper, R. 2006. *Daphnia magna* mortality when exposed to titanium dioxide and fullerene (C60) nanoparticles. *Environ Toxicol Chem*, 25, 1132–7.

Lovern, S. B., Strickler, J. R., and Klaper, R. 2007. Behavioral and physiological changes in *Daphnia magna* when exposed to nanoparticle suspensions (titanium dioxide, nano-C60, and C60HxC70Hx). *Environ Sci Technol*, 41, 4465–70.

Lu, C. M., Zhang, C. Y., Wen, J. Q., Wu, G. R., and Tao, M. X. 2002. Research of the effect of nanometer materials on germination and growth enhancement of Glycine max and its mechanism. *Soybean Sci*, 21, 168–172.

Lubick, N. 2008. Nanosilver toxicity: Ions, nanoparticles—or both? *Environ Sci Technol*, 42, 8617.

Ma, X. and Wang, C. 2010. Fullerene nanoparticles affect the fate and uptake of trichloroethylene in phytoremediation systems. *Environ Eng Sci*, 27, 989–92.

Madrid, E. N. and Friedman, W. E. 2010. Female gametophyte and early seed development in Peperomia (Piperaceae). *Am J Bot*, 97, 1–14.

Manabe, M., Tatarazako, N., and Kinoshita, M. 2011. Uptake, excretion and toxicity of nano-sized latex particles on medaka (Oryzias latipes) embryos and larvae. *Aquat Toxicol*, 105, 576–81.

Manusadzianas, L., Caillet, C., Fachetti, L., Gylyte, B., Grigutyte, R., Jurkoniene, S., Karitonas et al. 2012. Toxicity of copper oxide nanoparticle suspensions to aquatic biota. *Environ Toxicol Chem*, 31, 108–14.

McLaughlin, J. and Bonzongo, J. C. 2012. Effects of natural water chemistry on nanosilver behavior and toxicity to Ceriodaphnia dubia and Pseudokirchneriella subcapitata. *Environ Toxicol Chem*, 31, 168–75.

Meerburg, F., Hennebel, T., Vanhaecke, L., Verstraete, W., and Boon, N. 2012. Diclofenac and 2-anilinophenylacetate degradation by combined activity of biogenic manganese oxides and silver. *Microb Biotechnol*, 5, 388–95.

Meiring, J., Borm, P., Bagate, K., Semmler, M., Seitz, J., and Takenaka, S. 2005. The influence of hydrogen peroxide and histamine on lung permeability and translocation of iridium nanoparticles in the isolated perfused rat lung. *Part Fibre Toxicol*, 2, 3.

Mendonca, E., Diniz, M., Silva, L., Peres, I., Castro, L., Correia, J. B., and Picado, A. 2011. Effects of diamond nanoparticle exposure on the internal structure and reproduction of *Daphnia magna*. *J Hazard Mater*, 186, 265–71.

Mishra, R. R., Prajapati, S., Das, J., Dangar, T. K., Das, N., and Thatoi, H. 2011. Reduction of selenite to red elemental selenium by moderately halotolerant Bacillus megaterium strains isolated from Bhitarkanika mangrove soil and characterization of reduced product. *Chemosphere*, 84, 1231–7.

Moghimi, S., Hunter, A., and Murray, J. 2001. Long-circulating and target-specific nanoparticles: Theory to practice. *Pharmacol Rev*, 53, 283–318.

Monteiro-Riviere, N. 1990. Specialized technique: Isolated perfused porcine skin flap. In: Kemppainen, B. and Reifenrath, W. (eds.) *Methods Skin Absorption*. Boca Raton: CRC Press, pp. 175–89.

Monteiro-Riviere, N. and Riviere, J. 1999. Skin toxicology. In: Marquardt, H., Schafer, S., McCellan, R., and Welsch, F. (eds.) *Toxicology*. San Diego: Academic Press, pp. 439–57.

Monteiro, D. R., Silva, S., Negri, M., Gorup, L. F., De Camargo, E. R., Oliveira, R., Barbosa, D. B., and Henriques, M. 2012. Silver nanoparticles: Influence of stabilizing agent and diameter on antifungal activity against Candida albicans and Candida glabrata biofilms. *Lett Appl Microbiol,* 54, 383–91.

Mortimer, M., Kasemets, K., Heinlaan, M., Kurvet, I., and Kahru, A. 2008. High throughput kinetic Vibrio fischeri bioluminescence inhibition assay for study of toxic effects of nanoparticles. *Toxicol In Vitro,* 22, 1412–7.

Mortimer, M., Kasemets, K., and Kahru, A. 2010. Toxicity of ZnO and CuO nanoparticles to ciliated protozoa Tetrahymena thermophila. *Toxicology,* 269, 182–9.

Mortimer, M., Kasemets, K., Vodovnik, M., Marinsek-Logar, R., and Kahru, A. 2011. Exposure to CuO nanoparticles changes the fatty acid composition of protozoa Tetrahymena thermophila. *Environ Sci Technol,* 45, 6617–24.

Mouchet, F., Landois, P., Sarremejean, E., Dbernard, G., Puech, P., Pinelli, E., Flahaut, E., and Gauthier, L. 2008. Characterisation and *in vivo* ecotoxicity evaluation of double-wall carbon nanotubes in larvae of the amphibian *Xenopus laevis. Aquat Toxicol,* 87, 127–37.

Naha, P. C., Casey, A., Tenuta, T., Lynch, I., Dawson, K. A., Byrne, H. J., and Davoren, M. 2009a. Preparation, characterization of NIPAM and NIPAM/BAM copolymer nanoparticles and their acute toxicity testing using an aquatic test battery. *Aquat Toxicol,* 92, 146–54.

Naha, P. C., Davoren, M., Casey, A., and Byrne, H. J. 2009b. An ecotoxicological study of poly(amidoamine) dendrimers-toward quantitative structure activity relationships. *Environ Sci Technol,* 43, 6864–9.

Navalon, S., Martin, R., Alvaro, M., and Garcia, H. 2011. Sunlight-assisted Fenton reaction catalyzed by gold supported on diamond nanoparticles as pretreatment for biological degradation of aqueous phenol solutions. *ChemSusChem,* 4, 650–7.

Navarro, E., Baun, A., Behra, R., Hartmann, N. B., Filser, J., Miao, A. J., Quigg, A., Santschi, P. H., and Sigg, L. 2008a. Environmental behavior and ecotoxicity of engineered nanoparticles to algae, plants, and fungi. *Ecotoxicology,* 17, 372–86.

Navarro, E., Piccapietra, F., Wagner, B., Marconi, F., Kaegi, R., Odzak, N., Sigg, L., and Behra, R. 2008b. Toxicity of silver nanoparticles to Chlamydomonas reinhardtii. *Environ Sci Technol,* 42, 8959–64.

National Institute of Health. 2001. *Guidance Documentation on Using In Vitro Data to Estimate In Vivo Starting Doses for Acute Toxicity.* NIH publication NO. 01-4500.

Nemmar, A., Hoylaerts, M., Hoet, P., Dinsdale, D., Smith, T., and Xu, H. 2002. Ultrafine particles affect experimental thrombosis in an *in vivo* hamster model. *Am J Respir Crit Care Med,* 166, 998–1004.

Novak, S., Drobne, D., Valant, J., Pipan-Tkalec, Z., Pelicon, P., Vavpetic, P., Grlj, N., Falnoga, I., Mazej, D., and Remskar, M. 2012. Cell membrane integrity and internalization of ingested TiO(2) nanoparticles by digestive gland cells of a terrestrial isopod. *Environ Toxicol Chem,* 31, 1083–90.

O'Donnell, V. 2003. Free radicals and lipid signaling in endothelial cells. *Antioxid Redox Signal,* 5, 195–203.

Oberdorster, E. 2004. Manufactured nanomaterials (fullerenes, C60) induce oxidative stress in the brain of juvenile largemouth bass. *Environ Health Perspect,* 112, 1058–62.

Oberdorster, G. 2000. Toxicology of ultrafine particles: *In vivo* studies. *Phil Trans Roy Soc London Series,* 358, 2719–40.

Oberdorster, G., Ferin, J., and Lehnert, B. 1994. Correlation between particle size, *in vivo* particle persistence, and lung injury. *Environ Health Perspect,* 102, 173–79.

Oberdorster, G., Maynard, A., Donaldson, K., Castranova, V., Fitzpatrick, J., Ausman, K., Carter, J. et al. 2005a. Principles for characterizing the potential human health effects from exposure to nanomaterials: Elements of a screening strategy. *Part Fibre Toxicol,* 2, 8.

Oberdorster, G., Oberdorster, E., and Oberdorster, J. 2005b. Nanotoxicology: An emerging discipline evolving from studies of ultrafine particles. *Environ Health Perspect,* 113, 823–39.

Oberdorster, G., Sharp, Z., Atudorei, V., Elder, A., Gelein, R., and Kreyling, W. 2004. Translocation of inhaled ultrafine particles to the brain. *Inhal Toxicol,* 16, 437–45.

Oberdorster, G., Sharp, Z., Atudorei, V., Elder, A., Gelein, R., and Lunts, A. 2002. Extrapulmonary translocation of ultrafine carbon particles following whole-body inhalation exposure of rats. *J Toxicol Environ Health A,* 65, 1531–43.

Oughton, D. H., Hertel-Aas, T., Pellicer, E., Mendoza, E., and Joner, E. J. 2008. Neutron activation of engineered nanoparticles as a tool for tracing their environmental fate and uptake in organisms. *Environ Toxicol Chem,* 27, 1883–7.

Pace, H. E., Lesher, E. K., and Ranville, J. F. 2010. Influence of stability on the acute toxicity of CdSe/ZnS nanocrystals to *Daphnia magna. Environ Toxicol Chem,* 29, 1338–44.

Pakarinen, K., Petersen, E. J., Leppanen, M. T., Akkanen, J., and Kukkonen, J. V. 2011. Adverse effects of fullerenes (nC60) spiked to sediments on Lumbriculus varie-gatus (Oligochaeta). *Environ Pollut,* 159, 3750–6.

Panneerselvam, K. and Freeze, H. 1996. Mannose enters mammalian cells using a specific transporter that is insensitive to glucose. *J Biol Chem,* 271, 9417–21.

Parliament, E. 2006a. Corrigendum to Directive 2006/121/EC of the European Parliament and of the Council of 18 December 2006 amending Council Directive 67/548/EEC on the approximation of laws, regulations and administrative provisions relating to the classification, packaging and labelling of danger-ous substances in order to adapt it to Regulation (EC) No 1907/2006 concern-ing the Registration, Evaluation, Authorisation and Restriction of Chemicals (REACH) and establishing a European Chemicals Agency. *In:* Parliament, E. (ed.) *2006/121/EC.*

Parliament, E. 2006b. Corrigendum to Regulation (EC) No 1907/2006 of the European Parliament and of the Council of 18 December 2006 concerning the Registration, Evaluation, Authorisation and Restriction of Chemicals (REACH), establishing a European Chemicals Agency, amending Directive 1999/45/EC and repeal-ing Council Regulation (EEC) No 793/93 and Commission Regulation (EC) No 1488/94 as well as Council Directive 76/769/EEC and Commission Directives 91/155/EEC, 93/67/EEC, 93/105/EC and 2000/21/EC. *In:* Parliament, E. (ed.) *1907/2006.* European Parliament.

Parsons, J. G., Lopez, M. L., Gonzalez, C. M., Peralta-Videa, J. R., and Gardea-Torresdey, J. L. 2010. Toxicity and biotransformation of uncoated and coated nickel hydroxide nanoparticles on mesquite plants. *Environ Toxicol Chem,* 29, 1146–54.

Paterson, G., Ataria, J. M., Hoque, M. E., Burns, D. C., and Metcalfe, C. D. 2011. The toxicity of titanium dioxide nanopowder to early life stages of the Japanese medaka (Oryzias latipes). *Chemosphere,* 82, 1002–9.

Patra, M., Ma, X., Isaacson, C., Bouchard, D., Poynton, H., Lazorchak, J. M., and Rogers, K. R. 2011. Changes in agglomeration of fullerenes during ingestion and excretion in Thamnocephalus platyurus. *Environ Toxicol Chem,* 30, 828–35.

Pedroza, A. M., Mosqueda, R., Alonso-Vante, N., and Rodriguez-Vazquez, R. 2007. Sequential treatment via Trametes versicolor and UV/TiO2/Ru(x)Se(y) to reduce contaminants in waste water resulting from the bleaching process during paper production. *Chemosphere,* 67, 793–801.

Pereira, R., Rocha-Santos, T. A., Antunes, F. E., Rasteiro, M. G., Ribeiro, R., Goncalves, F., Soares, A. M., and Lopes, I. 2011. Screening evaluation of the ecotoxicity and genotoxicity of soils contaminated with organic and inorganic nanoparticles: The role of ageing. *J Hazard Mater,* 194, 345–54.

Perkel, J. M. 2011. What lies beneath: *In vivo* stem cell imaging. *Biotechniques,* 50, 223–7.

Perreault, F., Melegari, S. P., Fuzinatto, C. F., Bogdan, N., Morin, M., Popovic, R., and Matias, W. G. 2012a. Toxicity of pamam-coated gold nanoparticles in different unicellular models. *Environ Toxicol.* DOI: 10.1002/tox.21761. [Epub ahead of print].

Perreault, F., Oukarroum, A., Melegari, S. P., Matias, W. G., and Popovic, R. 2012b. Polymer coating of copper oxide nanoparticles increases nanoparticles uptake and toxicity in the green alga Chlamydomonas reinhardtii. *Chemosphere,* 87, 1388–94.

Petersen, E. J., Pinto, R. A., Mai, D. J., Landrum, P. F., and Weber, W. J., Jr. 2011. Influence of polyethyleneimine graftings of multi-walled carbon nanotubes on their accumulation and elimination by and toxicity to *Daphnia magna. Environ Sci Technol,* 45, 1133–8.

Petit, A. N., Eullaffroy, P., Debenest, T., and Gagne, F. 2010. Toxicity of PAMAM dendrimers to Chlamydomonas reinhardtii. *Aquat Toxicol,* 100, 187–93.

Pidgeon, N., Harthorn, B. H., Bryant, K., and Rogers-Hayden, T. 2009. Deliberating the risks of nanotechnologies for energy and health applications in the United States and United Kingdom. *Nat Nano,* 4, 95–8.

Pipan-Tkalec, Z., Drobne, D., Jemec, A., Romih, T., Zidar, P., and Bele, M. 2010. Zinc bioaccumulation in a terrestrial invertebrate fed a diet treated with particulate ZnO or ZnCl2 solution. *Toxicology,* 269, 198–203.

Poda, A. R., Bednar, A. J., Kennedy, A. J., Harmon, A., Hull, M., Mitrano, D. M., Ranville, J. F., and Steevens, J. 2011. Characterization of silver nanoparticles using flow-field flow fractionation interfaced to inductively coupled plasma mass spectrometry. *J Chromatogr A,* 1218, 4219–25.

Powell, J., Harvey, R., Ashwood, P., Wolstencroft, R., Gershwin, M., and Thompson, R. 2000. Immune potentiation of ultrafine dietary particles in normal subjects and patients with inflammatory bowel disease. *J Autoimmun,* 14, 99–105.

Poynton, H. C., Lazorchak, J. M., Impellitteri, C. A., Smith, M. E., Rogers, K., Patra, M., Hammer, K. A., Allen, H. J., and Vulpe, C. D. 2011. Differential gene expression in *Daphnia magna* suggests distinct modes of action and bioavailability for ZnO nanoparticles and Zn ions. *Environ Sci Technol,* 45, 762–8.

Quaroni, A. and Isselbacher, K. 1981. Cytotoxic effects and metabolism of benzo[a] pyrene and 7, 12-dimethylbenz[a]anthracene in duodenal and ileal epithelial cell cultures. *J Natl Cancer Inst,* 67, 1353–62.

Quinlan, T., Berube, K., Marsh, J., Janssen, Y., Taishi, P., and Leslie, K. 1995. Patterns of inflammation, cell-proliferation, and related gene-expression in lung after inhalation of chrysotile asbestos. *Am J Pathol,* 147, 728–39.

Răcuciu, M. and Creangă, D. E. 2009. Biocompatible magnetic fluid nanoparticles internalized in vegetal tissue. *Rom J Phys*, 54, 125–31.

Ramsden, C. S., Smith, T. J., Shaw, B. J., and Handy, R. D. 2009. Dietary exposure to titanium dioxide nanoparticles in rainbow trout, (Oncorhynchus mykiss): No effect on growth, but subtle biochemical disturbances in the brain. *Ecotoxicology*, 18, 939–51.

Raychowdhury, M., Ibarra, C., Damiano, A., Jackson, G., Smith, P., and Mclaughlin, M. 2004. Characterization of Na+-permeable cation channels in LLC-PK1 renal epithelial cells. *J Biol Chem*, 279, 20137–46.

Reeves, J. F., Davies, S. J., Dodd, N. J., and Jha, A. N. 2008. Hydroxyl radicals (*OH) are associated with titanium dioxide (TiO(2)) nanoparticle-induced cytotoxicity and oxidative DNA damage in fish cells. *Mutat Res*, 640, 113–22.

Renwick, L., Donaldson, K., and Clouter, A. 2001. Impairment of alveolar macro-phage phagocytosis by ultrafine particles. *Toxicol Appl Pharmacol*, 172, 119–27.

Ricardo, S., Bertram, J., and Ryan, G. 1994. Reactive oxygen species in puromycin aminonucleoside nephrosis: *In vitro* studies. *Kidney Int*, 45, 1057–69.

Rico, C. M., Majumdar, S., Duarte-Gardea, M., Peralta-Videa, J. R., and Gardea-Torresdey, J. L. 2011. Interaction of nanoparticles with edible plants and their possible implications in the food chain. *J Agric Food Chem*, 59, 3485–98.

Riviere, J., Bowman, K., Monteiro-Riviere, N., Dix, L., and Carver, M. 1986. The iso-lated perfused porcine skin flap (Ippsf). I. A novel *in vitro* model for percu-taneous absorption and cutaneous toxicology studies. *Fundam Appl Toxicol*, 7, 444–53.

Riviere, J. and Monteiro-Riviere, N. 1991. The isolated perfused porcine skin flap as an *in vitro* model for percutaneous absorption and cutaneous toxicology. *Crit Rev Toxicol*, 21, 329–44.

Robbens, J., Dardenne, F., Devriese, L., De Coen, W., and Blust, R. 2010. Escherichia coli as a bioreporter in ecotoxicology. *Appl Microbiol Biotechnol*, 88, 1007–25.

Rodea-Palomares, I., Boltes, K., Fernandez-Pinas, F., Leganes, F., Garcia-Calvo, E., Santiago, J., and Rosal, R. 2011. Physicochemical characterization and ecotoxi-cological assessment of CeO2 nanoparticles using two aquatic microorganisms. *Toxicol Sci*, 119, 135–45.

Romer, I., White, T. A., Baalousha, M., Chipman, K., Viant, M. R., and Lead, J. R. 2011. Aggregation and dispersion of silver nanoparticles in exposure media for aquatic toxicity tests. *J Chromatogr A*, 1218, 4226–33.

Rondeau-Mouro, C., Defer, D., Leboeuf, E., and Lahaye, M. 2008. Assessment of cell wall porosity in Arabidopsis thaliana by NMR spectroscopy. *Int J Biol Macromol*, 42, 83–92.

Rotaru, A. E., Jiang, W., Finster, K., Skrydstrup, T., and Meyer, R. L. 2012. Non-enzymatic palladium recovery on microbial and synthetic surfaces. *Biotechnol Bioeng*, 109, 1889–97.

Royal Society. 2004. *Nanoscience and Nanotechnologies: Opportunities and Uncertainties*. London.

Rustom, R., Wang, B., Mcardle, F., Shalamanova, L., Alexander, J., and Mcardle, A. 2003. Oxidative stress in a novel model of chronic acidosis in LLC-PK1 cells. *Nephron Exp Nephrol*, 95, e13–e23.

Ryan, M., Johnson, G., Kirk, J., Fuerstenberg, S., Zager, R., and Torok-Storb, B. 1994. HK-2: An immortalized proximal tubule epithelial cell line from normal adult human kidney. *Kidney Int*, 45, 48–57.

Saison, C., Perreault, F., Daigle, J. C., Fortin, C., Claverie, J., Morin, M., and Popovic, R. 2010. Effect of core-shell copper oxide nanoparticles on cell culture morphology and photosynthesis (photosystem II energy distribution) in the green alga, Chlamydomonas reinhardtii. *Aquat Toxicol*, 96, 109–14.

Saravanan, M., Vemu, A. K., and Barik, S. K. 2011. Rapid biosynthesis of silver nanoparticles from Bacillus megaterium (NCIM 2326) and their antibacterial activity on multi drug resistant clinical pathogens. *Colloids Surf B Biointerfaces*, 88, 325–31.

Sayes, C., Fortner, J., Guo, W., Lyon, D., Boyd, A., and Ausman, K. 2004. The differential cytotoxicity of water-soluble fullerenes. *Am Chem Soc*, 4, 1881–7.

Sayes, C. M., Wahi, R., Kurian, P. A., Liu, Y., West, J. L., Ausman, K. D., Warheit, D. B., and Colvin, V. L. 2006. Correlating nanoscale titania structure with toxicity: A cytotoxicity and inflammatory response study with human dermal fibroblasts and human lung epithelial cells. *Toxicol Sci*, 92, 174–185.

Schins, R. 2002. Mechanisms of genotoxicity of particles and fibers. *Inhal Toxicol*, 14, 57–78.

Schins, R. and Donaldson, K. 2000. Nuclear factor kappa-B activation by particles and fibres. *Inhal Toxicol*, 12, 317–26.

Schins, R., Knaapen, A., Cakmak, G., Shi, T., Weishaupt, C., and Borm, P. 2002. Oxidant-induced DNA damage by quartz in alveolar epithelial cells. *Mutat Res*, 517, 77–86.

Schreiner, K. M., Filley, T. R., Blanchette, R. A., Bowen, B. B., Bolskar, R. D., Hockaday, W. C., Masiello, C. A., and Raebiger, J. W. 2009. White-rot basidiomycete-mediated decomposition of C60 fullerol. *Environ Sci Technol*, 43, 3162–8.

Scott-Fordsmand, J. J., Krogh, P. H., Schaefer, M., and Johansen, A. 2008. The toxicity testing of double-walled nanotubes-contaminated food to Eisenia veneta earthworms. *Ecotoxicol Environ Saf*, 71, 616–9.

Scown, T. M., Santos, E. M., Johnston, B. D., Gaiser, B., Baalousha, M., Mitov, S., Lead, J. R. et al. 2010. Effects of aqueous exposure to silver nanoparticles of different sizes in rainbow trout. *Toxicol Sci*, 115, 521–34.

Scown, T. M., Van Aerle, R., Johnston, B. D., Cumberland, S., Lead, J. R., Owen, R., and Tyler, C. R. 2009. High doses of intravenously administered titanium dioxide nanoparticles accumulate in the kidneys of rainbow trout but with no observable impairment of renal function. *Toxicol Sci*, 109, 372–80.

Searl, A. 1994. A review of the durability of inhaled fibers and options for the design of safer fibers. *Ann Occup Hyg*, 38, 839–55.

Seda, B. C., Ke, P. C., Mount, A. S., and Klaine, S. J. 2012. Toxicity of aqueous C70-gallic acid suspension in *Daphnia magna*. *Environ Toxicol Chem*, 31, 215–20.

Seitz, F., Bundschuh, M., Dabrunz, A., Bandow, N., Schaumann, G. E., and Schulz, R. 2012. Titanium dioxide nanoparticles detoxify pirimicarb under UV irradiation at ambient intensities. *Environ Toxicol Chem*, 31, 518–23.

Sekar, D., Falcioni, M. L., Barucca, G., and Falcioni, G. 2011. DNA damage and repair following *in vitro* exposure to two different forms of titanium dioxide nanoparticles on trout erythrocyte. *Environ Toxicol*. Doi: 10.1002/tox.20778. [Epub ahead of print].

Semmler, M., Seitz, J., Erbe, F., Mayer, P., Heyder, J., and Oberdorster, G. 2004. Long-term clearance kinetics of inhaled ultrafine insoluble iridium particles from the rat lung, including transient translocation into secondary organs. *Inhal Toxicol*, 16, 453–9.

Shah, V. and Belozerova, I. 2009. Influence of metal nanoparticles on the soil microbial community and germination of lettuce seeds. *Water Air Soil Pollut*, 197, 143–8.

Shah, V., Dobiasova, P., Baldrian, P., Nerud, F., Kumar, A., and Seal, S. 2010. Influence of iron and copper nanoparticle powder on the production of lignocellulose degrading enzymes in the fungus Trametes versicolor. *J Hazard Mater*, 178, 1141–5.

Sharma, V. K. 2009. Aggregation and toxicity of titanium dioxide nanoparticles in aquatic environment—a review. *J Environ Sci Health A Tox Hazard Subst Environ Eng*, 44, 1485–95.

Shinohara, N., Matsumoto, T., Gamo, M., Miyauchi, A., Endo, S., Yonezawa, Y., and Nakanishi, J. 2009. Is lipid peroxidation induced by the aqueous suspension of fullerene C60 nanoparticles in the brains of Cyprinus carpio? *Environ Sci Technol*, 43, 948–53.

Shoults-Wilson, W. A., Reinsch, B. C., Tsyusko, O. V., Bertsch, P. M., Lowry, G. V., and Unrine, J. M. 2011a. Effect of silver nanoparticle surface coating on bioaccumulation and reproductive toxicity in earthworms (*Eisenia fetida*). *Nanotoxicology*, 5, 432–44.

Shoults-Wilson, W. A., Zhurbich, O. I., Mcnear, D. H., Tsyusko, O. V., Bertsch, P. M., and Unrine, J. M. 2011b. Evidence for avoidance of Ag nanoparticles by earthworms (*Eisenia fetida*). *Ecotoxicology*, 20, 385–96.

Shvedova, A., Castranova, V., Kisin, E., Schwegler-Berry, D., Murray, A., and Gandelsman, V. 2003. Exposure to carbon nanotube material: Assessment of nanotube cytotoxicity using human keratinocyte cells. *J Toxicol Environ Health A*, 66, 1909–26.

Sinyakov, M. S., Dror, M., Lublin-Tennenbaum, T., Salzberg, S., Margel, S., and Avtalion, R. R. 2006. Nano- and microparticles as adjuvants in vaccine design: Success and failure is related to host natural antibodies. *Vaccine*, 24, 6534–41.

Smith, C. B., Anderson, J. E., Edwards, J. D., and Kam, K. C. 2011. *In situ* surface-etched bacterial spore detection using dipicolinic acid-europium-silica nanoparticle bioreporters. *Appl Spectrosc*, 65, 866–75.

Smith, J., Johanesen, P., Wendt, M., Binion, D., and Dwinell, M. 2005. CXCL12 activation of CXCR4 regulates mucosal host defense through stimulation of epithelial cell migration and promotion of intestinal barrier integrity. *Am J Physiol Gastrointest Liver Physiol*, 288, G316–26.

Spohn, P., Hirsch, C., Hasler, F., Bruinink, A., Krug, H. F., and Wick, P. 2009. C60 fullerene: A powerful antioxidant or a damaging agent? The importance of an in-depth material characterization prior to toxicity assays. *Environ Pollut*, 157, 1134–9.

Stampoulis, D., Sinha, S. K., and White, J. C. 2009. Assay-dependent phytotoxicity of nanoparticles to plants. *Environ Sci Technol*, 43, 9473–9.

Stanley, J. K., Coleman, J. G., Weiss, C. A., Jr., and Steevens, J. A. 2010. Sediment toxicity and bioaccumulation of nano and micron-sized aluminum oxide. *Environ Toxicol Chem*, 29, 422–9.

Stringer, B., Imrich, A., and Kobzik, L. 1996. Lung epithelial cell (A549) interaction with unopsonized environmental particulates: Quantitation of particle-specific binding and IL-8 production. *Exp Lung Res*, 22, 495–508.

Stringer, B. and Kobzik, L. 1998. Environmental particulate-mediated cytokine production in lung epithelial cells (A549): Role of preexisting inflammation and oxidant stress. *J Toxicol Environ Health*, 55, 31–44.

Sun, H., Zhang, X., Zhang, Z., Chen, Y., and Crittenden, J. C. 2009. Influence of titanium dioxide nanoparticles on speciation and bioavailability of arsenite. *Environ Pollut*, 157, 1165–70.

Tan, C., Fan, W. H., and Wang, W. X. 2012. Role of titanium dioxide nanoparticles in the elevated uptake and retention of cadmium and zinc in *Daphnia magna*. *Environ Sci Technol*, 46, 469–76.

Tan, X.-M. and Fugetsu, B. 2007. Multi-walled carbon nanotubes interact with cultured rice cells: Evidence of a self-defense response. *J Biomed Nanotechnol*, 3, 285–8.

Tan, X.-M., Lin, C., and Fugetsu, B. 2009. Studies on toxicity of multi-walled carbon nanotubes on suspension rice cells. *Carbon*, 47, 3479–87.

Tao, X., Fortner, J. D., Zhang, B., He, Y., Chen, Y., and Hughes, J. B. 2009. Effects of aqueous stable fullerene nanocrystals (nC60) on *Daphnia magna*: Evaluation of sub-lethal reproductive responses and accumulation. *Chemosphere*, 77, 1482–7.

Teeguarden, J. G., Hinderliter, P. M., Orr, G., Thrall, B. D., and Pounds, J. G. 2007. Particokinetics *in vitro*: Dosimetry considerations for *in vitro* nanoparticle toxicity assessments. *Toxicol Sci*, 95, 300–12.

Templeton, R. C., Ferguson, P. L., Washburn, K. M., Scrivens, W. A., and Chandler, G. T. 2006. Life-cycle effects of single-walled carbon nanotubes (SWNTs) on an estuarine meiobenthic copepod. *Environ Sci Technol*, 40, 7387–93.

Thomas, K. V., Farkas, J., Farmen, E., Christian, P., Langford, K., Wu, Q., and Tollefsen, K. E. 2011. Effects of dispersed aggregates of carbon and titanium dioxide engineered nanoparticles on rainbow trout hepatocytes. *J Toxicol Environ Health A*, 74, 466–77.

Timblin, C., Guthrie, G., Janssen, Y., Walsh, E., Vacek, P., and Mossman, B. 1998. Patterns of c-fos and c-jun proto-oncogene expression, apoptosis, and proliferation in rat pleural mesothelial cells exposed to erionite or asbestos fibers. *Toxicol Appl Pharmacol*, 151, 88–97.

Unrine, J. M., Hunyadi, S. E., Tsyusko, O. V., Rao, W., Shoults-Wilson, W. A., and Bertsch, P. M. 2010a. Evidence for bioavailability of Au nanoparticles from soil and biodistribution within earthworms (Eisenia fetida). *Environ Sci Technol*, 44, 8308–13.

Unrine, J. M., Tsyusko, O. V., Hunyadi, S. E., Judy, J. D., and Bertsch, P. M. 2010b. Effects of particle size on chemical speciation and bioavailability of copper to earthworms (Eisenia fetida) exposed to copper nanoparticles. *J Environ Qual*, 39, 1942–53.

Urayama, S., Musch, M., Retsky, J., Madonna, M., Straus, D., and Chang, E. 1998. Dexamethasone protection of rat intestinal epithelial cells against oxidant injury is mediated by induction of heat shock protein. *J Clin Invest*, 102, 1860–5.

Valant, J., Drobne, D., and Novak, S. 2012. Effect of ingested titanium dioxide nanoparticles on the digestive gland cell membrane of terrestrial isopods. *Chemosphere*, 87, 19–25.

Valant, J., Drobne, D., Sepcic, K., Jemec, A., Kogej, K., and Kostanjsek, R. 2009. Hazardous potential of manufactured nanoparticles identified by *in vivo* assay. *J Hazard Mater*, 171, 160–5.

Van der Ploeg, M. J., Baveco, J. M., Van Der Hout, A., Bakker, R., Rietjens, I. M., and Van Den Brink, N. W. 2011. Effects of C60 nanoparticle exposure on earthworms (Lumbricus rubellus) and implications for population dynamics. *Environ Pollut*, 159, 198–203.

Van Hoecke, K., De Schamphelaere, K. A., Ramirez-Garcia, S., Van Der Meeren, P., Smagghe, G., and Janssen, C. R. 2011a. Influence of alumina coating on characteristics and effects of SiO2 nanoparticles in algal growth inhibition assays at various pH and organic matter contents. *Environ Int*, 37, 1118–25.

Van Hoecke, K., De Schamphelaere, K. A., Van Der Meeren, P., Lucas, S., and Janssen, C. R. 2008. Ecotoxicity of silica nanoparticles to the green alga Pseudokirchneriella subcapitata: Importance of surface area. *Environ Toxicol Chem*, 27, 1948–57.

Van Hoecke, K., De Schamphelaere, K. A., Van Der Meeren, P., Smagghe, G., and Janssen, C. R. 2011b. Aggregation and ecotoxicity of CeO nanoparticles in synthetic and natural waters with variable pH, organic matter concentration and ionic strength. *Environ Pollut*, 159, 970–6.

Van Hoecke, K., Quik, J. T., Mankiewicz-Boczek, J., Dw Schamphelaere, K. A., Elsaesser, A., Van Der Meeren, P., Barnes, C. et al. 2009. Fate and effects of CeO2 nanoparticles in aquatic ecotoxicity tests. *Environ Sci Technol*, 43, 4537–46.

Velzeboer, I., Hendriks, A. J., Ragas, A. M., and Van De Meent, D. 2008. Aquatic ecotoxicity tests of some nanomaterials. *Environ Toxicol Chem*, 27, 1942–7.

Verma, S., Das, S., and Khangarot, B. S. 2011. Toxicity of metallic oxides nanoparticle suspensions to a freshwater sludge worm Tubifex tubifex Muller. *J Biomed Nanotechnol*, 7, 216–7.

Vevers, W. F. and Jha, A. N. 2008. Genotoxic and cytotoxic potential of titanium dioxide (TiO2) nanoparticles on fish cells *in vitro*. *Ecotoxicology*, 17, 410–20.

Vickers, A., Rose, K., Fisher, R., Saulnier, M., Sahota, P., and Bentley, P. 2004. Kidney slices of human and rat to characterize cisplatin-induced injury on cellular pathways and morphology. *Toxicol Pathol*, 32, 577–90.

Wang, D., Hu, J., Forthaus, B. E., and Wang, J. 2011a. Synergistic toxic effect of nano-Al2O3 and As(V) on Ceriodaphnia dubia. *Environ Pollut*, 159, 3003–8.

Wang, D., Hu, J., Irons, D. R., and Wang, J. 2011b. Synergistic toxic effect of nano-TiO and As(V) on Ceriodaphnia dubia. *Sci Total Environ*, 409, 1351–6.

Wang, H., Kou, X., Pei, Z., Xiao, J. Q., Shan, X., and Xing, B. 2011c. Physiological effects of magnetite (Fe3O4) nanoparticles on perennial ryegrass (Lolium perenne L.) and pumpkin (Cucurbita mixta) plants. *Nanotoxicology*, 5, 30–42.

Wang, J., Zhang, X., Chen, Y., Sommerfeld, M., and Hu, Q. 2008. Toxicity assessment of manufactured nanomaterials using the unicellular green alga Chlamydomonas reinhardtii. *Chemosphere*, 73, 1121–8.

Warheit, D., Laurence, B., Reed, K., Roach, D., Reynolds, G., and Webb, T. 2004. Comparative pulmonary toxicity assessment of single-wall carbon nanotubes in rats. *Toxicol Sci*, 77, 117–25.

Warheit, D. B., Hoke, R. A., Finlay, C., Donner, E. M., Reed, K. L., and Sayes, C. M. 2007. Development of a base set of toxicity tests using ultrafine TiO2 particles as a component of nanoparticle risk management. *Toxicol Lett*, 171, 99–110.

Watanabe, T., Misawa, S., and Osaki, M. 2008. Root mucilage enhances aluminum accumulation in *Melastoma malabathricum*, an aluminum accumulator. *Plant Signaling Behavior*, 3, 603–05.

Werlin, R., Priester, J. H., Mielke, R. E., Kramer, S., Jackson, S., Stoimenov, P. K., Stucky, G. D., Cherr, G. N., Orias, E., and Holden, P. A. 2011. Biomagnification of cadmium selenide quantum dots in a simple experimental microbial food chain. *Nat Nanotechnol*, 6, 65–71.

Whitby, M. and Quirke, N. 2007. Fluid flow in carbon nanotubes and nanopipes. *Nat Nano*, 2, 87–94.

Wiench, K., Wohlleben, W., Hisgen, V., Radke, K., Salinas, E., Zok, S., and Landsiedel, R. 2009. Acute and chronic effects of nano- and non-nano-scale TiO(2) and ZnO particles on mobility and reproduction of the freshwater invertebrate *Daphnia magna*. *Chemosphere*, 76, 1356–65.

Wild, E. and Jones, K. C. 2009. Novel method for the direct visualization of *in vivo* nanomaterials and chemical interactions in plants. *Environ Sci Technol*, 43, 5290–4.

Wise, J. P., Sr., Goodale, B. C., Wise, S. S., Craig, G. A., Pongan, A. F., Walter, R. B., Thompson, W. D. et al. 2010. Silver nanospheres are cytotoxic and genotoxic to fish cells. *Aquat Toxicol*, 97, 34–41.

Worth, A. and Balls, M. 2002. Alternative (non-animal) methods for chemicals testing: Current status and future prospects. In: Andrew, P. W. (Ed.),. *Alternatives To Laboratory Animals (ATLA)*, Michael Balls Publisher FRAME, 30, Suppl. 1, pp. 125.

Wu, Y., Zhou, Q., Li, H., Liu, W., Wang, T., and Jiang, G. 2010. Effects of silver nanoparticles on the development and histopathology biomarkers of Japanese medaka (Oryzias latipes) using the partial-life test. *Aquat Toxicol*, 100, 160–7.

Xia, T., Zhao, Y., Sager, T., George, S., Pokhrel, S., Li, N., Schoenfeld, D. et al. 2011. Decreased dissolution of ZnO by iron doping yields nanoparticles with reduced toxicity in the rodent lung and zebrafish embryos. *ACS Nano*, 5, 1223–35.

Yan, D., Yin, G., Huang, Z., Li, L., Liao, X., Chen, X., Yao, Y., and Hao, B. 2011. Cellular compatibility of biomineralized ZnO nanoparticles based on prokaryotic and eukaryotic systems. *Langmuir*, 27, 13206–11.

Yang, F., Liu, C., Gao, F., Su, M., Wu, X., Zheng, L., Hong, F., and Yang, P. 2007. The improvement of spinach growth by nano-anatase TiO$_2$ treatment is related to nitrogen photoreduction. *Biol Trace Elem Res*, 119, 77–88.

Yang, W. W., Miao, A. J., and Yang, L. Y. 2012. Cd toxicity to a green alga chlamydomonas reinhardtii as influenced by its adsorption on TiO(2) Engineered Nanoparticles. *PLoS One*, 7, e32300.

Yang, X. Y., Edelmann, R. E., and Oris, J. T. 2010. Suspended C60 nanoparticles protect against short-term UV and fluoranthene photo-induced toxicity, but cause long-term cellular damage in *Daphnia magna*. *Aquat Toxicol*, 100, 202–10.

Zahir, A. A. and Rahuman, A. A. 2012. Evaluation of different extracts and synthesised silver nanoparticles from leaves of Euphorbia prostrata against Haemaphysalis bispinosa and Hippobosca maculata. *Vet Parasitol*. 187, 511–20.

Zaldivar, J. M. and Baraibar, J. 2011. A biology-based dynamic approach for the reconciliation of acute and chronic toxicity tests: Application to *Daphnia magna*. *Chemosphere*, 82, 1547–55.

Zhang, X., Sun, H., Zhang, Z., Niu, Q., Chen, Y., and Crittenden, J. C. 2007. Enhanced bioaccumulation of cadmium in carp in the presence of titanium dioxide nanoparticles. *Chemosphere*, 67, 160–6.

Zhang, X. Z., Sun, H. W., and Zhang, Z. Y. 2006. [Bioaccumulation of titanium dioxide nanoparticles in carp]. *Huan Jing Ke Xue*, 27, 1631–5.

Zhao, C. M. and Wang, W. X. 2010. Biokinetic uptake and efflux of silver nanoparticles in *Daphnia magna*. *Environ Sci Technol*, 44, 7699–704.

Zhao, C. M. and Wang, W. X. 2011a. Comparison of acute and chronic toxicity of silver nanoparticles and silver nitrate to *Daphnia magna*. *Environ Toxicol Chem*, 30, 885–92.

Zhao, C. M. and Wang, W. X. 2011b. Importance of surface coatings and soluble silver in silver nanoparticles toxicity to *Daphnia magna*. *Nanotoxicology*. 6, 361–70.

Zhao, J., Wang, Z., Liu, X., Xie, X., Zhang, K., and Xing, B. 2011. Distribution of CuO nanoparticles in juvenile carp (Cyprinus carpio) and their potential toxicity. *J Hazard Mater*, 197, 304–10.

Zhao, Q., Li, Y., Xu, J., Liu, R., and Li, W. 2005. Radioprotection by fullerenols of Stylonychia mytilus exposed to gamma-rays. *Int J Radiat Biol*, 81, 169–75.

Zheng, L., Hong, F., Lu, S., and Liu, C. 2005. Effect of nano-TiO$_2$ on strength of naturally aged seeds and growth of spinach. *Biol Trace Elem Res*, 104, 83–91.

Zhou, Y. and Yokel, R. 2005. The chemical species of aluminum influences its paracellular flux across and uptake into caco-2 cells, a model of gastrointestinal absorption. *Toxicol Sci*, 87, 15–26.

Zhu, H., Han, J., Xiao, J. Q., and Jin, Y. 2008a. Uptake, translocation, and accumulation of manufactured iron oxide nanoparticles by pumpkin plants. *J Environ Monit*, 10, 713–7.

Zhu, S., Oberdorster, E., and Haasch, M. L. 2006. Toxicity of an engineered nanoparticle (fullerene, C60) in two aquatic species, Daphnia and fathead minnow. *Mar Environ Res*, 62 Suppl, S5–9.

Zhu, X., Chang, Y., and Chen, Y. 2010a. Toxicity and bioaccumulation of TiO2 nanoparticle aggregates in *Daphnia magna*. *Chemosphere*, 78, 209–15.

Zhu, X., Zhu, L., Lang, Y., and Chen, Y. 2008b. Oxidative stress and growth inhibition in the freshwater fish Carassius auratus induced by chronic exposure to sublethal fullerene aggregates. *Environ Toxicol Chem*, 27, 1979–85.

Zhu, X. S., Zhu, L., Lang, Y. P., Li, Y., Duan, Z. H., and Yao, K. 2008c. Oxidative damages of long-term exposure to low level fullerenes (C60) in Carassius auratus. *Huan Jing Ke Xue*, 29, 855–61.

Zhu, Z. J., Carboni, R., Quercio, M. J., Jr., Yan, B., Miranda, O. R., Anderton, D. L., Arcaro, K. F., Rotello, V. M., and Vachet, R. W. 2010b. Surface properties dictate uptake, distribution, excretion, and toxicity of nanoparticles in fish. *Small*, 6, 2261–5.

Zuin, S., Pojana, G., and Marcomini, A. 2007. Effect-oriented physiocochemical characterization of nanomaterials. *In:* Monteiro-Riviere, N. A. and Ctran, C. L. (eds.) *Nanotoxicology: Characterization, Dosing and Health Effects*. 1st ed. New York: Informa Healthcare.

Index

A

AAO, *see* Anodic aluminum oxide (AAO)
ABC, *see* ATP-binding cassette (ABC)
Abraxane®, 10
  approved nanoparticles, 214
  FDA-approved nanopharmaceuticals, 242
ACI, *see* Andersen cascade impactor (ACI)
Acne vulgaris, 96
  antibiotics, 97
  benzoyl peroxide, 97
  NB-003, 98
  nodulocystic, 96
  retin-A-loaded microspheres, 98
  retinoids, 97–98
  salicylic acid, 97
  topical therapies, 96
  treatment, 97
Acquired immunodeficiency syndrome (AIDS), 134, 136
Active targeting, 18, 189, 219
  advantages, 189
  arginine–glycine–aspartate domains, 222
  HER2, 221
  mannose receptors, 223
  NLs, 318
Acute respiratory distress syndrome (ARDS), 78, 80
AD, *see* Atopic dermatitis (AD)
Adenoviruses, 83
AFM, *see* Atomic force microscope (AFM)
Age-related macular degeneration (AMD), 296
  FDA-approved nanopharmaceuticals, 242–244
  ocular nanogenomedicines, 323
  VEGF therapies, 314
AIDS, *see* Acquired immunodeficiency syndrome (AIDS)

Alginate, 53, 162
  nanoparticles, 9
  natural polymers, 246
  polymer, 245
Alternative nonanimal methods; *see also* Ecotoxicity models
  ecotoxicity, 369–372
  ENM safety aspects, 372
  ENM toxic effects, 368, 372
  plants models, 372–375
  in vitro and *in silico* approaches, 368
  in vitro models, 375–383
Alveolar, 50
  epithelium, 393–394
  macrophages, 341–342
AMD, *see* Age-related macular degeneration (AMD)
Amino acid transporters, 298, 299
Amphotericin B, 104, 106
  FDA-approved nanopharmaceuticals, 242–244
  liposomal, 309
  respiratory diseases, 44
Andersen cascade impactor (ACI), 59
Anodic aluminum oxide (AAO), 169
Anticancer drug delivery
  bioavailability enhancement, 214–219
  drug resistance, 223–227
  nanoparticles, 214
  targeting, 219–223
  theranostics, 228–230
Anticoagulants, 17
Antifungal encapsulated nanomaterials, 106
Anti-infective drugs, 50
Antimicrobial nanoemulsions, 105
Antisolvent method, 58
Antituberculosis drugs, 50, 53, 55
Antivascular endothelial growth factor (VEGF), 153, 314
  antibodies, 201
  fibroblasts, 164
  ODN, 317

Apoptosis, 346
    bcl-2 activity, 226
    deregulation, 226–227
    hypoxia, 227
    mitochondrial pathway, 346–347
Apoptosome, 347
ARDS, *see* Acute respiratory distress
        syndrome (ARDS)
ASGP-R, *see* Asialoglycoprotein receptor
        (ASGP-R)
Asialoglycoprotein receptor (ASGP-R), 78
Aspirin-triggered resolvin D1
        (AT-RvD1), 148
Asthma, 48
    AD, 98, 99–100
    BDP, 52
    respiratory diseases, 44
Atomic force microscope (AFM), 24,
        33, 34
    adhesive/cohesive forces, 60
    DNA fragment on mica, 34
    resolution measures, 34
Atopic dermatitis (AD), 98, 99
    barrier creams, 100
    calcium nanoparticles, 100
    clobetasol propionate, 100
    diagnosis, 99
    emollients, 100
    proteomic profiling, 99
    reactive oxygen species, 100
    tacrolimus, 99–100
    therapy, 99
ATP-binding cassette (ABC), 108, 225,
        299
AT-RvD1, *see* Aspirin-triggered resolvin
        D1 (AT-RvD1)
Attenuated bacteria, 77

B

BAB, *see* Blood–aqueous barrier (BAB)
Bacteria, 76; *see also* Cells
    attenuated bacteria, 77
    bacterial magnetic nanoparticles,
        77–78
    bactofection, 77
    as carrier to nanoparticles delivery,
        76–77
    molecular events, 78

Bacterial colonization, 151
Bacterial infections, 50
Bacterial magnetic nanoparticle (BMP),
        77–78
Bactofection, 77
BBB, *see* Blood–brain barrier (BBB)
BBMP, *see* Bifunctional bacterial
        magnetic nanoparticle
        (BBMP)
BCRP, *see* Breast cancer resistance
        proteins (BCRP)
BDP, *see* Beclomethasone dipropionate
        (BDP)
Beclomethasone dipropionate (BDP),
        52, 56
Benzoyl peroxide (BP), 96
Bifunctional bacterial magnetic
        nanoparticle (BBMP), 78
Bioavailability enhancement
    Blood–brain barrier crossing,
        217–218
    encapsulation, 214, 217
    fragile biomolecules, 218–219
    oral route, 215–217
    PTX degradation, 216
Biodegradable polymers, 246
Biofilm, 152
Biofunctional molecules, 13
Bioimaging
    computed tomography, 199–200
    international regulatory agencies,
        205–206
    magnetic resonance, 196–198
    magnetic substances, 187
    molecular imaging, 202–205
    nanoparticles, 188
    nanotechnology-oriented medical
        imaging, 189–191
    nuclear medicine, 191–193
    optical imaging, 205
    radioisotopes, 193–196
    ultrasonography, 200–202
Biological systems
    bacteria, 76–78
    cells, 78–80
    for nanoparticles delivery, 76
    virus, 80–84
Biopolymers, 166
Block copolymer micelles, 11

Blood, 15, 16, 385, 387
Blood–aqueous barrier (BAB), 288, 295, 296
Blood–brain barrier (BBB), 202, 288
    chemotherapies, 217
    PLGA, 218
Blood–retinal barrier (BRB), 288, 297–298
BMP, *see* Bacterial magnetic nanoparticle (BMP)
Bovine serum albumin (BSA), 139
BP, *see* Benzoyl peroxide (BP)
Brain uptake index (BUI), 288
BRB, *see* Blood–retinal barrier (BRB)
Breast cancer resistance proteins (BCRP), 225
Bronchial epithelium, 50
Brust–Schiffrin method, 6
BSA, *see* Bovine serum albumin (BSA)
Buckyballs, 6
BUI, *see* Brain uptake index (BUI)

C

Cadmium selenide (CdSe), 319
Candida albicans (*C. albicans*), 104
Carbon nanotube (CNT), 7, 338
Carbon-14, 194
Cardiac slices, 392
Carrier-mediated transport, 298–299
Carriers
    dual-mode carriers, 204
    single-mode carriers, 204
    triple-modality carriers, 205
Cascade impactors, 59
Cationic amino acid transporters (CATs), 299
Cationic lipid (CL), 135, 218, 310
Cationic liposomes, 56
CATs, *see* Cationic amino acid transporters (CATs)
CDKN, *see* Cyclin-dependent kinase inhibitor family (CDKN)
CdSe, *see* Cadmium selenide (CdSe)
Cell-penetrating peptide (CPP), 81
Cells; *see also* Virus
    ARDS, 78

as carrier to nanoparticles delivery, 78
    drug-delivery limitations, 79
    novel cell-mediated drug-delivery protocol, 80
    poor formulation stability, 78
    pre-loaded rat Sertoli cell, 79
    rat Sertoli cells isolation, 79
    SNAP, 80
CEN, *see* European Committee for Standardization (CEN)
Central nervous system (CNS), 131, 395–396
Centrifugation, *see* Cross-flow filtration
Ceramic nanoparticles, 5
CF, *see* Cystic fibrosis (CF)
CFA, *see* Complete Freund's adjuvant (CFA)
CH, *see* Cholesterol (CH)
Chemical methods, 25; *see also* Physical method
    emulsion polymerization, 25–26
    interfacial polymerization, 26
    polymerization process, 26
Chemical penetration enhancers, 94
Chitosan (CS), 104–105, 139, 153–154, 175, 176, 246, 304, 316
Chloroform, *see* Dichloromethane (DCM)
Cholesterol (CH), 56
Choroidal neovascularization (CNV), 314
Chronic obstructive pulmonary disease (COPD), 48
Cisplatin, 19
CL, *see* Cationic lipid (CL)
Clean technique; *see also* Rapid expansion of supercritical solution (RESS)
Clobetasol propionate, 100
CMV, *see* Cytomegalovirus (CMV)
CNS, *see* Central nervous system (CNS)
CNT, *see* Carbon nanotube (CNT)
CNV, *see* Choroidal neovascularization (CNV)
Collagen sandwich cultures, 391
Collagenoxidized regenerated cellulose (ORC)
Colloidal nanocarrier systems, 51–52

Complete Freund's adjuvant (CFA), 149
Computed tomography (CT), 48
    contrast agents, 199
    gold-loaded gelatin nanoparticle, 200
Conjunctiva pathways, 293–294
Constitutive proteins, 17
Conventional pharmaceuticals,
        302–303
COPD, *see* Chronic obstructive
        pulmonary disease (COPD)
Copper, 160
Copper nanoparticles (Cu-NPs), 160
Copper-64, 194
Cornea, 290–291
Corneal absorption, 301
Corneal endothelia cells, 292
Corneal endothelial monolayer, 292
Corneal epithelium, 291, 292
Corneal route, 301; *see also* Noncorneal
        route
    conjunctiva and sclera, 293
    corneal cellular organization, 291
    corneal epithelium, 291, 292
    corneal stroma, 292
    drug molecules, 292–293
    lipophilic drugs, 293
    transporters, 291
Corneal stroma, 292
Corticosteroids, 147
Cosmeceuticals, 109; *see also*
        Nanotechnology
    nanocleansers, 111–112
    nanocosmetics, 109, 110, 111
    nanoemollients, 111
    nanosunscreens, 112–113
Cowpea mosaic virus (CPMV), 80–81
CPMV, *see* Cowpea mosaic virus
        (CPMV)
CPP, *see* Cell-penetrating peptide (CPP)
Cremophor-EL, 10
Cross-flow filtration, 261
Cross-linked hydrogel nanoparticles, 13
CS, *see* Chitosan (CS)
CsA, *see* Cyclosporine A (CsA)
CT, *see* Computed tomography (CT)
Cubosomes, 319–320
Cu-NPs, *see* Copper nanoparticles
        (Cu-NPs)
Cutaneous drug delivery, 90

Cyclin-dependent kinase inhibitor
        family (CDKN), 102
Cyclosporine A (CsA), 57
CYP450, *see* Cytochrome P450
        (CYP450)
Cystic fibrosis (CF), 48–49
Cytochrome P450 (CYP450), 323, 390, 391
Cytomegalovirus (CMV), 303
Cytotoxicity tests, 161

D

D,L-hexamethylpropylene amine oxime
        (HMPAO), 55
DAPI staining, *see* 4′,6-diamidino-2-
        phenylindole staining (DAPI
        staining)
DCM, *see* Dichloromethane (DCM)
DDS, *see* Drug delivery systems (DDS)
Dendrimeric nanostructures
    for ocular drug delivery, 317, 318
Dendrimers, 11, 12
Deoxyribonucleic acid (DNA), 134, 240
Deposition, 397
    skin, 397–399
Dermatophytosis, 103
    antifungal encapsulated
        nanomaterials, 106
    chitosan, 104–105
    dermatophyte infection, 103
    mammalian cells, 103
    nanoparticles, 103
    nano-silver, 104
    soybean oil-derived nanoemulsions,
        105
    titanium dioxide, 105
DEX, *see* Dexamethasone (DEX)
Dexamethasone (DEX), 319
Dexamethasone palmitate incorporated
        in mannosylated liposomes
        (DPML), 57
Dialysis
    nanoparticles preparation, 267
    polymer solution, 264
    polymers and copolymers, 267
    schematic representation, 266
Dichloromethane (DCM), 247
Didodecyl dimethyl ammonium
        bromide (DMAB), 252

Diethylaminopropyl amine-poly(vinyl alcohol)-grafted-poly(lactide-*co*-glycolide) (DEAPA-PVAL-g-PLGA), 54
Differentiated thyroid cancer (DTC), 196
Diffusion-weighted imaging (DWI), 187
Dilauroyl phosphatidylcholine (DLPC), 56
Dimension, durability, and dose (three D's), 358
Dimethylformamide (DMF), 267
1,2-dioleyl-3-trimethylammonium-propane (DOTAP), 218
Dipalmitoyl phosphatidylcholine (DPPC), 56
DLPC, *see* Dilauroyl phosphatidylcholine (DLPC)
DLS, *see* Dynamic light scattering (DLS)
DMAB, *see* Didodecyl dimethyl ammonium bromide (DMAB)
DMF, *see* Dimethylformamide (DMF)
DNA, *see* Deoxyribonucleic acid (DNA)
DOTAP, *see* 1,2-dioleyl-3-trimethylammonium-propane (DOTAP)
Double-emulsion method
    nanoparticles preparation, 254
    PLGA and PCL particles, 255
    schematic representation, 253
    water-in-oil emulsion, 252
DOX, *see* Doxorubicin (DOX)
Doxorubicin (DOX), 78, 133, 226
DPI, *see* Dry powder inhaler (DPI); Dual polarization interferometry (DPI)
DPML, *see* Dexamethasone palmitate incorporated in mannosylated liposomes (DPML)
DPPC, *see* Dipalmitoyl phosphatidylcholine (DPPC)
Drug carrier systems, 1
Drug delivery systems (DDS), 1, 132, 288
    core–shell structure, 240
    formulation development, 241–246
    formulation techniques, 246–274
    GAS precipitation process, 172
    HMW and LMW, 174
    liposomes, 1
    nanoparticle-enabled, 19
    nanoparticles in, 3–20, 240
    nanotechnology products, 2
    using organic particles, 1–2
    polymeric nanoparticles, 171
    practitioners, 20
    rhEGF nanoparticles, 173
    virus-like particles, 83–84
Drug diffusion
    abnormal interstitial properties, 224
    tumor cell membrane, 225
    in vivo implanted tumors, 223
Drug release in action
    active internalization, 18
    Cisplatin, 19
    using Doxil, 18, 19
    initial release or burst, 17
    key goal, 18
    liposomes, 18
    membrane coating, 17
    nanospheres, 17
Drug resistance
    apoptosis deregulation, 226–227
    drug diffusion, 223–225
    efflux pump inhibition, 225–226
    tumor microenvironment, 224
Dry powder inhaler (DPI), 54
DTC, *see* Differentiated thyroid cancer (DTC)
Dual polarization interferometry (DPI), 24, 38
Dual-mode carriers, 204
Duplex System, 111
DWI, *see* Diffusion-weighted imaging (DWI)
Dynamic force mode, 33
Dynamic light scattering (DLS), 24, 34–35
Dynamic magnetic resonance imaging (Dynamic MRI), 187
Dynamic MRI, *see* Dynamic magnetic resonance imaging (Dynamic MRI)

E

EAU, *see* Experimental autoimmune uveoretinitis (EAU)
ECM, *see* Extracellular matrix (ECM)

Ecotoxicity models
   analytical technique range
      applicability, 365–366
   ENMs, 364
   nanosafety, 364, 367
   routes of exposure to ENMs, 367
ECVAM, *see* European Centre for the
      Validation of Alternative
      Methods (ECVAM)
EE, *see* Entrapment efficiency (EE)
Efflux pump inhibition
   PACA nanoparticle treatment, 226
   PgP, 225
Efflux transport machineries, 299
EFSA, *see* European Food Safety
      Authority (EFSA)
EGF, *see* Epidermal growth factor (EGF)
EGFR, *see* Epithelial growth factor
      receptor (EGFR)
Elan Pharmaceutical NanoCrystal®
      Technology, 4
Electron microscopy, 29–30
Electrospinning, 156, 165
Electrostatic interaction, 270
ELISA, *see* Enzyme-linked
      immunosorbent assay (ELISA)
Emollients, 111
Emulsion polymerization
   conventional emulsion
      polymerization, 271–272
   surfactant-free emulsion
      polymerization, 272–273
Emulsion polymerization, 25–26, 271–273
Emulsion solvent diffusion technique, 55
Endocytosis, 300–301
Endoplasmic reticulum
      aminopeptidase 1 (ERAP1), 107
Endothelial intracellular organelles, 292
Endothelium, 387, 390
Engineered nanomaterials (ENM), 356
   botanical concerns, 373
   evaluation, 367, 376–377
   routes of exposure to, 364, 367
   safety aspects of, 372
   toxic effects, 368, 372
Engineered nanoparticle (ENP), 338; *see
      also* Nanomaterial toxicity
   cellular uptake, 343, 344
   effects, 344

exposure routes to, 341, 342
source of exposure to environment,
      340
Enhanced permeability and retention
      effect (EPR effect), 189
ENM, *see* Engineered nanomaterials
      (ENM)
ENP, *see* Engineered nanoparticle (ENP)
Entrapment efficiency (EE), 249
Environmental Working Group (EWG),
      113
Enzyme-linked immunosorbent assay
      (ELISA), 159
Epidermal growth factor (EGF), 146
Epidermis, 144
Epithelial growth factor receptor
      (EGFR), 222
Epithelium, 393–394
EPR effect, *see* Enhanced permeability
      and retention effect (EPR
      effect)
ERAP1, *see* Endoplasmic reticulum
      aminopeptidase 1 (ERAP1)
ESF, *see* European Science Foundation
      (ESF)
European Centre for the Validation of
      Alternative Methods (ECVAM),
      368
European Committee for
      Standardization (CEN), 348
European Food Safety Authority
      (EFSA), 348
European Science Foundation (ESF), 44
   categories, 44, 45
EWG, *see* Environmental Working
      Group (EWG)
Experimental autoimmune uveoretinitis
      (EAU), 309
Extracellular matrix (ECM), 144
Eye, 288
   BAB, 295, 296
   barrier functions, 288, 290
   biological membranes, 289
   characteristics, 288
   corneal route and barrier, 290–293
   NPs and DDs, 288
   retina and BRB, 295–298
   structure, 289
   tear film, 290

F

FB, *see* Flurbiprofen (FB)
FDA, *see* Food and Drug Administration (FDA)
Fe₃O₄ nanoparticles, *see* Magnetite nanoparticles (Fe₃O₄ nanoparticles)
FGF, *see* Fibroblast growth factor (FGF)
Fibrin clot, 146
Fibroblast growth factor (FGF), 146
Fibroblasts, 394
Fick's law, 381
Fine particle fraction (FPF), 56
Flurbiprofen (FB), 320
Folate receptors, 222–223
Food and Drug Administration (FDA), 49, 241, 242, 243, 244
Fourier transform infrared spectroscopy (FTIR), 24, 36–37, 156
FPF, *see* Fine particle fraction (FPF)
Fragile biomolecules
  off-target effects, 219
  SiRNA, 218
FTIR, *see* Fourier transform infrared spectroscopy (FTIR)

G

GA, *see* Glutaraldehyde (GA)
GAG, *see* Glycosaminoglycan (GAG)
Gallium-68, 195
GALT, *see* Gastrointestinal associated lymphatic tissue (GALT)
γ-Fe₂O₃ nanoparticles, *see* Maghemite nanoparticles (γ-Fe₂O₃ nanoparticles)
Gamma photon emission images, 193
Ganciclovir (GCV), 315
GAS, *see* Gas antisolvent (GAS)
Gas antisolvent (GAS), 172
Gastrointestinal associated lymphatic tissue (GALT), 396
GCV, *see* Ganciclovir (GCV)
Gendicine®, 134
Gene delivery, 133–134; *see also* Vaccine delivery
  aspects, 136

carriers, 135
cationic lipids, 135
diseases, 134
DNA, 134
ideal nonviral gene delivery system, 135
serum nucleases, 134
SLN–DNA system, 136
viral and nonviral vectors, 134
Global pharmaceutical industry, 19
Glucose transporter expression, 298
Glucose transporters (Glut-1), 298
Glut-1, *see* Glucose transporters (Glut-1)
Glutaraldehyde (GA), 166
Glycosaminoglycan (GAG), 144, 167
GNP, *see* Gold nanoparticle (GNP)
Gold nanoparticle (GNP), 6, 319
Granulation tissue, 164
Growth factors, 170

H

HA, *see* Hyaluronic acid (HA)
HC nanosuspensions, *see* Hydrocortisone nanosuspensions (HC nanosuspensions)
HCG, *see* Hydrophobic chitosan glycol (HCG)
HDL, *see* High density lipoprotein (HDL)
Heart, 391–392
HIF, *see* Hypoxia-inducible factor (HIF)
High density lipoprotein (HDL), 199
High-molecular-weight (HMW), 174
High-pressure homogenization method, 58
High-speed agitation, 255
His, *see* Histidine (His)
Histidine (His), 133
HMEC-1, *see* Human dermal microvascular endothelial cells (HMEC-1)
HMPAO, *see* D,L-hexamethylpropylene amine oxime (HMPAO)
HMW, *see* High-molecular-weight (HMW)
Hollow silica nanoparticles, 5

Homogeneous nucleation, 272
Homogenization, 250
HPβCD, *see* Hydroxypropyl-β-
    cyclodextrin (HPβCD)
Human dermal microvascular
    endothelial cells (HMEC-1), 149
Human respiratory tract, 45
    active agent, 47
    clinical efficacy, 46
    diffusion, 48
    inhaled particles, 46–47
    sedimentation, 48
    transitional and respiratory zone, 45
Human telomerase reverse
        transcriptase promoter
        (m-hTERT promoter), 83
Hyaluronic acid (HA), 167–168, 316
Hybrid magnetic nanoparticles, 13
Hybridization, 13–14
Hydrocortisone nanosuspensions (HC
    nanosuspensions), 321
Hydrogel nanoparticles, 12, 13
Hydrophobic chitosan glycol (HCG), 133
Hydrophobic polymers, 28
Hydrothermal synthesis, 28–29
Hydroxypropyl-β-cyclodextrin
    (HPβCD), 53
Hypoxia-inducible factor (HIF), 227

I

ICAM-1, *see* Intracellular adhesion
    molecule-1 (ICAM-1)
ICP-MS, *see* Inductively coupled plasma
    mass spectroscopy (ICP-MS)
Ideal nonviral gene delivery system, 135
IGF, *see* Insulin-like growth factor (IGF)
IgG, *see* Immunoglobulin G (IgG)
IL, *see* Interleukin (IL)
IL-1β, *see* Interleukin-1β (IL-1β)
Immune system, 394–395
Immunoglobulin G (IgG), 17, 56, 139, 319
In vitro dosimetry metrics, 377
    calculation, 378, 380
    dose for nanoparticles *in vitro*, 379
    nominal media concentration, 380
    specificity levels for ENM dosing
        evaluation, 380

In vitro models, 375; *see also* Plants
        models
    cell type utilization, 376–377
    characteristics of, 375, 376
    particle transport rate influence,
        378
    particle/solution dynamics role, 377
    particokinetics, 380–383
    time and duration, 377
In vitro testing methods, 384; *see
        also* Alternative nonanimal
        methods
    deposition, 397–399
    exposure via translocation, 399
    generic issues, 384–385
    ingestion, 396–397
    inhalation, 393–395
    injection, 385, 387, 390–393
    for portal of entry testing, 386–387
    for potential target organs, 388–389
In vivo biodistribution, 204
Indio-111, 195
Indium phosphide-gallium (InP/Ga),
    319
Inductively coupled plasma mass
        spectroscopy (ICP-MS), 158
Inflammation, 145, 390
Inflammatory diseases, 102
Inflammatory phase
    A. baumannii, 161
    bacterial colonization, 151
    biofilm, 152
    copper, 160
    description, 145
    E. coli, 156
    fibrin clot formation, 146
    inhibitory effect, 150
    liposomes, 149
    nanoparticle-based drugs, 148
    nanoparticles applications, 147
    PVA, 156
    silver nanoparticles, 155
    silver toxicity, 158
    silver-resistant bacteria, 157
    skin discoloration, 159
    SNC's biosafety, 154
    SSD-treated group, 153
Influx transport machineries, 299

Ingestion, 396–397
   exposure route, 342–343
Inhalation aerosol particle deposition
   active agent, 47
   clinical efficacy, 46
   diffusion, 48
   inhaled particles, 46–47
   sedimentation, 48
   transitional and respiratory
      zone, 45
Inhalation therapy, 78, 393
   lungs, 393–395
   nervous system, 395–396
Inhaled drug aerosol particle deposition
      mechanisms, 47–48
Injection, 385
   blood, 385, 387
   endothelium, 387, 390
   heart, 391–392
   kidney, 392–393
   liver, 390–391
   spleen, 390
Inorganic nanoparticles, 2, 4; *see also*
      Lipid nanoparticles; Organic
      nanoparticles
   buckyballs, 6
   carbon nanotubes, 7
   ceramic nanoparticles, 5
   gold nanoparticles, 6
   health science field, 7
   metallic nanoparticles, 5–6
   Rapamune®, 5
   silica nanoparticles, 5
   silica precursors, 5
   soluble drugs, 4
   synthetic strategies, 7
   transmission electron microscope
      images, 6
InP/Ga, *see* Indium phosphide-gallium
      (InP/Ga)
Insulin-like growth factor (IGF), 146, 300
Integument, *see* Skin
Interfacial cross-linking reactions, 274
Interfacial polymerization, 26, 274
Interleukin (IL), 133, 308, 394
Interleukin-1β (IL-1β), 146
International regulatory agencies
   nanoparticles, 205

   quantum dots, 206
Intracellular adhesion molecule-1
      (ICAM-1), 149
Intraocular pressure (IOP), 309
Ionic gelation method, 270, 271
IOP, *see* Intraocular pressure (IOP)
IPPSF, *see* Isolated perfused porcine
      skin flap (IPPSF)
Isolated perfused porcine skin flap
      (IPPSF), 398–399

K

Keratin filaments, 91
Keratinocytes, 91
Keratohyalin granules, 91
Kidney, 392–393

L

Lancome®, 111
Langendorff, *see* Isolated perfused heart
Large porous particles (LPP), 53–54
LED device, *see* Light-emitting diode
      device (LED device)
Levovist agent, 201
LFA-1, *see* Lymphocyte function-
      associated antigen-1 (LFA-1)
Light-emitting diode device (LED
      device), 53
Lipid nanocapsules (LNC), 225; *see also*
      Polymeric nanoparticles
   liposomes, 7, 8
   solid, 8
Lipid precursors, 91
Lipid-based nanocarriers, 45, 54; *see also*
      Polymer-based nanocarriers
   liposomes, 55–57
   solid-lipid nanoparticles, 54–55
Lipoplexes, 56
Lipopolysaccharides (LPS), 149
Liposomal nanomedicines, 305–310
   application, 310
   CLs and SNLs, 310
   corneal permeation, 308
   DDS, 306–307
   IOP and EAU, 309
   liposomal formulations, 306, 309–310

Liposomal nanomedicines (*Continued*)
   liposomal nanoformulations, 307, 308
   liposomes, 306, 307
   nanoliposomes, 306
   in solvent evaporation method, 305, 306
   vesicular lipid bilayers, 305
   VIP and IL, 308, 309
Liposomes, 7, 18, 55, 106, 149, 306, 307
   amphotericin B, 309
   bacterial endotoxin inhalation, 57
   cationic, 56
   CH content, 56–57
   CsA, 57
   formulations, 8, 309
   MPS and RES, 56
   nanoformulations, 307
   nanomedicine delivery systems, 55–56
   NFκB, 57
   proliposomes, 56
   structure, 8
Listeria monocytogenes, 77
Liver, 390–391
LMW, *see* Low-molecular-weight (LMW)
LMWC, *see* Low-molecular-weight chitosan (LMWC)
LNC, *see* Lipid nanocapsules (LNC)
Low-molecular-weight (LMW), 174
Low-molecular-weight chitosan (LMWC), 105
LPP, *see* Large porous particles (LPP)
LPS, *see* Lipopolysaccharides (LPS)
Lung cancer-targeted nanomedicine, 55
Lung capillaries, 15
Lungs, 393
   cell lines *vs.* freshly derived cells, 395
   cocultures, 395
   epithelium, 393–394
   fibroblasts, 394
   immune system, 394–395
   macrophages, 394
   slices, 395
   whole heart–lung preparation, 395
Lymphocyte function-associated antigen-1 (LFA-1), 149

M

Macroaggregated albumin (MAA), 192
Macro-fold cells (M-cells), 137
Macromolecular antitumor drugs, 102
Macromolecules, 132
Macrophages, 175, 394
Maghemite nanoparticles (γ-Fe_2O_3 nanoparticles), 7
Magnesium oxide, 163
Magnetic resonance
   Ga-68-DOTA-NOC, 198
   nanoparticles, 196
   SPIO and USPIO agents, 197
Magnetite nanoparticles (Fe_3O_4 nanoparticles), 7
MALDI–TOF–MS, *see* Matrix-assisted laser desorption/ ionization time-of-flight mass spectrometry (MALDI–TOF–MS)
MAN microsphere, *see* Mannitol microsphere (MAN microsphere)
Mannitol microsphere (MAN microsphere), 50
Mannose receptors, 223
Mass median aerodynamic diameter (MMAD), 56
Matrix metalloproteinase (MMP), 145, 315
Matrix-assisted laser desorption/ ionization time-of-flight mass spectrometry (MALDI–TOF–MS), 37
M-cells, *see* Macro-fold cells (M-cells)
MCM-41, 5, 24
MCT, *see* Monocarboxylate transporter (MCT)
MDCT, *see* Multidetector computed tomography (MDCT)
MDR cells, *see* Multidrug-resistant cells (MDR cells)
Medical images, 188
Melanocyte stimulating hormone (MSH), 102
Melanoma, 101
Melanoma inhibitory activity (MIA), 107
Metallic nanoparticles, 5–6, 33

Methazolamide (MTA), 310
Methicillin-resistant *S. aureus* (MRSA), 151
Methyl methacrylic acid (MMA), 273
m-hTERT promoter, *see* Human telomerase reverse transcriptase promoter (m-hTERT promoter)
MIA, *see* Melanoma inhibitory activity (MIA)
Microbots, 76
Microbubbles, 202
Microemulsion polymerization, 273
    high surfactant concentration, 273
    water-soluble initiator, 274
Micrometer-sized iron oxide particles (MPIO particles), 198
Microparticle (MP), 148
Miniemulsion polymerization, 273
Mitochondria, 346, 347
MMA, *see* Methyl methacrylic acid (MMA)
MMAD, *see* Mass median aerodynamic diameter (MMAD)
MMP, *see* Matrix metalloproteinase (MMP)
Modified solvent diffusion method, *see* Spontaneous emulsification
Modified-release liposomal nanoformulations, 305
Molecular imaging
    carriers, 204–205
    in vivo and *ex vivo*, 204
    liposomatic radiolabeled nanoparticles, 203
    nanoparticles, 202
Monocarboxylate transporter (MCT), 298, 299
Mononuclear phagocyte system (MPS), 56, 220
MP, *see* Microparticle (MP)
mPEG-DSPE polymer, *see* Poly-(ethylene oxide)-block-distearoyl phosphatidyl-ethanolamine polymer (mPEG-DSPE polymer)
MPIO particles, *see* Micrometer-sized iron oxide particles (MPIO particles)

MPS, *see* Mononuclear phagocyte system (MPS)
MRP, *see* Multidrug resistance protein (MRP)
MRSA, *see* Methicillin-resistant *S. aureus* (MRSA)
MSH, *see* Melanocyte stimulating hormone (MSH)
MSLI, *see* Multi-stage liquid impingers (MSLI)
MTA, *see* Methazolamide (MTA)
Mucoadhesive microdiscs, 304–305
Mucosa, 396–397
Mucus hypersecretion, 49
Multicomponent hybrid nanoparticles, 14
Multidetector computed tomography (MDCT), 187
Multidrug resistance protein (MRP), 225, 294
Multidrug-resistant cells (MDR cells), 222
Multimodal functionality, 13–14
Multiwall nanotubes, 7
Multi-stage liquid impingers (MSLI), 59
Multi-walled carbon nanotube (MWCNT), 338

N

Nab-paclitaxel, *see* Abraxane®
NALT, *see* Nasalassociated lymphoid tissue (NALT)
Naltrexone (NTX), 311
Nanocapsules, 9, 25
Nanocleansers, 111–112
Nanocosmetics, 109
    antiaging products, 111
    dermatologic consumer products, 110
Nanodermatology, 90
Nanoemollients, 111
Nanoencapsulated drug particles
    atomic force microscope, 33, 34
    characterization, 24
    dual polarization interferometry, 38
    dynamic light scattering, 34–35
    electron microscopy, 29–30
    fourier transform infrared spectroscopy, 36–37

Nanoencapsulated drug particles
  (*Continued*)
  MALDI–TOF–MS, 37
  nuclear magnetic resonance, 38
  powder X-ray diffraction, 36
  scanning electron microscope, 31–33
  synthesis, 24
  techniques, 24
  transmission electron microscope,
    30–31
  ultraviolet–visible spectroscopy,
    37–38
  X-ray photoelectron spectroscopy,
    35–36
Nanoencapsulated drug synthesis
  chemical methods, 25–26
  drug-loaded particles, 24–25
  nanoencapsules, 25
Nanoencapsules, 25
Nanofibers, 156
Nanogenomedicines, 322
Nanoliposome (NL), 306
Nanomaterial characterization, 356–357
  alteration in physicochemical
    properties, 364
  analysis methods, 364–365
  biokinetics of nanosized particles,
    358
  biological activity of nanomaterial,
    362, 363–364
  characterization prioritization, 361,
    364
  direct risk to humans, 357, 358
  dose metrics, 360–361
  physicochemical characteristics,
    358–360
  recommendations on, 361, 362
Nanomaterial toxicity, 340
  on animal models, 340–341
  dermal route of exposure, 343
  drug-delivery route of exposure, 343
  exposure routes to ENPs, 341, 342
  ingestion route of exposure, 342–343
  respiratory route of exposure, 341, 342
  responsible factors for, 341
Nanomaterials (NM), 144, 338, 373
  alteration in optical properties of
    gold, 339
  applications of, 339, 340

dermal exposure to, 397
  primary route of potential exposure
    to, 398
  regulatory efforts, 348–349
  unique properties, 339
Nanomedicine, 15, 44, 144
Nanomedicine drug-delivery systems
  advantages, 43–44
  pulmonary, 44
  respiratory diseases, 44
Nano-milling method, 58
Nano-oligosaccharide factor (NOSF),
    150
Nanoparticle delivery
  oncolytic viruses, 83
  plant virus for, 82–83
Nanoparticle formulation
  chitosan, 246
  components, 241
  development, 241, 245
  polymerization methods, 270–274
  polymers, 245
  preformed polymers dispersion,
    247–270
Nanoparticle lung delivery systems;
    see also Targeted pulmonary
    nanomedicine
  lipid-based nanocarriers, 54–57
  polymer-based nanocarriers, 51–54
Nanoparticle toxicity mechanisms,
    344–345; *see also* Engineered
    nanoparticle (ENP)
  apoptosis, 346–347
  carcinogenesis, 347, 348
  developmental toxicity, 348
  ENPs-induced genotoxicity, 347, 348
  ENPs-induced inflammation, 347
  ENPs-induced reproductive toxicity,
    348
  oxidative stress, 345
  ROS production mechanisms,
    345–346
Nanoparticle-based drug delivery
    systems (NDDS), 2
  classification, 4
  journey in body, 14–17
Nanoparticles (NP), 1, 2, 24, 25, 76, 132,
    188, 214, 288, 373
  advantages, 132, 241

biotransformation pathway, 375
in blood vessel, 15
cellular uptake, 132
chemical characteristics, 2–3
coated with antibodies, 77
disadvantages, 241
for drug delivery, 132
efforts and targets, 132
endosomal degradation, 132–133
immunoglobulins, 17
impact, 19–20
inorganic, 4, 5, 6, 7
journey in body, 14–17
lipid, 7, 8
macromolecules, 132
passive tumor targeting, 16
using PEG, 133
PEG, 3
PEI, 133
plasma proteins, 16, 17
polymeric, 8–13
probable modes of cellular uptake
    of, 376
publications, 3
surface-to-mass ratio, 2
transferrin–PEG liposomes, 133
translocation, 375
types, 4
uptake, 373, 375
worldwide market consumption size,
    338
Nanoprecipitation, *see* Solvent
    displacement method
Nanosafety, 364, 367
Nano-silver, 104
Nano-sized counterparts, 112
Nanosized drug delivery system
    (NDDS), 213
Nanospheres, 240
Nanostructure lipid carrier (NLC), 54
Nanostructured biomaterials
    ECM deposition, 165
    Glycosaminoglycans, 167
    nanofiber matrix, 168
    PU, 169
    type I collagen, 166
Nanosunscreens, 112–113
Nanosuspensions, 320, 321
Nanosystems, 137

Nanotechnology, 75, 131, 144, 337–338;
    see also Cosmeceuticals
    acne vulgaris, 96–98
    atopic dermatitis, 98–100
    dermatophytosis, 103–106
    for diagnosis and treatment, 95–96
    products, 2
    psoriasis, 106–109
    skin cancer, 101–103
Nanotechnology-oriented medical
        imaging
    active targeting, 189
    liposomatic nanoparticles, 190
    nanoparticle surface, 190
    passive targeting, 189
    protection of agents, 191
Nanotitanium dioxide collagen artificial
        skin (NTCAS), 159
Nanotoxicity, treatment options for, 399
Nasal mucosa, 138
Nasal routes, 138
Nasalassociated lymphoid tissue
        (NALT), 138
National Institutes of Health (NIH), 45
Natural polymers, 8, 9, 246
Naturally derived polymers, 53
NB-003, 98
NDDS, *see* Nanoparticle-based drug
        delivery systems (NDDS);
        Nanosized drug delivery
        system (NDDS)
Near-infrared fluorescence (NIRF), 204
Necrosis, 390
Nervous system, 395
    central nervous system, 395–396
    peripheral nervous system, 396
Neuroblastoma-RAS (NRAS), 101
Neutral liposomes, 308
Next-generation impactor (NGI), 59
NF-κB, *see* Nuclear factor kappa B
        (NF-κB)
NGI, *see* Next-generation impactor
        (NGI)
NIH, *see* National Institutes of Health
        (NIH)
Niosomes, 311
NIRF, *see* Near-infrared fluorescence
        (NIRF)
Nitric oxide (NO), 394

NL, *see* Nanoliposome (NL)
NLC, *see* Nanostructure lipid carrier (NLC)
NM, *see* Nanomaterials (NM)
NMA, *see* N-methylolacrylamide (NMA)
N-methylolacrylamide (NMA), 274
NMR, *see* Nuclear magnetic resonance (NMR)
NO, *see* Nitric oxide (NO)
Nodulocystic acne vulgaris, 96
Noncorneal route, 301; *see also* Corneal route
    conjunctiva pathways, 293–294
    sclera pathways, 294–295
Non-steroidal anti-inflammatory drug (NSAID), 320
Nonviral vectors, 134, 134
NOSF, *see* Nano-oligosaccharide factor (NOSF)
Novel drug-delivery systems, 45
NP, *see* Nanoparticles (NP)
NRAS, *see* Neuroblastoma-RAS (NRAS)
NSAID, *see* Non-steroidal anti-inflammatory drug (NSAID)
NTCAS, *see* Nanotitanium dioxide collagen artificial skin (NTCAS)
NTX, *see* Naltrexone (NTX)
Nuclear factor kappa B (NF-κB), 57, 226, 394
Nuclear magnetic resonance (NMR), 24, 38
Nuclear medicine
    diagnostic functional images, 192
    scintigraphic images, 191
    ventilation–perfusion scintigraphy, 193

O

OB, *see* Oxidative burst (OB)
Ocular drug-delivery mechanisms, 298
    carrier-mediated transport, 298–299
    endocytosis and transcytosis, 300–301
    nanomedicine application, 288
    ocular transport machineries, 299–300
    simple passive transport, 298
    topical absorption, 301
Ocular nanogenomedicines, 321–322, 323
Ocular nanomedicines
    BAB and BRB, 324
    bioavailability, 322–324
    DDS, 324
    genomic/epigenomic pattern, 324–325
Ocular nanopharmaceuticals, 303, 304
    indomethacin-loaded CS NPs, 304
    for intraocular drug delivery, 304
    modified-release liposomal nanoformulations, 305
    mucoadhesive microdiscs, 304–305
    nanostructures, 305
    polymer-and lipid-based nanoformulations, 304
Ocular pharmacotherapy, 301–302
    bioavailability, 322–324
    conventional pharmacotherapy, 302–303
    cubosomes, 319–320
    dendrimeric nanostructures, 317, 318
    gold NPs, 319
    liposomal nanomedicines, 305–310
    nanosuspensions, 320, 321
    niosomes, 311
    ocular nanogenomedicines, 321–322, 323
    ocular nanopharmaceuticals, 303–305
    piroxicam nanosuspensions, 321
    polymer-based ocular nanomedicines, 311–317
    QD semiconductors, 318–319
Ocular transport machineries, 299–300
OECD, *see* Organization for Economic Co-operation and Development (OECD)
O-MALT, *see* Organized mucosa associated lymphoid tissue (O-MALT)
Oncolytic viruses, 83
Optical imaging, 205
Optison, 201
Oral routes, 138
    characteristics, 138

chemotherapies, 215
   NDDS, 217
   in vitro models, 216
Organic nanoparticles, 2; *see also*
   Inorganic nanoparticles
   transmission electron microscope
   image, 11
Organization for Economic
   Co-operation and
   Development (OECD), 338
Organized mucosa associated lymphoid
   tissue (O-MALT), 137
Oxidative burst (OB), 394

P

PACA, *see* Poly(alkylcyanoacrylate)
   (PACA)
Paclitaxel (PTX), 215
PAMAM, *see* Polyamidoamine
   (PAMAM)
PAN, *see* Poly(acrylonitrile) (PAN)
Particokinetics, 380
   degree of inaccuracy, 382, 383
   diffusion coefficient, 381
   metric uses, 383
   particle diffusion, 381
   particokinetic contribution, 382, 383
   principal deliverer mechanism,
     381–382
   terminal settling velocity, 382
Passive targeting, 18, 189
   CAELIX®/DOXIL® structure, 220
   EPR effect, 219
   pegylated nanoparticles, 221
Passive transport, 298
PBCA, *see* Poly(butyl cyanoacrylate)
   (PBCA)
PBS, *see* Phosphate-buffered solution
   (PBS)
PC4, *see* Phthalocyanine 4 (PC4)
PCA, *see* Poly(cyanoacrylate) (PCA)
PCL, *see* Poly(caprolactone) (PCL);
   Polycaprolactone (PCL)
PCS, *see* Photon correlation
   spectroscopy (PCS)
PDGF, *see* Platelet-derived growth factor
   (PDGF)
PDI, *see* Polydispersity index (PDI)

PDT, *see* Photodynamic therapy (PDT)
PDTC, *see* Pyrrolidine dithiocarbamate
   (PDTC)
PE, *see* Pulmonary embolism (PE)
PECA, *see* Poly(ethylcyanoacrylate)
   (PECA)
PEDF, *see* Pigment epithelium-derived
   factor (PEDF)
PEG, *see* Polyethylene glycol (PEG)
PEGylation, 16
PEI, *see* Polyethylenimine (PEI)
PEO–PPO–PEO, *see* Poly(ethyleneoxide)-
   poly(propyleneoxide)-
   poly(ethyleneoxide)
   (PEO–PPO–PEO)
PepT1, *see* Peptide transporter (PepT1)
Peptide GE11 sequence, 222
Peptide transporter (PepT1), 294
Perfusion magnetic resonance imaging
   (Perfusion MRI), 187
Perfusion MRI, *see* Perfusion magnetic
   resonance imaging (Perfusion
   MRI)
Peripheral nervous system, 396
Personalized medicine, 188
PET, *see* Positron emission tomography
   (PET)
PGA, *see* Poly glycolic acid (PGA)
P-glycoprotein (P-gp), 294
P-gp, *see* P-glycoprotein (P-gp)
Phase separation, 165
PHEA, *see* Poly(2-hydroxyethyl
   aspartamide) (PHEA)
Phosphate-buffered solution (PBS), 161
Photodynamic therapy (PDT), 102
Photon correlation spectroscopy
   (PCS), 35
Phthalocyanine 4 (PC4), 229
Physical method, 26; *see also* Chemical
   methods
   hydrothermal synthesis, 28–29
   plasma methods, 26–27
   spray synthesis, 29
   vapor deposition methods, 27–28
Pigment epithelium-derived factor
   (PEDF), 316
Piroxicam nanosuspensions, 321
PLA, *see* Poly lactic acid (PLA);
   Polylactide acid (PLA)

Plant virus, 82–83
Plants models, 372–373
   NP uptake into plants, 373, 375
   plant physiology and toxicology, 374
Plasma, 16
   methods, 26–27
Platelet-derived growth factor (PDGF), 146
PLG, *see* Poly(D,L-glycolide) (PLG)
PLGA, *see* Poly(lactic-*co*-glycolic) acid (PLGA)
PLLA, *see* Poly(L-lactic acid) (PLLA)
PLNP, *see* Polymerized lipid nanoparticle (PLNP)
PMMA, *see* Poly(methylmethacrylate) (PMMA); Polymethyl methacrylic acid (PMMA)
PMN elastase, *see* Polymorphonuclear elastase (PMN elastase)
PNPs, *see* Polymeric nanoparticles (PNPs)
Poly glycolic acid (PGA), 313
Poly lactic acid (PLA), 313
Poly(2-hydroxyethyl aspartamide) (PHEA), 133
Poly(acrylonitrile) (PAN), 169
Poly(alkylcyanoacrylate) (PACA), 226, 304
   nanoparticle synthesis, 26
Poly(butyl cyanoacrylate) (PBCA), 323–324
Poly(caprolactone) (PCL), 139, 169
Poly(cyanoacrylate) (PCA), 171
Poly(D,L-glycolide) (PLG), 171
Poly(ethylcyanoacrylate) (PECA), 26
Poly-(ethylene oxide)-block-distearoyl phosphatidyl-ethanolamine polymer (mPEG-DSPE polymer), 52
Poly(ethyleneoxide)-poly(propyleneoxide)-poly(ethyleneoxide) (PEO–PPO–PEO), 52
Poly(lactic-*co*-glycolic) acid (PLGA), 50, 53, 139, 171, 218, 246, 300
Poly(lactide-*co*-glycolide), *see* Poly(lactic-*co*-glycolic) acid (PLGA)
Poly(L-lactic acid) (PLLA), 171

Poly(methylmethacrylate) (PMMA), 26
Poly(vinyl alcohol) (PVA), 156
Poly(vinylidene fluoride-*co*-hexafluoropropene) (PVdF-HFP), 169
Polyacrylamide nanospheres, 25
Polyamidoamine (PAMAM), 215, 317, 318
Polycaprolactone (PCL), 53, 304
Polydispersity index (PDI), 254
Polyester-based polymers, 53
Polyethylene glycol (PEG), 3, 56, 133, 191, 306
Polyethylenimine (PEI), 133
Polylactide acid (PLA), 53
Polymer-based nanocarriers, 45, 51; *see also* Lipid-based nanocarriers
   polymeric micelles, 51–53
   polymeric nanoparticles, 53–54
Polymer-based ocular nanomedicines
   biodegradable PNPs, 315
   cellular biomarkers, 313–314
   GCV, 315
   ionotropic gelation technique, 316–317
   molecular structures, 312
   in nanomedicines, 313
   PLGA-PEDF nanospheres, 316
   PLGA-SF NPs, 315–316
   PNPs, 311, 312
   polymeric formulations, 312, 313
   VEGF and CNV, 314–315
Polymeric micelles, 10, 11, 51
   asthma and COPD, 52
   core of micelles, 51–52
   DNA encoding, 52–53
   inhalation gene delivery, 52
   using LED device, 53
   RES, 52
Polymeric nanoparticles (PNPs), 8, 53–54, 138, 171, 311; *see also* Inorganic nanoparticles
   Abraxane®, 10
   block copolymer micelles, 11
   dendrimers, 11, 12
   hydrogel nanoparticles, 12
   using in DDS, 9
   nanocapsules, 9
   natural, 9

NK911, 11
polymeric micelles, 10
polymersomes, 12
stimuli-responsive hydrogels, 12–13
structure, 10, 11
synthetic polymers, 10
Polymerization methods
emulsion polymerization, 271–273
interfacial polymerization, 274
microemulsion polymerization, 273–274
miniemulsion polymerization, 273
Polymerized lipid nanoparticle (PLNP), 48
Polymer dispersion
dialysis, 264–267
double-emulsion method, 252–255
emulsification solvent diffusion method, 259–261
ionic gelation method, 270
salting out, 261–262
single-emulsion solvent diffusion method, 255–258
single-emulsion solvent evaporation method, 247–251
solvent displacement method, 262–264
supercritical fluid technology, 267–270
Polymers, 8, 245
Polymersomes, 12
Polymethyl methacrylic acid (PMMA), 272
Polymorphonuclear elastase (PMN elastase), 147
poly-*N*-acetyl-glucosamine fibers (sNAG), 168
Polypropyleneimine octaamine dendrimers, 317
Polyurethane (PU), 168
Polyvinyl alcohol (PVA), 250
Poor drug–vehicle interaction, 95
Porous hollow silica nanoparticles, 5
Porous nanoparticles, 5
Positron emission tomography (PET), 187
Powder X-ray diffraction (Powder XRD), 24, 36
Powder XRD, *see* Powder X-ray diffraction (Powder XRD)

Primary human hepatocytes, 391
Profilaggrin, 91
Proliferative phase
drug-delivering, 171–174
ECM components, 164
nanostructured biomaterials, 165–169
nanotechnologies applications, 165
reepithelialization process, 164
surfaces modification, 169–171
Proliposomes, 56
Promordiale nanolotion, 111
Prostate-specific membrane antigen (PSMA), 189, 200
Proteomic profiling, 99
P-selectin antagonist, 48
PSMA, *see* Prostate-specific membrane antigen (PSMA)
Psoriasis, 106, 107
diagnosis, 107
genetic factors, 107
treatment, 108–109
PTX, *see* Paclitaxel (PTX)
PU, *see* Polyurethane (PU)
Pulmonary embolism (PE), 191
Pulmonary system, 45
PVA, *see* Poly(vinyl alcohol) (PVA); Polyvinyl alcohol (PVA)
PVdF-HFP, *see* Poly(vinylidene fluoride-*co*-hexafluoropropene) (PVdF-HFP)
Pyrrolidine dithiocarbamate (PDTC), 227

Q

Quantitative structural–activity relationship ((Q)SAR), 368
Quantum dot semiconductors (QD semiconductors), 318–319
Quantum dots (QDs), 17, 205, 338
Quasi-elastic light scattering (QELS), 35

R

RA, *see* Retinoic acid (RA)
Radio frequency (RF), 27
Radioguided occult lesion localization (ROLL), 192

Radioisotopes
    Carbon-14, 194
    gamma photon emission images,
        193
    sentinel node scintigraphy, 195
    SPECT image, 194
    Technetium-99 m, 193
    Tritium, 194
    whole-body scintigraphy, 196
Radiotracer
    Copper-64, 194
    Gallium-68, 195
    Indio-111 and technetium–99 m, 195
    Iodine-123, 124, 125, and 131, 195
Randomized controlled trial studies
        (RCT studies), 154
Rapamune®, 5
Rapid expansion of supercritical
        solution (RESS), 269
Rapid expansion of supercritical
        solution into liquid solvent
        (RESOLV), 269
RCE cells, *see* Retinal capillary
        endothelial cells (RCE cells)
RCT studies, *see* Randomized controlled
        trial studies (RCT studies)
REACH, *see* Registration, evaluation,
        authorization, and restriction
        of chemicals (REACH)
Reactive nitrogen species (RNS), 345
Reactive oxygen species, 100, 147, 345
recombinant human EGF (rhEGF), 170
Reepithelialization process, 164
Registration, evaluation, authorization,
        and restriction of chemicals
        (REACH), 367
Remodeling phase, 174
    nanotechnology applications, 175,
        176
    tissue proliferation, 174–175
RES, *see* Reticuloendothelial system
        (RES)
RESOLV, *see* Rapid expansion of
        supercritical solution into
        liquid solvent (RESOLV)
Respiratory diseases, 44, 48; *see also* Skin
        disease
    CF, 48–49
    COPD and asthma, 48

    infectious diseases, 50–51
    tuberculosis, 49–50
    vaccination, 51
Respiratory syncytial virus infection
        (RSV infection), 51
RESS, *see* Rapid expansion of
        supercritical solution (RESS)
Reticuloendothelial system (RES), 52,
        56, 196
Retin-A-loaded microspheres, 98
Retina, 295, 296
    BRB, 297–298
    drug delivery, 297
    RCE cells, 297
    in retinal physiology, 297
Retinal capillary endothelial cells
        (RCE cells), 297
Retinal pigment epithelium (RPE), 295,
        296–297
Retinal progenitor cell (RPC), 315
Retinal uptake index (RUI), 288
Retinoic acid (RA), 316
Retinoids, 97–98
Reverse transcription-polymerase chain
        reaction (RT PCR), 153
RF, *see* Radio frequency (RF)
rhEGF, *see* recombinant human EGF
        (rhEGF)
RIF, *see* Rifampicin (RIF)
Rifampicin (RIF), 50
RISC, *see* RNA-induced silencing
        complex (RISC)
RNA-induced silencing complex (RISC),
        218
RNS, *see* Reactive nitrogen species
        (RNS)
ROLL, *see* Radioguided occult lesion
        localization (ROLL)
RPC, *see* Retinal progenitor cell
        (RPC)
RPE, *see* Retinal pigment epithelium
        (RPE)
RSV infection, *see* Respiratory
        syncytial virus infection
        (RSV infection)
RT PCR, *see* Reverse transcription-
        polymerase chain reaction (RT
        PCR)
RUI, *see* Retinal uptake index (RUI)

S

Sacrificial nanoscale templates, 5
Salicylic acid, 97
Salting out
    aqueous solution, 262
    electrolyte salts, 261
    schematic representation, 263
SAS, *see* Supercritical antisolvent
        (SAS)
Scanning electron microscopy (SEM),
        24, 31, 59, 156
    development, 31
    electromagnetic fields and lenses,
        32, 33
    high-energy electrons, 32
    metallic nanoparticles, 33
    nanoparticles, 31–32
SCENIHR, *see* Scientific Committee
        on Emerging and Newly
        Identified Health Risks
        (SCENIHR)
Scientific Committee on Emerging and
        Newly Identified Health Risks
        (SCENIHR), 348
Sclera pathways, 294–295
SD method, *see* Spray drying method
        (SD method)
SDS, *see* Sodium dodecyl sulfate
        (SDS)
Self-assembly, 165
SEM, *see* Scanning electron microscopy
        (SEM)
Sentinel node and occult lesion
        localization (SNOLL), 192
Sentinel node scintigraphy, 195
Sertoli cell nanoparticle protocol
        (SNAP), 80
Sertoli cells, 80
Silica nanoparticles, 5
Silver dressings, 152
Silver nanoparticles and chitosan (SNC),
        153
Silver sulfadiazine (SSD), 151
Silver-resistant bacteria, 157
Single nucleotide polymorphism (SNP),
        107
Single photon emission computed
        tomography (SPECT), 187

Single-emulsion solvent diffusion
        method
    nanoparticles preparation, 257
    organic phase, 255
    rate of diffusion, 258
    schematic representation, 256
Single-emulsion solvent evaporation
        method
    drug entrapment, 251
    emulsion evaporation, 247
    homogenization and sonication, 250
    nanoparticles preparation, 249
    PVA concentration, 251
    schematic representation, 248
Single-mode carriers, 204
Single-walled carbon nanotube
        (SWCNT), 338
SIPP, *see* Superparamagnetic iron and
        platinum particle (SIPP)
SiRNA, *see* Small interfering RNA
        (SiRNA)
Skin, 90, 91, 144, 397–398
    cell culture, 398
    discoloration, 159
    histology, 91
    IPPSF, 398–399
    irritation testing, 399
    keratinocytes, 91
    stratum corneum, 91–92
    structure and function, 92
    in vivo starting doses, 398
Skin cancer, 101
    diagnosis, 101
    infrared spectrum, 101, 102
    macromolecular antitumor drugs,
        102
    melanoma, 101
    MSH, 102
    nanoscale optical fiber, 103
    theranostics, 102
    therapeutic compounds, 102–103
Skin disease
    acne vulgaris, 96–98
    atopic dermatitis, 98–100
    dermatophytosis, 103–106
    nanotechnology, 95–96
    psoriasis, 106–109
SLN, *see* Solid lipid nanoparticles (SLN)
Small interfering RNA (SiRNA), 218

Small molecules, 131
Small-sized nanoparticles, 137
sNAG, *see* poly-N-acetyl-glucosamine
        fibers (sNAG)
SNAP, *see* Sertoli cell nanoparticle
        protocol (SNAP)
SNC, *see* Silver nanoparticles and
        chitosan (SNC)
SNOLL, *see* Sentinel node and occult
        lesion localization (SNOLL)
SNP, *see* Single nucleotide
        polymorphism (SNP)
Sodium dodecyl sulfate (SDS), 255
Solid lipid nanoparticles (SLN), 8, 54, 95,
        136, 310
    lung cancer-targeted nanomedicine,
        55
    lymphatic uptake, 55
    pulmonary targeted delivery, 55
Solid nanoparticles, 3
Solid tumors, 76
Solid-lipid nanoparticles, 54–55
Solvent displacement method, 250, 265
    binary mixtures, 262
    nanocapsules, 264
    nanoparticle preparation, 266
    nanospheres, 264
Sonication, 250
SonoVue, 201
Soybean L-∞-phosphatidylcholine (SPC),
        56
Soybean oil-derived nanoemulsions, 105
SPC, *see* Soybean L-∞-
        phosphatidylcholine (SPC)
SPECT, *see* Single photon emission
        computed tomography
        (SPECT)
SPIO, *see* Superparamagnetic particles
        of iron oxide (SPIO)
SPION, *see* Superparamagnetic iron
        oxide nanoparticle (SPION)
Spleen, 390
Splenic filtration, 1
Spontaneous emulsification
    nanoparticles preparation, 261
    schematic representation, 260
    water-miscible solvents, 259
Spray drying method (SD method), 58
Spray freeze drying method, 58

Spray synthesis, 29
SSD, *see* Silver sulfadiazine (SSD)
SSM, *see* Superficial spreading
        melanoma (SSM)
Stem cells, 197
Stimuli-responsive hydrogels, 12–13
Stokes–Einstein relation, 381
Stratum basale, 91
Stratum corneum, 90, 91–92
Supercritical antisolvent (SAS), 270
Supercritical fluid technology, 58
    RESOLV, 269–270
    RESS, 269
    schematic representation, 268
    solvent-free particle, 267
Superficial spreading melanoma (SSM),
        101
Superparamagnetic iron and platinum
        particle (SIPP), 198
Superparamagnetic iron oxide
        nanoparticle (SPION), 228, 339
Superparamagnetic particles of iron
        oxide (SPIO), 196
Surfaces modification
    AAO, 169
    PVA, 170
    rhEGF effects, 171
    techniques, 27–28
SWCNT, *see* Single-walled carbon
        nanotube (SWCNT)
Synthetic polymers, 10, 168

T

Tacrolimus, 99–100
Targeted pulmonary nanomedicine,
        48; *see also* Nanoparticle lung
        delivery systems
    cystic fibrosis, 48–49
    infectious diseases, 50–51
    pulmonary disease and asthma, 48
    tuberculosis, 49–50
    vaccination, 51
Targeted pulmonary nanomedicine
        delivery systems, 44, 57
    active agent, 47
    aerosol inhalation deposition
        behavior, 58
    antibiotics, 50–51

cascade impactors, 59
CF airway, 51
characterization methods, 59
  experimental factors, 60
  in vitro characterization, 59
  in vitro pulmonary cell culture
      models, 60
  in vivo characterization, 59
  physiochemical and surface
      analytical techniques, 59
  preparation methods, 58
  sugar, polymer, lipid, and
      phospholipid, 46
Targeted pulmonary nanomedicines, 53
Targeting
  active targeting, 221–223
  passive targeting, 219–221
Taxol®, 19
TB, *see* Tuberculosis (TB)
Tear film, 290
Technetium–99 m, 195
TEM, *see* Transmission electron
      microscopy (TEM)
Temporomandibular joint (TMJ), 149
Tetanus toxoid (TT), 139
Tetrahydrofuran (THF), 257
TGF-beta1 molecule, *see* Transforming
      growth factor beta1 molecule
      (TGF-beta1 molecule)
TGF-α, *see* Transforming growth
      factor-α (TGF-α)
Theranostics, 102
  multifunctionalized nanoparticles
      imaging, 230
  therapeutics and diagnostics, 228
  tumors *in vivo* fluorescence imaging,
      229
Therapeutic utilities, 188
Thermal plasma method, 26
THF, *see* Tetrahydrofuran (THF)
three D's, *see* Dimension, durability, and
      dose (three D's)
Thrombin, 146
TIMP, *see* Tissue inhibitors of
      metalloproteinase (TIMP)
TiO$_2$–Ag nanoparticle (TiO$_2$–AgNP),
      105
TiO$_2$–AgNP, *see* TiO$_2$–Ag nanoparticle
      (TiO$_2$–AgNP)

TiO$_2$-NP, *see* Titanium dioxide
      nanoparticle (TiO$_2$-NP)
Tissue inhibitors of metalloproteinase
      (TIMP), 168
tissue plasminogen activator (tPA), 164,
      309
Titanium dioxide (TiO$_2$), 105, 112
Titanium dioxide nanoparticle
      (TiO$_2$-NP), 159
TMJ, *see* Temporomandibular joint
      (TMJ)
TNF-α, *see* Tumor necrosis factor-α
      (TNF-α)
Topical absorption, 301
Topical antibiotics, 96
Topical drug delivery, 92
  applications, 92
  challenges in, 94–95
  hydrophilic compounds, 93
  hydrophilic or lipophilic, 93
  kinetics, 94
  make-up and components, 94
  oral route, 92
  pilosebaceous unit, 93
  transappendageal penetration,
      92, 93
Topical pharmacotherapy, 303
Toxic solvents, 10
tPA, *see* tissue plasminogen activator
      (tPA)
Transcytosis, 300–301
Transdermal drug delivery, 92
Transferrin, 81
Transferrin–PEG liposomes, 133
Transforming growth factor-α (TGF-α),
      146
Transforming growth factor beta1
      molecule (TGF-beta1 molecule),
      205, 206
Transmission electron microscopy
      (TEM), 24, 30, 156, 319
  biological sample, 31
  magnetic nanoparticles, 32
  single-walled carbon nanotube, 31
Triple-modality carriers, 205
Tritium, 194
TSLI, *see* Twin-stage liquid impinger
      (TSLI)
TT, *see* Tetanus toxoid (TT)

Tuberculosis (TB), 49–50
Tumor extracellular matrix, 224
Tumor necrosis factor-α (TNF-α), 146, 394
Twin-stage liquid impinger (TSLI), 59
Type I collagen, 166

U

Ultrasmall superparamagnetic iron
    oxide particles (USPIO
    particles), 196
Ultrasonography, 200–202
    cardiac chamber ultrasound images,
        201, 203
    microbubbles, 202
    renal ultrasound images, 202
    transpulmonary contrast agents, 201
    ultrasound, 200
Ultrasound imaging (US imaging), 187,
    200
Ultraviolent photoelectron spectroscopy
    (UPS), 35
Ultraviolet–visible spectroscopy (UV–
    Vis spectroscopy), 24, 37–38
uPA, *see* urokinase plasminogen
    activator (uPA)
UPS, *see* Ultraviolent photoelectron
    spectroscopy (UPS)
urokinase plasminogen activator (uPA),
    164
US imaging, *see* Ultrasound imaging
    (US imaging)
USPIO particles, *see* Ultrasmall
    superparamagnetic iron oxide
    particles (USPIO particles)
UV–Vis spectroscopy, *see* Ultraviolet–
    visible spectroscopy (UV–Vis
    spectroscopy)

V

Vaccination, 51
Vaccine delivery, 136; *see also* Gene
    delivery
    chitosan, 139
    development, 136
    generation, 136–137
    immunogenicity, 137
    intestinal epithelium, 137

M-cells, 137–138
nanosystems, 137
oral and nasal routes, 138
polymeric nanoparticles, 138
small-sized nanoparticles, 137
vaccine and vaccine adjuvant, 139
Vapor deposition methods, 27–28
Vapor-phase fabrication process, 28
Vascular endothelial growth factor
    (VEGF), 153
Vasoactive intestinal peptide (VIP), 308
VEGF, *see* Antivascular endothelial
    growth factor (VEGF); Vascular
    endothelial growth factor
    (VEGF)
Vesicular lipid bilayers, 305
VIP, *see* Vasoactive intestinal peptide
    (VIP)
Viral infections, 50
Viral nanoparticle (VNP), 80
    CPMV, 80–81
    drug-delivery systems, 81–82
    future possibilities, 82
    oncolytic viruses, 83
    plant virus, 82–83
    virus-like particles, 83–84
Viral vectors, 134, 135
Virus; *see also* Bacteria
    as carrier to nanoparticles delivery,
        80–81
    CPMV, 80–81
    future possibilities, 82
    oncolytic viruses, 83
    plant virus, 82–83
    virus-like particles, 83–84
    VNP-based drug-delivery systems,
        81–82
Virus-like particle (VLP), 76, 83–84
Vivagel®, 12
VLP, *see* Virus-like particle (VLP)
VNP, *see* Viral nanoparticle (VNP)

W

Warburg effect, 204
Water-in-oil emulsion (w/o emulsion), 252
Water-soluble initiators, 273
Whole heart–lung preparation, 395
Whole-body scintigraphy, 196

Working Party on Manufactured
      Nanomaterials (WPMN), 338
Wound healing process
  local and systemic factors, 145
  nanomedicine applications, 144
  overlapping phases, 145
  therapies, 145
WPMN, *see* Working Party on
      Manufactured Nanomaterials
      (WPMN)

X

X-ray photoelectron spectroscopy (XRS),
    24, 35–36

Z

Zinc oxide (ZnO), 112
Zone inhibition tests, 161